Exercise and Sport Sciences Reviews

Volume 24, 1996

EXERCISE AND SPORT SCIENCES REVIEWS

Volume 24, 1996

Editor

JOHN O. HOLLOSZY, M.D.

Professor of Medicine
Department of Internal Medicine
Washington University School of Medicine
St. Louis, Missouri

American College of Sports Medicine Series

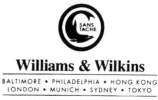

Williams & Wilkins

BALTIMORE • PHILADELPHIA • HONG KONG
LONDON • MUNICH • SYDNEY • TOKYO

A WAVERLY COMPANY

Accurate indications, adverse reactions, and dosage schedules for drugs are provided in this book, but it is possible that they may change. The reader is urged to review the package information data of the manufacturers of the medications mentioned.

RC
1200
. E94
V 24
July / 1999

Copyright © 1996
American College of Sports Medicine

Printed in the United States of America
(ISBN 0-683-18301-X)

96 97 98 99
1 2 3 4 5 6 7 8 9 10

Preface

Exercise and Sport Sciences Reviews, an annual publication sponsored by the American College of Sports Medicine, reviews current research concerning behavioral, biochemical, biomechanical, clinical, physiological, and rehabilitational topics involving exercise science. The Editorial Board for this series currently consists of 14 recognized authorities who have assumed responsibility for one of the following general topics: athletic medicine, biochemistry, biomechanics, environmental physiology, epidemiology, exercise physiology, gerontology, growth and development, metabolism, molecular biology, motor control, physical fitness, psychology and rehabilitation. The organization of the Editorial Board should help foster the commitment of the American College of Sports Medicine to publish timely reviews in areas of broad interest to clinicians, educators, exercise scientists, and students. The goal for this Editorial Board is to provide reviews in each of these 15 areas whenever sufficient new information becomes available on topics that are likely to be of interest to the readership of *Exercise and Sport Sciences Reviews.* Further, the Editor selects additional topics to be developed into chapters based on current interest, timeliness, and importance to the above audience. The contributors for each volume are selected by the Editorial Board members and the Editor.

John O. Holloszy, M.D.
Editor

Contributors

Donald A. Bailey, P.E.D.
College of Physical Education
University of Saskatchewan,
Saskatoon, Canada

Kenneth M. Baldwin, Ph.D.
Brain Research Institute and Physiological Science Department
University of California, Los Angeles
Los Angeles, California

Thomas J. Barstow
UCLA Medical Center
Department of Pediatrics
A-17 Annex Harbor
Torrance, California

Lawrence R. Brawley, Ph.D.
Department of Kinesiology and Health Studies and Gerontology
University of Waterloo
Waterloo, Ontario, Canada

Janet Buckworth, Ph.D.
Department of Health, Physical Education & Recreation
Georgia College
Milledgeville, Georgia

Vincent J. Caiozzo, Ph.D.
Departments of Orthopaedics and Physiology and Biophysics
College of Medicine
University of California
Irvine, California

Randal P. Claytor, Ph.D.
Department of Physical Education, Health & Sport Studies
Miami University
Oxford, Ohio

Dan Michael Cooper, M.D.
Professor of Pediatrics
UCLA School of Medicine
Chief, Division of Respiratory and Critical Care
Harbor-UCLA Medical Center
A-17 Annex Harbor
Torrance, California

Ron H. Cox, Ph.D.
Department of Physical Education, Health & Sport Studies
Miami University
Oxford, Ohio

Rod K. Dishman, Ph.D., FACSM
Department of Exercise Science
University of Georgia
Athens, Georgia

V. Reggie Edgerton, Ph.D.
Brain Research Institute and Physiological Science Department
University of California, Los Angeles
Los Angeles, California

David A. Essig, Ph.D.
Department of Exercise Science
School of Public Health
University of South Carolina
Blatt PE Center
Columbia, South Carolina

William J. Evans, Ph.D., Director
Noll Physiological Research Center
The Pennsylvania State University
University Park, Pennsylvania

Robert A. Faulkner
College of Physical Education
University of Saskatchewan
Saskatoon, Canada

Robert H. Fitts
Department of Biology
Wehr Life Sciences Building
Marquette University
Milwaukee, Wisconsin

Steven J. Fleck, Ph.D.
Sport Scientist
Sport Science and Technology Division
United States Olympic Committee
Colorado Springs, Colorado

Glenn A. Gaesser, Ph.D.
Department of Human Services
Health and Physical Education Program Area
University of Virginia
Charlottesville, Virginia

Gerald L. Gottlieb, Ph.D.
Research Professor
NeuroMuscular Research Center
Boston University
Boston, Massachusetts

Fadia Haddad, Ph.D.
Departments of Orthopaedics and Physiology and Biophysics
College of Medicine
University of California
Irvine, California

C.J. Heckman, Ph.D.
Department of Physiology
Northwestern University Medical School
Chicago, Illinois

Walter Herzog
Human Performance Laboratory
The University of Calgary
Calgary, Canada

William J. Kraemer, Ph.D.
Director of Research
Center for Sports Medicine
The Pennsylvania State University
University Park, Pennsylvania

I-Min Lee, M.B., B.S., Sc.D.
Brigham and Women's Hospital
Boston, Massachusetts

Wade H. Martin, III, M.D.
Division of Cardiology 111A/JC
John Cochran Hospital
St Louis, Missouri

Heather A. McKay
College of Physical Education
University of Saskatchewan
Saskatoon, Canada

Ralph S. Paffenbarger, Jr., M.D., Dr.P.H.
Stanford University, HRP Building
Room T213B
Stanford, California

David C. Poole, Ph.D.
Departments of Kinesiology and Anatomy/Physiology
Kansas State University
Manhattan, Kansas

W. Jack Rejeski, Ph.D.
Departments of Health and Exercise Science and Public Health Services
Wake Forest University
Winston-Salem, North Carolina

Roland R. Roy, Ph.D.
Brain Research Institute and Physiological Science Department
University of California, Los Angeles
Los Angeles, California

Thomas G. Sandercock, Ph.D.
Department of Physiology
Northwestern University Medical School
Chicago, Illinois

Sally A. Shumaker, Ph.D.
Department of Public Health Sciences
Bowman Gray School of Medicine of Wake Forest University
Winston-Salem, North Carolina

Mark S. Sothmann, Ph.D., FACSM
School of Allied Health Sciences
Indiana University Medical School
Indianapolis, Indiana

Jill E. White-Welkley, Ph.D.
Department of Health and Physical Education
Emory University
Atlanta, Georgia

Jeffrey J. Widrick
Department of Biology
Wehr Life Sciences Building
Marquette University
Milwaukee, Wisconsin

Contents

1
Muscle Compliance:
Implications for the Control of Movement
GERALD L. GOTTLIEB, PH.D.

COMPLIANCE AS A MECHANISM FOR MAKING THE HUMAN-ENVIRONMENT INTERFACE MORE PREDICTABLE

The observation that physical objects change their motion under the influence of external forces was formalized by Newton and is the basis of that field of physics known as classical dynamics. The "ease" with which an object is moved can be characterized by its compliance, an inherent property of any physical object that can quantitatively describe the motion resulting from the application of some force. An alternative form of description in terms of the "difficulty" of moving an object is its mechanical impedance (or stiffness) that describes the amount of force required to produce a particular motion. Compliance and impedance are equivalent, reciprocal ways of describing the mechanical properties of systems. Common experience informs us of three types of simple compliant objects: Inertia defines the relationship between acceleration and force. An object that is purely inertial, such as a mass in space, will neither start nor stop moving without the application of force according to Newton's first law of motion. Viscosity defines a relationship between velocity and force. Without the continued application of a force, viscosity will stop a moving object as occurs, for example, with motion in a liquid. Elasticity such as exhibited by springs defines a relation between location and force. It is, therefore, the only compliant characteristic that defines what is called a natural equilibrium position, a spatial location to which an object will return in the absence of another applied force.

Human movement involves the interaction of the limbs with compliant objects under continually changing conditions. Consider the task of grasping and lifting a wine glass from the perspective of the interaction of the fingertips with the external world. As the arm extends toward the glass, there is no force on the fingertips so that the perceived compliance is infinite (motion without force). At the instant that contact is made with the glass, motion of the fingertip stops while the force against the glass increases. Compliance drops to zero, and there is briefly force without motion. If the horizontal force rises enough to tip the glass, then for small angular displacements of the glass, force and displacement will be proportional, which describes an elastic compliance. When the glass is lifted, the

1

FIGURE 1.1.

When a hand reaches toward, grasps, and lifts a glass, the compliant interaction between the hand and the external object undergoes drastic and sudden changes. Before contact, there is no external resistance to movement of the hand (infinite compliance). Upon contact, there is initially no movement while contact forces rise (zero compliance.) If the glass is tilted slightly on one edge, the displacement force is proportional to the tilt (finite, elastic compliance). When the glass is lifted, displacement forces are proportional to acceleration (finite, inertial compliance).

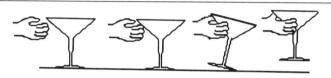

FIGURE 1.2.

The muscles, reflexes, and passive tissues of the limbs act together as a compliant interface between the neural control signal and external objects. This provides a uniformity to the interface between the nervous system and the physical environment that persists in spite of the complexities of the environment.

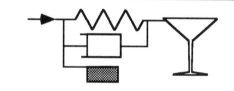

force in the fingertips will vary in proportion to the horizontal acceleration of the glass, which describes an inertial compliance (Fig. 1.1).

In each contact condition, a different mathematical equation is needed to characterize the force-motion relationship between the fingers and the glass. This would present a formidable problem if one had to design a robot to do this; yet, it is one of a class of tasks we perform daily without a moment's thought or difficulty (Fig. 1.2).

One of the reasons we can use our limbs to interact with the environment so easily is that the neuromuscular system itself is compliant, having its own inertial, viscous, and elastic properties. A major part of this intrinsic compliance lies immediately between the nervous system and the external world. It is created by the muscles, the limb, and the neural systems that control them. Intrinsic compliance thus makes the control problem much more uniform and predictable. Because of the intrinsic elastic compliance of the neuromuscular system, this also means that there are natural equilibrium positions of the body parts. This is termed posture, the configuration of the body when it is not moving. This chapter will describe the nature of these neuromusculoskeletal compliant properties, the mechanisms that underlie them, and the consequences they have for behavior.

COMPLIANT MECHANISMS

We can distinguish three different mechanisms that underlie compliant behavior of the joints: muscle properties, reflex circuits, and higher brain functions. One "simple" mechanical model of a neuromuscular system and its load can be seen in Figure 1.3. The classical three-element model in part A has been widely used as a descriptive model since Hill [23, 50]. In this model, the contractile element (CE) produces active force and lies in series with a series elastic element (SE) that resides partly in the cross-bridge structure and partly in the passive muscle attachments. The parallel elastic element (PE) is passive and only contributes significant force at longer muscle lengths. Because each element is complex, it is convenient to break them down into more but simpler elements. In this model shown in part B, the internal activation and contraction dynamics have been reduced to a set of simple mechanical components, each of which contributes specific properties. Within the muscle, actin-myosin molecules convert chemical energy from ATP to mechanical energy that is expressed in this figure by the force generator F. The output of F is an explicit and exclusive function of the neural activation command. Since the force produced by the contractile processes also depends upon the length of the muscle as well as the rate at which length is changing, we need elastic (Kp) and viscous (B) elements in parallel with F to provide that sensitivity. We also include a series elastic element (Ks) for the muscle and a second series elastic element (Kt) for the tendon and aponeurosis. The tendon attaches to the skeleton which, with the accompanying tissue, has an inertia M_{limb}. Muscle force only reaches an external load after being filtered by all of these intrinsic elements. Thus, muscle is an inherently compliant tissue.

The drawing is misleading because, for simplicity, we have shown only F to be controlled by neural activation of the muscle. In actually, B, K_p, and K_s are all increased by the strength of the neural activation signal. Neural activation of muscle arises in several structures of the brain and is also influenced by sensory inputs from muscle and tendon mechanoreceptors (to name only two). Both of these sources of activation vary with the values and rates of change of the mechanical output variables and thereby provide another mechanism by which compliant behavior will emerge. The K_t element is passive but nonlinear, becoming less compliant as tension in it increases [50].

Muscle Properties

Elastic behavior begins at the sarcomere level of the muscle fibers [16]. Figure 1.4A shows an idealized force-length diagram of a single sarcomere. If the normal operating length of muscle allows the sarcomeres to operate on

FIGURE 1.3.

A, A classical, three-element muscle model has a complex contractile element (CE) in parallel with a passive elastic element (PE) and in series with another elastic element (SE) that has both passive (tendon/aponeurosis) and active (cross-bridge) components. B, This model of the muscles and reflexes acting about the elbow joint partitions the three components in A into a more complex model made up of several, individually simpler elements. The model breaks down CE/PE/SE into elastic (K_s and K_p) and viscous (B) elements and a pure-force generating source of mechanical energy (F). The tendon/aponeurosis (K_t) is a nonlinear elastic element in series with the muscle and attaches it to an inertial limb segment. Superimposed upon these are length- and force-sensitive reflexes. All actions by the CNS to control external objects must be transmitted through and are filtered by the mechanical properties of these elements.

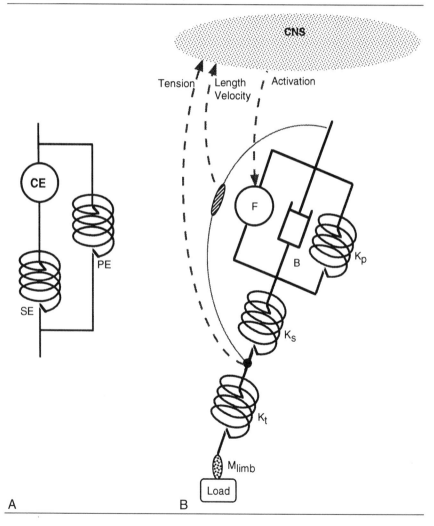

A   B

FIGURE 1.4.

A, The active tension developed in a single frog sarcomere as a function of sarcomere length. Spring-like behavior with positive stiffness is exhibited at lengths of less than 2 μm. The physiological process responsible for the dependence of tension over this range of lengths are not known. Redrawn from ref. 16. B, The net tension in a cat soleus reveals elastic behavior in two ways. Dashed lines show the tension produced when the muscle is held at a fixed length and stimulated at the indicated frequencies. Greater tension is generated at longer lengths, and the whole muscle acts similar to the single sarcomere at the left side of its length-tension curve. The continuous tracings show the changes in tension that ensue when the stimulated muscle is stretched an additional 6 mm at a speed of 1.2 mm/s. Tension increases more steeply at the onset of stretching which is consistent with an additional, viscous component. There is a rapid yielding of the muscle after only 1 or 2 mm of stretch in this areflexic preparation. Reproduced from ref. 29.

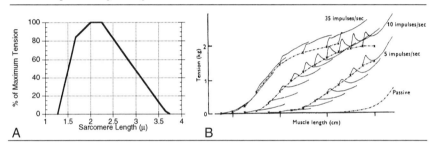

the left side of this diagram, then muscle acts, under static conditions, like a spring. It is not simple to directly extrapolate from the single sarcomere to the whole muscle, because even within one fiber, the sarcomeres are not uniform in length. In fact, questions have been raised as to whether sarcomeres operate on the left side of this curve. Operation on the right side of the curve presents theoretical problems because such a mechanical system could be unstable and the passive PE would be an important contributor to the net force in this region.

Studies of whole muscle preparations have shown that isometric muscle tension increases with length when constant frequency electrical stimulus trains are used to excite them. Figure 1.4B shows an example of four broken lines representing the isometric tension produced when muscle was held at various lengths and then stimulated at four different frequencies [29]. The active contractions correspond to the left side of Figure 1.4A. The higher the stimulation frequency, the greater the force at any muscle length. This kind of behavior is what would be produced by a spring when the spring parameters were controlled by the stimulus rate.

Were muscle such as "simple" spring, the same length-tension curves would be observed if the muscle were taken to some shorter length, stimulated at one of the frequencies and then gradually lengthened. That does not happen. The increase in tension produced by stretching a muscle while the stimulus rate is held constant is shown by the solid lines in Figure 1.4B. The force rises more steeply during the initial stretch but is followed by a yielding that varies in a complex manner with length, stimulating frequency and the rate of stretching. This kind of yielding is not seen, however, if activation occurs while the muscle is changing length. In general, "spring-like" behavior is exhibited by muscle under almost every kind of experimental condition.

The dependence of muscle force on its rate of change of length is conventionally described by the classical force-velocity relation [23] shown in Figure 1.5 [27]. When a muscle shortens (the right side of the figure) the amount of force available to move an external load diminishes with speed. Hill [23] empirically fit a curve described by Equation 1 to the measured points for shortening contractions in Figure 1.5. The effective viscosity is given by Equation 2 as the derivative of muscle force with respect to velocity. This viscosity is both nonlinear and dependent upon the strength of the muscle contraction.

FIGURE 1.5.

Force-velocity relation of a cat soleus muscle. The muscle was stimulated at a constant frequency while held at a constant length (velocity = 0). A step change in tension was imposed, and the velocity was measured 15 ms later. The muscle lengthened if the tension was increased and shortened if the tension was reduced. The resulting rate of change of length was proportional to the change in tension and the frequency of stimulation. Reproduced from ref. 27.

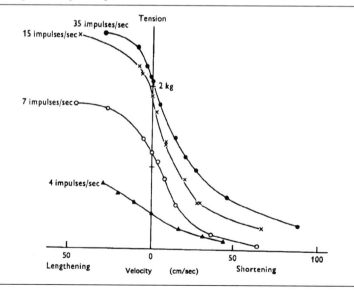

$$(F + a)\,v = (F_0 + F)\,b \qquad (1)$$

$$\frac{\delta F}{\delta v} = \frac{F + a}{b - v} \qquad (2)$$

In terms of the model shown in Figure 1.3, this happens because the viscous element (B) opposes shortening by the active force generator F. The strength of the viscous element, like that of the elastic element, depends upon the level of muscle activation.

The nonlinear and asymmetrical behavior of muscle viscosity under lengthening conditions is a striking feature of these curves. Muscles are much more compliant to rapid than to slow changes in length. The curves are especially flat for rapid lengthening where Equations 1 and 2 no longer apply. Since every muscle spends as much time lengthening as it does shortening and is often active during both roles, this is of considerable consequence when the energetics of contraction are being studied but probably much less so for biomechanics. The limitations of human experimental technique usually prevent us from separating the actions of agonist from antagonist by measurement. When working with net joint torque produced by the algebraic summation of agonists and antagonist, it will often make no difference whether the mechanical properties are unevenly distributed among the muscles, because only the combined properties can be measured. It is worth noting that the curves of Figure 1.5 are analogous to the constant stimulus length-tension curves on the right in Figure 1.4; that is, each marked point is from a separate measurement, and a smooth curve has been interpolated to show viscous-like behavior. There is no analog here to the insert figures of Figure 1.4 in which stretch has been applied and the force-time curve measured (but see section III on Viscous Damping below.)

The series elastic element in Figure 1.3 (K_s) is dependent upon the level of muscle activation, and its compliance is relatively small under physiological conditions of contraction. It does imply that it is not even theoretically possible to dissect a muscle down to the point where the force generator (F) could be directly measured without the interference of muscle compliance. In addition to this elastic element, many muscles have tendonous attachments to the skeleton that also function as a series elastic element. This is shown in Figure 1.3 as K_t. Although this is a passive element that is not directly affected by muscle activation, it is a highly nonlinear one that becomes less compliant as its tension increases [50]. It acts as an upper limit on how stiff the neuromuscular system can become, regardless of the level of muscle contraction. This property puts limits on how fast the muscle can move a load inasmuch as a compliant tendon must be stretched by substantial muscle shortening, which in turn is rate-limited by muscle viscosity, before large forces can be exerted externally.

This tendon elasticity is important when we consider how to model muscle and reflex action during experimentally measured movement. It is possible (and in fact probably common) for a flexor muscle to shorten while the limb segment to which it is attached is moving in the opposite direction because of lengthening of the muscle tendon. The most obvious way for this to happen is for an external torque to oppose muscle contraction, such as when catching a heavy object or when landing on the ball of the foot from a jump. Another way is during free movements of a limb when the motion of proximal limb segments can produce large interaction torques on distal segments. For example, Almeida et al. [3] show movements in which the shoulder is rapidly flexing and the elbow flexors are contracting strongly but the elbow joint is extending. The muscles' sensory receptors will inform the central nervous system (CNS) of the state of muscle shortening, but our most common measuring instruments will not. They will report the net lengthening of muscle plus tendon.

Reflex Properties

Although muscle itself is a complex compliant tissue, it is supported by segmental reflex circuits that augment and enhance this property. The muscle spindle lies in parallel with the muscle fibers and makes both monosynaptic and polysynaptic excitatory connections with the muscle in which the receptors lie. It also makes both excitatory and inhibitory polysynaptic connections with many other muscles. The response of a muscle spindle to imposed stretch is characterized as a weighted sum of spindle length and velocity, due in part to the viscoelastic dynamics of the spindles themselves [36–38]. Figure 1.6A illustrates, in diagrammatic form, spindle responses to a variety of stretch inputs. Figure 1.6B shows spindle recordings to ramp stretches of different speeds. The velocity component of the primary ending is large but nonlinear; thus results in scaling in a less than proportional manner for faster stretches [21].

The spindles lie within a negative feedback loop illustrated in Figure 1.7. Muscle activation by either central inputs or reflexes increases muscle force. This acts to decrease muscle length. If length decreases, reflex activation of muscle falls as does force output. Muscle force changes with length in a spring-like manner because its excitation by the muscle spindles increases with muscle length. A similar argument can be made for the viscous behavior of this loop, because of the velocity-sensitive component of spindle excitation. Externally applied forces that lengthen the muscle will be opposed by reflex-driven muscle forces, again in a spring/viscous-like manner.

The placing of a length- and velocity-sensitive receptor in a reflex arc such as this will augment the elastic and viscous behavior of the muscle itself. Both the muscles and the receptors are highly nonlinear and asymmetrical in their lengthening/shortening responses. It is striking that their combined action tends to be more linear than the action of either element alone [42], the nonlinearities of one tending to correct for the nonlinearities of the other. Figure 1.8B shows the asymmetrical lengthening and shortening behavior of a primary spindle afferent. Stretching is much more effective in al-

FIGURE 1.6.

A, A diagrammatic representation of primary and secondary spindle endings to different types of stretch inputs. Both endings increase their discharge rate when lengthened. Primary endings show a pronounced velocity sensitivity that can silence them during shortening. Reproduced from ref. 38. B, The responses of a primary spindle ending to a family of four ramp stretches. There is a highly nonlinear response to both the rate and degree of length change. The lower part of the figure shows the stretch waveform. Reproduced from ref. 21.

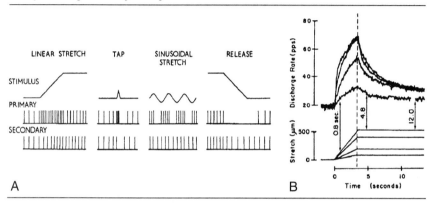

A   B

FIGURE 1.7.

A simplified block diagram of the stretch reflex. Muscle forces algebraically sum with external forces, and their net force alters muscle length. The spindles respond to length and velocity changes by altering muscle activity in a direction that opposes the change in length. This spindle-driven change of muscle activation in proportion to length and velocity changes creates elastic- and viscous-compliant behavior about the joint.

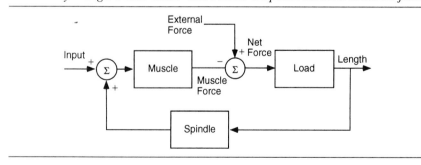

FIGURE 1.8.

The asymmetrical and linearizing nature of stretch reflex action is shown by the forces produced in response to imposed lengthening and shortening perturbations of the soleus muscle in a decerebrate cat. On the left are the forces produced with intact (RE-FLEX) and severed (MECHANICAL) reflex connections from the muscle spindles. The shaded areas represent the force added by the presence of functioning reflexes. On the right are the frequencies of firing recorded from primary spindle afferents under conditions similar to those on the left. The greater sensory response may help to compensate for the greater degree of yielding of the deafferent muscle seen during stretching. Reproduced from ref. 42.

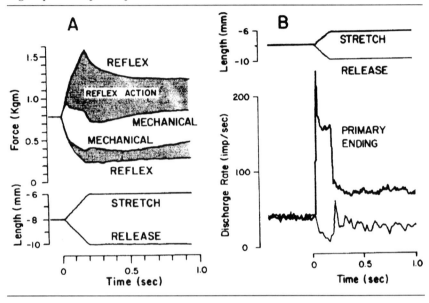

tering spindle output than shortening. Figure 1.8A shows the muscle forces produced by these imposed length changes. One set of curves, labeled "mechanical," shows the forces when the spindle's sensory nerves have been cut, and only the muscle, tonically excited over another reflex pathway, can resist the stretch. The other set of curves shows the forces produced when the reflex arc is left intact. The shaded area between the two sets of curves represents the reflex contribution. This contribution increases the effective stiffness of the joint, reduces the asymmetry of the response, and reduces the nonlinearity of the stiffness, especially to stretching.

This behavior illustrates a common observation. Taken individually, most of the elements of the neuromuscular control system exhibit profound nonlinearities. The "system," integrated to the level of a single joint, is much more linear. There must be many mechanisms contributing to this, the countervailing muscle-spindle nonlinearities being just one. It is also not certain to what extent all of a muscle's spindles experience the same length changes because of inhomogeneities within the muscle. For movements of more than a single joint, the fact that receptors act far more widely than their muscles of origin [41] has potentially profound consequences for motor behavior, but this problem has for the most part been unexplored (see Compliant Properties in Multidimensional Space below).

Although Figure 1.3 is a highly simplified mechanical model of one muscle's function within its reflex arc, it is too complex to work with directly to describe the integrated action of all the muscles about a single joint. Instead, it is far more useful to lump many elements together, somewhat like Figure 1.2. We will use a model that is described by a second-order linear differential equation given in Equation 3. In this equation, the viscosity, B, and the elasticity, K, represent the summed properties of all the muscle acting at the joint, and T_{active} is the algebraic sum of their torques. This kind of model has been extensively used as a descriptive tool for single joint and multijoint biomechanical studies. Two of the mechanical parameters on the right-hand side (B and K) depend upon the level of muscle activation but are usually treated as constants during an experimental procedure. T_{active} is a neurally controlled torque input. Note that B and K can be large, while T_{active} is small because the compliant coefficients of agonists and antagonists generally act as additive properties, whereas the net torque represents the difference between the torque generated by the two groups of muscles [24].

$$\tau = M \frac{d^2\theta}{dt^2} + B \frac{d\theta}{dt} + K\theta + T_{active} \qquad\qquad 3$$

where τ is externally expressed joint torque; θ is joint angle; M is effective moment of inertia; B is effective viscosity; K is effective elasticity; and T_{active} is net intrinsic muscle torque.

In the following sections we will assume that the neuromuscular system is approximately described by this equation. We will assume that the motion of the limb and its external load are identical and that the limb and the load both contribute to the effective movement of inertia, viscosity, and elasticity in an additive way.

MEASURING COMPLIANCE DURING MOVEMENT

When joint torques are generated by the voluntary contraction of the muscles acting about it or when external torques are applied to a limb segment (which can also be effectively generated by movement produced by the contractions of muscles at other joints), the compliant properties of the neuromuscular system about that joint determine in full or in part what the resulting motion will be. Quantification of these properties is complex because of the three distinct types of physiological properties that contribute to compliance that were described under Compliant Mechanisms above. In most human behavioral studies, all three are active so that the responses are a composite from the individual mechanisms.

The following section describes how Equation 3 can be used to characterize joint compliance using three different types of perturbing inputs. The ability of this equation to fit the data varies with the type of input, as do the magnitudes of the coefficients that describe the limb's mechanical properties. These results may be taken as a useful illustration of the fact that compliant behavior of a joint is strongly dependent upon the task the subject is performing when the measurements are made and the method used to make those measurements.

Movement Produced by External Torque

There are many ways to measure joint compliance by applying different perturbations and measuring the resulting torque and motion. Sinusoidal techniques have frequently been used to study the properties at the elbow [13, 28], wrist [46], thumb [12], jaw [14], neck [45], and ankle [2]. This is a simple approach to system characterization and, if the system is approximately linear (which is more often the case if the perturbations and the deviations they produce are small), it is a general approach that can predict responses to any input.

Figure 1.9 shows the torque and angle response as well as the principal muscle electromyograms (EMGs) for one frequency in an experiment in which a sinusoidal torque from a motor was applied to the ankle joint. Plots of the magnitude of joint compliance (the ratios of peak-to-peak angle to torque) as a function of frequency for two levels of tonic muscle contraction are illustrated. At low frequencies, the elastic properties are dominant so that compliance is constant below 2–5 Hz, depending on the contraction level. At high frequencies, inertial properties are dominant, and compliance falls as the square of frequency. In the middle frequencies, there is a complex interaction of all three elements. If these responses are modeled by the linear system described by Equation 3, the parameters can be estimated. Values for the viscous (B) and elastic (K) parameters are listed in the first two rows of Table 1.1. In one case the limb was relaxed (bias torque was zero), and in the other, there was a tonic contraction of 2.5 nm on which the perturbing oscillation was superimposed. The size of the peak depends upon the damping factor (ξ) that is defined for a linear system of this sort by Equation 4. Small values imply a large resonant peak in these middle frequencies around ω_0 (give by Eq. 5) and if perturbed, the tendency of the system to oscillate at a frequency given by ω_0, a property termed "underdamping." Values greater than 0.7 imply sluggish behavior, and the system is termed "overdamped."

$$\xi = \frac{B}{2\sqrt{KM}} \qquad\qquad 4$$

$$\omega_0 = \sqrt{K/M} \qquad\qquad 5$$

FIGURE 1.9.

A, Applying a sinusoidally varying torque to a human ankle joint results in oscillation with a phase lag and rhythmic excitation of the muscle EMGs. B, The magnitude of joint compliance depends upon the frequency of oscillation and upon the mean level of torque. Higher mean torque levels result in a stiffer joint at low frequencies but a very compliant joint for oscillation around 6 Hz where reflexes are producing muscle contractions that reinforce the motor torque. The smooth curves are fits of Equation 3. Reproduced from ref. 2.

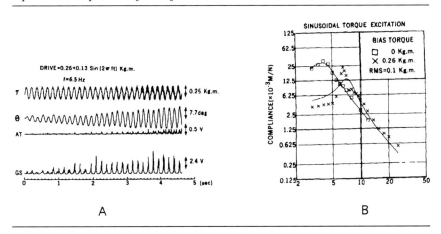

A   B

TABLE 1.1.
Estimates of Viscous and Elastic Stiffness and Damping Factor for Different Types of Torque Perturbations Applied to the Human Ankle Joint.

Bias Torque (nm)	B (nm/radians/s)	K (nm/radian)	ξ	Perturbation
0.0	0.31	16.5	0.25	Sinusoidal
2.5	0.39	57.4	0.15	Sinusoidal
0.0	0.43	12.0	0.38	Random
1.3	0.53	32.6	0.33	Random
2.5	0.58	48.0	0.31	Random
0.0	3.34	65.9	0.46	Step

Estimates are made assuming that Equation 3 describes the system.

Another method is to use random perturbations [1]. This has become a more widely used method because it is more efficient. It combines all the frequencies into a single input signal and then decomposes the responses into the individual frequency components by Fourier analysis. Figure 1.10 shows the same kinds of time series shown in Figure 1.9, as well as compliance as a function of frequency. The mechanical parameters for these data are shown

FIGURE 1.10.

A, Randomly varying torque produces motion that moves as though through a low-pass filter by the compliant characteristics of the joint. The EMG shows that the muscles are reflexively driven. Rhythmic activity is not present with this kind of driving signal. B, The magnitude of joint compliance depends upon the frequency of oscillation and upon the mean level of torque. Higher mean torque levels result in a stiffer joint at low frequencies. At higher frequencies where the curves merge, the compliance is dominated by the inertial properties of the joint and the measuring device. The smooth curves are fits of Equation 3. Reproduced from ref. 1.

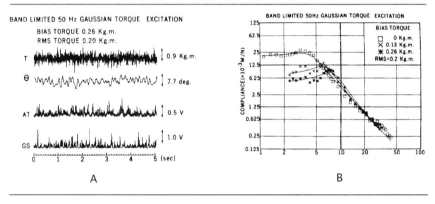

A   B

in the middle three rows of the table. Similar results have been reported over a considerably wider range of bias torque levels approaching maximal voluntary tonic isometric contraction [26, 30, 47]. These experiments found that both B and K scaled in proportion to the level of net torque so that their ratio, which defines the damping factor (ξ) of the system, remained relatively constant in the range of 0.3 as illustrated in Figure 1.11. The viscous and elastic parameters also change with joint angle [18, 48, 49].

Note that the method for the analysis of random perturbations *assumes* linearity and time invariance of the system. Nevertheless, the linear model of the system based on these mechanical parameters fits the data much better than for the sinusoidal case, as can be seen by the smooth curves fit to the data in Figure 1.10. A method to track time-varying parameters during voluntary contractions has been demonstrated [31, 35] although the method requires a large amount of data.

Perhaps the simplest way to measure joint compliance is to apply a step change in torque to a stationary limb and measure the resulting rotation. Because limb compliance has an elastic component, the limb will come to rest at a new equilibrium angle. The ratio of the change in angle to the change in torque is a measure of the elastic compliance. The lower portion of Figure 1.12 shows the estimated torques produced by the three mechanical components. The mechanical parameters used are given in the

FIGURE 1.11.
The parameters of a mechanical model (Eq. 3), fit to ankle compliance data for random perturbations, show effective elastic and viscous stiffness to be proportional to the level of muscle contraction over a wide range of joint torque up to maximal contraction. The inertial component is unchanged as expected. The damping ratio (Eq. 4) also remains approximately constant. Reproduced from ref. 30.

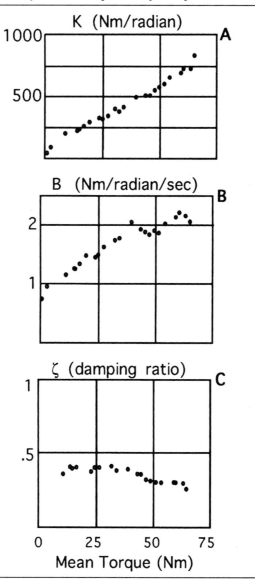

FIGURE 1.12.

The application of a step change in torque to the elbow produces a displacement. Using Equation 3 results in three mechanical torque components shown in the lower part of the figure. In the upper portion, the perturbing torque and the sum of the three components are compared.

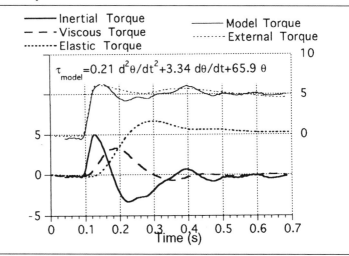

last row of Table 1.1. The upper portion of the graph shows the applied torque and the sum of the three components. For a perfect linear model, the two curves would be identical. The largest errors are in the interval from $t = 0.15$–0.25 s, which is where the reaction of stretch reflexes would be most apparent.

In contrast to the first two methods that used continuous perturbations delivered over 10–100 s, of seconds, this method needs much shorter data records. Note that this method gives the largest values of stiffness, although the bias torque was nominally zero. The reason for these large values may be found in the fact that these perturbations were delivered about 500 ms after the subject had completed a rapid elbow flexion to a target and was stationary at the target of the movement. Although the net joint torque was zero, he still had a high degree of cocontraction of both the flexors and extensors about the joint.

Voluntary Movement by a Compliant System

The compliance of the neuromuscular system also plays an important role during voluntary movement. This can be demonstrated by observing what happens when a person moves against an elastic load. The final position is one in which there is a stable equilibrium between the load and the motor system, both of which have elastic properties and which therefore both specify torque-angle relations that must be simultaneously satisfied. Figure 1.13, illustrates three movements in which a subject was asked to make a series of fast, 36° elbow flexions against a spring load that was usually 0.2 nm per degree of stiffness. This stiffness could be doubled or halved without the subject's knowledge, just before the start of the movement. The three trajectories show that the subject stopped short of the target when the spring was unexpectedly hardened and overshot when it was softened. The subject had been instructed not to correct these errors, but even if they had not been, corrections would not have begun before about $t = 0.5$ s or later.

This behavior can be explained in terms of the torque-angle diagram shown in Figure 1.14. The three lines leading out from the origin show the torque-angle properties of the three load springs. When the subject moved, spring force started from zero and increased along one of those lines. The limb came to rest about 300 ms later at one of the torque-angle equilibrium points indicated by the open circles (corresponding to about $t = 0.55$ s in Fig. 1.13).

Let us consider three types of hypothetical controllers illustrated in Figure 1.15. Were the neuromuscular system an ideal controller of joint position (Fig. 1.15A), all three movements would have reached the same final angle and the circles would lie along the vertical dotted arrow in Figure 1.14. The CNS would have specified the angle θ_d that was desired, and the neuromuscular controller would have generated muscle torque sufficient

FIGURE 1.13.

Voluntary elbow flexions made against an elastic load, the stiffness of which cannot be anticipated by the subject, stop at a final equilibrium position that depends upon the load stiffness. Three average trajectories are shown. On two-thirds of the movements, the load stiffness was 11.5 nm/radian (0.2 nm/degree). On one-sixth of the movements the stiffness was doubled, and on the remaining one-sixth it was halved without the prior knowledge of the subject.

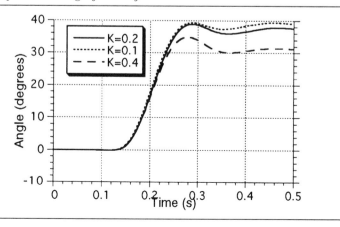

to exactly match the spring torque at 36° for each of the three springs. In this simple model, θ_d is the controlling input signal, and F_m is the resulting muscle torque described by Equation 6. This type of controller is, by definition, capable of producing whatever value of F_m is needed.

$$F_m = K_1\theta_d \qquad\qquad 6$$

This kind of perfect position control is of course an extreme and unachieved behavior. At the opposite extreme would be an ideal torque con-

FIGURE 1.14.

The external spring load defines a relation between joint angle and torque that is described by one of the three lines originating at the origin of the graph. When the movements shown in this figure reached equilibrium, the spring torque was equal and opposite to net joint torque at the positions indicated by the open circles. This implies that the intrinsic stiffness of the limb is proportional to the slope of the regression line drawn through those three points.

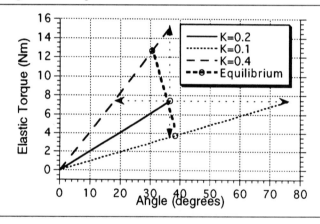

FIGURE 1.15.

Three idealized models for controlling the position of an elastic load. A, An ideal position control system is by definition capable of generating whatever forces are required by the load. Therefore, it will always produce the correct, intended position. B, An ideal force generator will produce any desired force. This will only produce a correct position if that force is properly matched to the compliant characteristics of the load. C, A compliant force controller consists of an ideal force generator in parallel with an intrinsic compliance. The force applied to the load is the sum of the forces of these two elements. If the intrinsic compliance is much less than the external compliance, most of the work done by the force generator is on the internal element, and, therefore, changes in the external compliance have a smaller effect.

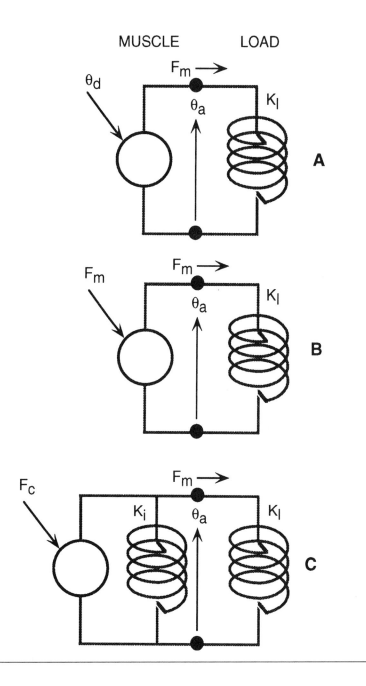

trol system (Fig. 1.15B). The CNS would have specified the desired muscle torque, and all of the final positions would lie on the horizontal arrow in Figure 1.14. Because the load stiffness was not known in advance (and could not have become known for some period of time after the movement started) the control system would have been forced to guess what torque would be needed, and that guess would probably be the torque appropriate to move the most likely value of the spring load to 36°. In this case, F_m is the controlling input and θ_a is the resulting output:

$$\theta_a = F_m/K_1 \qquad\qquad 7$$

The resulting movement would have been accurate when the guess was correct (most of the time) but would have produced large position errors for the other two springs. If the subject expected the load to have some value K_e, the input torque to produce a desired movement of θ_d would be $K_e\theta_d$. If the load turned out to be K_a, then the actual movement produced (θ_a) would be

$$\theta_a = \theta_d K_e/K_a \qquad\qquad 8$$

The neuromuscular system is neither a perfect position nor torque controller. What we see can be described by a compliant torque control system (Fig. 1.15C), one that has its own intrinsic stiffness (K_i) that lies in parallel with the force controller (or equivalently in series with a position controller). We must introduce the idea of an internal variable, F_c, that represents the torque produced by intrinsic contractile mechanisms that is required to shorten both the external spring and the intrinsic spring. The torque that is actually applied to the load spring still satisfies Equation 7, and the internally generated torque is given by Equation 9.

$$F_c = (K_1 + K_i)\theta \qquad\qquad 9$$

Suppose that through practice, the CNS has learned that commanding the neuromuscular apparatus to generate a torque $F_c = (K_i + K_e)\theta_d$ will produce a desired movement of θ_d where K_e is the value of the load that has been encountered during that practice. If on a subsequent movement this expected load is not met and the actual load is K_a, then the actual movement distance resulting from F_c will be

$$\theta_a = \theta_d (K_i + K_e)/(K_i + K_a) \qquad\qquad 10$$

The intrinsic stiffness of K_i corresponds to the slope of the heavy dashed line in Figure 1.14 and has a value of about 1 nm per degree. Because this stiffness is significantly greater than that of the load springs, the errors in final position produced by a system described by Equation 10 are much smaller than those produced by a system described by Equation 8 (which is Equation 10 with $K_i = 0$). This system appears to act much more like an ideal position control system than an ideal force control system, but this is a consequence of our choice of external loads. This is a compliant control system, and its behavior is in effect a form of automatic load compensation that is an intrinsic property of a compliant controller.

Inertial Dynamics

Were real loads merely elastic, the movement could be controlled simply by choosing a trajectory. Inasmuch as position and force would always be connected by algebraic relations, specifying one would specify both. For movements involving more than one joint, these would in general not be linear relations, but the problem of generating the right forces in order to get the desired movements would still be relatively simple. The presence of inertia, however, complicates the relationship between force and motion in all but the slowest movements. Figure 1.16 shows what the net joint torques must be in order to perform the single-joint movements shown in Figure 1.14. All we have done is add to the spring torque the torque necessary to accelerate and decelerate the moment of inertia of the moving limb segment. The result is a torque pattern that bears little resemblance to the angular trajectory.

At the onset of a movement, displacement and velocity are by definition close to zero. Therefore, compliant torques that are proportional to these variables will be small. Acceleration is the first variable to become significant, so at movement onset, inertial torques are likely to be the dominant components of the dynamic torque produced by the muscles. Because every movement is loaded by the inertia of the limb, even if nothing else is added, these torques can be anticipated and planned for as part of any general

FIGURE 1.16.
The muscle torques are sufficient to oppose both external elastic and inertial loads and the inertial load of the limb itself. This figure shows the sum of the inertial and elastic components for the three movements shown in Figure 1.13.

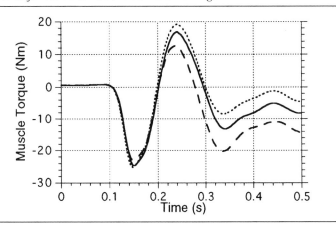

strategy for controlling a movement. Before discussing the consequences of this, we must also consider the viscous properties of the neuromuscular controller.

Viscous Damping

The viscous properties of the neuromuscular system, while recognized in the force-velocity characteristics of the muscle tissue and in the velocity sensitivity of the stretch reflexes, have received the least attention from investigators. Studies that applied sinusoidal torques to the limb (see section entitled Movement Produced by External Torque above [2, 28]) can characterize elastic and inertial properties but do not accurately capture the viscous ones. The reason is that sinusoidal oscillation of a limb can evoke strong reflex responses if delivered at the proper frequency. For example, with sinusoidal oscillation, the compliance of the ankle at 6 Hz may be double the 2-Hz compliance and may become extremely nonlinear at 12 Hz [2]. At both 6 and 12 Hz, strong reflex activation is seen as bursts of EMG at 6 Hz. Although from the frequency response measurements produced by these types of experiments the joint seems highly underdamped, this is a characterization that is limited to the type of stimulus used, not a general description of the joint mechanical properties.

These kinds of resonances and nonlinearities are not evoked by aperiodic inputs as illustrated by the responses to random torque disturbances shown above. Those studies have shown that limbs are only slightly underdamped. The damping is sufficient to prevent them from oscillating uncontrollably when perturbed while not slowing voluntary movement excessively.

The behavioral consequences of this viscosity can also be demonstrated by examining discrete perturbations of limb during voluntary movement. The angles and velocities of two movements are shown in the first two panels of Figure 1.17. The experiment was designed so that 80% of the movements were made with a light inertial load, and these are illustrated by the solid lines. On the other 20% of the movements, the inertia was increased without informing the subject, and these are shown by the dotted lines. Because the subject did not know the actual inertia until the movement was already underway, we assume that the subject generated the same central command to initiate all of the movements. Thus, any differences in the EMG patterns must result from reflex or voluntary reactions to the changes in the trajectory and the joint torques that follow from encountering the occasionally larger load.

Consistent with that assumption is the fact that the EMG patterns are essentially identical for about the first 120 ms of the contraction (to $t = 0.3$), as shown in the third panel. The net muscle torques for the two movement conditions are shown in the fourth panel. Larger torques were produced for the larger load, but this was not sufficient to prevent the movement from slowing by almost a factor of two.

FIGURE 1.17.
*Elbow flexion of an inertial load is slowed by increases in load magnitude. In this ex-
periment the increase was not known in advance of the movement. The top four graphs
show the angle, velocity, muscle torque, and biceps and triceps muscle EMGs for movements against the smaller (solid line) and heavier (dotted line) loads. The bottom
graph shows the difference between the angle, velocity, and torque of the two movements. Muscle torque differs before the EMG has changed because of muscle compliance. The first 100 ms of the difference in torque is paralleled by the difference in movement velocity. This implies that it is the viscous rather than the elastic property of joint
compliance that is important in the early phases of a fast voluntary movement.*

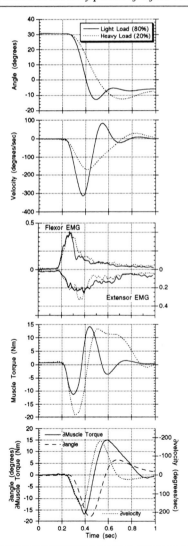

To explain why the forces and kinematics change in this way, it is useful to examine the differences between the two movement series. In the fifth panel we have subtracted the angle and velocity variables obtained with the smaller load from those obtained with the larger and plotted these as the dashed and dotted curves, respectively. The heavier load is moved more slowly; therefore, these curves are initially negative. The solid line is the difference between the two muscle torque curves. The muscle torques are initially identical for both loads and begin to differ from each other about 75 ms after the start of the agonist EMG burst. The graph has been scaled to illustrate that the torque divergence begins at about the same time that the velocities of the two movements diverge and well before the two angles diverge. We have chosen scales such that the torque and velocity almost exactly overlap for about 100 ms, after which the torque difference is greater than that of the scaled velocity difference. Further note that in most of this interval when the torque and velocity differences overlap, the EMG patterns of the two movements are identical. The torque and velocity difference curves separate slightly after the time the agonist EMG for the larger load exceeds that for the smaller.

In terms of the mechanical model described by Equation 3, we can explain these differences by two hypotheses. The first is to assume that T_{active} is identical for both movements for the duration that the EMGs of the two movements are identical. This load-invariant activation interval is about 120 ms from the onset of the agonist burst. The second hypothesis is that effective muscle viscosity is about 4.6 nm/radian/s. The earliest torque differences between the two movements result from the velocity differences and are independent of any changes in the central control signal or in reflex compensation because those mechanisms have not had time to act. In mechanistic terms, against the smaller load the limb can move faster during the interval when the muscle torques are identical. As the movements diverge in velocity, a greater fraction of the muscles' mechanical output for the lighter load is absorbed by the intrinsic viscosity. Hence, the net torque expressed against the smaller load is less than against the larger load.

Reflexes do act, after $t = 0.3$ s, as evidenced by detectable differences in the EMG pattern. After this point in the trajectories, the larger load is moved by a larger torque produced in part by greater muscle activation. Note that substantial differences between the angular trajectories of the two movements do not develop until later, so that we would not attribute the torques to muscle or reflex elastic properties (that by definition scale with angular differences) until much later in the trajectory.

These viscous estimates are made during an interval of considerable muscle activity. They are about double the estimates we made previously by much more indirect methods that were based on the entire movement [20]. They are about an order of magnitude greater that those found by random perturbations of the stationary ankle [1, 26] or slowly moving elbow [6], which were made at lower, static or quasistatic contraction levels (Table 1.1). This emphasizes the point made earlier that one cost of using a simple mechanical model expressed by Equation 3 is that the parametric values of that model are not general but depend strongly on the conditions of behavior and stimulus under which they were measured.

Compliant Properties in Multidimensional Space

All of the studies described above have been performed on single joints or with the movements constrained to a single degree of freedom. Our natural movements are seldom constrained in this way. Experiments that show compliant behavior of the arm when the hand is free to move in two dimensions have also been performed. Mussa Ivaldi [40] and colleagues [32] used a two-dimensional manipulandum which could produce small, step-like displacements of the hand (analogous to the step displacement experiments described in the section Movement Produced by External Torque above) and used the ratio of the restoring forces to the perturbing displacements as the measure of limb stiffness at equilibrium. Figure 1.18 shows how such data were analyzed. In two dimensions, force is a vector having both magnitude and direction. In the figure, the hand is located at the central dot noted by the letter "P." It was displaced in eight different directions either 4 or 8 mm, and the resulting force was measured. This force was partitioned into two components. One was radial, pointing toward P, and the other was the residual force, orthogonal to the radial component, pointing in a tangential direction. On the left are shown the radial components, the length of each drawn vector representing the magnitude of the restoring force. On the right are shown the magnitudes of the circumferential components. These forces would tend to make the hand rotate about the original point.

The existence of this radially directed force "field" demonstrates the spring-like behavior of the neuromuscular system at equilibrium in two spatial dimensions. This is not entirely surprising, because it means no more (and no less) than that any displacement of the hand is opposed by forces produced by muscle and reflex mechanisms. The absence of significant rotational components is more remarkable, however. Were a limb made up of muscles that spanned only a single joint and reflexes that did not act across muscles (or at least acted symmetrically), then there could be no rotational components [25]. Because neither of these conditions is satisfied, the absence of torsional components could represent a specific adaptation of reflex mechanisms to avoid their occurrence.

An interesting property of this elastic force field is illustrated by Figure 1.19. The shoulder (indicated by "S") is fixed. Rotation can occur about both the shoulder and elbow. Five L shapes indicate the arm configuration to hold the hand at different points on the horizontal plane in front of the subject. The ellipses represent the magnitude of the restoring force gener-

FIGURE 1.18.

Perturbation of the arm in the horizontal plane produces forces that are proportional to the magnitude of displacement. The resulting force vector can be decomposed into two components, one acting in the radial direction (left) and the other circumferentially (right). On the left are shown the force components that act in opposition to the displacement. The arrows point in the direction of the force vector, and their length is proportional to the size of the force. Forces that act toward the initial position of the hand (at P) are indicative of a spring-like, two-dimensional force field. On the right are shown the remaining, orthogonal force components. These could be generated by the muscular and reflex linkages that extend over more than a single joint. These components appear to be quite small. Reproduced from ref. 25.

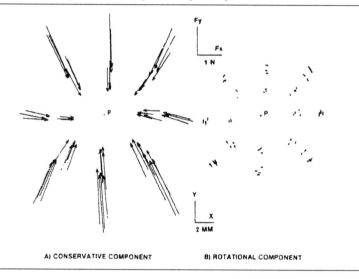

A) CONSERVATIVE COMPONENT   B) ROTATIONAL COMPONENT

ated to a fixed amplitude of hand displacement in different directions. The arm is stiffer along the long axis of the ellipse and more compliant along its short axis. The symmetrical, elliptical shape oriented toward the shoulder was a consistent finding [40]. Like the absence of rotational force components, this is a compliant property of the system that is not physically inevitable. Reflex mechanisms can easily be imagined that would produce different results.

VOLUNTARY MOVEMENT BY A COMPLIANT CONTROLLER

In controlling movements, it is not obvious what the brain is "thinking" about. Because of the compliant properties of the physical systems being moved, net force and limb trajectory are inescapably linked by the dynamical equations of motion. A priori, from the point of view of system control,

FIGURE 1.19.

The spring-like force field is not uniform. It demonstrates a relatively symmetrical behavior, being stiffest along the long axis of the ellipses. This figure shows the relative stiffness of the arm measured at five different hand positions. The orientation of the ellipses tends to always be with the long axis pointing toward the shoulder. Reproduced from ref. 40.

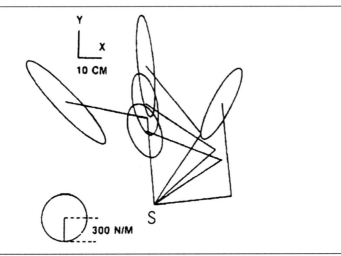

either force or trajectory could be the independent variable. This has led to two very different approaches to models for voluntary control.

Force Control Models

There is an intuitive appeal to the notion that movement is controlled by a central plan for the production of muscle force. This is evident from the long history of such models in the motor control literature [11, 22, 32, 43]. Such a control scheme postulates that the CNS can work backwards from its desired movement to specify the levels of muscle activation that will generate the appropriate forces. These models are able to describe how the CNS can control movement when knowledge of the relationship between force and motion is easily known [17]. One source of such knowledge is prior experience. This is consistent with the universal observation that motor skill requires practice.

In general, however, determining the forces necessary to produce a particular movement, especially with multiple degrees of freedom and interacting limb segments, is an extremely difficult task, called the inverse dynamics problem [5]. Although this approach has been used in robotic applications, it is unlikely to be one used by the CNS.

Force control models do not explicitly address either the role of reflexes, nor do they provide a basis for postural equilibrium. On both counts, they fail to account for the effects of either external perturbations or equivalently, of an incorrect program that has not been accurately matched to the external requirements of the task. Muscle forces and joint torques vary with the position of the limb, so that for a force controller to perform even so simple a task as slowly (so that we might ignore acceleration-dependent forces) lifting a suitcase requires precise knowledge of the load and complex computations. Errors in the joint torque will produce errors in final joint position that will oscillate or grow until the limb or the suitcase reach some mechanical limit, such as full flexion/extension or the floor.

In defense of such models, however, is the fact that compliant neuro-muscular mechanisms are present. "Motor program" models for force control always operate in parallel with additional mechanisms that could allow kinematic success in spite of apparent errors in force production [19].

Equilibrium Point Models

The fact that a posturally stable equilibrium position (EP) for a compliant limb exists suggests that these properties in themselves could also be the basis for the control of voluntary movement. Gradually shifting a centrally defined EP from one position in space to another would produce motion of the limb from one location to another. This is a parsimonious and elegant hypothesis that combines both posture and movement in a single mechanism. It also avoids the problems of dealing with inverse dynamics that plague force control models.

Asatryan and Feldman [4] proposed that for each muscle of an agonist-antagonist pair, a variable, λ, would define an equilibrium length for each such that a net force could be generated according to Equations 11–13 [33].

$$\tau = f(c)\ (\theta - r) \tag{11}$$

$$r = (\lambda_{ag} + \lambda_{ant})/2 \tag{12}$$

$$c = (\lambda_{ag} - \lambda_{ant})/2 \tag{13}$$

The variable c controls the effective stiffness of the joint, whereas r controls the equilibrium position. Figure 1.20 below illustrates how position (θ) could be controlled for two different constant loads (weights, for example) by specifying r alone. Assuming for simplicity that λ_{ant} and $f(c)$ remain constant, λ_{ag} has some value λ_1 to hold the limb at rest at an initial equilibrium (θ_1, τ_1). To change position to θ_2 with the same load, it is only necessary to change λ_{ag} to λ_2 and to change the torque to τ_2 without changing position it is only necessary to change λ_{ag} to λ_4. The time course of the variable r (or in the single muscle case λ) can be regarded as describing a virtual trajectory that the actual position of the limb will approximate. In the absence of an external load, it would be identical with the actual position.

FIGURE 1.20.

The position of the limb is established by an equilibrium relationship between the compliant characteristics of the neuromuscular system (Eq. 11) and the external load. The S-shaped curves show four different compliant characteristics, distinguished by their x-axis intercept labeled λ. By regulating λ, the nervous system can control the position of the limb or maintain a constant position when the load changes. For a constant load τ_1, the limb can be moved from θ_1 to θ_2 by changing λ_1 to λ_2. The limb can be held at θ_1 when the load changes to τ_2 by changing λ_1 to λ_4.

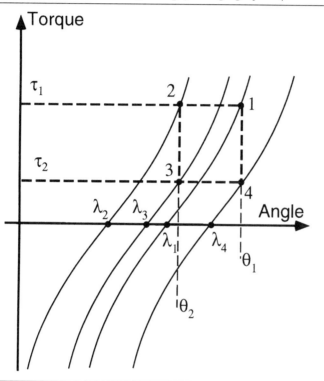

This hypothesis further proposes that the motor neuron pools of each muscle are driven by the difference between its current length (as reported by sensor receptors) and its centrally specified value of λ [15]. Thus, the errors between the actual and virtual trajectories produce the forces for movement through length-sensitive spinal reflexes.

A variant approach described by Bizzi and colleagues [8, 9, 39] also relies upon the creation of an EP by the cocontraction of elastic, antagonistic muscle pairs. Figure 1.21 shows how an equilibrium state may be defined by varying the relative degree of activation of the agonist and antagonist muscle groups. Each muscle is represented by one of the two oppositely

FIGURE 1.21.

The torque of a limb can be described by two opposing springs that represent the opposing flexor and extensor muscles. The limb is in equilibrium with no external load when the muscle torques are equal and opposite at the point of intersection of the two lines. Changing the relative activation of the muscles allows the equilibrium point to move over the range of movement. This kind of control in which only the slope and not the intercept of the joint "spring" is controllable would not be a very efficient or accurate mechanism at the extreme ends of its range.

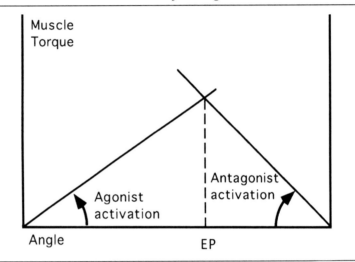

slanting lines. Assuming no external load, at equilibrium muscle forces are equal and opposite, therefore, the EP is at the intersection of the two lines. Simultaneously increasing contraction in both muscles steepens the lines and decreases joint compliance without movement. The limb can be moved by unequal cocontraction. This model implies very high and unrealistic levels of contraction for muscles operating at short lengths and has been revised in recent versions [8, 9, 39]. The hypothesis assumes that more of the patterning of muscle activity arises from central programming and that reflex activation plays a supplementary rather than an exclusive role in creating the compliant behavior of the limb.

Equilibrium point models are congruent with some simpler biomechanical experiments. Transient torque perturbations do not change final position [10, 34]. As shown above, changes in external inertial loads (which impose only a transient change in net joint torque for movements in the horizontal plane) also do not prevent the limb from achieving its intended target.

Both EP models are adequate for slow movement, but neither have been shown to be able to produce the forces or the EMG patterns that are associated with fast movements against different dynamic loads. One problem they face is in accounting for the large forces required to accelerate and decelerate inertial loads during fast movements that are difficult to produce by a moving EP. Both models have attempted to address this issue with arguably limited success [15, 39].

Partitioning the Relative Contributions of Compliant Mechanisms

It would be of interest to be able to partition the compliant force produced by the neuromuscular system among its three contributing members; muscle, reflex, and central. The central contribution is the most problematic because the brain is capable of controlling the neuromuscular apparatus in so many different ways, depending both upon intention and knowledge. Figure 1.22 illustrates the displacements of the elbow to three identical, small (1-nm) steps of torque under three instructional conditions. In all three cases, the subject was stationary and exerted a small constant flexion torque prior to the stimulus. The largest displacement occurred when the subject was told not to react to the torque and simply maintain a constant level of effort. This might be taken as a measure of combined muscle and reflex stiffness, about 10.3 nm/radian in this case. The intermediate displacement occurred when the subject was told to stop the movement as quickly as possible, without returning the arm to its original position. This

FIGURE 1.22.
The elbow is displaced by the application of a 1-nm step change in torque. The larger dotted curve starting at about 100 ms shows the displacement when the subject was instructed not to react to the step. The solid curve shows the approximate doubling in effective stiffness of the joint by instructing the subject to "catch" the manipulandum and stop it as soon as possible without returning it to the initial position. The smallest displacement was produced when an audio warning tone preceded the perturbation by 500 ms.

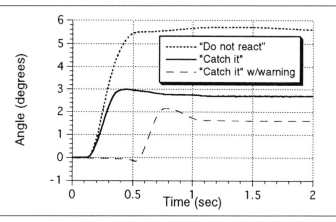

illustrates the ability of the higher nervous centers to double the effective stiffness of the arm to 21 nm/radian by cocontraction of the muscles in response to the perturbation. The limiting factor on stiffness in this condition is the reaction time of the subject rather than the strength of the response. The smallest displacement was produced when the subject was provided with a warning sound, 500 ms before the presentation of the torque. Here he increased the stiffness 3 1/2 times (36 nm/radian) over the first condition by coactivating the elbow muscles in anticipation of the perturbation. It is likely that in this case, performance is limited by the amount of practice the subject has had and that considerably "stiffer" behavior could have been obtained. Thus, although this measure of joint stiffness gives a simple description of behavior, it is realized by very complex and adaptable mechanisms.

Separating muscle contributions from those of the reflexes is perhaps a realistic task but has thus far proven impossible by direct measurement. Using indirect methods supplemented by simulations, investigators have suggested that at the elbow, the reflexes act to approximately double the stiffness of the muscles alone [7]. Stein et al. [44] have concluded from simulation studies that the gain of the reflex arcs are as high as they can be without making the neuromuscular system unstable.

SUMMARY

We suggest in this review that compliant properties of the neuromuscular system influence and must be considered at every level of motor function. These properties emerge from the combined operation of many physiological mechanisms. At the behavioral level, no aspect of the compliant response can be attributed to muscles or reflexes alone. Furthermore, for all but the slowest movements, all three mechanical properties must be taken into account. Although we have considered only reactions to external forces and the implications for normal voluntary movements, there are many other areas of relevance that we have not discussed. In particular, clinically important problems such as the control of orthotic/prosthetic devices, functional electrical stimulation, and the effects on muscle tone of neuromuscular pathologies like Parkinsonism are all issues in which compliant behavior is either the cause of problems or must at least be well characterized to allow successful treatment. These are all issues worthy of further study.

ACKNOWLEDGEMENTS

This work was supported in part by NIH Grants RO1-AR 33189 and RO1-NS 28176.

REFERENCES

1. Agarwal, G. and G. L. Gottlieb. Compliance of the human ankle joint. ASME J. *Biomech. Eng.* 99:166–170, 1977.
2. Agarwal, G., and G. L. Gottlieb. Oscillation of the human ankle joint in response to applied sinusoidal torque on the foot. *J. Physiol.* (Lond.), 268:151–176, 1977.
3. Almeida, G. L., D. H. Hong, D. M. Corcos, and G. L. Gottlieb. Organizing principles for voluntary movement: extending single joint rules. *J. Neurophysiol.* in press, 1995.
4. Asatryan, D. G., and A. G. Feldman. Functional tuning of the nervous system with control of movement or maintenance of a steady posture—I. Mechanographic analysis of the work of the joint or execution of a postural task. *Biofizika* 10:837–846, 1965 (English translation 925–935).
5. Atkeson, C. G., and J. M. Hollerbach. Kinematic features of unrestrained vertical arm movements. *J. Neurosci.* 5:2318–2330, 1985.
6. Bennett, D. J., et al. Time-varying stiffness of human elbow joint during cyclic voluntary movement. *Exp. Brain Res.* 88:433–442, 1992.
7. Bennett, D. J., M. Gorassini, and A. Prochazka. Catching a ball: contributions of intrinsic muscle stiffness, reflexes and higher order responses. *Can. J. Physiol. Pharmacol.* 72:525–534, 1994.
8. Bizzi, E., N. Accornero, W. Chapple, and N. Hogan. Arm trajectory formation in monkeys. *Exp. Brain Res.* 46:139–143, 1982.
9. Bizzi, E., N. Hogan, F. A. Mussa-Ivaldi, and S. Giszter. Does the nervous system use equilibrium-point control to guide single and multiple joint movements? *Behav. Brain Sci.* 15:603–613, 1992.
10. Bizzi, E., A. Polit, and P. Morasso. Mechanisms underlying achievement of final head position. *J. Neurophysiol.* 39:434–444, 1976.
11. Bock, O. Scaling of joint torque during planar arm movements. *Exp. Brain. Res.* 101:346–352, 1994.
12. Brown, T. I. H., P. M. H. Rack, and H. F. Ross. Forces generated at the thumb during imposed sinusoidal movements. *J. Physiol.* 332:69–85, 1982.
13. Cannon, S., and G. I. Zahalak. The mechanical behavior of active human skeletal muscle in small oscillations. *J. Biomech.* 15:111–121, 1982.
14. Cooker, H. S., C. R. Larson, and E. S. Luschei. Evidence that the human jaw stretch reflex increases the resistance of the mandible to small displacements. J. Physiol. 308:61, 1980.
15. Feldman, A. G., and M. F. Levine. Positional frames of reference in motor control: the origin and use. *Behav. Brain Sci.* in press, 1995.
16. Gordon, A. M., A. F. Huxley, and F. J. Julian. The variation in isometric tension with sarcomere length in vertebrate muscle fibres. *J. Physiol. (Lond.)* 184:170–192, 1966.
17. Gottlieb, G. L. A computational model of the simplest motor program. *J. Motor Behav.* 25:153–161, 1993.
18. Gottlieb, G. L., and G. Agarwal. Dependence of human ankle compliance on joint angle. *J. Biomech.* 11:177–181, 1978.
19. Gottlieb, G. L., D. M. Corcos, and G. Agarwal. Strategies for the control of single mechanical degree of freedom voluntary movements. *Behav. Brain Sci.* 12:189–210, 1989.
20. Gottlieb, G. L., M. L. Latash, D. M. Corcos, T. J. Liubinskas, and G. Agarwal. Organizing principles for single joint movements: V. Agonist-antagonist interactions. *J. Neurophysiol.* 67:1417–1427, 1992.
21. Hasan, Z., and J. Houk. Analysis of response properties of deferented mammalian spindle receptors based on frequency response. *J. Neurophysiol.* 38:663–673, 1975.
22. Henry, F. M., and D. E. Rogers. Increased response latency for complicated movements and a memory drum theory of neuromotor reaction. *Res. Q.* 31:448–458, 1960.
23. Hill, A. V. The heat of shortening and the dynamic constants of muscle. *Proc. R. Soc. (Lond.) [Biol]* B126:136–195, 1938.
24. Hogan, N. Adaptive control of mechanical impedance by coactivation of antagonist muscles. *IEEE Trans. Auto. Control* AC-29:681–690, 1984.

25. Hogan, N. The mechanics of multi-joint posture and movement control. *Biol. Cybern.* 52:315–331, 1985.

26. Hunter, I. W., and R. E. Kearney, Dynamics of human ankle stiffness: variation with mean ankle torque. *J. Biomech.* 15:747–752, 1982.

27. Joyce, G., and P. M. H. Rack. Isotonic lengthening and shortening movements of cat soleus muscle. *J. Physiol.* (Lond.), 204:475–491, 1969.

28. Joyce, G., P. M. H. Rack, and H. F. Ross. The forces generated at the human elbow joint in response to imposed sinusoidal movements of the forearm. *J. Physiol. (Lond.)* 240:351–374, 1974.

29. Joyce, G., P. M. H. Rack, and D. R. Westbury. The mechanical properties of cat soleus muscle during controlled lengthening and shortening movements. *J. Physiol.* (Lond.) 204:461–474, 1969.

30. Kearney, R. E., and I. W. Hunter. System identification of human joint dynamics. *Crit. Rev. Biomed. Eng.* 18:55–87, 1990.

31. Kirsch, R. F., R. E. Kearney, and J. B. MacNeil. Identification of time varying dynamics of the human triceps surae stretch reflex. I. Rapid isometric contraction. *Exp. Brain Res.* 97:115–127, 1993.

32. Lashley, D. S. The accuracy of movement in the absence of excitation from the moving organ. *Am. J. Physiol.* 43:169–194, 1917.

33. Latash, M. L. Virtual trajectories of single-joint movements performed under two basic strategies. *Neuroscience* 47:357–365, 1992.

34. Latash, M. L., and G. L. Gottlieb. Compliant characteristics of single joints: preservation of equifinality with phasic reactions. *Biol. Cybern.* 62:331–336, 1990.

35. MacNeil, J. B., R. B. Kearney, and I. W. Hunter. Identification of time-varying biological systems from ensemble data. *IEEE Trans. Biomed. Eng.* 39:1213–1225, 1992.

36. Matthews, B. H. Nerve endings in mammalian muscle. *J. Physiol.* (Lond.) 78:1–53, 1933.

37. Matthews, P. B. Muscle spindles and their motor control. *Physiol. Rev.* 44:219–288, 1964.

38. Matthews, P. B. *Mammalian Muscle Receptors and Their Central Actions.* Baltimore: Williams & Wilkins, 1972.

39. McIntyre, J., and E. Bizzi. Servo hypotheses for biological control of movement. *J. Motor Behav.* 25:193–202, 1993.

40. Mussa Ivaldi, F. A., N. Hogan, and E. Bizzi. Neural, mechanical, and geometric factors subserving arm posture in humans. *J. Neurosci.* 5:2732–2743, 1985.

41. Nichols, T. R. A biomechanical perspective on spinal mechanisms of coordinated muscular action: an architectural principle. *Acta Anat. (Basel)* 151:1–13, 1994.

42. Nichols, T. R., and J. Houk, Improvement in linearity and regulation of stiffness that results from actions of stretch reflex. *J. Neurophysiol.* 39:119–142, 1976.

43. Schmidt, R. A., et al. Motor-output variability: a theory for the accuracy of rapid motor acts. *Psychol. Rev.* 86:415–451, 1979.

44. Stein, R. B., et al. Analysis of short-latency reflexes in human elbow flexor muscles. *J. Neurophysiol.* 73:1900–1911, 1995.

45. Viviani, P., and A. Berthoz. Dynamics of the head-neck system in response to small perturbations: analysis and modeling in the frequency domain. *Biol. Cybern.* 19:19, 1985.

46. Walsh, E. G. Motion at the wrist induced by rhythmic forces. *J. Physiol. (Lond.),* 230:44P–45P, 1973.

47. Weiss, P. L., I. W. Hunter, and R. E. Kearney. Human ankle joint stiffness over the full range of muscle activation levels. *J. Biomech.* 21(7):539–544, 1988.

48. Weiss, P. L., R. E. Kearney, and I. W. Hunter. Position dependence of ankle joint dynamics—I. Passive mechanics. *J. Biomech.* 19:727–735, 1986.

49. Weiss, P. L., R. E. Kearney, and I. W. Hunter. Position dependence of ankle joint dynamics—II. Active mechanics. *J. Biomech.* 19:737–751, 1986.

50. Zajac, F. E. Muscle and tendon: properties, models, scaling and application to biomechanics and motor control. *CRC Crit. Rev. Biomed. Eng.* 17:359–411, 1989.

2
The Slow Component of Oxygen Uptake Kinetics in Humans

GLENN A. GAESSER, Ph.D.
DAVID C. POOLE, Ph.D.

Despite considerable evidence to the contrary, it is common dogma that exercise oxygen uptake increases as a linear function of work rate (WR) to the maximal level (Fig. 2.1, upper panel). In reality, however, the linearity of the $\dot{V}O_2$-WR relation pertains only for exercise tests performed exclusively below the lactate threshold (T_{Lac}) or where the WR is incremented rapidly to the maximum. Thus, for all constant-load exercise tests which incur a sustained lactic acidosis (i.e., $>T_{Lac}$), a slowly developing component of the $\dot{V}O_2$ kinetics is superimposed upon the rapid phase of $\dot{V}O_2$ initiated at exercise onset. The magnitude of this slow component increases with WR $>T_{Lac}$ and, if it cannot be stabilized, will drive $\dot{V}O_2$ to its maximum and signal imminent fatigue. Conceptually, it is crucial to appreciate that this slow component represents an additional energetic requirement (amounting to >1.0 liters O_2/min, in the extreme) *above* that predicted on the basis of the $<T_{Lac}$ $\dot{V}O_2$-WR relation.

In general, there has been a marked reluctance to acknowledge the presence of the $\dot{V}O_2$ slow component in the physiological literature, particularly in textbooks of exercise physiology [2, 36, 44, 74, 81, 91, 126]. One reason for this may stem from the fact that the slow component undermines some of the more fundamental concepts in exercise physiology, such as the steady state and oxygen deficit, which are deeply rooted in the exercise physiology literature [2, 36, 44, 55, 58, 59, 66, 74, 81, 91]. Without a steady state, our notion of a caloric equivalent for exercise becomes eroded. Furthermore, the $\dot{V}O_2$ slow component presents a challenge to our understanding of muscle energetics. It is our contention, however, that resolving the mechanistic basis for this phenomenon will provide valuable insights into muscle function and dysfunction.

The purpose of this chapter is to : 1) establish the historical precedence for the $\dot{V}O_2$ slow component; 2) characterize its occurrence with respect to the domains of exercise intensity; 3) define its physiological significance; 4) review the evidence for its mechanistic bases; 5) define the slow component adaptations to exercise training; and 6) present potential practical applications whereby modification of the submaximal exercise $\dot{V}O_2$ response may be altered as a means of improving exercise tolerance and thus mobility in patient populations.

FIGURE 2.1.

Upper panel, A schematic representation of the relationship between $\dot{V}O_2$ and time and $\dot{V}O_2$ and work rate (WR) for one subject. Note the attainment of a steady state depicted within 2–3 min for all WRs, the absence of a slow component for WR >T_{Lac} (i.e., WR $\geq$ 150 W), and the linearity of the $\dot{V}O_2$-WR relationship throughout the entire range of WR. Lower panel, Version of the upper panel, revised to portray the true physiological response. Note the slow component of $\dot{V}O_2$ manifest for >T_{Lac} WR and the resulting impact on the $\dot{V}O_2$-WR relationship. See Figure 2.2 for further analysis. Reproduced from ref. 2.

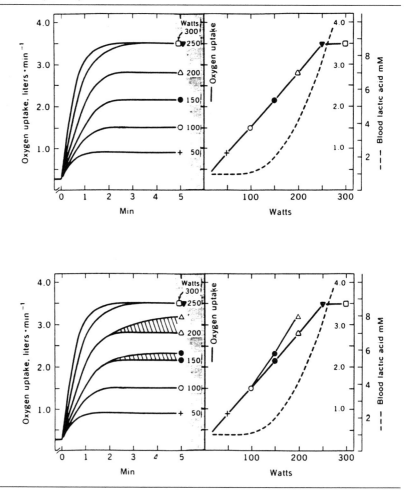

THE $\dot{V}O_2$ SLOW COMPONENT:
DEFINITION AND HISTORICAL PRECEDENCE

The $\dot{V}O_2$ slow component we address in this chapter is not to be confused with the "O_2 drift" that is typically seen during moderate exercise of a prolonged duration [30, 54, 64]. In those instances, the gradual rise in $\dot{V}O_2$ over the course of perhaps an hour or more of exercise is typically $<\sim 200$ ml of O_2. This rise in $\dot{V}O_2$ is not usually associated with an elevated, or rising, blood lactate concentration. The slow component of $\dot{V}O_2$ that we address is a different phenomenon, usually of much greater magnitude, and is observed only during $>T_{Lac}$ work rates where this extra $\dot{V}O_2$ component either stabilizes within ~ 20 min or drives $\dot{V}O_2$ to the maximum. Typically, the slow component is defined as the continued rise in $\dot{V}O_2$ beyond the 3rd min of exercise [6, 24, 45, 87, 93, 118, 123].

Thus, we purposely have avoided using the term "O_2 drift." Furthermore, the word "drift" (according to Webster's) connotes moving "in a random or casual way; to become carried along subject to no guidance or control." There is no evidence which refutes the notion that the $\dot{V}O_2$ slow component represents a controlled or regulated process. It's just that precise knowledge of the specific mechanisms has yet to be elucidated. Moreover, the pattern of $\dot{V}O_2$ response certainly cannot best be described as "random" or "casual." Thus, we contend that the term "O_2 drift" should not be used, certainly not to describe the $\dot{V}O_2$ slow component of heavy or severe exercise.

We also wish to make the distinction between the $\dot{V}O_2$ slow component, which has for the most part been identified using cycle ergometry [6–11, 18, 19, 22–25, 28, 35, 52, 56, 70, 83, 87–89, 93, 101, 128], and the slight, gradual rise in $\dot{V}O_2$ typically seen during submaximal negative work, such as downhill running [37, 65, 115, 116]. It is likely that the two phenomena have different mechanistic bases.

Published evidence for a slow component of $\dot{V}O_2$ during heavy intensity cycle ergometry has existed since at least 1961. Astrand and Saltin [3] presented data for five subjects who performed three to six bouts of exhausting, or near-exhausting, exercise for durations lasting up to ~ 8 min. Data for one of these subjects is presented in Figure 2.2. It is clear that a slow component of $\dot{V}O_2$ is evident for the two less intense work rates. The subject was not fatigued after 8 min of exercise at the lightest work rate (275 W), and the $\dot{V}O_2$ was still rising. The trajectory suggests that this subject's $\dot{V}O_{2max}$ of just over 4 L/min (which was attained at all higher work rates) might have been attained had the exercise duration at 275 W been extended for another 2–3 min. Eliciting $\dot{V}O_{2max}$ with "submaximal" work rates is a consequence of the $\dot{V}O_2$ slow component. Each of the other four subjects in that study exhibited similar response patterns for $\dot{V}O_2$. The surprising feature of these findings, and of this figure in particular, is that it appears in Astrand and Rodahl's *Textbook of Work Physiology* [2] just two pages

FIGURE 2.2.

$\dot{V}O_2$ responses for one subject during five different high-intensity exercise bouts. Arrows indicate point of fatigue. The subject was not fatigued after 7–8 min at 275 W. Note the existence of a slow component of $\dot{V}O_2$ (i.e., continued increase in $\dot{V}O_2$ after the 3rd min of exercise) at 275 and 300 W. See text and refer to Figure 2.1 for further discussion. Reproduced from ref. 2.

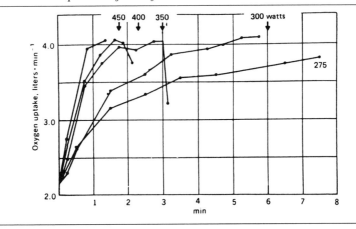

after the $\dot{V}O_2$-time and $\dot{V}O_2$-work rate relationships presented in the upper panel of Figure 2.1 (which shows no evidence of a slow component and depicts $\dot{V}O_2$ rising linearly to the maximum). Thus, it is likely that a truer representation of the $\dot{V}O_2$-time and $\dot{V}O_2$-work rate relationships depicted in Figure 2.1 is that which is presented in the lower panel of that figure, showing the slow component for work rates above T_{Lac} and the corresponding upward curvature to the $\dot{V}O_2$-work rate relationship.

Since the unequivocal findings of Astrand and Saltin [3], many others, particularly Whipp and associates [117–123], have demonstrated the existence of a slow component. It is important to recognize that this phenomenon presents itself in a range of exercise modalities, including cycling [6–11, 18, 19, 22–25, 28, 52, 56, 70, 83, 87–89, 93, 95, 101, 128], running [29, 80, 103], and isometric exercise [110].

CHARACTERIZATION OF $\dot{V}O_2$ WITH RESPECT TO EXERCISE INTENSITY DOMAINS

With respect to their attendant $\dot{V}O_2$ and blood lactate responses, three domains of exercise intensity can usefully be discriminated (Fig. 2.3). These are defined as follows: The domain of *moderate exercise* encompasses all work rates which can be accomplished without induction of a sustained lactic aci-

FIGURE 2.3.

Schematic representation of the $\dot{V}O_2$ response to incremental exercise (left panel) and the $\dot{V}O_2$ and blood lactate responses to constant-load exercise in each exercise intensity domain (center and right panels). Each panel is demarcated into moderate ($<T_{Lac}$), heavy ($>T_{Lac}<W_a$), and severe ($>W_a$) exercise domains, where T_{Lac} and W_a denote the lactate threshold and asymptote of the power-time relationship, respectively. Notice that for the rapid incremental test the $\dot{V}O_2$-work rate is linear to the maximum, with the classic plateau at $\dot{V}O_{2max}$. For constant-load exercise within the moderate domain, $\dot{V}O_2$ increases rapidly with first order kinetics in the face of unchanged blood [lactate]. Work rates above the lactate threshold within the heavy domain induce an additional slow component of $\dot{V}O_2$, which delays attainment of a steady state and elevates the $\dot{V}O_2$ above that predicted on the basis of the sub-T_{Lac} energetics. Blood [lactate] remains elevated and plateaus in concert with the $\dot{V}O_2$. For severe-intensity exercise, both $\dot{V}O_2$ and blood [lactate] increase to achieve a maximum exercise value at fatigue. For constant-load exercise, the shaded panels denote $\dot{V}O_2$ slow component. In each panel, fatigue is noted by the arrow. See text for further details.

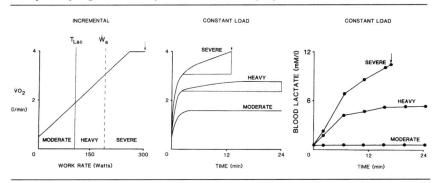

dosis i.e., below the lactate threshold (T_{Lac}). As was recognized initially by Hill and Lupton [59], at the onset of constant-load exercise, $\dot{V}O_2$ increases monoexponentially with a time constant, τ, of ~45 s, to achieve a steady state within about 3 min in health individuals:

$$\dot{V}O_2(t) = \dot{V}O_2(ss)\ (1-e^-[t-\delta]/\tau])\qquad 1$$

where $\dot{V}O_2(t)$ is the increase of $\dot{V}O_2$ at time t above that at rest, $\dot{V}O_2(ss)$ is the increase of $\dot{V}O_2$ at steady state, and δ represents an early delay-like phase (Phase 1) which precedes the exponential rise (Phase 2) to the steady state (Phase 3) [121]. These 3 phases of the $\dot{V}O_2$ on-response reflect the underlying physiology of the transient phase. In *Phase 1*, increases of $\dot{V}O_2$ within the early delay-like component have been attributed principally to augmented cardiac output and thus pulmonary blood flow [66, 112], with smaller contributions likely arising from changes in lung gas stores [9] and mixed venous O_2 content [23]. *Phase 2* is initiated by the arrival at the lung of venous blood from the exercising muscle, and increased $\dot{V}O_2$ in this phase represents augmented O_2 extraction and any continued increase of pulmonary blood flow. The notion that pulmonary $\dot{V}O_2$ in Phase 2 reflects closely muscle $\dot{V}O_2$ is supported strongly by modeling studies [8] and also the temporal correspondence between Phase 2 pulmonary $\dot{V}O_2$ changes and those of phosphocreatine within the exercising muscle [6]. Recently, Grassi and colleagues [51], have developed a method which enables essentially continuous determination of leg blood flow and hence $\dot{V}O_2$ across the transition from unloaded pedaling to a moderate work rate. During Phase 2, both alveolar and muscle $\dot{V}O_2$ increased exponentially with statistically indistinguishable kinetics (i.e., half-times for muscle $\dot{V}O_2$ averaged 27.9 s and those for alveolar $\dot{V}O_2$, 25.5 s, $P > 0.05$). These results substantiate the conclusions developed on the basis of less direct Magnetic Resonance Spectroscopy (MRS) and modeling approaches presented above.

Within the domain of moderate intensity exercise, the Phase 2 time constant is relatively invariant with work rate but is faster in highly fit subjects and for a given subject can be reduced by training (e.g., ref. 52). In *Phase 3* the steady-state $\dot{V}O_2$ response increases as a linear function of work rate within the moderate intensity domain, having a gain of 9–11 ml $O_2/W/min$ [56, 117, 122].

The domain of *heavy exercise* is initiated at the lowest work rate at which blood lactate appearance exceeds its rate of removal (i.e., T_{Lac}) and there is a sustained elevation of blood lactate for the duration of the work. The upper boundary to this domain is defined as the highest work rate at which blood lactate can be stabilized (also termed the maximum lactate steady state). Thus, lactate appearance and removal rates are once again balanced, but at an elevated blood lactate concentration. This work rate corresponds to the power(W)-time(t) asymptote (W_a) [88, 89; please refer to PHYSIOLOGICAL SIGNIFICANCE below for a detailed analysis of the W-t relationship]. However, it has been argued that the W-t asymptote may overestimate slightly the upper limit for the heavy exercise domain [75]. One compelling feature within this domain is the tight coherence between blood lactate and $\dot{V}O_2$ profiles. With rare exception [97, 103], the temporal profiles of blood lactate and $\dot{V}O_2$ are qualitatively and quantitatively related [88, 93, 117].

Thus, following 80–110 s after exercise onset [10, 83], the slow component of $\dot{V}O_2$ becomes superimposed upon the rapid initial increase associated with exercise onset. For exercise in this domain, the slow component appears to develop most rapidly early in the exercise bout (i.e., minutes 3–10) [24, 87–89, 93, 120]. Some uncertainty exists as to whether this rapid component is slowed $>T_{Lac}$ [83] or not [10]. What is certain is that the slow component represents an additional or excess $\dot{V}O_2$ above that predicted from sub-T_{Lac} $\dot{V}O_2$-work rate considerations [56, 87, 88, 93, 117, 120] (Fig. 2.4). Thus, within the domain of heavy exercise, the $\dot{V}O_2$ cost per unit of work (i.e., $\dot{V}O_2/W$) rises substantially above the 9–11 ml found in the moderate intensity domain, and thus for increments of heavy exercise, calcu-

FIGURE 2.4.

Upper panel, Temporal response profile of $\dot{V}O_2$ to different levels of constant-load exercise. Shaded panels correspond to the increase of $\dot{V}O_2$ above that predicted from sub-T_{Lac} $\dot{V}O_2$-work rate relationship (i.e., slow component). Notice that $\dot{V}O_2$ rises above that predicted solely for work rates which elicit a $\dot{V}O_2 > T_{Lac}$. Lower panel, Comparison of $\dot{V}O_2$ responses to constant-load (open circles) and incremental (closed circles) exercise. For incremental exercise (15 W/min), $\dot{V}O_2$ for each work rate is the average value of $\dot{V}O_2$ for all breaths during the final 30 s of each 60-s interval at that work rate. For constant-load exercise, $\dot{V}O_2$ is the average $\dot{V}O_2$ for all breaths in minutes 9 and 10 or at fatigue. Arrows denote elevation of $\dot{V}O_2$ above that predicted from the sub-T_{Lac} $\dot{V}O_2$-work rate relationship. Notice that for $> T_{Lac}$ constant-load work rates, work efficiency (η) is reduced considerably. Reproduced from ref. 56.

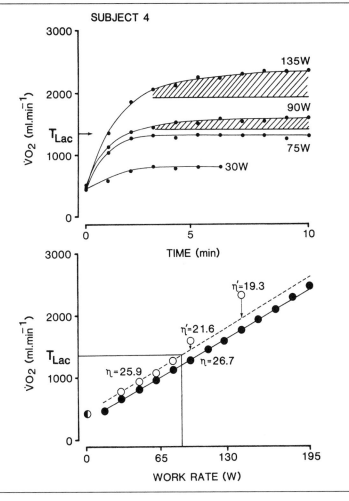

erate intensity domain, and thus for increments of heavy exercise, calculated work efficiency is reduced [56] (Fig. 2.5).

All available evidence demonstrates that the $\dot{V}O_2$ slow component presents only above T_{Lac}, irrespective of the absolute metabolic rate at which this occurs [56, 93, 122]. Henson and colleagues [56] demonstrated this most clearly when they exercised subjects with a broad range of fitness and $\dot{V}O_{2max}$ levels (i.e., $\dot{V}O_{2max}$ 1.6 to 5.3 L/min). Notice in Figure 2.6, that slow-component behavior is in evidence exclusively at work rates above T_{Lac} (as estimated using "v-slope" gas exchange criteria) and drives the $\dot{V}O_2$ at a given work rate above that found in the fitter individual. Thus, in the least fit subject (no. 2: T_{Lac}, 1.2; $\dot{V}O_{2max}$, 1.8 L/min) 75 W is supra-T_{Lac}, and the slow component drives $\dot{V}O_2$ higher than that found for this work rate in the fitter subject, no. 4 (T_{Lac}, 1.4; $\dot{V}O_{2max}$, 2.4 L/min), for whom this work rate is sub-T_{Lac}. This is seen again at 135 W where the much fitter subject, no. 11 (T_{Lac}, 2.3; $\dot{V}O_{2max}$, 4.7 L/min), has a far lower $\dot{V}O_2$ than subject no. 4 who exhibits a large slow component.

FIGURE 2.5.

$\dot{V}O_2$/watt (upper panel) and efficiency of work (lower panel) measured during constant-load exercise at or below T_{Lac} and for two work rates $>T_{Lac}$. Different symbols denote individual subjects. Reproduced from ref. 56.

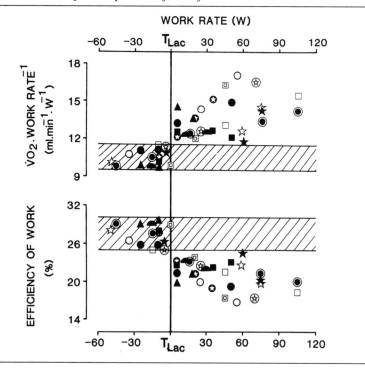

FIGURE 2.6.

Temporal response profiles of $\dot{V}O_2$ during constant-load exercise for three subjects of widely disparate fitness levels. As previously, shaded panels portray increase of $\dot{V}O_2$ above that predicted from sub-T_{Lac} $\dot{V}O_2$-work rate relationship. See text for further details. Reproduced from ref. 56.

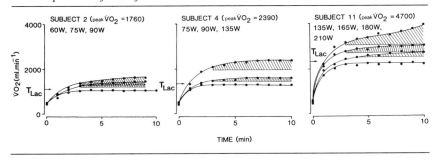

Within the domain of *severe-intensity* exercise, neither $\dot{V}O_2$ nor blood lactate can be stabilized; rather, both rise inexorably until fatigue ensues, at which point $\dot{V}O_2$ achieves its maximum (Fig. 2.7). Because $\dot{V}O_2$ rises as a function of both time and power within the heavy- and severe-exercise intensity domains, it is not appropriate to identify discrete work rates with respect to $\dot{V}O_2$. Thus, the common practice of reporting exercise intensity as a percentage of $\dot{V}O_{2max}$ is fundamentally flawed within these upper domains. As a consequence of the lower boundary to the severe-exercise domain corresponding to the W-t asymptote, which commonly occurs at close to 50% of the work rate difference between T_{Lac} and $\dot{V}O_{2max}$ on an incremental ramp test [89], there exists a broad range of work rates over which $\dot{V}O_2$ will increase with time to achieve its maximum. Work rates in the severe-exercise intensity domain which are close to the W-t asymptote will exhibit a particularly large $\dot{V}O_2$ slow component which develops progressively over the tolerable duration of the work (typically 10–20 min). To date, there is experimental evidence that in the extreme the $\dot{V}O_2$ slow component may account for as much as 1.0–1.5 L/min [10, 18, 88, 93, 117]. Remarkably, constant-load exercise performed at just a few W below the W-t asymptote presents an entirely different metabolic scenario. Specifically, $\dot{V}O_2$ stabilizes within 10–20 min, reflecting slow-component kinetics, blood lactate ceases to increase, and the exercise load can be sustained for a considerable period.

Modeling the $\dot{V}O_2$ Slow Component

To date, the dynamics of the $\dot{V}O_2$ slow component have eluded formal characterization [10, 83, 123]. Thus, there is no consensus as to whether the data conform best to an exponential or linear process. It is possible that the $\dot{V}O_2$ slow component exhibits fundamentally different dynamics for heavy- as opposed to severe-intensity exercise. Linnarsson [70] fitted slow-compo-

FIGURE 2.7.

Left panel, $\dot{V}O_2$-work rate relationship for incremental exercise (solid symbols) and constant-load exercise bouts at and above the power-time asymptote (W_a, hollow circles) for one subject. Note that for the exercise at W_a, this represents the upper limit of the heavy domain, and the $\dot{V}O_2$ stabilizes at a submaximal value in marked contrast to the 5 bouts performed $>W_a$, which all result in a maximum $\dot{V}O_2$ at fatigue (arrows). Right panel, $\dot{V}O_2$ response for constant-load exercise at W_a, just a few watts $>W_a$ and at the work rate which gave a maximum $\dot{V}O_2$ on the incremental test (n = 7). For W_a exercise, the plateau value at 24 min is given; both of the higher work rate tests were by definition in the severe-intensity domain and consequently induced fatigue at <24 min. Similar to the subject depicted in the left panel, note that for each of the seven subjects, exercise at just a few watts $>W_a$ produced a maximum $\dot{V}O_2$ at fatigue. Reproduced from data from refs. 88 and 89.

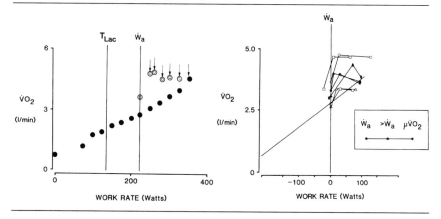

nent data to an exponential model; however, he found that the time constant for individual subjects was excessively long i.e., 30–60 min or more. Using short exercise bouts of just 8 min Barstow and Mole [10] found evidence for both exponential (6 of 8) and linear (1 of 8) slow-component behavior. Similarly, Paterson and Whipp [83] were unable to distinguish between exponential and linear fits. One feature of the response that is visually compelling is that within the severe exercise intensity domain, beyond 3 min of exercise onset, $\dot{V}O_2$ projects to the maximum with what appears to be a linear trajectory (see Fig. 2 of ref. 88 and Fig. 4 of ref. 10). However, in this domain, assessing the fit of an exponential model to the data is critically dependent upon estimation of an appropriate theoretical asymptote which lies beyond the physiological limits. Thus, exponential behavior cannot rigorously be discounted. What may be more useful in future studies is to investigate slow-component kinetics strictly within the domain of heavy-intensity exercise and continue the exercise until an unequivocal asymptote of $\dot{V}O_2$ is achieved.

PHYSIOLOGICAL SIGNIFICANCE

The W-t relationship for exhausting, high-intensity exercise depicted in Figure 2.8 was initially described by Hill in 1927 [58]. This relationship conforms to a rectangular hyperbola [78, 79, 88, 89, 119]:

$$W' = (W - W_a) \cdot t \qquad\qquad 2$$

where t is time in seconds and W' denotes a constant amount of work which can be performed above the asymptote of power, W_a (Fig. 2.8). This relationship can be transformed into its linear formulation:

$$W = (W'/t) + W_a \qquad\qquad 3$$

in which W' and W_a are given by the slope and intercept, respectively. The precise physiological determinants of parameters W' and W_a remain to be defined. However, W_a may reasonably be considered to represent a sustainable rate of adenosine triphosphate (ATP) repletion defined either in terms of work rate or O_2 cost of exercise, i.e., $W_a\{O_2\}$. In contrast, W' comprises a finite store of energetic equivalents consisting of the available phosphagen pool, O_2 stores in venous blood, and myoglobin and anaerobic glycolysis leading to production and accumulation of lactate. Thus, W' may be considered to be equivalent to the O_2 deficit. Exercise at or below W_a may be continued beyond the initial transient, without continued depletion of the energy stores (W'). In contrast, exercise $>W_a$ draws continuously upon the W' compartment at a rate given by $W-W_a$, and fatigue ensues in time t as predicted from Equations 2 and 3 above.

That the form of the W-t relationship is hyperbolic is supported empirically [21, 63, 78, 79, 88, 89, 119] and by a solid theoretical foundation, unlike exponential formulations [124]. Thus, if one makes the tenable assumption that the factor(s) ultimately inducing fatigue (e.g., accumulation of H^+, $H_2PO_4^-$, lactate, or depletion of the high-energy phosphate pool) change as either an exponential or linear monotonic function of time toward some limiting level for all work rates $>W_a$, the parameter characterizing this rate of change (i.e., time constant or slope) should be a function of $W-W_a$. Accordingly, for all constant-load exercise tests $>W_a$, the exercise time to fatigue will decrease hyperbolically as W increases.

This W-t relationship is powerful because for high-intensity exercise that leads to fatigue within 1–30 min, knowing parameters W_a and W' for a given subject, the tolerable duration of exercise can be estimated with precision. Beyond this range, additional considerations come into play which distort the underlying physiology. Specifically, at extremely high work rates that lead to exhaustion within 60 s, mechanical force generation may become limiting. At the other end of the spectrum, beyond 30 min, the tolerable duration of work may become limited by substrate (carbohydrate) depletion, fluid imbalance, or thermoregulatory shortcomings.

FIGURE 2.8.

Upper panel, the power-time relationship for severe-intensity exercise. Lower panel, Linear formulation of the power-time relationship which allows precise determination of parameters W_a (intercept) and W' (slope). The excellent linear fit demonstrates the truly hyperbolic nature of the power-time relation. See text for further details. Reproduced from ref. 89.

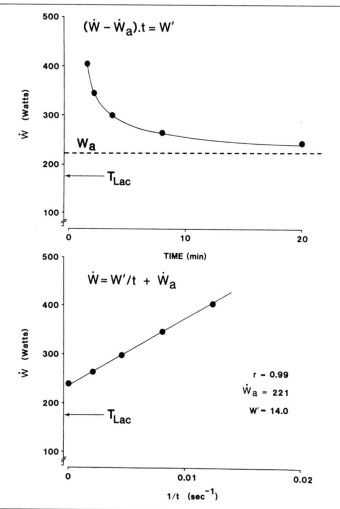

The etiology of muscle fatigue (i.e., failure to sustain a required power output) is complex, potentially involving one or more of several sites between excitatory input to higher motor sensors and the actual contractile process itself [16, 43]. Obviously, the precise nature of the fatigue process will be influenced by the type of exercise, its intensity, and the condition of the subject. It is well accepted that factors inducing fatigue during high-intensity exercise for which the tolerable duration is only several minutes (i.e., severe-intensity exercise) will be different from those found during lower intensity exercise which can be sustained for up to several hours (moderate- and heavy-intensity exercise). Whereas the W-t relationship cannot isolate specific causes of fatigue, it does provide a tight conceptual framework in which to study the fatigue process and attendant physiological changes.

Thus, for exercise in the severe-intensity domain (i.e., $>W_a$), no gas exchange or metabolic steady state can be achieved. Rather, blood lactate, lactate-to-pyruvate ratio, and $[H^+]$ continue to rise (presumably reflecting intramuscular changes), bicarbonate falls, and $\dot{V}O_2$ rises inexorably toward the maximum at fatigue [88, 89]. The augmented $\dot{V}O_2$ reflects an increase in both exercising muscle blood flow and O_2 extraction, with each process contributing in approximately equal proportion to the "excess" $\dot{V}O_2$ above that predicted [12, 87]. Such exercise likely recruits all three major fiber Types (I, IIa, IIb), and generates high intracellular concentrations of H^+ and $H_2PO_4^-$ which inhibit the contractile mechanism [e.g., 39, 41, 76, 82]. It is also possible that the lactate ion itself reduces muscle tension [60]. Glycogen depletion has been largely dismissed as a putative mediator at these intensities on the basis that muscle biopsies reveal substantial glycogen stores remaining at fatigue [14]. However, consistent with the finding that IIb fibers do become selectively depleted of glycogen within several minutes at these work rates [108], glycogen supercompensation does improve exercise tolerance in the severe-intensity domain [72]. Therefore, it is possible that selective fiber glycogen depletion may reduce power output and promote fatigue even at severe exercise intensities. In marked contrast to the above, exercise at work rates $\leq W_a$ in the heavy-intensity domain allows all these metabolic variables to reach approximately stable levels within 20 or so minutes from exercise onset, and consequently the exercise can be continued for a prolonged period [88]. In this domain, where $\dot{V}O_2$ typically plateaus at 60–85% $\dot{V}O_{2max}$, and there is presumably little alteration in intracellular H^+ and $H_2PO_4^-$ concentrations beyond the initial transient, it is difficult to conceive that these factors are an integral part of the fatigue process. Indeed, at these work rates exercise tolerance has been linked strongly to initial muscle glycogen levels, with fatigue closely related to muscle glycogen depletion. Within the domain of heavy-intensity exercise (i.e., $>T_{Lac} < W_a$), it is likely that the rate of glycogen depletion increases proportionally with work rate, and this is reflected by maintenance of augmented blood lactate concentrations which stabilize at progressively higher values up to W_a.

For heavy and severe-intensity exercise, the evidence presented above indicates that continually increasing profiles of blood lactate and $\dot{V}O_2$ are sentinel processes signaling imminent fatigue. This raises the issue of whether constraining the rise of $\dot{V}O_2$ and blood lactate during severe-intensity exercise delays the onset of fatigue. Ribiero et al. [92] found that by progressively lowering cycle ergometer power output to ~85% of the initial value, $\dot{V}O_2$ could be maintained at 75–80% of maximum for 40 min (without fatigue) and blood lactate at ~5 mM, on average. In the same vein, by systematically reducing treadmill velocity during 30 min of running, subjects studied by Stoudemire and colleagues [104] were able to maintain $\dot{V}O_2$ at $\geq 90\%$ $\dot{V}O_{2max}$ and keep the blood lactate level relatively constant (in the 3–6 mM range) for the latter 25 min of the run (Fig. 2.9). These observations support the notion that for exercise $>W_a$ in the severe-intensity domain, the slow component of $\dot{V}O_2$ projects to the maximum; however, by systematic attenuation of power output or running velocity, fatigue can be deferred and the metabolic and gas exchange profiles revert to those seen $<W_a$ in the heavy-intensity domain. The data of Stoudemire et al. [104] also show that $\dot{V}O_2$ close to, and in some instances equal to, $\dot{V}O_{2max}$ can be maintained for periods of time much longer than generally assumed [17]. This can only occur, of course, with a systematic reduction in the absolute running velocity (or, presumably, power output).

O₂ Deficit Considerations

The O_2 deficit concept first proposed by Hill in the early part of this century provides a conceptually useful framework for understanding exercise energetics. However, complexities associated with $\dot{V}O_2$ slow-component behavior may confound accurate calculation and interpretation of the O_2 deficit.

FIGURE 2.9.

Velocity, $\dot{V}O_2$, and blood lactate during 30 min of running for one male subject (solid circles) and one female subject (open circles). Treadmill velocity was systematically adjusted downward to maintain each subject's rating of perceived exertion (RPE) constant (~ 17 on the Borg Scale) throughout the 30-min run and at a level commensurate with the RPE associated with a blood lactate concentration of ~ 4 mM obtained during an incremental treadmill test for determination of $\dot{V}O_{2max}$. The dashed lines on the top two panels represent the velocity associated with the 4 mM of blood lactate obtained in incremental testing and the $\dot{V}O_{2max}$ of each subject. Both subjects attained 99–100% of age-predicted maximum heart rate during the incremental test. Over the last 25 min of the run, the male subject maintained ~ 93% of $\dot{V}O_{2max}$, and the female subject maintained ~ 100% $\dot{V}O_{2max}$. This occurred in the face of decreases in velocity of 34 m/min and 49 m/min for the male and female subjects, respectively. From N. M. Stoudemire et al., unpublished data.

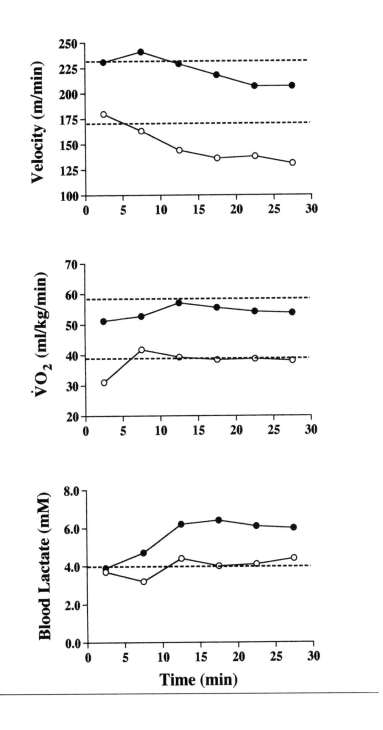

At the onset of moderate-intensity exercise ($<T_{Lac}$), $\dot{V}O_2$ increases with finite kinetics, whereas that of ATP turnover rate presumably achieves its steady-state level instantaneously. One necessary consequence of this behavior is that an O_2 deficit will be incurred. Thus, for moderate-intensity exercise the O_2 deficit is the product of the increment in steady-state $\dot{V}O_2$ above resting, $\dot{V}O_2(ss)$, and the effective time constant, τ, such that:

$$O_2 \text{ deficit} = \dot{V}O_2(ss) \cdot \tau \qquad\qquad 4$$

For moderate-intensity exercise, the O_2 deficit is comprised principally of reductions in the high-energy phosphate pool (PCr) and O_2 stores depletion, with a minor contribution from anaerobic glycolysis. For moderate-intensity exercise bouts of limited duration, the $\dot{V}O_2$ on- and off-kinetics are virtually symmetrical in this domain, and thus the notion that the excess postexercise O_2 uptake repletes stores drawn upon at exercise onset is valid.

One fundamental precept for calculation of the O_2 deficit is that the O_2 requirement of the exercise be known, and, as seen above, for moderate exercise this is straightforward. However, for heavy- and severe-intensity exercise, the appropriate frame of reference is not intuitively obvious. Specifically, is the O_2 requirement for a given heavy work rate that predicted on the basis of the sub-T_{Lac} energetics, or does the slow component represent a legitimate portion of the O_2 requirement from exercise onset and therefore should be included? Pertinent to this issue, two studies, published almost simultaneously, demonstrate that the $\dot{V}O_2$ response to heavy exercise is best characterized by a rapid primary single exponential followed by a secondary slow component of delayed onset [10, 83]. This is also true for severe-intensity exercise when a substantial slow component is present. At yet higher work rates, $\dot{V}O_2$ increases monoexponentially to the maximum, and fatigue becomes manifest before a slow component can develop. For these latter exercise bouts, the O_2 deficit conforms to the relationship:

$$O_2 \text{ deficit} = \dot{V}O_{2max} \cdot \tau \qquad\qquad 5$$

As developed by Whipp [118], this formulation indicates that the O_2 deficit will be the same for all work rates for which the rapid initial kinetics project to a $\dot{V}O_2 > \dot{V}O_{2max}$. The notion of the independence of work rate and O_2 deficit in this instance supports the theoretical foundation for the hyperbolic W-t curve. Furthermore, it suggests that the $\dot{V}O_2$ projected on the basis of the rapid $\dot{V}O_2$ kinetics represents the appropriate frame of reference for calculation of the O_2 deficit for all work rates $>W_a$. Whether this is also true for work rates $\leq W_a$ but $>T_{Lac}$ is, at present, speculative.

CAUSES OF THE $\dot{V}O_2$ SLOW COMPONENT

A number of factors have been postulated to contribute to the slow component of $\dot{V}O_2$ observed during heavy and severe exercise. These include the effects of: lactate [6, 23, 86, 88, 89, 93, 105, 111, 123], epinephrine [49, 88, 128], cardiac and ventilatory work [24, 53,128], temperature [53, 87], potassium [129], less efficient mitochondrial P-O coupling [125], reduced chemical-mechanical coupling efficiency [87, 118, 125], and recruitment of lower-efficiency fast-twitch motor units [31, 61, 101]. Each of these will be addressed. Before doing so, however, it must be emphasized that although the mechanism(s) underlying the phenomenon remain speculative, the primary origin of the $\dot{V}O_2$ slow component appears to be the working limbs [77, 85, 87, 95, 110].

By simultaneously measuring both pulmonary and leg $\dot{V}O_2$ during cycle ergometry, Poole and associates [87] demonstrated that ~86% of the increment in pulmonary $\dot{V}O_2$ beyond the third minute of exercise could be accounted for by the increase in leg $\dot{V}O_2$ (Figs. 2.10, 2.11). These data indicate that the majority of the $\dot{V}O_2$ slow component is attributable to factors within the working limbs. As such, factors having an effect outside the working musculature likely contribute minimally to the slow component of $\dot{V}O_2$.

Of all the factors hypothesized to play a role in this phenomenon, *lactate* has received the most attention [6, 23, 86, 88, 89, 93, 105, 111, 123]. At least for cycle ergometry, the magnitude of the slow component has been shown to be highly correlated with the rise in blood lactate during exercise [88, 93, 123]. In humans, infusion of lactate has been reported to elevate $\dot{V}O_2$ at rest [106] and during exercise [96]. Ryan et al. [96], for example, demonstrated that infusion of sodium L-(+)-lactate in humans during exercise elevated blood lactate concentration (from 3.9 mM to 5.3 mM) and raised $\dot{V}O_2$ by 129 ml/min. Lactate may stimulate gluco/glyconeogenesis during exercise, and although the energetic cost of this process is likely to be small, it can occur within the active muscle [107, 118]. Wasserman and colleagues [105, 111], however, have contended that it is not lactate per se, but rather the accompanying acidosis that causes the slow component of $\dot{V}O_2$ during heavy exercise. They postulated that the reduction in pH accompanying lactic acidosis, via the Bohr effect, shifts the oxyhemoglobin dissociation curve to the right, in effect raising capillary PO_2 and allowing $\dot{V}O_2$ to continue to rise. It is crucial to appreciate, however, that this hypothesis cannot explain why $\dot{V}O_2$ rises above that projected from the sub-T_{Lac} $\dot{V}O_2$-WR relationship. Furthermore, there are several lines of evidence that cast doubt on the hypothesis that lactate, or lactic acidosis, is the cause of the $\dot{V}O_2$ slow component.

In some instances blood lactate has been shown to be elevated and rising progressively even when $\dot{V}O_2$ is in a steady state [97]. In treadmill running, it is possible to see a significant $\dot{V}O_2$ slow component even when the blood lactate concentration remains unchanged, near resting levels [103]. Moreover, blood lactate can be elevated significantly during exercise by infusion of epinephrine without any change in exercise $\dot{V}O_2$ [45, 49, 98, 99, 128], even in the face of a reduced blood pH [45]. Additionally, Poole et al. [86] recently demonstrated that L-(+)-lactate infusions into the arter-

FIGURE 2.10.

Mean response of pulmonary and leg V̇O₂ to light (upper panel) and severe (lower panel) constant-load cycle ergometer exercise. Total exercise (100%) was 26 min for light exercise and an average of 20.8 min for severe exercise. "Twice-one-leg" V̇O₂ represents the product of 2 × blood flow and arteriovenous O₂ difference. Lines represent exponential fits. The slow component is only evident for severe exercise, during which the pulmonary and twice-one-leg V̇O₂ responses closely parallel each other. Reproduced from ref. 87.

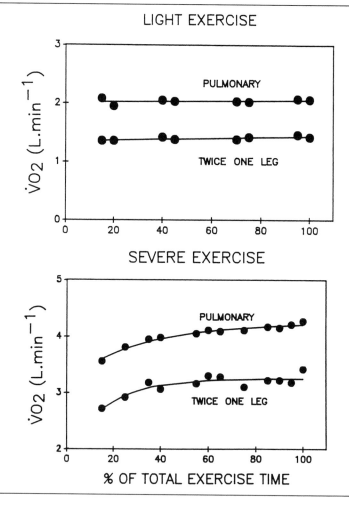

FIGURE 2.11.

Relationship between mean pulmonary and twice-one-leg $\dot{V}O_2$ during severe exercise. Each value represents actual $\dot{V}O_2 - \dot{V}O_2$ at min 3 of exercise. Solid line is the regression line (r = 0.91). Dashed line represents the line of identity. Numbers indicate sampling time as a percentage of the total exercise time. These data demonstrate that ~86% of the slow component arises from the exercising muscles. Reproduced from ref. 87.

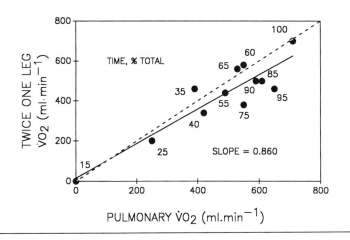

ial supply of electrically stimulated dog gastrocnemius muscle did not increase $\dot{V}O_2$, despite significantly elevating the concentrations of blood (by ~10 mM) and muscle (to >9 mM) lactate. In sum, these observations suggest that lactate is correlated with, but not causal to, the $\dot{V}O_2$ slow component.

The $\dot{V}O_2$ cost of respiratory muscle work necessary to increase *pulmonary ventilation* undoubtedly contributes to the progressive rise in $\dot{V}O_2$ seen during exercise >T_{Lac}. Quantifying the percentage of the slow component that can be assigned to the additional O_2 requirements for ventilation depends upon the values selected to estimate the energy cost of breathing. Aaron et al. [1] determined that the O_2 cost of ventilations ranged from 1.79 ml/L (for ventilations in the range of ~63–79 L/min) to 2.85 ml/L (for ventilation in the range of ~117–147 L/min). During heavy and severe exercise, pulmonary ventilation may rise by ~20–60 L/min during the time the $\dot{V}O_2$ slow component is elicited [24, 25, 87, 123]. Thus, the O_2 cost of this rise in ventilation may range from ~36 to ~171 ml/min. It is not uncommon to observe $\dot{V}O_2$ slow components in the range of 500 ml/min to >1,000 ml/min [56, 87, 93, 123]. In the study by Poole et al. [87], for example, mean ventilation for the subjects rose from 95.5 L/min at 3 minutes to 152.3 L/min at the end of exercise, during which time mean pulmonary $\dot{V}O_2$ increased by 710 ml/min. Using a value of 2.85 ml/L, the 56.8 L/min increase in ventilation required an additional O_2 uptake of 162 ml/min. This represented $\sim$23% of the 710 ml/min slow component that was evident by the end of exercise. Other published data [128] are consistent with this value and suggest that ventilation probably accounts for a relatively small percentage of the total $\dot{V}O_2$ slow component.

Epinephrine has been suggested as a possible mediator of the slow component [45, 49, 128]. It is well documented that epinephrine infusion increases resting metabolic rate [42, 71, 102]. Furthermore, plasma epinephrine concentration increases considerably during heavy and severe exercise [87, 88]. It has also been shown that β-adrenergic blockade with propranolol has the potential to alter the $\dot{V}O_2$ response found during 90 min of moderate exercise [64]. However, more recent evidence suggests that the β-adrenergic system does not play a role in the slow component of O_2 uptake during heavy or severe exercise. Infusion of epinephrine into humans during exercise has no appreciable effect on $\dot{V}O_2$ [49, 72, 98, 99, 128], despite raising the plasma epinephrine concentration to levels seen in supramaximal exercise [49] (Fig. 2.12). Additionally, a preliminary report by Davis et al. [34] suggests that β-adrenergic blockade with propranolol does not diminish the magnitude of the slow component of O_2 uptake during severe exercise.

Core and muscle temperatures increase during exercise [25, 38, 53, 87, 88, 94] and thus may, via the "Q_{10}" effect, contribute to the progressive rise in $\dot{V}O_2$ during heavy exercise. If the Q_{10} effect increases $\dot{V}O_2$ in proportion to the attendant metabolic rate and the working muscles are generating 80–90% of that metabolic rate, then the Q_{10} effect of any exercising muscle has the potential to increase the $\dot{V}O_2$ 5–10 times that occurring in the rest of the body. Also, by deduction, with the majority of the slow component arising from the working limbs, any effect of temperature is most likely to predominate within the exercising muscles. Poole et al. [87] estimated (assuming a Q_{10} of 2.5) that, during heavy exercise in which leg $\dot{V}O_2$ rose from 2.72 L/min at 3 minutes to 3.42 L/min at the end of exercise, a 1°C-rise in muscle temperature (femoral venous blood temperature rose by $\sim$0.8°C during this time) could account for $\sim$272 ml/min of the 700 ml/min ($\sim$39%) slow component arising from the exercising limbs. This assumes, of course, that venous blood temperature accurately reflects the temperature of the exercising muscles. If so, the Q_{10} effect in working muscles theoretically could account for a significant portion of the $\dot{V}O_2$ slow component. However, rising muscle temperature has been observed in the face of constant leg $\dot{V}O_2$ [87], and elevating body (and likely also muscle) temperature did not increase pulmonary $\dot{V}O_2$ in exercising humans [94]. This conclusion is also supported by the data of Dill et al. [38] and Poole et al. [88].

During heavy exercise, muscle releases *potassium,* and the plasma concentration of potassium increases [69, 129]. When incubated with a Ringer's solution containing a high (18-mM) concentration of potassium,

FIGURE 2.12.

Mean (± SE; n = 6) arterialized venous plasma epinephrine concentration (top panel) and V̇O$_2$ (bottom panel) responses prior to and during 20 min of constant-load cycle ergometer exercise for control (solid circles) and epinephrine-infusion (open circles) trials. Epinephrine infusion (100 ng/kg/min) began at the end of the 10th min of exercise. Epinephrine infusion significantly increased arterialized venous plasma epinephrine concentration but had no effect on V̇O$_2$. Reproduced from ref. 49.

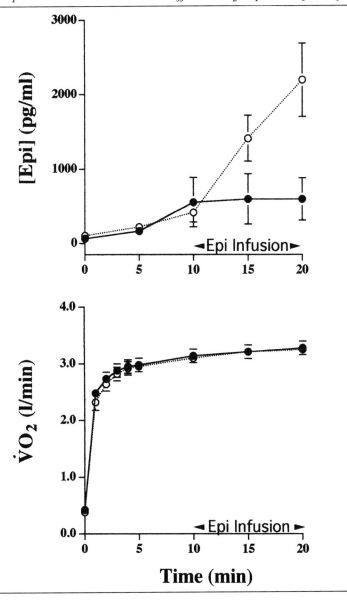

the metabolic rate of isolated frog muscle has been shown to be greatly increased [5]. Yasuda et al. [129] reported high correlations (0.93–0.98) between exercise $\dot{V}O_2$ and blood potassium concentration in six subjects exercising at two intensities. However, these investigators did not examine the temporal relationship between the changes in blood potassium and the slow component of $\dot{V}O_2$. Poole et al. [87] reported that venous plasma potassium concentration rose initially at the onset of constant-load, heavy exercise but remained stable from 3 minutes to the end of exercise, during which time pulmonary and leg $\dot{V}O_2$ continued to rise by $\sim$700 ml/min.

With the majority of the $\dot{V}O_2$ slow component arising from the working limbs, the mechanisms responsible must, therefore, have their effect predominantly on the exercising skeletal muscles. Several possibilities exist, in addition to the potential impact of factors previously discussed (most notably temperature). An increase in muscle temperature, for example, may compromise P-O coupling efficiency [125]. During exercise at work rates $\gg T_{Lac}$, a decrease in muscle pH may impair contractile function [27, 60], thereby necessitating recruitment of additional motor units to maintain power output.

A large body of evidence suggests that the $\dot{V}O_2$ slow component may primarily be attributable to *motor unit recruitment* patterns during exercise, namely the recruitment of lower efficiency, fast-twitch fibers. The energetic differences between slow- and fast-twitch motor units are well documented [26, 32, 50, 67, 68, 100, 114]. Shinohara and Moritani [101] demonstrated that between the 4th and 7th min of high-intensity cycle ergometry, the integrated electromyogram (iEMG) of the working muscles was positively ($r = 0.53$, $P < 0.01$) correlated with the rise in pulmonary $\dot{V}O_2$. The authors contended that because the iEMG largely reflects changes in motor unit recruitment and/or firing frequency, the slow component of $\dot{V}O_2$ may have been due to recruitment of more motor units, particularly fast-twitch ones, during the exercise bout. With this in mind, it is noteworthy that Coyle and associates [31, 61] have demonstrated in trained cyclists that constant-power exercise $\dot{V}O_2$ is strongly correlated with the percentage of fast-twitch fibers in the vastus lateralis muscles of these athletes; that is, the greater the percentage of fast-twitch fibers, the higher the $\dot{V}O_2$ cost and the lower the cycling efficiency. Additionally, preliminary findings of Gaesser et al. [46] indicate that the slow component of $\dot{V}O_2$ is significantly higher in untrained men cycling at 100 rpm compared to 50 rpm. This observation is consistent with the notion of an optimal velocity of shortening which may dictate that more fast-twitch motor units must be recruited at higher cadences. Taken together, these findings suggest that motor-unit recruitment patterns during exercise, possibly reflecting the additional recruitment of fast-twitch motor units for all power outputs $>T_{Lac}$, explain a large part of the $\dot{V}O_2$ slow component.

Whether *substrate* availability and utilization have the potential to impact O_2 uptake kinetics significantly is unclear. The gradual, slow increase in $\dot{V}O_2$

observed during prolonged moderate exercise can be abolished by glucose infusion [54]. Cappon et al. [19], on the other hand, reported that ingestion of a glucose polymer solution 45 min prior to a 10-min exercise bout in the severe-intensity domain significantly increased pulmonary $\dot{V}O_2$ by 10% (~300 ml) compared to control conditions. Preliminary work by Carmines et al. [20] suggests that, compared to a normal mixed diet, consuming either a high-carbohydrate or high-fat meal for 4 days prior to heavy exercise does not alter the $\dot{V}O_2$ slow component, although the absolute level of $\dot{V}O_2$ throughout the exercise period tended to be highest with the high-fat diet.

We are aware of no published information suggesting that any hormone can alter the $\dot{V}O_2$ slow component. However, the preliminary work conducted by Weltman et al. [113] indicates that *testosterone* may alter the O_2 uptake kinetics in response to heavy exercise in men. In five normal men, blood testosterone levels were manipulated by 3 weeks of treatment with leuprolide (testosterone = 22 ng/dl), saline (testosterone = 713 ng/dl), and testosterone (testosterone = 1554 ng/dl) in a double-blind randomized manner, with a 6-week washout between trials. Mean ($\pm$ SD) end-exercise $\dot{V}O_2$ (testosterone = 2.53 $\pm$ 0.99 L/min; saline = 2.36 $\pm$ 0.94 L/min; leuprolide = 2.13 $\pm$ 0.98 L/min), as well as the $\dot{V}O_2$ slow component (testosterone = 423 $\pm$ 149 ml/min; saline = 392 $\pm$ 177 ml/min; leuprolide = 264 $\pm$ 142 ml/min), were highest in the elevated testosterone condition and lowest in the depressed testosterone condition ($P < 0.05$ for end-exercise $\dot{V}O_2$; $P < 0.08$ for $\dot{V}O_2$ slow component). The mechanism for this apparent effect of testosterone remains unknown.

ATTENUATION OF THE $\dot{V}O_2$ SLOW COMPONENT WITH ENDURANCE TRAINING

It is well documented that endurance exercise training results in faster $\dot{V}O_2$ kinetics at exercise onset [52, 57, 90]. For a given absolute work rate, however, the level of $\dot{V}O_2$ eventually attained after exercise onset may either be unchanged [33, 47, 52, 57] or decreased [13, 15, 24, 25, 45, 89, 128]. For work rates in the moderate-intensity domain ($<T_{Lac}$), steady-state $\dot{V}O_2$ after endurance training is not appreciably different for work rates below the pretraining T_{Lac} [33]. For work rates above the pretraining T_{Lac} but below the posttraining W_a, $\dot{V}O_2$ in the steady state (if the duration is sufficiently long that it is attained) or at the end of exercise is invariably lower [24, 128]. This lower $\dot{V}O_2$ is due to attenuation of the $\dot{V}O_2$ slow component [24, 128].

Casaburi et al. [24] were the first to examine the influence of endurance training on the slow component of $\dot{V}O_2$. Before and after 8 weeks of endurance training, 10 subjects performed constant-load exercise bouts at intensities corresponding to 90% of the pretraining ventilatory threshold (used as a proxy for T_{Lac}), and 25, 50, and 75% of the difference between the pretraining ventilatory threshold and $\dot{V}O_{2max}$. After training, the slow components were reduced by ~150–200 ml/min for the three highest exercise intensities. Expressed as a percentage of the pretraining slow component, these reductions ranged between ~50–90%, with the largest relative reduction occurring for the work rate that corresponded to 25% of that difference between the pretraining ventilatory threshold and $\dot{V}O_{2max}$. This was attributable to the fact that, after training, this work rate fell below the post-training ventilatory threshold (which was increased by 38%). This observation underscores the general finding that, at least for cycle ergometry, a pronounced slow component of $\dot{V}O_2$ is only observed for work rates above T_{Lac}.

Reductions in the $\dot{V}O_2$ slow component and end-exercise $\dot{V}O_2$ have been documented after 7 [89] or 8 [13, 15, 130] weeks of training. Womack et al. [128], however, recently demonstrated that the $\dot{V}O_2$ slow component is attenuated within the very first few weeks after endurance training begins. For the seven subjects trained by Womack et al. [128], significant reductions in the slow component of $\dot{V}O_2$ and end-exercise $\dot{V}O_2$ were observed after just 2 weeks of training (Fig. 2.13). In fact, no further statistically significant reduction in constant-load exercise $\dot{V}O_2$ occurred during the succeeding 4 weeks of the 6-week training program; a slow component is

FIGURE 2.13.
Mean $\dot{V}O_2$ for seven subjects during 20 min of constant-load heavy exercise prior to endurance training and after 3 and 6 weeks of training. The horizontal line indicates the $\dot{V}O_2$ at min 3 for the pretraining trial. The slow component (0.42 L/min pre-training) was reduced by ~50% after 3 weeks of training. The lack of any additional reduction in the slow component after 3 weeks may have been attributable to the fact that the absolute training workload remained unchanged (and thus the relative workload decreased) throughout the 6 weeks of training. Reproduced from ref. 128.

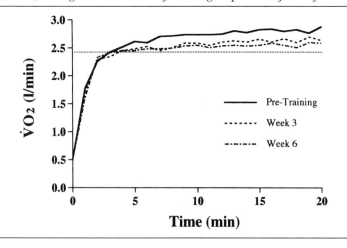

still evident after 6 weeks of training (Fig. 2.13). This perhaps was due to the fact that: 1) the mean constant-load work rate (184 W) was still above the mean power output associated with posttraining T_{Lac} (132 W), and 2) the absolute training workload remained constant for each subject throughout the 6 weeks of training. Had the workload been increased each week to coincide with the subjects' improved exercise capacity, greater increases in T_{Lac} may have occurred, with further attenuation of the slow component. Nevertheless, the magnitude of the reduced $\dot{V}O_2$ ($\sim$220 ml/min, $\sim$50% reduction) is similar to, or greater than, that reported by Casaburi et al. [24] after 8 weeks of training. This indicates that most, if not all, of the adaptation occurs very early in the training program.

The mechanism of the reduced $\dot{V}O_2$ slow component after training remains unknown. Many factors, essentially those discussed in the previous section, have been hypothesized to play a role. Again, lactate certainly has received the most attention. Casaburi et al. [24] found that the reductions in $\dot{V}O_2$ slow component and end-exercise blood lactate concentration were significantly correlated (r = 0.64, P < 0.001). However, other evidence strongly suggests that the reduction in blood lactate observed after training is not the cause of the attenuated slow component, despite the fact that the two adaptations have been reported to be highly correlated. In contrast to the data of Casaburi et al. [24], it is possible to observe marked reductions in blood lactate concentrations after training without any change in exercise $\dot{V}O_2$ [47].

More compelling evidence is supplied by the study of Womack et al. [128], which was designed to examine the effect of lactate and epinephrine on the training-induced reduction in the $\dot{V}O_2$ slow component. Blood lactate and plasma epinephrine concentrations during constant-load exercise for >T_{Lac} WR have been documented to be reduced significantly within the first few weeks of training [47, 48, 127], similar to the rapid attenuation of the $\dot{V}O_2$ slow component [128]. However, the decrease in blood lactate and plasma epinephrine appear to play no causal role in the reduced $\dot{V}O_2$ requirement for heavy exercise. In addition to the constant-load exercise tests performed prior to and after each of the 6 weeks of training, the subjects in the study of Womack et al. [128] performed one additional constant-load exercise bout (same absolute power output as all previous constant-load bouts), during which epinephrine was infused during the last 10 min of the 20-min exercise bout. The infusion raised plasma epinephrine concentration 12-fold, from 0.20 ng/ml up to 2.42 ng/ml. The end-exercise concentration of 2.42 ng/ml was 16-fold higher than that observed during the "control" trial (after 6 weeks of training) and 6-fold higher than the end-exercise concentration elicited during the pretraining exercise bout. Epinephrine infusion increased the blood lactate concentration by 2.4 mM (4.2–6.6 mM). This increase represented $\sim$50% of the training-induced reduction in end-exercise blood lactate concentration that occurred (end-exercise blood lactate for pretraining = 8.8 mM; for week 6 = 4.3 mM). Despite this increase in blood lactate, exercise $\dot{V}O_2$ was unaffected, a finding that supported previous epinephrine infusion studies without the training intervention [45, 72, 98, 99]. These data of Womack et al. [128] also show convincingly that the reduced $\dot{V}O_2$ slow component accompanying endurance training is in no way caused by the reduction in plasma epinephrine levels.

The reduction in pulmonary ventilation with training has been postulated to account for some of the observed decrease in the exercise $\dot{V}O_2$. Casaburi et al. [24] found that the reduction in $\dot{V}O_2$ slow component after 8 weeks of endurance training was significantly correlated (r = 0.51, P < 0.01) with the reduction in ventilation. However, in that study, the attenuated $\dot{V}O_2$ slow components of ~150–200 ml/min were associated with reductions in pulmonary ventilation of ~5–20 L/min. Using an average O_2 cost of ventilation of 2 ml/L (from the data of Aaron et al. [1] discussed in the previous section), the reduced ventilation is likely to account for only ~5–27% of the reduction in exercise $\dot{V}O_2$. After training, the reduced ventilation during heavy or severe exercise has been reported to vary considerably, between 6 and 40 L/min [13, 24, 25, 47]. Reductions of this magnitude would be expected to reduce $\dot{V}O_2$ by ~12–114 ml/min, depending upon the absolute ventilation [1]. Accordingly, these values could account for between 14 and 30% of the reported reductions in exercise $\dot{V}O_2$ after training.

As discussed in the previous section, it is likely that the slow rise in $\dot{V}O_2$ during heavy exercise and the progressive increase to maximum $\dot{V}O_2$ during severe exercise are due to the recruitment pattern of motor units. It is also possible, if not probable, that an alteration in motor-unit recruitment pattern, perhaps reflecting activation of fewer fast-twitch fibers, can explain much of the reduction in $\dot{V}O_2$ slow component observed after endurance training. The fact that the $\dot{V}O_2$ slow component can be reduced within the first 2 weeks of training [128] and that the majority of the slow component is attributable to $\dot{V}O_2$ within the working limbs [87] suggests that this may be the case. The definitive answer to this unresolved issue will require use of methods to document the change in neuromuscular activity during constant-load exercise before and after training, preferably in a manner that can clarify the time course of the neuromuscular adaptations.

PRACTICAL APPLICATIONS

Assessment of $\dot{V}O_{2max}$

The presence of a slow component which projects $\dot{V}O_2$ to its maximum for all work rates $>W_a$ provides for considerable freedom in designing exercise tests to measure $\dot{V}O_{2max}$ [88]. Specifically, rather than progressively increasing the work rate to the maximum as done in the increasingly popular incremental or ramp protocols, any constant-load work rate $>W_a$ will achieve a similar $\dot{V}O_2$. By judicious selection of a work rate which can be sustained for only 4–6 minutes or so, a rapid assessment of $\dot{V}O_{2max}$ can be made. This rationale emphasizes again the impropriety of characterizing work rates within the domain of severe-intensity exercise with respect to $\%\dot{V}O_{2max}$. With the sole condition that exercise is performed to fatigue within the severe-intensity domain (i.e., $>W_a$), all work rates will yield the same end-point $\dot{V}O_2$, i.e., $\dot{V}O_{2max}$.

Functional Significance with Respect to Patient Populations

As emphasized previously, one fundamental tenet of the $\dot{V}O_2$ slow component is that it represents an "excess" metabolic cost above that calculated for the work rate on the basis of linear first-order muscle energetics [56, 88, 120]. Irrespective of the precise mechanistic basis for this effect, it is clear that exercise training substantially reduces $\dot{V}O_2$ at supra-T_{Lac} work rates [24, 88, 128]. Also, by elevating the work rate at T_{Lac} [46], training serves to increase the range of work rates achievable before slow-component behavior manifests itself. For absolute work rates which remain $>T_{Lac}$ even after training, the magnitude of the slow component is reduced concomitant with diminished cardiac and ventilatory [25] demands and also a lowered degree of intra- and extracellular metabolic perturbation [24, 25, 40, 89]. For the healthy individual, these changes are associated with increased $\dot{V}O_{2max}$, maximal cardiac output, exercising ventilation, and peripheral adaptations (increased capillarity, mitochondrial oxidative enzymes) that enhance the ability of the muscle to achieve a greater O_2 flux. This training response is depicted schematically in Figure 2.14, which is constructed from a *series of constant-load square wave exercise bouts* performed by a healthy individual (left panels), a cardiac function-limited patient (upper right), and a ventilatory function-limited patient (lower right). In the healthy individual, $\dot{V}O_2$ increases linearly with work rate up to T_{Lac}, beyond which there is a $\dot{V}O_2$ "excess" which eventually drives $\dot{V}O_2$ to the maximum that occurs close to the maximum cardiac output. At maximum exercise, ventilation does not approach the maximum voluntary ventilation (MVV). After training, T_{Lac} increases, and the $\dot{V}O_2$ slow component obtains at a substantially higher work rate, where again it elevates $\dot{V}O_2$ to its new maximum at a higher cardiac output. Although maximum exercising ventilation is elevated, it still does not attain the MVV. Consider now patient populations that are limited by a low ceiling of cardiac or ventilatory function that cannot be elevated by training because of irreversible pathology. For the *cardiac function-limited patient* whose T_{Lac} and $\dot{V}O_{2max}$ occur at very low work rates, as with the healthy subject, the $\dot{V}O_2$ slow component increases $\dot{V}O_2$ toward the maximum. However, for this patient, the presiding cardiomyopathy prevents augmented cardiac function with training. In this instance, the only opportunity for enhancing work performance is raising T_{Lac} and offsetting the occurrence

FIGURE 2.14.

Schematic illustration of the response of $\dot{V}O_2$ and $\dot{V}E$ evoked by a series of individual, constant-load exercise tests performed below (solid lines) and above (dashed lines) the lactate threshold (T_{Lac}). Notice that for healthy subjects (left panels) the increase of $\dot{V}O_2$ and $\dot{V}E$ below T_{Lac} is approximately linear. In contrast, at $>T_{Lac}$ the $\dot{V}O_2$ and $\dot{V}E$ requirement per unit of work is increased. The highest work rate produces a level of ventilation ($\dot{V}E_{max}$) which is below the maximum voluntary ventilation (MVV). After training, T_{Lac} is increased, and there is a corresponding increase in the linear portion of the $\dot{V}O_2$ and $\dot{V}E$ responses. At the highest work rate, $\dot{V}O_{2max}$ is increased, and $\dot{V}Emax$ approaches the MVV more closely. For patients with cardiac and ventilatory limitations, this scenario occurs at much lower work rates. For the cardiac-limited patient (upper right), the maximum work rate is limited by the abnormally low $\dot{V}O_{2max}$. For the ventilatory-limited patient (lower right), it is the pathologically decreased MVV which constrains exercise tolerance. In those patients in whom the pathophysiology sets a low and immovable ceiling on their achievable $\dot{V}O_{2max}$ or MVV, the only way to improve the exercise tolerance is to lower the $\dot{V}O_2$ (or $\dot{V}E$) demand $>T_{Lac}$ by reduction of the excess $\dot{V}O_2$ associated with the slow component of the $\dot{V}O_2$ kinetics. Reproduced from Poole, D. C., T. J. Barstow, G. A. Gaesser, W. T. Willis, and B. J. Whipp. $\dot{V}O_2$ slow component: physiological and functional significance. Med. Sci. Sports Exerc. 26:1354–1358, 1994.

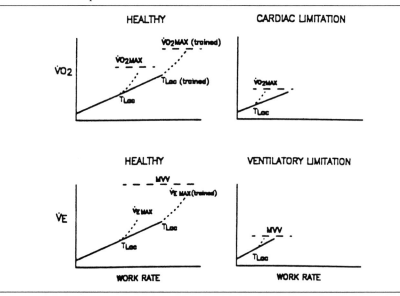

of the slow component such that the $\dot{V}O_2$-work rate relation retains its linearity over a greater range of work rates. The maximum benefit for this patient would be achieved by pushing T_{Lac} up to $\dot{V}O_{2max}$. Similarly, for the *ventilatory function-limited patient* whose MVV occurs at maximal exercise and cannot be enhanced by training, the opportunity to increase work rate depends crucially on lowering the ventilatory demands of the work. As with the cardiac patient, this can be achieved by elevating T_{Lac} and increasing the range of work rates for which the $\dot{V}O_2$-WR relation is linear. Thus, after training $\dot{V}CO_2$ is reduced due to a lowered $\dot{V}O_2$ (slow component), reduced HCO_3^- buffering of lactic acid, and reduced H^+ stimulation of the peripheral chemoreceptors. Whereas the ability of exercise training to increase T_{Lac} and to reduce the $\dot{V}O_2$ slow component is firmly established, the efficacy of this strategy to benefit these patient populations remains to be substantiated.

CONCLUSION

Despite an extensive body of evidence demonstrating the existence of the $\dot{V}O_2$ slow component, this phenomenon generally has gone unacknowledged in textbooks of exercise physiology. The slow component, which in the extreme can drive $\dot{V}O_2$ to its maximum even during "submaximal" exercise, is integrally related to the fatigue process. Thus, it has applications to our understanding of endurance performance and may be useful in clinical settings as well. To date, neither the kinetics nor the precise mechanism(s) have been fully elucidated.

The majority ($>\sim80\%$) of the slow component appears to be localized to the exercising limbs. Thus, the additional $\dot{V}O_2$ attributable to processes outside the exercising limbs, such as ventilation, cardiac and accessory muscle work, glyco/gluconeogenesis, and elevation of body temperature, are likely to be relatively small. Of these, ventilation appears to be quantitatively the most significant. Although the blood lactate profile is well correlated with the time course and magnitude of the slow component, the relationship is coincidental rather than causal.

The most likely mechanism accounting for the slow component is muscle fiber (motor unit) recruitment. The integrated EMG data of Shinohara and Moritani [101] suggest that during heavy and severe exercise a change in motor unit firing frequency and/or recruitment may give rise to the slow phase of the $\dot{V}O_2$ response in these intensity domains. This altered recruitment pattern may reflect fatigue within selected muscle fibers during heavy and severe exercise; within the first few minutes of repeated isometric exercise, for example, Vollestad et al. [109] have demonstrated significant muscle fatigue. Studies both in vitro [5, 26, 32, 50, 114] and in vivo [31, 61] show that fast-twitch muscle is less efficient than slow-twitch muscle. Also, the time constant for $\dot{V}O_2$ is appreciably slower in fast-twitch muscle [32, 67]. If both fast-twitch and slow-twitch motor units are recruited at the onset of heavy or severe exercise, then the $\dot{V}O_2$ response during exercise in these intensity domains may potentially be explained in large part by the energetic and kinetic differences between these motor unit types.

Whipp and Mahler [120; see also ref. 10 for review] hypothesized that the $\dot{V}O_2$ kinetics are limited by mitochondrial content. In humans, mitochondrial content of slow-twitch fibers has been reported to be 50% greater than that in fast-twitch oxidative glycogenolytic fibers and three times greater than that in fast-twitch glycogenolytic fibers [62]. Thus, recruitment of fast-twitch motor units during heavy and severe exercise would be expected from the linear extrapolation of the $\dot{V}O_2$-WR relationship in the sub-T_{Lac} domain. Both of these observations have been well documented. However, the direct participation of a specific fiber population in the $\dot{V}O_2$ slow component remains to be established.

On the other hand, the slow component has been judged to be a discrete process which is only initiated some 80–100 s after exercise onset [10, 83]. This would argue against the simultaneous recruitment of both fast- and slow-twitch motor unit types. If, however, we consider that there is a spacial and temporal heterogeneity of blood flow within the exercising muscle [84], the $\dot{V}O_2$ response of some muscle fibers, particularly fast-twitch, that are recruited at exercise onset may lag behind that of others, depending upon the time required for blood flow to increase in their adjacent capillaries. These unresolved issues require additional research.

The increased mitochondrial content in all fiber types which is documented to occur with endurance training [62] may play a role in the attenuation of the $\dot{V}O_2$ slow component. This could conceivably occur as a result of either less reliance on the recruitment of fast-twitch motor units during a given absolute WR after training or, alternatively, recruitment of a population of fast-twitch motor units with a higher oxidative capacity and hence faster $\dot{V}O_2$ kinetics. These possibilities also require further research.

ACKNOWLEDGMENTS

We wish to acknowledge the contributions of Drs. Thomas Barstow, Wayne Willis, Edward Coyle, and especially those of Dr. Brian Whipp. Some of the material presented in this chapter was supported in part by grants from the National Heart, Lung, and Blood Institute of the National Institutes of Health (HL 17731 and 50306), and the Cigarette and Tobacco Surtax Fund of the State of California through the Tobacco-Related Disease Research Program of the University of California (2KT 0066).

REFERENCES

1. Aaron, E. A., K. C. Seow, B. D. Johnson, and J. A. Dempsey. Oxygen cost of exercise hyperpnea: implications for performance. *J. Appl. Physiol.* 72:1818–1825, 1992.
2. Astrand, P.-O., and K. Rodahl. *Textbook of Work Physiology: Physiological Basis of Exercise.* New York: McGraw-Hill, 1986, pp. 299–303.
3. Astrand, P.-O., and B. Saltin. Oxygen uptake during the first minutes of heavy exercise. *J. Appl. Physiol.* 16:971–976, 1961.

4. Barany, M. ATPase activities of myosin correlated with speed of muscle shortening. *J. Gen. Physiol.* 50:197–216, 1967.

5. Barnes, W. S. Depressing effect of calcium antagonists on oxygen consumption in isolated skeletal muscle during potassium depolarization. *Can. J. Physiol. Pharmacol.* 66:836–840, 1988.

6. Barstow, T. J. Characterization of $\dot{V}O_2$ kinetics during heavy exercise. *Med. Sci. Sports Exerc.* 26:1327–1334, 1994.

7. Barstow, T. J., R. Casaburi, and K. Wasserman. O_2 uptake kinetics and O_2 deficit as related to exercise intensity and blood lactate. *J. Appl. Physiol.* 75:755–762, 1993.

8. Barstow, T. J., N. Lamarra, and B. J. Whipp. Modulation of muscle and pulmonary oxygen uptakes by circulatory dynamics. *J. Appl. Physiol.* 68:979–989, 1990.

9. Barstow, T. J., and P. A. Mole. Simulation of pulmonary oxygen uptake during exercise in humans. *J. Appl. Physiol.* 63:2253–2261, 1987.

10. Barstow, T. J., and P. A. Mole. Linear and nonlinear characteristics of oxygen uptake kinetics during heavy exercise. *J. Appl. Physiol.* 71:2099–2106, 1991.

11. Bason, R., C. E. Billings, E. L. Fox, and R. Gerke. Oxygen kinetics for constant work loads at various altitudes. *J. Appl. Physiol.* 35:497–500, 1973.

12. Bellardinelli, R., T. J. Barstow, J. Porszasz, and K. Wasserman. Skeletal muscle oxygenation during constant work rate exercise. *Med. Sci. Sports Exerc.* 27:512–519, 1995.

13. Belman, M. J., and G. A. Gaesser. Exercise training below and above the lactate threshold in the elderly. *Med. Sci. Sports Exerc.* 23:562–568, 1991.

14. Bergstrom, J., L. Hermansen, E. Hultman, and B. Saltin. Diet, muscle glycogen and physical performance. *Acta Physiol. Scand.* 71:140–150, 1967.

15. Bhambhani, Y., and M. Singh. The effects of three training intensities on $\dot{V}O_{2max}$ and $\dot{V}E/\dot{V}O_2$ ratio. *Can. J. Appl. Spt. Sci.* 10:44–51, 1985.

16. Bigland-Ritchie, B. Muscle fatigue and the influence of changing neural drive. *Clin. Chest. Med.* 5:21–34, 1984.

17. Billat, V., J. C. Renoux, J. Pinoteau, B. Petit, and J. P. Koralsztein. Reproducibility of running time to exhaustion at $\dot{V}O_{2max}$ in subelite runners. *Med. Sci. Sports Exerc.* 26:254–257, 1994.

18. Camus, G., G. Atchou, J. C. Brucker, D. Giezendanner, and P. E. di Prampero. Slow upward drift of $\dot{V}O_2$ during constant-load cycling in untrained subjects. *Eur. J. Appl. Physiol.* 58:197–202, 1988.

19. Cappon, J. P., E. Ipp, J. A. Brasel, and D. M. Cooper. Acute effects of high fat and high glucose meals on the growth hormone response to exercise. *J. Clin Endocrinol. Metab.* 76:1418–1422, 1993.

20. Carmines, A. A., L. Wideman, J. Y. Weltman, M. L. Hartman, A. Weltman, and G. A. Gaesser. High-carbohydrate and high-fat diets do not alter slow component of $\dot{V}O_2$ during heavy exercise (Abstract). *Med. Sci. Sports Exerc.* 27:S9, 1995.

21. Carnevale, T. J., and G. A. Gaesser. Effects of pedalling speed on the power-duration relationship for high-intensity exercise. *Med. Sci. Sports Exerc.* 23:242–246, 1991.

22. Casaburi, R., T. J. Barstow, T. Robinson, and K. Wasserman. Influence of work rate on ventilatory and gas exchange kinetics. *J. Appl. Physiol.* 67:547–555, 1989.

23. Casaburi, R., J. Daly, J. E. Hansen, and R. M. Effros. Abrupt changes in mixed venous blood gas composition after the onset of exercise. *J. Appl. Physiol.* 67:1106–1112, 1989.

24. Casaburi, R., T. W. Storer, I. Ben-Dov, and K. Wasserman. Effect of endurance training on possible determinants of $\dot{V}O_2$ during heavy exercise. *J. Appl. Physiol.* 62:199–207, 1987.

25. Casaburi, R., T. W. Storer, and K. Wasserman. Mediation of reduced ventilatory response to exercise after endurance training. *J. Appl. Physiol.* 63:1533–1538, 1987.

26. Close, R. I. Dynamic properties of fast and slow skeletal muscles of the rat during development. *J. Physiol. (Lond.)* 175:74–95, 1964.

27. Cooke, R., K. Franks, G. B. Luciani, and E. Pate. The inhibition of rabbit skeletal muscle contraction by hydrogen ions and phosphate. *J. Physiol. (Lond.)* 395:77–97, 1988.

28. Cooper, D. M., C. Berry, N. Lamarra, and K. Wasserman. Kinetics of oxygen uptake and heart rate at onset of exercise in children. *J. Appl. Physiol.* 59:211–217, 1985.
29. Costill, D. L. Metabolic responses during distance running. *J. Appl. Physiol.* 28:251–255, 1970.
30. Coyle, E. F., M. T. Hamilton, J. G. Alonso, S. J. Montain, and J. L. Ivy. Carbohydrate metabolism during intense exercise when hyperglycemic. *J. Appl. Physiol.* 70:834–840, 1991.
31. Coyle, E. F., L. S. Sidossis, J. F. Horowitz, and J. D. Beltz. Cycling efficiency is related to the percentage of type I muscle fibers. *Med. Sci. Sports Exerc.* 24:782–788, 1992.
32. Crow, M. T., and M. J. Kushmerick. Chemical energetics of slow- and fast-twitch muscles of the mouse. *J. Gen. Physiol.* 79:147–166, 1982.
33. Davis, J. A., M. H. Frank, B. J. Whipp, and K. Wasserman. Anaerobic threshold alterations caused by endurance training in middle-aged men. *J. Appl. Physiol.: Respirat. Environ. Exerc. Physiol.* 46:1039–1046, 1979.
34. Davis, S. E., C. J. Womack, M. Gutgesell, E. Barrett, A. Weltman, and G. A. Gaesser. Effects of B-blockade on slow component (SC) of $\dot{V}O_2$ during moderate and heavy exercise (Abstract). *Med. Sci. Sports Exerc.* 26:S208, 1994.
35. Denis, C., D. Dormois, J. Castells, R. Bonnefoy, S. Padilla, A. Geyssant, and J. R. Lacour. Comparison of incremental and steady state tests of endurance training. *Eur. J. Appl. Physiol.* 57:474–481, 1988.
36. DeVries, H. A., and T. J. Housh. *Physiology of Exercise: For Physical Education, Athletics and Exercise Science.* Madison, WI: Brown & Benchmark, 1994, pp. 216–222.
37. Dick, R. W., and P. R. Cavanaugh. An explanation of the upward drift in oxygen uptake during prolonged sub-maximal downhill running. *Med. Sci. Sports Exerc.* 19:310–317, 1987.
38. Dill, D. B., H. T. Edwards, P. S. Bauer, and E. J. Levenson. Physical performance in relation to external temperature. *Arbeitsphysiologie* 4:508–518, 1931.
39. Donaldson, S. K., and L. Hermansen. Differential, direct effects of H^+ on Ca^{2+}-activated force of skinned fibers from the soleus, cardiac and adductor magnus muscle of rabbits. *Pfleugers Arch.* 376:55–65, 1978.
40. Dudley, G. A., P. C. Tullson, and R. L. Terjung. Influence of mitochondrial content on the sensitivity of respiratory control. *J. Biol. Chem.* 262:9109–9114, 1987.
41. Fabiato, A., and F. Fabiato. Effects of pH on the myofilaments and the sarcoplasmic reticulum of skinned cells from cardiac and skeletal muscles. *J. Physiol. (Lond.)* 276:233–255, 1978.
42. Fellows, I. W., T. Bennett, and I. A. Macdonald. The effect of adrenaline upon cardiovascular and metabolic functions in man. *Clin. Sci.* 69:215–222, 1985.
43. Fitts, R. H. Cellular mechanisms of muscle fatigue. *Physiol. Rev.* 74:49–94, 1994.
44. Fox, E. L., R. W. Bowers, and M. L. Foss. *The Physiological Basis of Physical Education and Athletics,* 4th Ed. Philadelphia: W. B. Saunders, 1988, pp. 32–33.
45. Gaesser, G. A. Influence of training and catecholamines on exercise $\dot{V}O_2$ response. *Med. Sci. Sports Exerc.* 26:1341–1346, 1994.
46. Gaesser, G. A., R. J. Cooper, and L. A. Wilson. Blood [lactate] and "excess" O_2 uptake during high intensity cycling at slow and fast cadences (Abstract). *Physiologist* 35:210, 1992.
47. Gaesser, G. A., and D. C. Poole. Lactate and ventilatory thresholds: disparity in time course of adaptations to training. *J. Appl. Physiol.* 61:999–1004, 1986.
48. Gaesser, G. A., and D. C. Poole. Blood lactate during exercise: time course of training adaptation in humans. *Int. J. Sports Med.* 9:284–288, 1988.
49. Gaesser, G. A., S. A. Ward, V. C. Baum, and B. J. Whipp. Effects of infused epinephrine on slow phase of O_2 uptake kinetics during heavy exercise in humans. *J. Appl. Physiol.* 77:2413–2419, 1994.
50. Gibbs, C. L., and W. R. Gibson. Energy production of the rat soleus muscle. *Am. J. Physiol.* 223:864–871, 1972.
51. Grassi, B., D. C. Poole, R. S. Richardson, D. R. Knight, B. K. Erickson, and P. D. Wagner. Muscle O_2 kinetics in humans: implications for metabolic control. *J. Appl. Physiol.* (In Press)

52. Hagberg, J. M., R. C. Hickson, A. A. Ehsani, and J. O. Holloszy. Faster adjustment to and recovery from submaximal exercise in the trained state. *J. Appl. Physiol.: Respirat. Environ. Exerc. Physiol.* 48:218–224, 1980.

53. Hagberg, J. M., J. P. Mullin, and F. J. Nagle. Oxygen consumption during constant-load exercise. *J. Appl. Physiol.* 45:381–384, 1978.

54. Hamilton, M. T., J. G. Alonso, S. J. Montain, and E. F. Coyle. Fluid replacement and glucose infusion during exercise prevent cardiovascular drift. *J. Appl. Physiol.* 71:871–877, 1991.

55. Henry, F. M. Aerobic oxygen consumption and alactic debt in muscular work. *J. Appl. Physiol.* 3:427–438, 1951.

56. Henson, L. C., D. C. Poole, and B. J. Whipp. Fitness as a determinant of oxygen uptake response to constant-load exercise. *Eur. J. Appl. Physiol.* 59:21–28, 1989.

57. Hickson, R. C., H. A. Bomze, and J. O. Holloszy. Faster adjustment of O_2 uptake to the energy requirement of exercise in the trained state. *J. Appl. Physiol.: Respirat. Environ. Exerc. Physiol.* 44:877–881, 1978.

58. Hill, A. V. *Muscular Movement in Man.* New York: McGraw-Hill, 1927.

59. Hill, A. V., and H. Lupton. Muscular exercise, lactic acid, and the supply and utilization of oxygen. *Q. J. Med.* 16:135–171, 1923.

60. Hogan, M. C., L. B. Gladden, S. Kurdak, and D. C. Poole. Increased [lactate] in working dog muscle reduces tension development independent of pH. *Med. Sci. Sports Exerc.* 27:371–377, 1995.

61. Horowitz, J. F., L. S. Sidossis, and E. F. Coyle. High efficiency of type I muscle fibers improves performance. *Int. J. Sports Med.* 15:152–157, 1994.

62. Howald, H., H. Hoppeler, H. Claasen, O. Mathieu, and R. Straub. Influences of endurance training on the ultrastructural composition of the different muscle fiber types in humans. *Pfluegers Arch.* 403:369–376, 1985.

63. Hughson, R. L., C. J. Orok, and L. E. Staudt. A high velocity treadmill running test to assess endurance running potential. *Int. J. Sports Med.* 5:23–25, 1984.

64. Kalis, J. K., B. J. Freund, M. J. Joyner, S. M. Jilka, J. Nitolo, and J. H. Wilmore. Effect of B-blockade on the drift in O_2 consumption during prolonged exercise. *J. Appl. Physiol.* 64:753–758, 1988.

65. Klausen, K., and H. Knuttgen. Effect of training on oxygen consumption in negative muscular work. *Acta Physiol. Scand.* 83:319–323, 1971.

66. Krogh, A., and J. Lindhard. The regulation of respiration and circulation during the initial stages of muscular work. *J. Physiol. (Lond.)* 47:112–136, 1913.

67. Kushmerick, M. J. Energetics of muscle contraction. L. E. Peachy, R. H. Adrian, and S. R. Geiger (eds). *Handbook of Physiology, Section 10: Skeletal Muscle.* Bethesda, MD: American Physiological Society, 1983, pp. 189–236.

68. Kushmerick, M. J., R. A. Meyer, and T. R. Brown. Regulation of oxygen consumption in fast- and slow-twitch muscle. *J. Appl. Physiol. (Cell Physiol.)* 263:C598–C606, 1992.

69. Lindinger, M. I., R. S. McKelvie, and G. J. F. Heigenhauser. K^+ and Lac^- distribution in humans during and after high-intensity exercise: role in muscle fatigue attenuation? *J. Appl. Physiol.* 78:765–777, 1995.

70. Linnarsson, D. Dynamics of pulmonary gas exchange and heart rate changes at start and end of exercise. *Acta Physiol. Scand. Suppl.* 415:1–68, 1974.

71. Lundholm, L., and N. Svedmyr. Studies on the stimulating effects of adrenaline and noradrenaline on respiration in man. *Acta Physiol. Scand.* 67:65–75, 1989.

72. Marshall, R. J., and J. T. Shepherd. Effects of epinephrine on cardiovascular and metabolic responses to leg exercise in man. *J. Appl. Physiol.* 18:1118–1122, 1963.

73. Maughan, R. J., and D. C. Poole. The effects of a glycogen-loading regimen on the capacity to perform anaerobic exercise. *Eur. J. Appl. Physiol.* 46:211–219, 1981.

74. McArdle, W. D., F. I. Katch, and V. L. Katch. *Exercise Physiology: Energy, Nutrition, and Human Performance,* 3rd Ed. Philadelphia: Lea & Febiger, 1991, pp. 127–134.

75. McLellan, T. M., and K. S. Cheung. A comparative evaluation of the individual anaerobic threshold and the critical power. *Med. Sci. Sports Exerc.* 24:543–550, 1992.

76. Metzger, J. M., and R. L. Moss. Greater hydrogen ion-induced depression of tension and velocity in skinned single fibers of rat fast than slow muscles. *J. Physiol. (Lond.)* 393:727–742, 1987.

77. Mole, P., and R. L. Coulson. Energetics of myocardial function. *Med. Sci. Sports Exerc.* 17:538–545, 1985.

78. Monod, H., and J. Scherrer. The work capacity of a synergic muscular group. *Ergonomics* 8:329–338, 1965.

79. Moritani, T., A. Nagata, H. A. DeVries, and M. Muro. Critical power as a measure of physical work capacity and anaerobic threshold. *Ergonomics* 24:339–350, 1981.

80. Nagle, F. J., D. Robinhold, E. Howley, J. Daniels, G. Baptista, and K. Stoedefalke. Lactic acid accumulation during running at submaximal aerobic demands. *Med. Sci. Sports* 2:182–186, 1970.

81. Noble, B. J. *Physiology of Exercise and Sport.* St. Louis, MO: Times Mirror/C. V. Mosby, 1986, pp. 107–109.

82. Nosek, T. M., K. Y. Fender, and R. E. Godt. It is deprotonated inorganic phosphate that depresses force in skinned skeletal muscle fibers. *Science* 236:191–193, 1987.

83. Paterson, D. H., and B. J. Whipp. Asymmetries of oxygen uptake transients at the on- and offset of heavy exercise in humans. *J. Physiol. (Lond.)* 443:575–586, 1991.

84. Piiper, J. Modeling of oxygen transport to skeletal muscle: blood flow distribution, shunt, and diffusion. *Adv. Exp. Med. Biol.* 316:3–10, 1992.

85. Poole, D. C. Role of exercising muscle in slow component of $\dot{V}O_2$. *Med. Sci. Sports Exerc.* 26:1335–1340, 1994.

86. Poole, D. C., L. B. Gladden, S. Kurdak, and M. C. Hogan. L-(+)-Lactate infusion into working dog gastrocnemius: no evidence lactate per se mediates $\dot{V}O_2$ slow component. *J. Appl. Physiol.* 76:787–792, 1994.

87. Poole, D. C., W. Schaffartzik, D. R. Knight, T. Derion, B. Kennedy, H. J. Guy, R. Prediletto, and P. D. Wagner. Contribution of exercising legs to the slow component of oxygen uptake kinetics in humans. *J. Appl. Physiol.* 71:1245–1253, 1991.

88. Poole, D. C., S. A. Ward, G. W. Gardner, and B. J. Whipp. Metabolic and respiratory profile of the upper limit for prolonged exercise in man. *Ergonomics* 31:1265–1279, 1988.

89. Poole, D. C., S. A. Ward, and B. J. Whipp. The effects of training on the metabolic and respiratory profile of high-intensity cycle ergometer exercise. *Eur. J. Appl. Physiol.* 59:421–429, 1990.

90. Powers, S. K., S. Dodd, and R. E. Beadle. Oxygen uptake kinetics in trained athletes differing in $\dot{V}O_{2max}$. *Eur. J. Appl. Physiol.* 54:306–308, 1985.

91. Powers, S. K., and E. T. Howley. *Exercise Physiology: Theory and Application to Fitness and Performance,* 2nd Ed. Madison, WI: Brown & Benchmark, 1994, pp. 52–62.

92. Ribiero, J. P., V. Hughes, R. A. Fielding, W. Holden, W. Evans, and H. G. Knuttgen. Metabolic and ventilatory responses to steady state exercise relative to lactate thresholds. *Eur. J. Appl. Physiol.* 55:215–221, 1986.

93. Roston, W. L., B. J. Whipp, J. A. Davis, D. A. Cunningham, R. M. Effros, and K. Wasserman. Oxygen uptake kinetics and lactate concentration during exercise in humans. *Am. Rev. Respir. Dis.* 135:1080–1084, 1987.

94. Rowell, L. B. Cardiovascular limitations to work capacity. E. Simonsen (ed). *Physiology of Work Capacity and Fatigue.* Springfield, IL: Charles C Thomas, 1971, pp. 132–169.

95. Rowell, L. B., B. Saltin, B. Kiens, and N. J. Christensen. Is peak quadriceps blood flow in humans even higher during exercise with hypoxemia? *Am. J. Physiol.* 251:H1038–H1044, 1986.

96. Ryan, W. J., J. R. Sutton, C. J. Toews, and N. L. Jones. Metabolism of infused L(+)-lactate during exercise. *Clin. Sci.* 56:139–146, 1979.

97. Scheen, A., J. Juchmes, and A. Cession-Fossion. Critical analysis of the "anaerobic threshold" during exercise at constant workloads. *Eur. J. Appl. Physiol.* 46:367–377, 1981.
98. Scheen, A., J. Juchmes, A. Cession-Fossion, and G. Volon. Perfusion intraveineuse d'adrénaline et adaptation à l'exercice musculaire chez l'homme. *Arch. Int. Physiol. Biochim. Biophys.* 87:575–584, 1979.
99. Scheen, A., and P. Lemaire. Abaissement du seuil d'hyperventilation par perfusion intraveineuse d'adrenaline lors d'un exercice trianglaire. *Arch. Int. Physiol. Biochim. Biophys.* 91:187–196, 1983.
100. Sejersted, O. M., and N. K. Vollestad. Increased metabolic rate associated with muscle fatigue. P. Marconnet, P. V. Komi, B. Saltin, and O. M. Sejersted (eds). *Muscle Fatigue Mechanisms in Exercise and Training. Med. Sports Sci.,* Basel; Switzerland: S. Karger, 1992, pp. 115–130.
101. Shinohara, M., and T. Moritani. Increase in neuromuscular activity and oxygen uptake during heavy exercise. *Ann. Physiol. Anthropol.* 11:257–262, 1992.
102. Sjostrom, L., Y. Schutz, F. Gudinchet, L. Hegnell, P. G. Pittet, and E. Jequier. Epinephrine sensitivity with respect to metabolic rate and other variables in women. *Am. J. Physiol.* 245:E431–E442, 1983.
103. Steed, J., G. A. Gaesser, and A. Weltman. Rating of perceived exertion and blood lactate concentration during submaximal running. *Med. Sci. Sports Exerc.* 26:797–803, 1994.
104. Stoudemire, N. M., L. Wideman, K. A. Pass, C. L. McGinnes, G. A. Gaesser, and A. Weltman. Validity of regulating blood [Hla] during running by ratings of perceived exertion (Abstract). *Med. Sci. Sports Exerc.* 27:S15, 1995.
105. Stringer, W., K. Wasserman, R. Casaburi, J. Pórszász, K. Maehara, and W. French. Lactic acidosis as a facilitator of oxyhemoglobin dissociation during exercise. *J. Appl. Physiol.* 76:1462–1467, 1994.
106. Svedmyr, N. Metabolic effects of infused L-(+)-lactate in man before and after triiodothyronine treatment. *Acta Physiol. Scand.* 67:229–235, 1966.
107. Talmadge, R. J., J. I. Scheide, and H. Silverman. Glycogen synthesis from lactate in a chronically active muscle. *J. Appl. Physiol.* 66:2231–2238, 1989.
108. Thompson, J. A., H. J. Green, and M. E. Houston. Muscle glycogen depletion patterns in fast twitch subgroups of man during submaximal and supramaximal exercise. *Pfluegers Arch.* 379:105–108, 1979.
109. Vollestad, N. K., O. M. Sejersted, R. Bahr, J. J. Woods, and B. Bigland-Ritchie. Motor drive and metabolic responses during repeated submaximal contractions in humans. *J. Appl. Physiol.* 64:1421–1427, 1988.
110. Vollestad, N. K., J. Wesche, and O. M. Sejersted. Gradual increase in leg oxygen uptake during repeated submaximal contractions in humans. *J. Appl. Physiol.* 68:1150–1156, 1990.
111. Wasserman, K., J. E. Hansen, and D. Y. Sue. Facilitation of oxygen consumption by lactic acidosis during exercise. *News Physiol. Sci.* 6:29–34, 1991.
112. Wasserman, K., B. J. Whipp, and J. Castagna. Cardiodynamic hyperpnea: hyperpnea secondary to cardiac output increase. *J. Appl. Physiol.* 36:457–464, 1974.
113. Weltman, A., J. Y. Weltman, L. Jahn, J. D. Veldhuis, G. A. Gaesser, and D. A. Fryburg. Effects of varying plasma testosterone (T) concentrations on the growth hormone (GH) and $\dot{V}O_2$ response to acute exercise. (Abstract). *Med. Sci. Sports Exerc.* 27:S131, 1995.
114. Wendt, I. R., and C. L. Gibbs. Energy production of rat extensor digitorum longus muscle. *Am. J. Physiol.* 224:1081–1086, 1973.
115. Westerlind, K. C., W. C. Byrnes, C. Harris, and A. R. Wilcox. Alterations in oxygen consumption during and between bouts of level and downhill running. *Med. Sci. Sports Exerc.* 26:1144–1152, 1994.
116. Westerlind, K. C., W. C. Byrnes, and R. S. Mazzeo. A comparison of the oxygen drift in downhill vs. level running. *J. Appl. Physiol.* 72:796–800, 1992.

117. Whipp, B. J. Dynamics of pulmonary gas exchange. *Circulation* 76(Suppl. VI):18–28, 1987.
118. Whipp, B.J. The slow component of O_2 uptake kinetics during heavy exercise. *Med. Sci. Sports Exerc.* 26:1319–1326, 1994.
119. Whipp, B. J., D. J. Huntsman, N. Stoner, N. Lamarra, and K. Wasserman. A constant which determines the duration of tolerance to high-intensity work. *Fed. Proc.* 41:1591, 1982.
120. Whipp, B. J., and M. Mahler. Dynamics of pulmonary gas exchange during exercise. J. B. West (ed). *Pulmonary Gas Exchange*, Vol. II. New York: Academic Press, 1980, pp. 33–96.
121. Whipp, B. J., S. A. Ward, N. Lamarra, J. A. Davis, and K. Wasserman. Parameters of ventilatory and gas exchange dynamics during exercise. *J. Appl. Physiol.* 52:1506–1513, 1982.
122. Whipp, B. J., and K. Wasserman. Oxygen uptake kinetics for various intensities of constant-load work. *J. Appl. Physiol.* 33:351–356, 1972.
123. Whipp, B. J., and K. Wasserman. Effect of anaerobiosis on the kinetics of O_2 uptake during exercise. *Fed. Proc.* 45:2942–2947, 1986.
124. Wilkie, D. R. Equations describing power input by humans as a function of duration of exercise. P. Cerretelli and B. J. Whipp (eds). *Exercise Bioenergetics and Gas Exchange.* Amsterdam: Elsevier, 1980, pp. 75–80.
125. Willis, W. T., and M. R. Jackman. Mitochondrial function during heavy exercise. *Med. Sci. Sports Exerc.* 26:1347–1354, 1994.
126. Wilmore, J. H., and D. L. Costill, *Physiology of Sport and Exercise.* Champaign, IL: Human Kinetics, 1994, p. 108.
127. Winder, W. W., J. M. Hagberg, R. C. Hickson, A. A. Ehsani, and J. A. Mclane. Time course of sympathoadrenal adaptation to endurance exercise training in man. *J. Appl. Physiol.* 45:370–374, 1978.
128. Womack, C. J., S. E. Davis, J. L. Blumer, E. Barrett, A. L. Weltman, and G. A. Gaesser. Slow component of O_2 uptake during heavy exercise: adaptation to endurance training. *J. Appl. Physiol.* 79:838–845, 1995.
129. Yasuda, Y., K. Ishida, and M. Miyamura. Effects of blood gas, pH, lactate, potassium on the oxygen uptake time courses during constant-load bicycle exercise. *Japanese J. Physiol.* 42:223–237, 1992.
130. Yoshida, T., Y. Suda, and N. Takeuchi. Endurance training regimen based on arterial blood lactate: effects on anaerobic threshold. *Eur. J. Appl. Physiol.* 49:223–230, 1982.

3
Physical Activity and Health-related Quality of Life

W. JACK REJESKI, Ph.D.
LAWRENCE R. BRAWLEY, Ph.D.
SALLY A. SHUMAKER, Ph.D.

For more than a decade, our culture has experienced a growing interest in exercise and various other forms of physical activity. This trend is evident in the rapidly growing fitness industry, in which the focus is on the development and marketing of health and fitness products, the integration of physical fitness with corporate America, and television programs that offer fitness instruction for a variety of audiences and modes of training. Whereas the impetus for many of these developments comes from entrepreneurial motives, it is also spurred by federal policy statements, such as Healthy People 2000 [17]. Indeed, there are accumulating data that demonstrate that exercise and physical activity are related to the prevention of, and successful rehabilitation from, several chronic diseases. For example, epidemiological data show that physical activity reduces the incidence of cardiovascular diseases [70] and is a viable treatment option in the fight against essential hypertension [71]. Research links exercise to the normalization of fat metabolism [82, 86] and increased caloric expenditure is now well accepted as a key feature of weight-control programs [10, 11]. Other research suggests that exercise is a viable therapy for persons with chronic obstructive pulmonary disease (COPD) [3] and may help to prevent the loss of independence in elderly patients with knee osteoarthritis (OA) (W. H. Ettinger et al., manuscript in preparation, 1995). Finally, a growing body of literature demonstrates that participation in various forms of physical activity is associated with positive mental health [67, 76].

Although the traditional medical outcomes in clinical research are morbidity and mortality, recent developments in the literature underscore the importance of augmenting these endpoints with assessments of the participants' health-related quality of life (HRQL) [39]. Indeed, functional status or participants' HRQL is instrumental to a complete understanding of the disease process and various preventive behaviors, as they effect both the individual person and society. HRQL is now generally accepted as an appropriate measure of treatment efficacy in most clinical research. For example, in the United States, the National Institutes of Health now mandates the inclusion of HRQL in most clinical trials, and the Federal Drug Administration accepts HRQL measures in the approval process for new cancer treatments.

The focus of this chapter is on HRQL [40] and not on the broader concept of quality of life [2]. As Fries and Spitz [29] indicate, HRQL represents a restricted concept of quality of life: "We do not mean happiness, satisfaction, living climate, or environment. Rather, we are speaking of health-oriented quality of life: those aspects that might be affected positively or negatively in clinical studies and the clinical situation." Exercise and various other forms of physical activity offer promising interventions for the enhancement of HRQL. For example, Ewart and his colleagues demonstrate that exercise testing and training can enhance cardiac patients' psychological well-being and their self-confidence toward various activities of daily living (ADLs) [21, 22], and our data suggest that exercise training has a positive influence on the disability of patients with knee OA (W. H. Ettinger et al., manuscript in preparation, 1995).

Specific objectives for this chapter are defined and met in three distinct sections. First, we discuss key elements of the HRQL concept and discuss several debates on this emerging field of study, which is essential to understanding what is known about HRQL and physical activity, as well as to developing an appreciation for the direction of future study. Second, we examine existing research concerning relationships between physical activity and HRQL. We present selected studies from gerontology, cardiovascular diseases, arthritis, and pulmonary disease to characterize the types of questions asked, the answers provided, and the methodologies used in this area of research. In our third and final section, we explore the use of social psychological models to examine health behavior and cognition as intermediary outcomes, leading to perceived HRQL, and to discriminate HRQL outcomes from their determinants.

WHAT IS HEALTH-RELATED QUALITY OF LIFE?

Over the years, a number of definitions of HRQL have been proposed, with consensus emerging only recently. Schipper et al. [85] state that HRQL ". . . represents the functional effects of an illness and its consequent therapy upon a patient, as perceived by the patient." Alternatively, Wenger and Furberg [99] provide a more detailed description of HRQL that is consistent with most current views of this concept. In their definition, HRQL encompasses ". . . those attributes valued by patients, including: resultant comfort or sense of well-being; the extent to which they were able to maintain reasonable physical, emotional, and intellectual function; and the degree to which they retained their ability to participate in valued activities with the family, in the workplace, and in the community."

HRQL Represents Patient-defined Outcomes

In the definition given by Wenger and Furberg [99], it is clear that HRQL involves participants' subjective appraisals of function. Although an investigator might employ a stair climbing task to evaluate how (COPD) influences participants' abilities to *perform* activities of daily living, ultimately it is patients' assessments of their abilities that define this aspect of HRQL. Those of us involved in clinical programs are well-aware of the mismatches that exist between actual ability and perceptions of function. It is common for people to be more or less competent than they believe themselves to be, which is a human characteristic that figures prominently in social cognitive theories of behavior [4]. Moreover, patients may meet or exceed some criterion defined by the medical community, yet be unhappy with limitations that exceed this standard. This is certainly true when patients meet the minimal insurance standards of physical disability, yet are displeased with symptoms experienced during their occupational or leisure activities. As Shumaker et al. [84] point out, subjective appraisals in HRQL involve not only an evaluation of perceived function but also satisfaction with a particular level of function.

Finally, a number of investigators emphasize that an additional dimension of HRQL is the importance that people attribute to different areas of function. As Feinstein and colleagues [23] note:

> ". . . some patients might gladly accept an impairment in continence in exchange for improved mental function; other patients might prefer the reverse. A woman with severe deformity of multiple joints caused by rheumatoid arthritis might be marked as *essentially unimproved* by her physician because the joints remain deformed after therapy, but she might be delighted by having regained the desired ability to sew or hold playing cards. Conversely, a women who is marked as *improved* because she has gained the latter ability might regard herself as *unimproved* because she remains unable to walk without aid."

The Multidimensional Nature of HRQL

A second major feature of HRQL is the multidimensional nature of the concept. Although there are some differences in the specific dimensions discussed by various authors, close inspection reveals that there is more agreement than disagreement. For example, Fries and Spitz [29] provide a hierarchy of health outcomes that includes five dimensions: death, disability, discomfort, iatrogenic conditions (side effects from drug therapy or other medical intervention), and economic factors. As shown in Figure 3.1, their model goes from general to specific, with measurement conducted at the level of the specific components. The health assessment questionnaire (HAQ), which was developed from this model, has a disability subscale that

FIGURE 3.1.
The hierarchy of patient outcome. Reproduced from ref. 29.

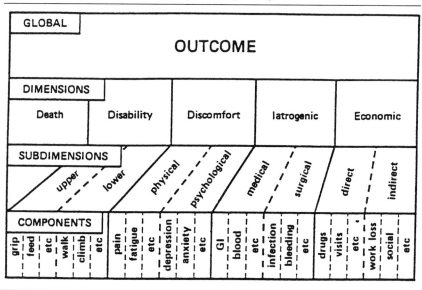

evaluates difficulty with eight different categories of function (e.g., dressing and walking), a simple analog subscale for pain, fatal and nonfatal indices for iatrogenic conditions that involve self-report and audit of hospital records, and subscales that evaluate both the direct and indirect economic impact of disease [30]. Fries et al. [30] admit that the HAQ does not provide evaluation of social interaction or patient satisfaction; it is also noticeably weak in the areas of physical and psychological discomfort.

Shumaker et al. [84] provide an integrated overview of how different investigators conceptualize the dimensions of HRQL. As they indicate, core dimensions include physical functioning, emotional well-being, social functioning, and role activities, as well as life satisfaction and health perceptions. They also note that many investigators include, in addition to the core dimensions, cognitive (or neuropsychological) functioning, sexual functioning and intimacy, and productivity (subsuming work-related issues), as well as factors associated with perceived and actual symptoms of illness, adverse effects of treatment, energy and vitality (and their converse, fatigue), pain, self-esteem/body image, and sleep/rest. Although social support is sometimes included within the context of social functioning, it is usually treated as a moderator of the HRQL concept.

A major issue related to the dimensions that characterize HRQL is the confusion between potential *causes* or *moderators* of HRQL and *patient-defined outcomes*. For example, in Fries and Spitz's [29] model of health outcomes discussed earlier, iatrogenic conditions and the economics of disease represent antecedents, as opposed to outcome dimensions, of HRQL. This distinction is salient when we consider events that occur in exercise therapy such as muscular soreness. Although this physical symptom represents a potential negative outcome, it should be viewed as an antecedent to the participants' view of their HRQL; that is, muscular soreness could elicit feelings of incompetence or negative affect which, in turn, influence HRQL. Our intent is not to undermine any hierarchical organizational model, such as that proposed by Fries and Spitz [29]. On the other hand, it is important to differentiate concepts so that conceptual distinctions exist between various dimensions of HRQL. This conceptual distinctiveness is critical if the multidimensional HRQL construct is to be useful with respect to: 1) developing knowledge about health outcomes, 2) being operationally defined for purposes of assessment, and 3) predicting which dimensions of HRQL are most likely to be affected by rehabilitative treatment (e.g., exercise or life-style change).

The importance of providing distinctions in models becomes clearer with a specific example. Suppose a disease state produces an associated reduction in cognitive function in some individuals. Deficits in memory and comprehension, when examined with existing models, would be classified under the cognitive dimension of HRQL [91]. However, such a classification does not speak to how these changes have influenced patients' perceptions. When loss of memory or comprehension detracts from a person's perception of retaining personal control over his or her affairs, it is the individual's *recognition of this loss* that defines quality. When the deficit is of a magnitude in which loss goes unrecognized, then is patient-defined HRQL diminished? This position fits in nicely with the conceptual distinction between impairments and functional limitations that is found in the disability literature [62]; that is, deficits in cognitive function represent *impairments,* whereas the perceived influence of these changes on the patient's life constitute *functional limitations.*

The issue of clarity in conceptual distinctions is not simply confined to the level of models but also to the measurement of factors in these models. This is not a problem unique to the study of HRQL, but it is common to the measurement of variables presumed to represent perceptions, cognitions, and affect. However, the essence of accurately representing patient-defined HRQL outcomes in research is the strength of the measurement link between a concept and its operational definition. The next section concerns the key problems associated with measures used in HRQL research.

HRQL Measures

A major issue in the HRQL measurement literature concerns the use of composite scores vs. dimension-specific test batteries [39]. The most extreme position with composite scores has been adopted by Kaplan and Bush [40]; these investigators have developed the Quality of Well Being Scale

(QWB) that "... combines preference weighted measures of symptoms and functioning to provide a numerical point-in-time expression of well-being that ranges from zero (0) for death to one (1.0) for asymptomatic optimal functioning; that is, higher scores represent better health." However, there are several problems with this approach. First, the QWB offers a very restricted representation of the individual HRQL factors. For example, the physical activity subscale focuses on very low levels of function. Of the three categories described in the QWB, two involve the use of a wheelchair or severe physical limitations. Also, concern has been expressed over the instability in the weights assigned to the different factors. Fries and Spitz [29] have noted that "... the value judgements required are known to differ substantially among individuals, in the same individual at different points in time, and between patients sick with a particular problem and those without the problem." Third, the QWB places a heavy emphasis on mortality/morbidity. This approach suppresses the contribution of limitations in other dimensions of HRQL and, by design, does not allow one to discriminate among dimensions.

Dimension-specific test batteries can also be problematic. Using an exercise trial as an example, suppose an investigator assesses participants' difficulties with ADLs, their social functioning, and their physical symptom reporting. The investigator finds that exercise improves self-report of function in the performance of ADLs but has little effect on social functioning or on the experience of pain and discomfort. One can then conclude that exercise therapy directly influences the HRQL dimension of perceived physical functioning. However, this change may or may not be meaningful or important to the patients in question. One solution to the problem has been to add single-item scales that assess patients' perceptions of their overall HRQL. In this approach, weighting is done on an idiographic level via each patient's phenomenology.

HRQL measures can also be classified as either generic (i.e., instruments designed to assess HRQL in a broad range of populations) or population/condition-specific (i.e., instruments designed for use with specific diseases, age groups, or ethnic groups). Within these two categories are single items, indices, health profiles (single instruments measuring several different aspects of HRQL), and instruments designed to assess each dimension of HRQL that are combined to create a battery of measures [84,93]. In addition, types of responses can vary considerably across measures, and this variation is directly related to the underlying conceptualization of HRQL. Even within a particular HRQL domain (e.g., satisfaction with function), the actual level of measurement and response categories can vary. For example, there are four levels of measurement (nominal, ordinal, interval, and ratio), each yielding different types of information. In terms of response categories, items range from simple dichotomous yes/no responses to those that have three to more ranked categories to items that are treated as interval scales on a single dimension (e.g., agree/disagree, always/never, or visual analogs). A single profile might use different response categories or might be consistent across various dimensions [92].

The primary advantage of generic health status measures is that they permit comparisons across a broad range of diseases and groups of patients. The RAND Medical Outcome Study measure was developed from such a model and offers a classic example of the usefulness of this type of instrument. Conversely, most diseases have their own unique symptoms and create a vast array of impairments and subsequent functional limitations. Thus, specific measures are also necessary. In this regard, Rejeski and Shumaker [80] outline issues that are specific to knee osteoarthritis. For example, knee pain and associated coping strategies are critical to understanding activity patterns. Furthermore, activity patterns are believed to be the key to understanding the progression of knee OA. The implication here is that a full HRQL assessment in patient populations requires the selection of measures that are both generic and population specific.

Summary

Our purpose in this initial section of the chapter was to explore the conceptual basis of HRQL. We believe that a clear understanding of this concept is essential to the systematic growth of knowledge in this domain. From the literature reviewed and from our own analysis of research on *physical activity*, we propose an organizational framework for HRQL outcomes that involves six content dimensions. These include: global indices of HRQL, physical function, physical symptoms/states, emotional function, social function, and cognitive function (Table 3.1). As indicated previously, measures can be generic or condition/disease-specific. Furthermore, despite a lack of supporting data, when assessing either perceptions or behaviors within specific content domains, it may be important to evaluate both the associated value and level of satisfaction that patients' report for particular attributes/abilities. Finally, we want to underscore the importance of identifying antecedents, moderating variables, mediating variables, and outcome measures in HRQL research. Too often these distinctions are not made, leading to confusion concerning the effects of a particular treatment on HRQL. As we review existing HRQL research on physical activity in the next section, we will use the framework presented above to organize what is known and to reflect on lessons learned from this research.

PHYSICAL ACTIVITY AND HRQL: DIRECT AND INDIRECT EVIDENCE

First, we will review studies that constitute direct support for a relationship between physical activity and HRQL. These include studies examining several HRQL concepts concurrently (e.g., emotional, physical, and social

TABLE 3.1.
Content Dimensions for Physical Activity and Health-related Quality of Life

I. Global indices of HRQL
II. Physical function
    Difficulties with ADLs and other performance-related domains
    Physical self-concept
    Health-related perceptions
III. Physical symptoms/states
    Pain discomfort
    Fatigue
    Energy
    Sleep
IV. Emotional function
    Depression
    Anxiety
    Anger/hostility
    Self-esteem
    Mood/affect
V. Social function
    Social dependency
    Leisure-time pursuits
    Family/work roles
VI. Cognitive function
    Memory
    Attention
    Problem-solving/decision making

function) and those which target HRQL as a primary outcome. Second, we will present representative studies and the results of previous reviews in the physical activity literature relevant to specific domains that contribute to HRQL. For example, there are studies limited to the investigation of physical or emotional function. Third, we will present lessons learned from the review of these literatures and use these lessons as a platform to suggest targets for improvement in future studies of physical activity and HRQL.

Direct Relationships between Physical Activity and HRQL

Of the 28 studies we located that constitute direct evidence for a relationship between physical activity and HRQL, 10 of them involved asymptomatic adults. In the case of the elderly, however, degree of health was sometimes compromised by frailty and weakened physical states. The remaining 18 studies involved patient populations from three broad areas: cardiovascular disease (i.e., hypertension, myocardial infarction, and angina), pulmonary disease (i.e., COPD, emphysema, bronchitis, asthma, lung transplant, and chronic respiratory disease), and arthritis (i.e., rheumatoid arthritis, OA, and fibromyalgia).

Two chronic diseases that we excluded from detailed review were cancer and diabetes. Existing studies with cancer were omitted because of measurement limitations and other shortcomings in study design. On the other hand, a detailed review of the diabetes literature was not considered, because physical activity typically plays a central role in most treatment regimens, making it difficult to isolate the unique contribution of these interventions to HRQL. It is instructive, however, to highlight the results of a large 2-year observational study of physical activity and HRQL that included diabetics in the sampling frame [90]. In this study, older Type I diabetics (mean age, 56 yr) with higher levels of physical activity enjoyed better physical functioning, greater energy/less fatigue, less pain, greater psychosocial well-being, and less distress than those low in physical activity. Because the HRQL scores for both high- and low-active participants were in the healthy range, these data suggest that when exercise influences HRQL, it does so by enhancing an already healthy state.

The principle HRQL studies in the physical activity literature involving cardiovascular disease, pulmonary disease, and arthritis are summarized in Tables 3.2–3.7. Eleven of these investigations were randomized control trials (RCTs), and another seven were exercise training studies. The remaining 10 studies were correlational and, in several instances, involved program evaluations. All of the studies concerned either young to middle-aged adults (14 studies: mean age range, 40–55+ yr) or older adults (14 studies: mean age range 60–80+ yr). A majority of the studies (n = 19) had a strong supervised component, where individuals both participated in or learned about exercise for varying periods of time (i.e., a few weeks to several months). The RCTs and exercise training studies are in the majority, although some of these studies had both supervised and self-regulated exercise treatment conditions. The correlational and program evaluation studies dealt with both supervised and individually self-regulated exercises (i.e., leisure time pursuits, organized sports, other "free-living or active-living" physical activity). Furthermore, most intervention studies that were designed to improve fitness and physical performances (e.g., the 6-min walk) were successful in doing so; however, the exercise prescription underlying these changes varied as a function of participants' ages, initial levels of fitness, and disease status. The majority of the interventions reported had a clear aerobic component that was in excess of 20 min long (~ range, 20–50 min), with intensities that varied from as low as 45% to as high as 85% of peak heart rate. Thus, the physiological demands of these training programs range from low to moderate.

In general, physical activity/exercise is associated with improvements in various aspects of HRQL, regardless of the age, activity status, or health of the participants. For example, only two of ten studies that dealt with sedentary healthy participants or sedentary, frail, older persons failed to find positive associations between physical activity and HRQL outcomes. Similar trends were observed in studies with chronically diseased populations. There are, however, some qualifications regarding this literature that should be kept in mind. Specifically, there is a relatively heterogeneous mixture of

TABLE 3.2.
Healthy Sedentary Adults

Authors	Participants	Design and Dose	Measures	Major Results	Comments
Brown et al.[9]	• 66 men and 69 women • Mean age: men = 50.6 yr, women = 54.8 yr	• Exercise training study • Random assignment to 16 wk of low-intensity walk, low-intensity walk + relaxation, moderate-intensity walk, or Tai chi • Dose: low intensity = 45–55% HRR, 40–50 min, 3× wk; moderate intensity walk = 65–75% of HRR, 30–40 min, 3× wk	• STAI (anxiety)[a] • POMS (mood) • PANAS (affect) • STAXI (anger) • Global self-esteem • Physical competence • Body acceptance • LSES (life satisfaction; most like HRQL)	• Women experienced significant reductions in mood disturbance and greater satisfaction with body • Men experienced increased positive affect • No differences for HRQL or related measures • $\dot{V}o_{2max}$ improved more in walking conditions than other conditions for both genders	None
King et al.[43]	• 60 men and women • Mean age = 48 yr	• Exercise training study • Random assignment to 24-wk home-based program or assessment only control • Dose: Rx=65% baseline-peak HR, 5 × per week, men 47 min and women 54 min each session	• 14-item measure assessing multiple aspects of HRQL (e.g., depression, anxiety, stress, mood, and sense of control)	• Increase in $\dot{V}o_{2max}$ for M/F exercisers • Weight loss for M exercisers • HRQL items changing: satisfaction with exercise-induced changes in physical parameters • HRQL changes unrelated to Δfitness	Exercise adherence exceeded 75%
Norris et al.[66]	• Males, 20–50 yr • Initial pool, n = 150; final adherers, n = 77	• Exercise training study • Assigned to aerobic, anaerobic, control group • Dose: 10 wk, 2 Center and 1 self-regulated each wk; 30–40-min sessions, including 20–30 min jogging	• Job stress • Life situation (HRQL) • General health questionnaire	• Aerobic exercise had strongest + effects on life quality • Both aerobic and anaerobic better than control • HRQL not related to Δfitness	56% adherence in aerobic, 48% in anaerobic, and 50% in control

[a]HRR, heart rate reserve; HR, heart rate; STAI, State-Trait Anxiety Inventory; POMS, Profile of Mood States; PANAS, Positive Affect-Negative Affect Schedule; STAXI, State-Trait Anger Expression Inventory; LSES, Life Satisfaction in the Elderly Scale; M/F, male/female; Δ, change.

TABLE 3.3.
Healthy Sedentary Elderly

Author	Participants	Design and Dose	Measures	Major Results	Comments
Hawkins and Duncan [34]	• 30 men and 96 women • Mean age: 78 yr	• Correlational • Cross-sectional • Structural equation modeling	• Personal health practices • Self-evaluation of life function (HRQL measure)	• Physical activity (current and past) was related to HRQL factors: physical symptoms/disabilities, health status and depression	None
King et al. [42]	• 197 men and 160 women • Mean age: men = 56 yr, women = 57 yr	• RCT • Four conditions: high-intensity, group-based; high-intensity, home-based; low-intensity, home based; assessment-only control • 4–8-wk program • Dose: high-intensity = 40 min walk/job, $3\times$ wk $\approx$ 73–88% peak HR; low-intensity = 30-min walk, $5\times$ wk, $\approx$ 60–73% peak HR	• Beck Depression • TMAS (anxiety) • Perceived Stress • Perceived change in mental and physical functioning	• Greater participation was related to lower anxiety and depression independent of fitness • Reduction in body weight was related to lower 12-month depressive symptoms • Greater reduction in anxiety in women than men • Significant increase in $\dot{V}O_{2max}$	75% adherence to home-based and 53% to group-based
McMurdo and Burnett [56]	• Men and women (n=87) • Mean age: 65 yr	• Exercise training study • Random assignment to exercise or health education control	• Geriatric Depression • Life Satisfaction Index • Health Status	• Improved perceived health status and life satisfaction for exercise group	83% adherence in exercise group and 71% in health

TABLE 3.3.—*continued*

Author	Participants	Design and Dose	Measures	Major Results	Comments
		• Dose: 25 min of endurance and resistance training, 3× wk		• Greater decrease in depression for exercise group	education control group
Stephens [89]	• 2407 men and 3325 women, 40+ years old	• Epidemiological study • Four survey data bases from U.S. and Canada	• General Well-Being Schedule • CES Depression • Bradburn's Affect Balance • Health opinion survey • Positive/negative self-description	• Level of physical activity related positively to mental health (i.e., upbeat mood, general WB, low frequency of anxiety/depression • Above findings independent of education and physical health • Strongest effects for older women	• Relationships generalized across populations and measures • Choice of activity and quality of activity time may be important for psychological benefits

[a]HR, heart rate; TMAS, Taylor Manifest Anxiety Scale; CES, Center for Epidemiologic Studies; WB, well-being.

TABLE 3.4.
Frail, Sedentary, and Chronically Diseased Elderly

Author	Participants	Design and Dose	Measures	Major Results	Comments
McMurdo and Rennie [57]	• 8 men and 33 women • Mean age: 81 yr • Residents of nursing homes	• RCT: Random assignment of four homes to exercise or reminiscence control; • Dose: 2× wk, 35 min of strengthening exercises; baseline and 7-month assessments	• ADL • Geriatric Depression • Life satisfaction • Minimental	• Decreased depression for both groups, but exercise had a significantly greater increase than control • ADLs of exercise group improved • Improved grip strength, spinal flexion in favor of exercise group	91% attendance to exercise and 84% attendance to control
Morey et al. [60]	• n = 75, men and women • Mean age=68 yr	• 5-yr observational study • Subsample of 75 out of 500 for longitudinal study • Dose: 1.5 hr, 3× wk (15-min stationary bike, 5-min stair climb, 20-min floor exercise, 25-min brisk walk; goal 65–75% HRR	• Sickness Impact Profile • General Well-Being	• At baseline, persons with low MET capacity (<6) had poorer psychosocial and physical function on the SIP • Adherers over 5 yr (n=19) had a 22% increase in METs at year 2 and a 10% decrease at year 5 • Well-being lower for dropouts	43% dropout in 1st year
Stewart et al. [90]	• 1758 men and women with chronic disease • Mean age=56.1 yr	• Observational, 2-yr longitudinal • Cross-sectional • Dose: self-reported frequency and time walking and leisure activity	• Physical/role function • Social activity limitation due to 1) pain, energy, and fatigue, 2) sleep problems, 3) health distress, 4) health perceptions, 5) psychological distress/well-being	• At baseline, higher levels of physical activity associated with better physical functioning and health • Higher levels of physical activity associated with better psychological well-being at 2 yr	Patterns of findings most consistent for hypertension, MI, CHF, and Type I diabetes

TABLE 3.5.
Chronic Disease: Hypertension, Myocardial Infarction and Angina

Author	Participants	Design and Dose	Measures	Major Results	Comments
Dubbert et al. [19]	• Sedentary men with hypertension (n = 28); no meds • Mean age: 42 yr • 68% white and 32% black	• Exercise training study • Random assignment to exercise or control; 10 wk • Dose: 4× wk, 30 min ~ 65–80% max HR; used preferred mode of aerobics; two sessions staff monitored and two self-monitored; control group performed nonaerobic activity for same frequency/duration but <60% max HR	• Jenkins Activity Survey • STAI (state anxiety) • Global mood rating	• JAS: speed and impatience decreased significantly for moderate-intensity exercise • Mood improved for both groups • Significant reduction in SBP and DBP	93% adherence with supervised session and 85% median attendance for all four sessions
Holmback et al. [37]	• 33 men and 34 women • Mean age = 55 yr; acute MI patients	• Exercise training study • Random assignment to exercise or usual care control, 12 wk training with 1 yr follow-up • Dose: 45-min aerobic sessions, 2× wk; ~ 70–85% peak HR	• Self-report of physical performance and well-being (e.g., ADLs w/o fatigue, self-confidence, anxiety, depression, insomnia, relaxation)	• Improvement in fitness immediately after training, but no difference at 1-yr follow-up • At 1-yr follow-up no differences in self-reports	No self-report data on immediate training effects
Lavie and Milani [46]	• 120 men and 31 women who completed phase II cardiac rehab (subgroup from a larger sample of 83 women and 375 men) • Mean age: men=61 yr, women=63 yr	• Observational, retrospective, no control group • Dose: 12-wk program, 3× wk • No long-term follow-up	• Anxiety, depression and hostility • MOS (SF-36) • Energy, general health, pain, function and well-being	• Almost all measures significantly improved for both genders; the only difference was that women have lower %Δ for perceived function and total HRQL	Multivariate analyses revealed no omnibus gender effect

				Results	Comments
				• Reductions in body fat and estimated exercise capacity for both genders	
Oldridge et al. [70]	• 201 acute MI patients (87% men and 13% women) selected because they manifested moderate anxiety and depression (elevated but not to clinical levels) • Mean age: 53 yr	• RCT, stratified parallel group design • Dose: 8-wk program plus behavioral counseling or usual care control; 50-min exercise 2× wk, including 20–30 min aerobics ~ 65% max HR, behavioral counseling 90 min 1× wk • Multiple assessments	• Time trade-off utility measure • HRQL after MI (piloted and content validated) • Quality of Well-Being, including symptoms, mobility, physical activity, social activities	• All disease-specific and general HRQL measures improved in both groups over 12 mo • Significant but modest 8-wk effect, favoring program group for improved emotion and decreased state of anxiety • No evidence that treatment had a differential effect for those more anxious or depressed	Short-term benefits of rehabilitation not maintained at 12-mo follow-up
Pierce et al. [74]	• 90 mild hypertensives, 61% men and 39% women • Mean age: 45 yr; 75% white and 25% black	• RCT involving aerobics, strength training, or waitlist control • Dose: 16 wk supervised exercise, 3× wk, 35 min walking or 30 min strength training • No long-term follow-up	• STAI (anxiety) • CES-D (depression) • Cook Medley Hostility • Social support • Health Locus of Control • Emotional reactivity • Cognitive function • Perceived change in health and psychological function	• No differences on psychosocial measures but a multivariate effect for perceived-change questions with both aerobic and strength groups improving more than control group • 16% change in aerobic power for aerobic group only	Over 80% compliance in both aerobic and weight training group; no exercise in control group; authors suggest that impact may have been better if groups had had lower initial fitness levels

TABLE 3.5.—*continued*

Author	Participants	Design and Dose	Measures	Major Results	Comments
Stern and Cleary [87]	• 651 male volunteers who had MIs • Mean age: 52 yr	• Multicenter controlled trial; randomized to exercise or control • This report was on preparatory program of physical activity prior to randomization • Dose: 3× wk for 6 wk; minimum of 20 min on aerobics @ 72% of age-predicted max HR	• Internal/External Control • Life Events Scale • MMPI • Taylor Manifest Anxiety and Depression Scale • Katz Adjustment Scale	• Significant improvements in short-term responses to preparatory program in reducing problems of psychosocial adjustment, depression, sexual activity and vocational adjustment • Improvement in work capacity	• 78% compliance with preparatory exercise program; these data came from a short-term observation phase of the major study
Stern and Cleary [88]	• 651 male volunteers who had MIs • Mean age: 52 yr	• Multicenter controlled trial; randomized to exercise of control • Assessments at baseline, 6mo, 1 yr and 2 yr • Dose: 3× wk for 8 wk; @ 70–85% peak HR; long term program = 3× wk, 15 min aerobics and 30 min games and skills	• Internal/External Control • Life Events Scale • MMPI • Taylor Manifest Anxiety and depression Scale • Katz Adjustment Scale	• No differences between group at any testing period; same when blocking on depression, anxiety or work capacity • The exercise group always had higher work capacity than the controls; however, it was greatest at 6 mo	Compliance was 90% for 8-wk program, but it decreased to 48% at 18 months; 30% of controls reported self-regulated exercise

Reference	Sample	Design/Dose	Measures	Results	Comments
Wiklund et al. [100]	• 42 men and 8 women with stable angina • Had angina pectoris for a median of 27 mo (range: 4–207 months)	• Correlational study • Relationship between patients' performance on a standard Bruce Test and self-reported measures of HRQL	• Psychological well-being • Angina-related HRQL (disease-specific problems, cardiac symptoms, emotions, physical limitations, and life satisfaction)	• Exercise tolerance was related to physical dimensions of AP HRQL measure in the expected positive directions	None
Worchester et al. [102]	• 224 men, age = 54.4 yr • Post-MI patients	• RCT, randomized to either high-intensity or low-intensity exercise • Dose: 8 wk, 60 min (walk/jog), 3× wk for high-intensity group and 60 min, 2× wk of light exercise and calisthenics; both groups told to walk 30 min/day at comfortable pace.	• STAI (anxiety) • IPAT (depression) • Sense of well-being scale plus measures of social, marital, and occupational adjustment	• No differences between groups at baseline, 4 or 12 months on almost all measures • Improvements in occupational adjustment better for high-intensity group at 4 but not 12 mo • Work capacity high for high-intensity group at 4 but not 12 mo; 12-mo values higher than baseline	Compliance was 83% in high-intensity and 87% in low-intensity programs; no data on exercise behavior between termination of 8-wk program and follow-up testing; patients anxiety levels were normal at entry

aMI, myocardial infarction; HR, heart rate; STAI, State-Trait Anxiety Inventory; MOS, Medical outcome studies; CES-D, Center for Epidemiological Depression Scale; MMPI, Minnesota Multiphasic Personality Inventory; IPAT, Institute for Personality and Ability Testing; JAS, Jenkins Activity Survey; SBP, systolic blood pressure; DBP, diastolic blood pressure;

TABLE 3.6
Chronic Disease: Pulmonary

Authors	Participants	Design and Dose	Measures	Major Results	Comments
Atkins et al. [3]	• 28 men and 48 women • Mean age: = 64.8 yr • Could walk 100 yd without severe dypsnea	• RCT to increase exercise • Randomly assigned to one of five groups: behavioral modification only, cognitive/behavioral modification, cognitive modification only, attention control, or no treatment control • Dose: five progressive levels of walking (Stage 1, 60% max treadmill speed for 5 min, 2× daily to stage 5, 70% max treadmill speed for 20 min 2× daily); lasted 3 mo	• Health status index (functional scales for mobility, physical activity, social activity, symptom disturbances) • Quality of well-being • Efficacy expectations for walking	• At 3 mo, mean QWB scores higher for three experimental groups than for control groups: Δ in exercise tolerance significantly related to Δ in QWB; self-efficacy for walking higher in treatment than in attention control group; efficacy also related to changes in exercise tolerance and QWB • At 6-mo follow-up, QWB of exercise groups higher than controls (differences larger at 6 months); compliance was related to gains in QWB and exercise groups experienced significant greater exercise tolerance, compared to controls • No evidence of change in physiologic function	The cognitive behavioral treatment approach led to better compliance than in other treatment groups; there was 74% compliance with 6-mo assessments; all exercise groups walked more than controls, however, cognitive behavioral treatment walked significantly more than other groups; change in pulmonary function not expected with this disease

Study	Sample	Design/Intervention	Measures	Results	Comments
Guyatt et al. [32]	• 23 men and 8 women • Mean age: 64.6 yr	• 6 month postdischarge from 4–6 wk multidisciplinary rehab program • Assessments made at baseline, then at a minimum 2 and 24 weeks postprogram • Dose: Rx based on graded cycle ergometer test (symptom-limited)	• HRQL measure specific to this population (CRQ)[a]; assesses physical function and symptoms, as well as emotional function	• HRQL improved 2 wks postprogram • At 24 wk there was considerable attenuation for study adherers (of 24 patients improved at 2 wks, only 11 remained improved at 24 wk • Trend toward significant 6-min walk times at 2 wk • Spirometry unchanged	Patients who completed HRQL measures at baseline and 24 wk were far superior in HRQL at baseline than dropouts; 90% compliance with rehab program (68% compliance with 24-wk assessment and 54% exercised 6 wk postprogram)
Manzetti et al. [51]	• 7 men and 2 women • Mean age: 40 yr • Awaiting lung transplant; no medication would influence exercise tolerance	• Random assignment to education or education + exercise (pilot study) • Groups stratified so that each had equal number of obstructive or restrictive disease • Dose: education 3× weekly for 6 wk, Exercise group went 2× wk at 80% max ventilation for 30 min (treadmill, bike, light aerobics, weight training)	• Quality of Well-Being • Quality of life index • Symptom frequency & symptom distress scale	• QWB improved in both groups over time; no differences between groups over time • 6-min walk time improved for both groups over time	Results are qualified by small n and large variances
Vale et al. [97]	• 19 men and 32 women • Mean age was 64.2 yr • COPD patients in rehab	• Retrospective design with two groups: structured outpatient rehab exercise maintenance (EM) or no structured exercise maintenance (NEM)	• HRQL specific to COPD (CRQ)	• HRQL improved from pre- to postrehab for both groups; also, both groups' HRQL decreased at follow-up but was significantly higher than baseline; no	Poorer baseline exercise endurance was predictive of greater decline in follow-up

TABLE 3.6—*continued*

Authors	Participants	Design and Dose	Measures	Major Results	Comments
		• 3 assessments: baseline, postrehab, and follow-up • Dose: Rehab involved 6 wk of health education + aerobic and light strength training, 2× wk; postrehab EM involved similar protocol 1× week w/o health education		• differences between groups • 12-min walk improved pre- to postrehab in both groups • 12-min walk decreased at follow-up but higher than baseline	testing on exercise endurance; not true for HRQL; 100% compliance for follow-up assessment

[a]CRQ, Chronic Respiratory Disease Questionnaire

TABLE 3.7.
Chronic Disease: Arthritis

Author	Participants	Design and Dose	Measures	Major Results	Comments
Buckelew et al. [12]	• 3 men and 76 women • Mean age: 44 yr • Fibromyalgia	• Correlational • Studied relationship between self-reported activity from AIMS with HRQL	• Arthritis Impact Measurement Scale (AIMS) • Arthritis Self-Efficacy Scale; physical function, pain self-efficacy, and self-efficacy for controlling arthritis symptoms	• Positive relationship between HRQL and physical activity • Self-efficacy for pain, function and symptoms predicted physical activity scores (7–12% of variance) • Self-efficacy was best predictor of reported pain	Full models using demographics, disease severity, AIMS, and self-efficacy accounted for 21–26% variance in pain and 14–23% in AIMS physical activity scores
Kovar et al. [45]	• 17 men and 85 women • Mean age: 69 yr • OA of knee	• RCT • Random assignment to either fitness walk + education or usual medical care • 8 wk • Dose: Supervised 3× wk, about 30 min walking, some counseling (re: adherence to walking)	• AIMS	• Intervention group significantly improved over control in pain reduction and physical activity • Trend toward improved psychosocial function in intervention group • Intervention group made significantly better improvement in 6-min walk than in control group	90% compliance with study; treatment group increased 18.4% in 6-min walk, whereas there was a 5% decrease in the control group
Lorig and Holman [48]	• Study 1: n = 707; mean age: 64 yr; 84% women and 16% men; 75% OA and 25% other	• Review of arthritis self-management program: subjects randomized to program or control;	• Self-report: pain, disability, CES-Depression and Beck Depression Scale	• Study 1: Compared to controls', ASMP treatment significantly reduced pain and increased weekly	Changes in self-efficacy had stronger associations with

TABLE 3.7.—*continued*

Author	Participants	Design and Dose	Measures	Major Results	Comments
	• Study 2: n=127; similar characteristics	• baseline and 4-month assessment • 1× education each wk for 2hr; 12 sessions; 15 patients per group; instruction involved pain management and self-designing an exercise program	• Self-Efficacy for Arthritis Scale • Self-report of exercise	exercises; no effects for disability or depression • Study 2: Compared to controls, efficacy-enhancing ASMP treatment resulted in increased no. of blocks walked, reduced pain, increased self-efficacy	changes in health status than in exercise behavior; analyses involved covarying baseline measures
Minor et al. [59]	• 80 with OA and 40 with RA; 18% men and 82% women • Mean age: for OA=63.8 yr; RA=54.3 yr	• RCT with follow-up; random assignment to aerobic walk, aerobic aquatics, usual care control • 12-wk programs with testing at baseline, 3, 6, and 12 mo • Dose: 3× wk for 60 min ~ 60–80% max HR; gradual progression from 10–35 min within the 60 min	• Tennessee Self-Concept Scale • AIMS	• Compared to control, at 12 wk, both exercise groups improved in aerobic capacity, physical activity, physical symptoms, anxiety and depression; no change in self-concept • Exercise groups had better improvement than controls for time on exercise test • HRQL effects for walk group were maintained at 6 months, except for depression; aquatics group was similar, except that they did not maintain improvement with anxiety; the only difference between groups was in aerobic capacity	85% compliance with 12-wk program; after 6 mo, 63% reported 60 min of exercise per wk and at 12 mo this decreased to 57%; After 24 wk, the control group made a steady increase in improvement for symptom-oriented HRQL outcomes; they also experi-

			enced improvement in aerobic capacity and other measures of physical function; lack of differences between groups appears to be due to improvement in control group, rather than to a large decrease in the treatment effect
			• At 12 months, aquatics group had a significant increase over baseline for self-concept, anxiety and pain; there were no between group differences
			None
Minor and Brown [58]	• Same sample Minor et al. paper above	• Measures described above in Minor et al.	• Predictors of self-reported exercise behavior at 3 mo: aerobic capacity, depression, and anxiety, change in depression and anxiety (R^2adj=0.41)
	• Study design described above in Minor et al.		• At 9 mo initial anxiety, prior exercise for 1st 3 mo (R^2 adj = 0.31)
	• The only addition is that they follow subjects for an additional 9 mo, so that now they have 3-, 9-, and 18-month data posttreatment		• At 18 mo: prior exercise for first 3 months, exercise for 1st 9 mo, baseline aerobic capacity; change in pain (R^2 adj = 0.39)
	• Goal of study is to examine predictors of exercise adherence after leaving the formal 12-wk program		

^{a}R^2adj = R^2 adjusted.

study designs (e.g., treatment alone vs. treatment plus follow-up), treatment durations (e.g., 6 wk vs. 32 wk), and disease characteristics (e.g., types of disease and time since onset). Furthermore, there are two important features of measurement that need to be underscored. First, because of differences in populations studied and investigator preferences, outcomes measured typically varied from one study to another. In fact, one of the most striking features of the HRQL studies reviewed is that there is no common pattern to the measures used. Second, HRQL assessment involves a test battery consisting of both individual dimensions and a global index of HRQL. For a number of reasons, investigators do not always include every dimension in their test battery, and global assessments do not always make the distinction between quality of life and *health-related* quality of life.

Despite the aforementioned limitations, it is reasonable to conclude that some positive change in HRQL does occur when people elect to be more physically active on their own (e.g., Stewart et al. [90]), or when they receive exercise therapy as part of a structured intervention. However, these relationships are *not* detected in *every facet* of HRQL. For example, in those areas in which an older individual is functioning at or above the norm (e.g., is able to perform ADLs like younger adults), the impact of exercise is apt to be less dramatic (i.e., a ceiling effect). However, when exercise is perceived as broadly adding to an already healthy state, change might be detected in overall HRQL.

Finally, the associations reported in many of these studies tend *not* to be dependent upon changes in fitness. At first glance, this observation is confusing, given that fitness changes are typically observed as standard, valid indicants of physiologic status. However, the correlations between measures of fitness and HRQL tend to be much weaker than the correlations between performance-based measures of dysfunction and HRQL. The most likely reason for this pattern in the data is that performance measures are more observable and thus are more salient to peoples' lives than changes in $\dot{V}O_{2max}$.

Indirect Evidence on Physical Activity and HRQL

In contrast to HRQL studies, we now direct our attention to several areas of related research that constitute indirect evidence of a link between physical activity and HRQL. These include psychological well-being (PWB); physical, cognitive, and social function; and reports of physical symptoms.

PWB EMOTIONAL FUNCTION. PWB or emotional function is a term that has been used to describe a cluster of negative and positive affective states. In the physical activity literature, these states include the following constructs: depression, anxiety or tension, positive affect, and self-esteem. There have been several recent reviews of the exercise literature on depression and anxiety [8, 13, 55, 61, 67, 76]. The conclusions from these reports are similar and support a positive relationship between exercise and the reduction of depressive and anxiety/tension-related symptoms. This conclusion applies to both men and women of various ages and is independent of health status. North et al. [67] found that the largest effect sizes for depression were for programs of 17 weeks or longer, whereas in the anxiety/tension literature, the effect sizes were largest for programs of 16 weeks or longer [76]. At this time, it is difficult to discern whether the therapeutic effects of physical activity for depression and anxiety/tension are dependent on activity intensity; however, there are RCTs that have found beneficial effects for low-intensity activity. A corollary to this observation is the failure to demonstrate that improvements seen in depression and anxiety/tension with exercise are dependent on changes in fitness. Also, although study designs dealing with anxiety/tension reduction have been largely restricted to aerobic-type activity [76], anaerobic exercise appears to be as effective as aerobic exercise in countering depressive symptomatology [67].

In a review prepared for the Second International Consensus Symposium on Physical Activity, McAuley [53] concluded that there is a positive relationship between exercise habits and self-esteem for both young adults and children. This correlation increases when exercise is personally valued and when measures of PWB are specific vs. general. For example, there is a strong positive relationship between exercise and PWB when self-efficacy (i.e., exercise-related self-confidence) is used as a specific PWB index. This occurs with long-term training (chronic dose) and single bouts of exercise (acute dose) in both normal and clinical samples, as well as for adults of both genders. However, it should be noted that improved self-efficacy may be more reflective of the process variables that encourage changes in HRQL than HRQL itself [73, 77] and, as we will see below, it is more appropriately associated with the dimension of physical functioning. In addition, when positive affect is the main variable used to represent PWB, the correlation between exercise and PWB increases. There is no such evidence for this relationship among the overtrained.

In another recent review of studies of elderly participants (mean age, 56.7 yr), McAuley and Rudolph [54] found correlations between involvement in physical activity and PWB that were similar to those patterns observed in younger samples. Furthermore, the strength of these relationships was directly related to the length of time that the elderly were involved in activity programs. This moderator effect requires cautious interpretation because of the possibility of selective adherence. Although McAuley and Rudolf's [54] review of 38 studies involved thousands of subjects, large and small samples, formal and informal programs, and a program duration from 10 to more than 20 wk, there was little evidence that the physical activity-PWB relationship was moderated by either gender or age. Finally, although improvements in the physical fitness and in the PWB of the elderly were observed in a number of studies, these improvements were not necessarily related, suggesting that *involvement* or changes in cognition/perception may be as important to increased PWB as changes in training status.

PHYSICAL, COGNITIVE, AND SOCIAL FUNCTION. Data from a number of studies on older populations and chronically diseased groups suggest that physical activity is related to improvement in both physical and cognitive function [7]. Furthermore, there are studies in the developmental disability literature that argue that physical activity can have a positive influence on the social behavior of mentally retarded individuals [31]. In addition, studies in the workplace and with various disabled populations indicate that physical activity holds promise as an intervention to enhance work-related behavior [24].

Physical Function. One might surmise that enhanced physical function is the most pronounced consequence of involvement in physical activity. In this context, and consistent with our definition of HRQL, we restrict our attention to *perceptions* of function, as opposed to improvements in objective outcomes (i.e., performance or physiologic parameters). Although objective and subjective indices of physical function are related, there is clear evidence that the two domains are distinct [78]. Moreover, a focus on perception is consistent with our previous discussion of the conceptual basis of HRQL. We should also point out that perceptions related to physical function involve both 1) physical self-concept and 2) self-reports of having difficulties with ADL. These two content areas parallel the objective domains represented by physiologic and performance-based outcomes, respectively.

In examining the literature on physical activity and self-concept, the most sophisticated area of study concerns a related topic known as self-efficacy. Although McAuley [53] has conceptualized the research on physical self-efficacy under the rubric of PWB, it is more akin to a self-system or state-like self-concept variable about an individual's abilities than to self-esteem, because there is no affective dimension to these beliefs. As mentioned in the section on PWB, McAuley [53] has shown that self-efficacy beliefs are favorably related to both short-term and long-term exercise programs. Ewart [21], in studying cardiac patients, found that strength training led to enhanced-efficacy beliefs which, in turn, were linked to improvement in related ADLs. Other research on cardiac patients by Roviaro and his colleagues [83], using a more trait-like index (the Tennessee Physical Self-Concept Scale), found that aerobic exercise improved body concept. What is interesting in the self-concept research with physical activity is that changes in beliefs about physical abilities/qualities do not always covary with objective measures of fitness [38]. Thus, some of the psychological benefits of physical activity appear to be as much cognitive or involvement-related as they are related to changes in physiological systems [3]. Finally, physical activity may be linked to other more specific dimensions of self-concept, such as health perceptions or feelings of increased coordination [52].

In addition to the work on self-concept, there is a growing body of literature in medicine demonstrating that physical training programs enhance patients' perceptions of their abilities to perform ADLs. Modes of training have involved aerobic exercise [6, 15, 45, 59, 65, 69], muscular strengthening [25–27] and Tai-Chi Chuan [44]. ADLs have ranged from very basic tasks such as dressing oneself to more instrumental tasks (IADLs) such as going to the grocery store or doing laundry. Because there is a strong ceiling effect with ADLs in the population at large, this research is largely restricted to investigations in patients with chronic diseases [6, 15, 25–27, 44, 45, 59, 63] and older, frail adults [57, 69]. In other words, most daily tasks or activities can be performed with a minimal degree of physical fitness. Three of the above studies involving ADLs were RCTs involving knee OA [45, 59], congestive heart failure [3], or the frail elderly [69]. Data from these investigations suggest that even *slight* improvements in physical fitness can be successful in causing a positive change in ADLs. For example, in a study with nursing home participants, ADLs were enhanced with very low intensity activity (e.g., seated exercises). Furthermore, when Dekhuijzen et al. [15] studied COPD, they reported that changes in ADLs were not linked to changes in physiologic function.

Cognitive Function. A relatively small number of cross-sectional human studies consistently show that physical activity has a strong positive association with cognitive/neuropsychological performance [20]. These data are in agreement with conclusions reached by Thomas et al. [96] in the International Proceedings Consensus Statement where they reported that chronic exercise produced modest improvements in the performance of a limited number of cognitive tasks. According to Dustman et al. [20], data from longitudinal training studies (2+ yr) are required to confirm whether aerobic exercise has a pronounced long-term effect on cognitive function. It is not known whether the effects of aerobic exercise generalize to low-intensity physical activities. Additionally, the question remains as to whether improvements in objective measures of cognitive function (i.e., neuropsychological and performance improvements) translate into improved mental activity when one is performing ADLs [20]. For example, does increased involvement in physical activity or improvement in physical fitness aid in the storage or recall of information that is used on a day-to-day basis? This latter point is critical to the operational definition of HRQL in that the concept involves both perception of change and the associated meaning of this change for the quality of an individual's life.

Social Function. The most extensive literature on physical activity and social function is in the area of developmental disabilities; however, these findings are largely limited to case study reports and static group designs. Notwithstanding these shortcomings, results are promising. For example, aerobic activities in persons with mild-to-severe mental disabilities lead to reductions in stereotypic (e.g., intense staring or repeated vocalizations) and maladaptive behaviors (e.g., class disruptions). For a review of this literature, interested readers should refer to Gabler-Halle and Chung [31]. In the only controlled study of which we are aware, Beasley [5] found that aerobic exercise led to increased work performance (rate of production) in mildly to moderately retarded adults. There was no evidence that exercise reduced absenteeism.

To our knowledge, the only other research on social function has been in work-related contexts or research on chronic diseases, in which the emphasis was on outcome measures, such as social dependency/acceptance, employment-related stress, and involvement in leisure activity. Limited study suggests that exercise in the workplace is related to reduced absenteeism and improved output among workers without disabilities [18, 24]. There are also reports of reduced job stress with aerobic training in persons with chronic diseases [66, 83]. However, other than a single group design created by Fisher ét al. [27], focusing on strength training, there is no evidence that exercise reduces social dependence [25], social inhibition [16], or social inadequacy [15]. One study, by Roviaro et al. [83], found that an exercise program in cardiac rehabilitation resulted in more active use and enjoyment of leisure-time pursuits.

PHYSICAL SYMPTOMS/STATES. There are data from studies on chronic diseases that various forms of physical activity can reduce symptoms such as pain, swollen joints, breathlessness, and fatigue and can increase perceptions of vigor and energy. For example, investigations of both rheumatoid arthritis [75] and knee OA [14, 26, 28, 45, 59] suggest that both strength training [14, 25, 27] and aerobic conditioning [45, 59, 75] are effective in reducing joint pain. Furthermore, Lyngberg et al. [49] found that increased physical activity in patients with rheumatoid arthritis led to a 35–45% decrease in swollen joints. For yet another chronic disease, Fishman et al. [28] reported that physical activity is linked to decreased breathlessness in individuals with COPD (see also Table 3.6).

When Nordemar et al. [64] studied patients with rheumatoid arthritis, they reported that increased physical activity also has the potential to reduce feelings of tiredness. This conclusion is similar to that of studies on congestive heart failure [6, 90], as well as those studies of hypertension and diabetes [90]. Interestingly, in the general exercise literature, it is argued that one of the most dramatic effects following acute bouts of aerobic activity is an increase in energy [80, 95], effects that appear limited to participants with low baseline energy values [1, 79]. Also, despite reservations with the quality of extant data, O'Connor and Youngstedt [68], in reviewing research on physical activity and sleep, concluded the following: "Epidemiological studies show that exercise is perceived as helpful in promoting sleep and suggest that regular physical activity may be useful in improving sleep quality and reducing daytime sleepiness."

Summary of the Major Lessons Learned from the Review

In this section, we discussed both direct and indirect research supporting the position that physical activity is a viable nonpharmacologic intervention with HRQL. Before concluding our discussion of this evidence, it would be helpful to review the 10 major lessons learned.

- HRQL test batteries should include both generic and condition/population-specific measures. It is important to be able to contrast different conditions/diseases on a common measure of HRQL; however, specific conditions/diseases also have unique symptoms and characteristics that demand focused methods of assessment.
- The degree of change observed in HRQL outcomes with physical activity depends on initial (baseline) test values (e.g., participants who already exhibit normal levels of functioning will not improve as much as those who are in weakened states and are responsive to the stimulus properties of exercise).
- Investigators mistakingly equate change in a single dimension of assessment with improved HRQL (e.g., statistically significant changes in ADL scores may not substantially effect participants' perceptions of their overall HRQL).
- Change in various HRQL outcomes should not be expected to follow a common time course (e.g., increased physical activity can have short-term effects on the reduction of pain or fatigue that may not be reflected in changing social roles until some later point in time).
- The impact of physical activity on HRQL depends not only on the physiological dynamics of treatment but also on the social and behavioral characteristics of specific interventions (e.g., participants may experience improvement in various physiological capacities without recognizing or learning how these capacities might be used to facilitate ADLs and roles).
- Although RCTs are well-designed to examine the effects of short-term treatments, there is a lack of conceptual rigor in the design of follow-up testing (e.g., 6-month post-treatment, testing typically occurs without any assessment of intervening processes/behavior).
- In general, investigators fail to draw clear distinctions among moderator, mediator, and outcome variables [e.g., a case in which enhanced self-efficacy to overcome pain (mediator) does not improve social role functioning (a dimension-specific outcome measure), yet enhances a global outcome index of HRQL].
- The selection of HRQL test batteries are frequently devoid of any conceptual basis (e.g., measures are chosen without any consideration given to their relevance or sensitivity to change with a given population or treatment).
- There has been a failure to evaluate the "costs" associated with intervention as they contribute to HRQL (e.g., the time demands and discomfort of exercise therapy may negate potential positive effects of physical therapy on HRQL).
- The majority of the studies reviewed assumed that improved physical

function at a variety of levels will be perceived similarly by all participants; however, it is well known that people vary in the extent to which they value various aspects of their physical selves (e.g., the value placed on an incremental change in leg strength may have no meaning in a participant's life; thus, functional value may be an important moderator variable to consider in judging treatment effects).

EXERCISE: PREDICTING ITS IMPACT ON PATIENT-DEFINED OUTCOMES

Although HRQL is considered an important outcome in clinical trials that evaluate the efficacy of physical activity and exercise interventions [91, 93], its links to causal antecedents and cognitive/behavioral processes continues to be limited. Specifically, in most of the studies we reviewed, HRQL measures were treated as medical outcomes with little or no attention given to the process of change. Issues to consider whether exercise-related HRQL research is to advance include:

- What specifically was responsible for the change in HRQL?
- How great a role do social psychological processes play in influencing HRQL outcomes?
- When did the treatment have its most pronounced effect on HRQL?
- Which dimensions of HRQL changed? What was the rate of change?

Earlier in this chapter we dealt with the challenge of defining HRQL, and it was evident that much of the struggle came from the lack of a clear conceptual model. A similar problem arises in studying processes of change. In the absence of a conceptual blueprint, one readily becomes "dazzled" by the complexity inherent in the HRQL concept [33]. A means of addressing this problem of studying processes is to use existing theoretical models in the field of health psychology as potential foundations and as one means of avoiding the reinvention of the theoretical wheel. This idea is not novel and has been suggested, in part, by Patrick and Erickson [73]. Theories of health behavior can be useful in building a testable framework in which health behaviors are viewed as intermediary outcomes, en route to HRQL outcomes. Similarly, other self-oriented theories (e.g., subjective well-being, self-presentation) may be useful in this regard. Note that in defining healthy actions and behaviors as intermediary outcomes, we are not confusing this behavior with HRQL. Because most social-cognitive theories are reciprocal and, thus, dynamic, they fit well with the idea of predicting process variables and downstream HRQL outcomes as a function of more global moderating variables (e.g., social support).

In addition to the conceptual advantages of using empirically supported theories to link various antecedent factors to perceived HRQL, there are also measurement advantages. For several theories, measurement of theoretical variables has received careful scrutiny and may provide a basis for helping to construct and validate measures of various aspects of perceived positive or negative health [73]. An example may be useful in illustrating the links proposed. When the categorization proposed earlier in this chapter is kept in mind, the basic blueprint can be described as follows:

		Intermediary		
Antecedents	➡	HRQL variables	➡	Downstream
		(mediators)		HRQL outcomes

When we use self-efficacy theory as one example of intermediary HRQL outcomes, it can be shown that gains in one's confidence to carry out various ADL skills lead to increases in behavior which, when successful, strengthen confidence for future ADL behavior. Because personal control (or limitation on it) is an important aspect of various parts of physical and social functioning, expressing personal control in terms of self-efficacy allows us to examine causal links between antecedents and HRQL outcomes. Using self-efficacy as an indicant of perceived control is not in conflict with psychological theory [4, 50, 98], and there is clinical, empirical evidence that suggests that this model is a viable link to HRQL. For example, Keefe and his associates [41] examined the effectiveness of a pain-coping skills program in knee OA patients, as compared to that using a usual care control condition. Patients who experienced the greatest change in pain control via coping training also showed the greatest improvement in ADLs. Furthermore, Rejeski and his colleagues [77a] have shown that, even after controlling for cardiovascular fitness and strength, efficacy beliefs are important predictors of performance-related ADL behavior.

Other recent examples reflect both the influence of intermediary outcomes and the confusion of these outcomes with the assessment of HRQL. Leedham et al. [47], recently explored the relationship among preoperative positive expectations and adjustment, adherence, and postoperative health in heart transplant patients. Positive expectations were drawn from a quality of life scale, yet were actually measured as "specific beliefs about the efficacy of treatment and chances for future health and survival as well as general feelings about the self and future." The majority of items on the scale concern future expectations about treatment and survival which, in our classification, would be HRQL antecedents. In addition, adherence behavior can be conceptualized as part of an intermediary outcome process that leads to later health outcomes and psychological adjustment. The findings of Leedham et al. suggest a positive association between positive expectations (PE) and adherence behavior (e.g., dietary changes, exercise, monitoring, avoidance of overexertion), and between PE and psychological adjustment, postoperative health, and HRQL. The relationships between antecedents (PE), treatment adherence (intermediary outcome), and psychological adjustment (a dimension of HRQL) could have been conceptualized with existing expectancy-value theoretical frameworks (e.g., self-efficacy theory and the theory of planned behavior). Furthermore, the separation of antecedents such as PEs from an individual's perception of HRQL leads to more concise conceptualization and operational definitions that constitute valid conceptual measures for the latter concept.

The importance of basing the study of HRQL in theory is found in a recent example from the work of Heidrich et al. [35]. Patients' adjustments to cancer are thought to reflect their quality of life. However, the investigators emphasize that there is little in the way of theoretical explanation concerning how individuals manage to regain or retain psychological well-being when confronted with the specter of cancer and its treatment. In this study, the investigators hypothesized and found that self-discrepancy (between ideal and actual self) *mediates* the relationship between physical health status perceptions and PWB. Health status perceptions (HRQL) in this investigation were concerned with a number of measures of symptomatology and function (i.e., do/do not have pain, nausea and only degree of ability to perform ADLs), disease time-line (self-perceived as acute, episodic, or chronic), and health status (present-past comparison). Use of the self-discrepancy concept was proposed as the theoretical mediator between HRQL measures of function and psychosocial adjustment to illness, a second, and different, HRQL concept. The theoretical issue examined was based on conceptualizations, such as Taylor's [93] theory of cognitive adaptation (i.e., adjustment to threatening events), Rosenberg's [81] notions of the adaptive capacity of the self, and Higgins' [36] ideas about self-discrepancy. Although the theoretical proposals offered by the study require additional validation in the future, it underscores the use of a conceptual framework in examining HRQL. The authors introduced a testable explanatory process of the way in which individuals lose, maintain, or enhance facets of HRQL (i.e., indicants of psychological adjustment, well-being, and distress).

If HRQL research is to move beyond simple outcomes and offer some explanation as to why treatments do or do not work, greater investment must be made in studying intermediary outcomes—the process variables that link antecedents to eventual HRQL outcomes. Future HRQL research using various modes of physical activity and exercise as a treatment modality must reflect what we have learned from preceding investigations of HRQL in a variety of areas. An indication of learning involves the inclusion of intermediate theory-based outcomes. Positive results hold promise for the use of frameworks to both plan interventions and provide conceptual clarification, a quality badly needed in the growing literature on exercise and HRQL.

CONCLUSIONS

In concluding this chapter, we want to point out that there have been major battles within clinical research to simply accent HRQL as an outcome.

Hence, until very recently, the theory-based approach we present would have been unacceptable to the medical community. Now that HRQL is recognized as important to medical science, an opportunity exists to move the field forward. Our plea for the development and use of a strong theoretical basis for HRQL research is not unique to the study of physical activity. Wilson and Cleary [101] recently called for the use of conceptual models in linking clinical and medical outcome variables with HRQL. One of their primary criticisms is that the principal goal of the HRQL field to date has been to validly and comprehensively describe health status, not to *understand* HRQL. They argue that few existing conceptual models include the full range of HRQL variables typically assessed. Furthermore, consistent with our suggestions, they emphasize the importance of the individual as an active agent in HRQL and call for the study of intermediary processes. Although we would characterize their model as organizational, one including multiple levels of factors that impinge on HRQL (i.e., biological, psychological, social, and environmental), we agree regarding the need for the future study of HRQL as an outcome variable in clinical care and health promotion.

ACKNOWLEDGMENTS

This chapter was supported, in part, by Grant AG10484-01 from the National Institute of Aging.

REFERENCES

1. Abele, A., and W. Brehm. Mood effects of exercise versus sports games: findings and implications for well-being and health. *Int. Rev. Health Psychol.* 2:53–80, 1993.
2. Andrews, F. M., and S. B. Withey. *Social Indicators of Well-Being: Americans' Perceptions of Life Quality.* New York: Plenum, 1976.
3. Atkins, C. J., R. M. Kaplan, R. M. Timms, S. Reinsch, and K. Lofback. Behavioral exercise programs in the management of chronic obstructive pulmonary disease. *J. Consult. Clin. Psychol.* 52:591–603, 1984.
4. Bandura, A. *Social Foundations of Thought and Action: A Social Cognitive Theory.* Englewood Cliffs, NJ: Prentice-Hall, 1986.
5. Beasley, C. R. Effects of a jogging program on cardiovascular fitness and work performance of mentally retarded adults. *Am. J. Ment. Defic.* 86:609–613, 1982.
6. Blackwood, R., R. A. Mayou, J. C. Garnham, C. Armstrong, and B. Bryant. Exercise capacity and quality of life in the treatment of heart failure. *Clin. Pharmacol. Ther.* 48:325–332, 1990.
7. Bouchard, C., R. J. Shephard, and T. Stephens (eds). *Physical Activity, Fitness, and Health: International Proceedings and Consensus Statement.* Champaign, IL: Human Kinetic, 1994.
8. Brown, D. R. Physical activity, ageing, and psychological well-being. *Can. J. Sport Sci.* 17:185–193, 1992.
9. Brown, D. R., Y. Wang, and A. Ward, et al. Chronic psychological effects of exercise and exercise plus cognitive strategies. *Med. Sci. Sports Exerc.* 27:765–775, 1995.
10. Brownell, K. D. Exercise and obesity. *Behav. Med. Update* 4:7–11, 1982.

11. Brownell, K. D. When and how to diet. *Psychol. Today* June:41–46, 1989.
12. Buckelew, S. P., S. E. Murray, J. E. Hewett, J. Johnson, and B. Huyser. Self-efficacy, pain, and physical activity among fibromyalgia subjects. *Arthritis Care Res.* 8:43–50, 1995.
13. Byrne A, and D. G. Byrne. The effects of exercise on depression, anxiety, and other mood states. *J. Psychosom. Med.* 37:565–574, 1993.
14. Chamberlain, M. A., G. Care, and B. Harfield. Physiotherapy in osteoarthritis of the knees. *Int. Rehabil. Med.* 4:101–106, 1982.
15. Dekhuijzen, P. N. R., M. M. L. Beek, H. T. M. Folgering, and C. L. A. Van Herwaarden. Psychological changes during pulmonary rehabilitation and target-flow inspiratory muscle training in COPD patients with a ventilatory limitation during exercise. *Int. J. Rehabil. Res.* 13:109–117, 1990.
16. Dixhoorn, J. V., H. J. Duivenvoorden, J. Pool, and F. Verhage. Psychic effects of physical training and relaxation therapy after myocardial infarction. *J. Psychosom. Med.* 34:327–337, 1990.
17. Department of Health and Human Services. *Healthy People 2000, National Health Promotion and Disease Prevention Objectives.* Washington, D.C.: U.S. Government Printing Office, DDHS (PHS) 91-50212, 1991, p. 107.
18. Donoghue, S. The correlation between physical fitness, absenteeism and work performance. *Can. J. Public Health* 68:201–203, 1977.
19. Dubbert, P. M., J. E. Martin, W. C. Cushman, E. F. Meydrech, and R. G. Carroll. Endurance exercise in mild hypertension: effects on blood pressure and associated metabolic and quality of life variables. *J. Hum. Hypertens.* 8:265–272, 1994.
20. Dustman, R. E., R. Emmerson, and D. Shearer. Physical activity, age, and cognitive-neuropsychological function. *J. Aging Phys. Act.* 2:143–181, 1994.
21. Ewart, C. K. Psychological effects of resistive weight training: implications for cardiac patients. *Med. Sci. Sports Exerc.* 21:683–688, 1989.
22. Ewart, C. K., C. Barr Taylor, L. B. Reese, and R. F. DeBusk. Effects of early postmyocardial infarction exercise testing on self-perception and subsequent physical activity. *Am. J. Cardiol.* 51:1076–1080, 1983.
23. Feinstein, A. R., B. R. Josephy, and C. K. Wells. Scientific and clinical problems in indexes of functional disability. *Ann. Intern. Med.* 105:413–420, 1986.
24. Fielding, J. E., and K. K. Knight. Cost-benefit analysis of workplace active living programs: the employer perspective. H. A. Quinney, L. Gauvin, and A. E. T. Wall (eds). *Toward Active Living: Proceeding of the International Conference on Physical Activity, Fitness, and Health.* Champaign, IL: Human Kinetics, 1994, pp. 187–192.
25. Fisher, N. M., and D. R. Pendergast. Effects of a muscle exercise program on exercise capacity in subjects with osteoarthritis. *Arch. Phys. Med. Rehabil.* 75:792–797, 1994.
26. Fisher, N. M., D. R. Pendergast, G. E. Gresham, and E. Calkins. Muscle rehabilitation: its effect on muscular and functional performance of patients with knee osteoarthritis. *Arch. Phys. Med. Rehabil.* 72:367–374, 1991.
27. Fisher, N. M., G. E. Gresham, M. Abrams, J. Hicks, D. Horrigan, and D. R. Pendergast. Quantitative effects of physical therapy on muscular and functional performance in subjects with osteoarthritis of the knee. *Arch. Phys. Med. Rehabil.* 74:840–847, 1993.
28. Fishman, D. B., and T. L. Petty. Physical, symptomatic and psychological improvement in patients receiving comprehensive care for chronic airway obstruction. *J. Chronic Dis.* 24:775–785, 1971.
29. Fries, J. F., and P. W. Spitz. The hierarchy of patient outcomes. B. Spilker (ed). *Quality of Life Assessments in Clinical Trials.* New York: Raven Press, 1990, pp. 25–35.
30. Fries, J. F., P. W. Spitz, R. G. Kraines, and H. R. Holman. Measurement of patient outcome in arthritis. *Arthritis Rheum.* 23:137–145, 1980.
31. Gabler-Halle, D., J. W. Halle, and Y. B. Chung. The effects of aerobic exercise on psychological and behavioral variables of individuals with developmental disabilities: a critical review. *Res. Dev. Disabil.* 14:359–386, 1991.

32. Guyatt, G. H., L. B. Berman, and M. Townsend. Long-term outcome after respiratory rehabilitation. *Can. Med. Assoc. J.* 137:1089–1095, 1987.

33. Hall, C. S., and G. Lindzey. *Theories of Personality,* 2nd Ed. New York: Wiley, 1970.

34. Hawkins, W. E., and T. Duncan. Structural equation analysis of an exercise/sleep health practices model on quality of life in elderly persons. *Percept. Mot. Skills* 72:831–836, 1991.

35. Heidrich, S. M., C. A. Forsthoff, and S. E. Ward. Psychological adjustment in adults with cancer: the self as a mediator. *Health Psychol.* 13:346–353, 1994.

36. Higgins, E. T. Self-discrepancy: a theory relating self and affect. *Psychol. Rev.* 94:319–340, 1987.

37. Holmback, A. M., U. Sawe, and B. Fagher. Training after myocardial infarction: lack of long-term effects on physical capacity and psychological variables. *Arch. Phys. Med. Rehabil.* 75:551–554, 1994.

38. Jasnoski, M. L., D. S. Holmes, S. Solomon, and C. Aguiar. Exercise, changes in aerobic capacity, and changes in self-perceptions: an experimental investigation. *J. Res. Personality* 15:460–466, 1981.

39. Kaplan, R. M., J. P. Anderson, A. W. Wu, W. Mathews, F. Kozin, and D. Orenstein. The quality of well-being scale. *Med. Care* 27:S27–S43, 1989.

40. Kaplan R. M., and J. W. Bush. Health-related quality of life measurement for evaluation research and policy analysis. *Health Psychol.* 1:61, 1982.

41. Keefe, F. J., D. S. Caldwell, D. A. Williams, et al. Pain coping skills training in the management of osteoarthritis knee pain: a comparative study. *Behav. Ther.* 21:49–62, 1990.

42. King, A. C., C. B. Taylor, and W. L. Haskell. Effects of differing intensities and formats of 12 months of exercise training on psychological outcomes of older adults. *Health Psychol.* 12:292–300, 1993.

43. King, A. C., C. B. Taylor, W. L. Haskell, and R. F. DeBusk. Influence of regular aerobic exercise on psychological health: a randomized, controlled trial of healthy middle-aged adults. *Health Psychol.* 8:305–324, 1989.

44. Kirsteins, A. E., F. Dietz, and S. M. Hwang. Evaluating the safety and potential use of a weight bearing exercise: Tai-Chi Chuan for rheumatoid arthritis patients. *Am. J. Phys. Med. Rehabil.* 70:136–141, 1991.

45. Kovar, P. A., J. P. Allegrante, C. R. MacKenzie, M. G. Peterson, B. Gutin, and M. E. Charlson. Supervised fitness walking in patients with osteoarthritis of the knee: a randomized control trial. *Ann. Intern. Med.* 116:529–534, 1992.

46. Lavie, C. J., and R. V. Milani. Effects of cardiac rehabilitation and exercise training on exercise capacity, coronary risk factors, behavioral characteristics, and quality of life in women. *Am. J. Cardiol.* 75:340–343, 1995.

47. Leedham, B., B. E. Meyerowitz, J. Muirhead, and W. H. Frist. Positive expectations predict health after heart transplantation. *Health Psychol.* 14:74–79, 1995.

48. Lorig, K., and H. Holman. Arthritis self-management studies: a twelve-year review. *Health Educ. Q.* 20:17–28, 1993.

49. Lyngberg, K., B. Danneskiold-Samsoe, and O. Halskov. The effect of physical training on patients with rheumatoid arthritis, changes in disease activity, muscle strength and aerobic capacity: a clinically controlled minimized cross-over study. *Clin. Exp. Rheumatol.* 6:253–260.

50. Maddux, J. E., L. R. Brawley, and A. Boykin. Self-efficacy and healthy behavior: Protection, promotion and detection. J. E. Maddux (ed). *Self-Efficacy, Adaptation, and Adjustment: Theory, Research, and Application.* New York: Plenum, pp. 173–196, 1995.

51. Manzetti, J. D., L. A. Hoffman, S. M. Sereika, F. C. Sciurba, and B. P. Griffith. Exercise, education, and quality of life in lung transplant patients. *J. Heart Lung Transplant.* 13:297–305, 1994.

52. Marsh, H. W., G. E. Richards, S. Johnson, L. Roche, and P. Tremayne. Physical self-description questionnaire: psychometric properties and a multitrait-multimethod analysis of relations to existing instruments. *J. Sport. Exerc. Psychol.* 16:270–305, 1994.

53. McAuley, E. Physical activity and psychosocial outcomes. C. Bouchard, R. J. Shephard, and T. Stephens (eds). *Psychical Activity, Fitness, and Health: International Proceedings and Consensus Statement.* Champaign, IL: Human Kinetics, 1994, pp. 851–867.
54. McAuley, E., and D. Rudolph. Physical activity, aging and psychological well-being. *J. Aging Phys. Act* 3:67–96, 1995.
55. McDonald, D. G., and J. A. Hodgdon. *The Psychological Effects of Aerobic Fitness Training: Research and Theory.* New York: Springer-Verlag, 1991.
56. McMurdo, M. E. T., and L. Burnett. Randomized controlled trial of exercise in the elderly. *Gerontology* 38:292–298, 1992.
57. McMurdo, M. E. T., and L. Rennie. A controlled trial of exercise by residents of old people's homes. *Age Ageing* 22:11–15, 1993.
58. Minor, M. A., and J. D. Brown. Exercise maintenance of persons with arthritis after participation in a class experience. *Health Educ. Q.* 20:83–95, 1993.
59. Minor, M. A., Hewett, J. E., R. R. Webel, et al. Efficacy of physical conditioning exercise in patients with rheumatoid arthritis and osteoarthritis. *Arthritis Rheum.* 32:1396–1405, 1989.
60. Morey, M. C., G. M. Crowley, M. S. Robbins, R. A. Cowper, and R. J. Sullivan. The Gerofit Program: A VA innovation. *South. Med. J.* 87:S83–S87, 1994.
61. Morgan, W. P. Physical activity, fitness, and depression. C. Bouchard, R. J. Shephard, and T. Stephens (eds). *Physical Activity, Fitness, and Health: International Proceedings and Consensus Statement.* Champaign, IL: Human Kinetics, 1994, pp. 851–867.
62. Nagi, S. Z. Disability concepts revisited: Implications for prevention. A. M. Pope, and A. R. Tarlov (eds). *Disability in America: toward a National Agenda for Prevention.* Washington, D.C.: National Academy Press, 1991, pp. 309–327.
63. Nordemar, R. Physical training in rheumatoid arthritis: a controlled long-term study. II: Functional capacity and general attitudes. *Scand. J. Rheumatol.* 10:25–30, 1981.
64. Nordemar, R., U. Berg, B. Ekblom, and L. Edstrom. Changes in muscle fiber size and physical performance in patients with rheumatoid arthritis after 7 months' physical training. *Scand. J. Rheumatol.* 5:233–238, 1976.
65. Nordemar, R., B. Ekblom, L. Zachrisson, and K. Lundquist. Physical training in rheumatoid arthritis: a controlled long-term study. I. *Scand. J. Rheumatol.* 10:17–23, 1981.
66. Norris, R., D. Carroll, and R. Cochrane. The effects of aerobic and anaerobic training on fitness, blood pressure, and psychological stress and well-being. *J. Psychosom. Res.* 34:367–375, 1990.
67. North, T. C., P. McCullagh, and Z. Vu Tran. Effects of exercise on depression. *Exerc. Sport Sci. Rev.* 18:379–415, 1990.
68. O'Connor, P. J., and S. D. Youngstedt. Influence of exercise on human sleep. *Exerc. Sport Sci. Rev.* 23:105–134, 1995.
69. O'Hagan, C. M., D. M. Smith, and K. L. Pileggi. Exercise classes in rest homes: effect on physical function. *N. Z. Med. J.* 107:39–40, 1994.
70. Oldridge, N., G. Guyatt, N. Jones, et al. Effects of quality of life with comprehensive rehabilitation after acute myocardial infarction. *Am. J. Cardiol.* 67:1084–1089, 1991.
71. Paffenbarger, R. S., and R. T. Hyde. Exercise adherence, coronary heart disease and longevity. R. K. Dishman (ed). *Exercise Adherence: Its Impact on Public Health.* Champaign, IL: Human Kinetics, 1988, pp. 41–73.
72. Paffenbarger, R. S., A. L. Wing, R. T. Hyde, and D. L. Jung. Physical activity and incidence of hypertension in college alumni. *Am. J. Epidemiol.* 117:245–256, 1983.
73. Patrick, D. L., and P. Erickson. *Health Status and Health Policy: Quality of Life in Health Care Evaluation and Resource Allocation.* New York: Oxford Press, 1993.
74. Pierce, T. W., D. J. Madden, W. C. Siegel, and J. A. Blumenthal. Effects of aerobic exercise on cognitive and psychosocial functioning in patients with mild hypertension. *Health Psychol.* 12:286–291, 1993.
75. Perlman, S. G., K. J. Connell, A. Clark, et al. Dance-based aerobic exercise for rheumatoid arthritis. *Arthritis Care Res.* 3:29–35, 1990.

76. Petruzzello, S. J., D. M. Landers, B. D. Hatfield, K. A. Kubitz, and W. A. Salazar. A meta-analysis on the anxiety-reducing effects of acute and chronic exercise. *Sports Med.* 11:143–182, 1991.
77. Rejeski, W. J., and L. R. Brawley. *Surgeon General's Report: Relationships between Physical Activity and Health-related Quality of Life*, in press, 1995.
77a. Rejeski, W. J., T. Craven, W. H. Ettinger, S. Shumaker, and M. McFarlane. Self-efficacy and pain in disability with knee OA. *J. Gerontol.*, in press, 1995.
78. Rejeski, W. J., W. H. Ettinger, S. Shumaker, P. James, R. Burns, and J. T. Elam. Assessing performance-related disability in patients with knee osteoarthritis. *Osteoarthritis Cartilage*, in press, 1995.
79. Rejeski, W. J., L. Gauvin, M. L. Hobson, and J. L. Norris. Effects of baseline responses, in-task feelings, and duration of activity on exercise-induced feeling states in women. *Health Psychol.* 14:1–10, 1995.
80. Rejeski, W. J., and Shumaker, S. Knee-osteoarthritis and health-related quality of life. *Med. Sci. Sports Exerc.* 26:1441–1445, 1994.
81. Rosenberg, M. *Conceiving the Self.* Malabar, FL: Kreiger, 1986.
82. Rosenthal, M., W. L. Haskell, R. Solomon, A. Widstrom, and G. M. Raven. Demonstration of a relationship between level of physical training and insulin stimulated utilization in normal humans. *Diabetes* 32:408–411, 1983.
83. Roviaro, S., D. S. Holmes, and R. D. Holmsten. Influence of a cardiac rehabilitation program on the cardiovascular, psychological, and social functioning of cardiac patients. *J. Behav. Med.* 7:61–81, 1984.
84. Shumaker, S. A., R. T. Anderson, and S. M. Czajkowski. Psychological tests and scales. B. Spilker (ed). *Quality of Life Assessments in Clinical Trials.* New York: Raven Press, 1990, pp. 95–113.
85. Schipper, H., J. Clinch, and V. Powell. Definitions and conceptual issues. B. Spilker (ed). *Quality of Life Assessments in Clinical Trials.* New York: Raven Press, 1990, pp. 11–24.
86. Seals, D. R., J. M. Hagberg, Z. B. F. Hurley, A. A. Ehsani, and J. O. Holloszy. Effects of endurance training on glucose tolerance and plasma lipid levels in older men and women. *J.A.M.A.* 252:645–649, 1984.
87. Stearn, M. J., and P. Cleary. National exercise and heart disease project: psychosocial changes observed during a low-level exercise program. *Arch. Intern. Med.* 141:1463–1467, 1981.
88. Stearn, M. J., and P. Cleary. National exercise and heart disease project: long-term psychosocial outcomes. *Arch. Intern. Med.* 142:1093–1097, 1982.
89. Stephens, T. Physical activity and mental health in the United States and Canada: evidence from four population studies. *Prev. Med.* 17:35–47, 1988.
90. Stewart, A. L., R. D. Hays, K. B. Wells, W. H. Rogers, K. L. Spritzer, and S. Greenfield. Long-term functioning and well-being outcomes associated with physical activity and exercise in patients with chronic conditions in the medical outcomes study. *J. Clin. Epidemiol.* in press, 1995.
91. Stewart, A. L., and A. C. King. Evaluating the efficacy of physical activity for influencing quality of life outcomes in older adults. *Ann. Behav. Med.* 13:108–116, 1991.
92. Stewart, A. L., and A. C. King. Conceptualizing and measuring quality of life in older populations. R. P. Abeles, H. C. Gift, and M. G. Ory (eds). *Aging and Quality of Life.* New York: Springer, in press, 1995.
93. Stewart, A. L., A. C. King, and W. L. Haskell. Endurance exercise and health-related quality of life in 50–65 year-old adults. *Gerontologist* 33:782–789, 1993.
94. Taylor, S. E. Adjustment to threatening events: a theory of cognitive adaptation. *Am. Psychol.* 38:1161–1173, 1983.
95. Thayer, R. E. *The Biopsychology of Mood and Arousal.* New York: Oxford University Press, 1989.
96. Thomas, J. R., D. M. Landers, W. Salazar, and J. Etnier. Exercise and cognitive function.

C. Bouchard, R. J. Shephard, and T. Stephens (eds). *Physical Activity, Fitness, and Health: International Proceedings and Consensus Statement.* Champaign, IL: Human Kinetics, 1994, pp. 521–529.

97. Vale, F., J. Z. Reardon, and R. L. ZuWallack. The long-term benefits of outpatient pulmonary rehabilitation on exercise endurance and quality of life. *Chest* 103:42–45, 1993.

98. Weinstein, N. D. Testing for competing theories of health-protective behavior. *Health Psychol.* 12:324–333, 1993.

99. Wenger, N. K., and C. D. Furberg. Cardiovascular disorders. B. Spilker (ed). *Quality of Life Assessments in Clinical Trials.* New York: Raven Press, 1990, pp. 335–345.

100. Wiklund, I., M. B. Comerford, and E. Dimenas. The relationship between exercise tolerance and quality of life in angina pectoris. *Clin. Cardiol.* 14:204–208, 1991.

101. Wilson, I. B., and P. D. Cleary. Linking clinical variables with health-related quality of life: a conceptual model of patient outcomes. *J.A.M.A.* 273:59–65, 1995.

102. Worchester, M. C., D. L. Hare, R. G. Oliver, M. A. Reid, and A. J. Goble. Early programmes of high and low intensity exercise and quality of life after acute myocardial infarction. *Br. Med. J.* 307:1244–1247, 1993.

4
From Motor Unit to Whole Muscle Properties During Locomotor Movements

C. J. HECKMAN, Ph.D.
THOMAS G. SANDERCOCK, Ph.D.

Muscle has been studied with several different goals, including understanding of molecular mechanisms of force generation, comparative analysis of basic muscle properties across different animal species, detailed investigations of nonlinear behaviors, and assessment of the role of muscle properties in the neural control of movement by the central nervous system (CNS). This review primarily considers the last of these goals. It is unlikely that the CNS is in any way directly informed of molecular interactions within a given sarcomere. Rather, it is the functional result, the macroscopic muscle mechanical behaviors, that are important. Even at this level, muscle appears to be highly complex. Which of these properties is most important for control of movement? This same question applies for the construction of models of muscle that are needed to understand control of movement: Which muscle properties are most important for a model of a given movement?

The appropriate context for addressing this question is defined by the neural and mechanical conditions that actually exist in normal motor behaviors. These conditions can be strikingly different from the controlled conditions that are typical in the laboratory. Consider first the normal neural activation pattern. The fundamental element of motor control is the motor unit. Increasing neural activation produces a complex overlapping pattern of recruitment and rate modulation of a large population of motor units with highly heterogeneous properties. This natural activation pattern stands in marked contrast to the usual techniques applied in the lab, such as activation of a single skinned muscle fiber via Ca^{2+} or stimulation of an entire muscle by electrical pulses applied to its nerve. At the same time, the muscle is often experiencing mechanical conditions that are highly dynamic. The primary measurement of muscle dynamic behavior in the lab, the force-velocity relationship, is made during constant-activation and constant-velocity conditions. In contrast, in a natural movement such as locomotion, both activation and velocity undergo dramatic and continuous variations.

The goal of this review is to consider the recent advances in our understanding of how the force generated by muscle in natural activation and mechanical conditions arises from its fundamental neuromechanical properties. The design of these studies to be considered is generally one in which the data from the controlled conditions of the laboratory experiment are directly related to data obtained during normal movement patterns. Specifically, this chapter will: 1) review the basic functional properties of muscle; 2) examine studies showing how a whole muscle's properties can arise from natural recruitment and rate modulation patterns of a population of motor units with highly heterogeneous properties; and 3) examine studies that have made direct measurements from muscle during normal locomotion and then contrasted those measurements with known basic properties of muscle to determine the muscle's normal operating range and possible design principles for muscle use. Goals 2 and 3 sharply limit the scope and length of this review, for there are, as yet, few studies of these fundamental issues, and those have primarily been done in animal preparations.

SUMMARY OF BASIC MUSCLE NEUROMECHANICAL PROPERTIES

In this section a brief overview of basic neuromechanical properties of muscle are presented. This is not meant to be an in-depth review of this enormous body of literature but rather to provide a basis for consideration of how muscle force is generated in natural movement conditions. For a discussion of basic muscle properties, the review by McMahon [48] is suggested. For a catalog of the functional complexities of muscle, the strong-hearted reader should consult the review by Partridge and Benton [52].

Basic Muscle Properties and the Hill Model

Muscle has three basic properties. Muscle receives neural input in the form of discrete action potentials. The rate at which the action potentials arrive at the muscle determines the degree of muscle activation. The steady-state relation between stimulus rate and force is defined as an approximately sigmoidal rate-force (R-F) function. Muscle force is also strongly affected by length because of changing filament overlap within the sarcomere. The force-length (F-L) relationship has an ascending limb, a plateau region of optimal force generation (defining an optimal length, L_O), and a descending limb (see Fig. 4.1C below). When a muscle is activated during movement, the resulting force is greatly affected by velocity. Hill [32] characterized the force-velocity (F-V) relationship during shortening movements with a hyperbolic function that intersects both force and velocity axes (see Fig. 4.3 below), giving a maximal velocity (V_{max}) at which force falls to zero. During lengthening, the dependency of muscle force on velocity is more complex: initially it increases quite steeply with velocity, but then this slope of the function declines, and a plateau is reached at moderate lengthening velocities (37, 47, 58).

These three relationships (R-F, F-L, and F-V) plus muscle stiffness are often used to form the basis of mathematical models described as Hill-type models. Originally, the Hill-model contractile element consisted solely of the F-V function during shortening, which was placed in series with a spring representing tendon and in parallel with a spring representing passive tissue [32]. Recent models sometimes add the lengthening F-V function and use the F-L and R-F relationships to scale the F-V curve in order to achieve more realistic behavior. The stiffness of the tendon is usually constant, but an exponential increase is used sometimes also. See Zajac [67] or Winter [65] for a thorough treatment of Hill-type models.

Complex Muscle Mechanical Behaviors

Muscle is a complex nonlinear system that so far has resisted a concise mathematical description. Muscle exhibits a number of behaviors that are not captured by the R-F, F-L, and F-V functions in-series with a tendon stiffness and thus are not captured in Hill-type muscle models. The following is a brief review intended to provide a flavoring of the complexity that muscle can exhibit under certain conditions.

In the Hill model, the in-series stiffness of muscle is primarily determined by tendon characteristics, but it is now clear that in-series stiffness varies with muscle excitation (e.g., see Ref. 49). When little of the muscle is active, whole muscle stiffness is low and depends primarily on how many cross-bridges are attached. When muscle is fully active, the stiffness of a tendon may become the primary determinant of whole muscle stiffness. The stiffness of the tendon is also believed to play a key role in energy storage and release in some modes of locomotion [3]. Rapid stretch of an active muscle often elicits the phenomenon of yielding, in which muscle initially responds with a nearly linear force increase to the imposed stretch (the so-called short-range stiffness) but then undergoes a sudden transition to a lower slope or, in slow-twitch muscles, a precipitous drop in force [37].

Muscle also exhibits a number of behaviors that can be thought of as being history dependent, in that their occurrence depends on a particular sequence of events. Perhaps the R-F function is most influenced by muscle history, because its shape is highly sensitive to the measurement protocol [6]. As simple a change as reversing the order of the test frequencies has a profound effect. In addition, in isometric conditions, muscle force can be strongly potentiated by a brief high-frequency activation (posttetanic potentiation) or even by a single pair of closely spaced stimuli (doublet potentiation) [11]. Of course, if stimulation is prolonged, fatigue ensues. The effect of history is so severe, the R-F function should be viewed as a qualitative, rather than a quantitative, measure of muscle function.

The phenomenon of excess tension is another example of history dependence. Muscle generates a greater isometric force when it has been stretched during activation, compared to when it has been stretched passively and then activated [1]. The converse phenomenon is also often seen: less isometric force after shortening of an active muscle. The stretch to elicit excess tension is usually quite slow.

An additional complexity exists in that there are interactions between the

R-F, F-L, and F-V functions. Perhaps the most important interaction is that between the R-F and F-L functions. Rack and Westbury [56] showed that as stimulation rate is reduced below that needed to achieve maximal force, the L_O point of the F-L function progressively shifts to longer lengths. Thus, the F-L function at low stimulation rates is not simply a scaled-down version of that at high rates. The possible interactions between the F-V and R-F functions have not yet been studied, but it appears that, at least for lengthening, there is an FL-FV interaction. At longer lengths, lengthening at a given velocity produces more force [58].

Muscle Architecture

The sarcomere is the basic contractile unit of muscle. Sarcomeres within a fiber are linked in series and contract together, so any property dependent on length, such as the F-L and F-V curves, is proportional to the number of sarcomeres [59, 64]. Laterally, the muscle is composed of myofilaments that are grouped together to form muscle fibers. In general, muscle is composed of many long, thin muscle cells or fibers that run parallel to each other. The parallel arrangement suggests that the total force a muscle can produce is proportional to the number of fibers multiplied by the cross-sectional area of each fiber. Therefore, provided that the sarcomeres in a muscle are identical, and provided that the fibers in a muscle are the same length and are parallel to each other, the whole muscle can be viewed as a scaled version of the sarcomere (see ref. 67 for more details on a dimensionless muscle model).

Few, if any, mammalian muscles fit the idealized profile above. Muscles come in a vast array of sizes and shapes, and complex architecture is more the rule than the exception (for reviews, see Refs. 3, 18, 51, 62). Muscle fibers often lie at an angle to the direction in which the entire muscle shortens. This angle, called the angle of pennation, allows more muscle tissue to be packed into a volume and thus increase the power to weight ratio [3]. Assuming that the pennate fibers are attached to two bony surfaces that slide by but do not approach each other, muscle force and length can be calculated by scaling fiber force and length by the cosine of the angle of pennation. This is the correction most models use to compensate for pennation. The true effects of pennation are more complex when the fibers are attached to connective tissue sheets (called aponeurosis) that show local deformation [18].

Muscles are often composed of fibers of different lengths to accommodate skeletal dimensions (e.g., the jaw muscles, where fiber length increases with distance from the axis of rotation) [18]. Recent studies have also shown that many seemingly long-fibered muscles do not have fibers that run the length of the muscle (from tendon insertion to the tendon of origin) but rather are composed of fibers connected serially [13, 61]. The functional implications of serial fibers are uncertain. They are likely to add compliance to the muscle beyond that attributed to the muscle fiber and tendon.

The function of the connective tissue within a muscle is incompletely understood. At the muscle-tendon junction, the fibers terminate in collagen fibrils which, a short distance from the muscle-tendon junction, blend to form the aponeurosis or tendon. Muscle fibers are also enveloped in a connective tissue layer composed of fine collagen fibers, the endomysium [61]. In series-fibered muscles, the fiber end is tapered, and tension is transmitted from the contractile proteins to the endomysium. It is not clear to what extent the fibers within a muscle are mechanically linked—that is, to what extent does the shortening of one fiber pull on its neighboring fiber? Clearly, the serial fibers must transmit force to either the endomysium or other fibers. The mechanical linkage of fibers is likely to impact force production in a partially activated muscle. It may also influence linear summation of force between fibers (see later sections).

MUSCLE HETEROGENEITY: DIFFERENCES IN MOTOR UNIT PROPERTIES

Muscle heterogeneity creates problems in understanding muscle function during volitional movements. A single muscle has multiple inputs that are the action potential trains to each of its constituent motor units. In the context of locomotion, a muscle is usually assumed to operate as a single functional unit, which creates a profound problem. What is the input to a single muscle? Can a lumped-parameter model be used to express whole muscle output, even though the motor units and fibers within a muscle have markedly different contractile properties? Perhaps such a model will be shown to be too simplistic, and muscle will need to be modeled at the motor unit level.

Isometric Properties of Motor Units and Their Neural Control

The mechanical properties of motor units have been most thoroughly studied in the isometric state, allowing relatively clear resolution of their tiny forces, which are 2–4 orders of magnitude smaller than the whole muscle force. Even in these restricted conditions, the differences in the motor units within a single muscle are extraordinary, with the range of unit tetanic forces varying as much as 100-fold, contraction times varying as much as 5-fold, and fatigue resistances varying greater than 10-fold (reviewed in ref. 9). Furthermore, it is important to realize that all of these differences exhibit systematic covariances: force is directly proportional to contraction speed and inversely proportional to fatigue resistance. These patterns have been used to classify units into categories that closely correspond to those based on histochemical analyses. In this review, we will rely on the classification scheme of Burke and colleagues (see ref. 9 for a review). Based on mechanical unit properties: Type S units—slow twitch, low force, and highly fatigue resistant; FR units—fast twitch, medium force, and moderately fatigue resistant, and FF units—fast twitch, high force, and easily fatigued. Type S units are composed of fibers exhibiting an histochemical profile with low myosin ATPase and high oxidative enzymes (Type I), whereas FR has a high myosin ATPase and oxidative enzyme profile (Type IIA) and FF has a high myosin ATPase and glycolytic enzyme profile (Type IIB) [9].

The degree to which these classifications reflect true categories vs. an arbitrary grouping among a continuous range of variation is still not entirely clear. In this review, the S, FR, and FF terminology is largely used to provide a convenient way of summarizing the wide differences in mechanical properties, and it should be kept in mind that the key variables, such as force and contraction speed, vary continuously in the motor unit population without clear grouping.

In natural conditions, motor units are activated by the synaptic input applied to their motoneurons. Because motoneurons that innervate a single muscle (i.e., a motoneuron pool) have a wide range of thresholds for generation of action potentials, they are not all activated simultaneously but instead tend to be recruited in a sequential fashion (reviewed in ref. 5). The rate of discharge of a motor unit at its recruitment threshold is low, about 5–15 Hz. Its rate then rapidly increases as the synaptic drive to the motoneuron is increased above its threshold. At the same time, higher threshold units are being recruited and then also undergoing rate modulation. The result is a complex overlapping pattern, whereby increases in force are mediated simultaneously by recruitment and rate modulation across the motor unit population.

The fundamental organizing principle for control of muscle force and, indeed, one of the most striking organizing features in the CNS in general, is that the recruitment thresholds for motor units are systematically correlated with their mechanical properties. Thus, the motoneurons of Type S motor units tend to have low thresholds, whereas Type FR and FF motoneurons have progressively higher thresholds [16]. Henneman and colleagues (reviewed in ref. 28) were the first to realize the full significance of these correlations and suggested that the differences in threshold resulted from differences in motoneuron size. Thus, the normal pattern of orderly recruitment (i.e., S>FR>FF) is often referred to as Henneman's "size principle" [5]. Recent work has shown that only a portion of the differences in motoneuron thresholds is because of size per se [10, 23, 40], but because motor units with large forces do generally have the highest thresholds, the term "size principle" conveys the essential features of the normal recruitment process. It should be kept in mind that recruitment order is not perfectly rigid and that, in fact, there is a considerable degree of randomness in the overall orderly pattern.

Henneman and colleagues were also the first to fully understand the functional implications of the size principle (e.g., ref. 29). They pointed out that, because the normal S>FR>FF recruitment scheme is ordered according to increasing force and decreasing fatigue resistance, use of this sequence for force generation maximizes precision and fatigue resistance. Furthermore, they emphasized that having a single recruitment sequence meant that the CNS could view the entire motoneuron pool as a single functional entity. Thus, instead of having to individually calculate the activation pattern and force output of each of the hundreds of motor units within each muscle, the CNS can just "apply" an overall synaptic drive to the pool to generate a proportional amount of force output.

Rate-Force and Force-Length Properties of Motor Units

The initial studies of motor unit properties focused on the most basic mechanical parameters: maximal force, contraction time, and fatigue resistance (see ref. 9 for a review). Studies of the R-F and F-L properties of motor units are fewer in number but provide essential information for assessing whether normal recruitment of motor units in the isometric state can be adequately captured by a lumped, Hill-type model.

The systematic differences in twitch contraction time in S vs. F motor units are matched by corresponding differences in their R-F relations studies, with S units achieving maximal force at much lower rates than S units [8, 39]. For example, FR and FF units require rates about 30 spikes/s higher than S units to achieve 50% of maximal force [8, 39].

The first studies of F-L relations in single motor units found that unit L_Os exhibited a surprisingly large range [4, 60], perhaps because of differences in the anatomical territory of the motor units. In addition, studies of the interaction between motor unit R-F and F-L functions [27] have shown that single units exhibit the same effect that was originally seen by Rack and Westbury [56] in the whole cat soleus. That is, as stimulus rate decreases, L_O shifts to a longer length. The exact effect of this shift in L_O during natural activation is difficult to predict, because of the overlapping nature of the recruitment and rate pattern. Computer simulations that address this issue are presented below.

Dynamic Mechanical Properties of Motor Units

Single motor unit forces were first systematically measured by Henneman and colleagues in the middle 1960s (reviewed in ref. 28). For more than 20 years, these measurements were confined to isometric conditions to ease the technical difficulties of single-unit force resolution. A major difficulty is that dynamic response of the muscle's passive tissue can generate forces that are much greater than the forces generated by an active single motor unit. The initial studies of motor units in dynamic conditions focused on small stretches at relatively short lengths to minimize this problem. Petit et al. showed that Type S units actually appear to be stiffer to quick stretch than F units [54], which they suggested might be another advantage of recruitment of S units during postural tasks. Powers and Binder [55] found that small shortening or stretching movements alter the amplitude of subsequent isometric forces by as much as 40%, which, potentially, is a serious history-dependent effect. However, it is not yet clear as to what degree these changes reflect interactions between active and passive muscle fibers (see Linearity of Summation of Force from Muscle Fibers and Motor Units.)

Studies of the F-V function require large changes in length, in which large passive forces are unavoidable. Three recent studies have successfully resolved unit forces on this passive background [14, 27, 53]. In part, this was accomplished by studying small muscles [14, 53], but computer-controlled muscle pullers were also highly advantageous, mainly because they can provide precisely repeatable intertrial intervals, which make passive force sufficiently consistent to allow it to be measured on alternate trials and, subsequently, to be subtracted, to reveal the unit force.

Overall, the results correspond to what would be expected on the basis of studies of whole muscles with unit populations that are either dominantly slow twitch or fast twitch (e.g., Ref. 59). This is, Type S units have much lower V_{max} than FF units [53], yielding at least a 5-fold range. Distinct groupings of F-V behavior for the different motor unit types were not apparent. Rather, both V_{max} and F-V slope at moderate velocities strongly correlate with maximal isometric force and isometric contraction time [27, 53]. However, Devasahayam and Sandercock [14] found much weaker correlation between the F-V function characteristics and isometric properties, perhaps because they studied the rat soleus muscle, which is predominantly slow twitch and, thus, has a restricted range of properties.

Linearity of Summation of Force from Muscle Fibers and Motor Units

When force is normally generated by the recruitment and rate modulation of motor units, then the linearity of the summation of these forces is an important determinant of the control of force. At least three factors affect the linearity of motor unit force summation: the muscle anatomy, the in-series compliance in aponeurosis and tendon; and the mechanical interactions between individual muscle fibers. As mentioned above, some muscles are composed of fibers that do not run the length of the muscle [61], which would tend to generate nonlinear force summation. In some architecture, the angle of pennation will change as more of the fibers are recruited, altering the way forces are summated. In static conditions, the increased tendon stretch as force increases should produce a shift in the F-L relationship of individual motor units. Thus, the force of a unit activated by itself in an otherwise passive muscle may be at L_O but, when the unit is recruited at 50% of maximal force in normal conditions, the muscle fibers of this unit will be operating at a length that is shorter than L_O. The quantitative effect of these various factors on linear summation is not known, but the effect of the shift in the F-L function can be estimated for muscles whose F-L functions and tendon compliances are known. For example, the cat medial gastrocnemius muscle has a tendon compliance of about 0.06 mm/newton (N) [64]. Thus, at 50% of maximum medial gastrocnemius force (~50 N), internal shortening of about 3 mm can be expected to occur. The corresponding shift in the medial gastrocnemius F-L function could alter motor unit force by as much as 30–40%.

Linearity of summation at very low levels of force has been investigated by studying summation of combinations of 2–5 single motor units. In every case, there is nonlinear summation, but it is a positive nonlinearity in that the actual sum of the motor unit forces is greater than the calculated sum based on each unit's force measured in isolation [15, 55]. This positive nonlinearity appears to be the result of nonlinear viscous interactions between the active fibers of the motor unit and the passive fibers of the rest of the muscle [27, 55]. That is, the isolated isometric forces of the units are actually reduced by these fiber-fiber interactions, whereas the combination of motor unit forces is sufficient to overcome those interactions and generate slightly more force at the tendon. This interpretation is based on two findings: first, slow movements, which should break the filament interactions, sharply reduce nonlinear summation [55] and, second, slow movement also actually potentiates the forces of small motor units above their isometric values [26]. Heckman et al. [26] showed that in the cat medial gastrocnemius, this movement potentiation only occurred in units with force less than 200 mN. As this is far less than 1% of the tetanic force of this muscle (~100N), this suggests that filament-filament interaction forces are, at best, of minor importance in normal movements.

In summary, at present it appears that nonlinearities resulting from filament interactions are probably unimportant. However, it should be kept in mind that these interactions may be more important in large muscles with complex architecture. The effects of architecture and tendon compliance have not been systematically studied and may induce substantial nonlinearities.

Mechanical Consequences of Natural Recruitment and Rate Patterns

How important are the systematic differences in motor unit properties that exist within each muscle? Most muscle models assume a single lumped function, which is essentially the same as assuming a single, uniform muscle fiber. Yet, as the brief review above showed, a long history of studies in the isometric state have established the existence of a high degree of mechanical heterogeneity among the units within a single muscle, while neurophysiological studies have established the existence of orderly recruitment of these units. The result is that, as the synaptic drive to a muscle increases, units with different mechanical properties are progressively recruited. Are these changes significant for the CNS or for muscle models? The following paragraphs consider how the mechanical properties of the muscle vary during the recruitment and rate modulation of its constituent population of motor units. Essentially, this constitutes a consideration of the fundamental input-output properties of the motoneuron pool and the muscle it innervates.

Experimental measurements of this whole system input-output function have proved to be extremely difficult to achieve. In humans, force control is excellent, but synaptic input cannot be measured. Moreover, the response of the muscle to shortening or lengthening will be strongly affected by the reflex input from muscle spindles and Golgi tendon organs. In animal preparations, synaptic input can be measured in individual motoneurons, and reflexes can be eliminated, but gradation of input across the full range needed to reach maximal force is not yet possible.

Recent studies have instead adopted a computer simulation approach [17, 25]. The feasibility of this approach primarily results from the availability of extensive experimental studies of the electrical properties of single motoneurons and the mechanical properties of single motor units. In steady-state conditions, the input-output function of a single motoneuron can be described by means of a relatively simple relationship between current injected via a microelectrode and rate of spike discharge (reviewed in ref. 5). This relationship primarily consists of a threshold and then a remarkably linear suprathreshold relationship between current and rate (I-R function). The slope of this relation changes at higher rates, but most of the force generation of the muscle fibers innervated by the motoneuron occurs within this initial linear segment, which is called the primary range [38]. Normally, of course, motoneurons are activated by synaptic input, not by injected currents. Although the electrical structure of the motoneuron is highly complex, it appears that synaptic and injected currents are essentially equivalent in their effect on the primary range of steady-spike discharge rate (reviewed in ref. 5). The full input-output function in steady-state conditions for a single motor unit is obtained by coupling the motoneuron I-R function to the R-F function of the muscle fibers it innervates, giving the overall transformation of synaptic current to isometric force, i.e., the motor unit I-F function (see Fig. 4-1A).

A realistic simulation of the input-output function of the whole motor neuron pool and its muscle can be obtained by constructing a set of realistic motor unit I-F functions, using the available experimental data to specify an appropriate range of differences among S, FR and FF functions (Fig. 4.1A shows examples for the cat medial gastrocnemius). Various levels of synaptic currents are applied to each single unit in the simulated pool, and the resultant force outputs are summated together to yield whole muscle force. When all motor units receive the same proportion of the synaptic input and linear force summation is assumed, the result is a whole pool function that is roughly sigmoidal, as shown in Figure 4.1-B for the cat medial gastrocnemius [25]. This is the most basic input-output function of the motoneuron pool and its muscle. Analysis of the simulations showed that the initial up-

FIGURE 4.1.

Computer simulations of the input-output function of the mammalian motoneuron pool. A, Representative single-unit I-F functions, which result from the combination of the motoneuron I-R function and the R-F of the muscle fibers it innervates. B, The whole pool input-output function that results when a uniform input is applied to the single-unit I-F functions, and their forces are linearly summated. C, The whole pool F-L relations at various levels of synaptic input, with realistic recruitment and rate patterns. The dashed lines indicate the function that would result from simply scaling the F-L curve that occurs at maximal activation. D, The whole pool F-V functions at various levels of input, with realistic recruitment and rate patterns. Data in A and B from ref. 25; in C and D from ref. 27 and 53). Modified from ref. 5.

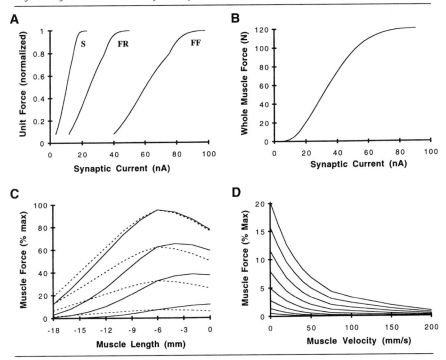

wards curvature is largely a result of the orderly recruitment of units with increasing forces, while the final smooth approach to maximum comes from the R-F functions of the largest motor units. The substantial linear range in between results from a mixture of recruitment and rate modulation.

Because experimental data using intracellular recording techniques are available on the effects of various synaptic inputs on S and F motoneurons (reviewed in ref. 5), it has been possible to reconstruct the effects of different synaptic organizations on the input-output function. This is not a major topic of this review, but it should be noted that the overall sigmoid shape of the function is preserved remarkably well during large variations in the organization of the synaptic input [24]. It should also be noted, however, that some synaptic inputs, especially the neuromodulatory ones that can alter the electrical properties of motoneurons, can increase the slope of the function. In particular, inputs that use the monoamines serotonin and noradrenaline as neurotransmitters can substantially increase input-output gain. In addition, feedback from muscle sensory receptors would be expected to profoundly influence this function, but the exact nature of that influence for a wide range of input-output levels is as yet unknown.

This simulation approach can also be used to understand the F-L and F-V functions of the pool change as motor units undergo recruitment and rate modulation [27]. As noted above, the L_O point for the F-L function of single motor units shifts to shorter lengths as stimulation rate increases. Figure 4.1C shows that this shift persists in the entire population undergoing normal recruitment and rate modulation (solid lines). This may be functionally important, because it tends to increase the steepness (i.e., stiffness) of the F-L function, in comparison to what would be expected when the submaximal F-L functions were simply scaled versions of the maximal function (compare dashed to solid lines). The key issue for the F-V function is the shift in V_{max} as recruitment proceeds from S to F units. Figure 4.1D illustrates that, because S units generate very small forces, in comparison to F units, most of the shift in V_{max} occurs at very low forces—in this case, less than 5% of maximum. It should be noted that Figure 4.1D is based on the motor units in the cat medial gastrocnemius muscle, which contains only 25% Type S units. The shift would be expected to occur over a larger fraction of total force in muscles with higher percentages of slow-twitch units.

MUSCLE PROPERTIES AND LOCOMOTOR MOVEMENTS

There are many demands placed on the muscles involved in locomotion. We use this term in its broadest sense, including posture, walking, running, swimming, and jumping. During standing, the efficient maintenance of muscle length is of primary importance. A muscle with slow F-V and R-F relationships is energetically the most efficient. On the other hand, sprinting places a premium of muscle speed and power, requiring muscle with fast characteristics. As mentioned previously, there are many different types of muscle architecture and, therefore, different ways, with different trade-offs, to meet basic functional criteria. The goal of this section is to consider how muscle force in locomotion arises from muscle mechanical properties. Therefore, we will focus on the relatively few studies that have made direct measurements from muscle during normal locomotion and the contrasted those direct measurements with known basic properties of muscle to determine the muscles' normal operating range and possible design principles for muscle use. Some of the best direct measurements come from studies in which devices to measure force and length of individual muscles have been chronically implanted (for a review, see refs. 7 and 44). However, it should be emphasized that because the number of studies in this area is as yet limited because of technical difficulties, our understanding is still quite incomplete.

Operating Range on the Rate-Force Relationship

The electromyogram (EMG) is a relatively easy signal to measure, and it is used frequently to estimate activation to a muscle. The EMG is used in two fundamentally different ways. First, when the EMG is recorded intramuscularly, using an electrode with a small recording surface, it can be used to distinguish the action potential train from a single motor unit. However, the movements in locomotion usually seriously degrade the selectivity needed for reliable single-unit measurements. The second way an EMG is used is in providing a rough index of the general excitation to a muscle. Large intramuscular or surface electrodes measure the complex sum of the action potentials from multiple motor units. This signal is usually rectified and filtered. Unfortunately, the relationship between the rectified EMG and force varies in different muscles, for different recording electrodes, or even with placement of the electrodes (see refs. 12 and 44). This signal is usually rectified and filtered. However, the relationship between rectified, filtered EMG and the recruitment and rate modulation of active motor units remains unclear. Therefore, EMG measurements must be carefully obtained and interpreted with caution [12, 44].

Nonetheless, it is quite clear that the neural activation of muscle undergoes large and dynamic changes in locomotion, implying that rates of single units undergo substantial modulations. The only direct confirmation of this inference is the study of Hoffer et al. [33, 34], who recorded single motor unit discharge patterns in locomotion in the freely moving cat, using electrodes chronically implanted in spinal ventral roots. The normal pattern of recruitment was seen, with all units displaying a wide range of rate modulation, whose overall pattern closely correlated with the envelope of the rectified, smoothed EMG. However, it should be emphasized that these changes in rate were highly dynamic. Thus, the resulting forces cannot be predicted from studies of motor unit R-F relationships, which so far have only been measured in steady-state conditions. Furthermore, R-F relations are highly sensitive to potentiation and fatigue (see above), and the degree to which these factors contribute to locomotor force is unknown.

Operating Range on the Force-Length Relationship

One fundamental issue is to establish how changes in muscle length in normal movements are positioned on a muscle's F-L function. One hypothesis is that the range of lengths associated with locomotor movements should fall within a region of the F-L function centered around L_O, because this is where efficiency and power are maximized. Studies of swimming in fish and jumping in frogs performed by Rome and colleagues [45, 57] indicate that muscle lengths do stay near L_O. In locomotion in the cat, this issue has been investigated in the ankle extensors [31, 60] and, generally speaking, the highest forces in locomotion also occurred near L_O.

However, a number of findings indicate that substantial force generation often occurs on either side of L_O—that is to say, on either the ascending or descending limbs of the F-L function. For example, the positions of the cat ankle extensor F-L functions in relation to the physiological range of motion is skewed, such that L_O occurs is at a relatively long length [31, 60, 64]. While the peak force occurs during the stretch at the onset of the stance phase and is thus at a relatively long length near L_O, after this point, the ankle extensor exert substantial forces while rapidly shortening, and most of this occurs on the ascending limb of the F-L function [31, 60]. In addition, studies of F-L functions in the hindlimbs of frogs suggest that much of the normal range of motion for thigh muscles can occur on the descending limb [41]. A recent study in humans used laser diffraction to measure actual sarcomere lengths during surgery for carpal tunnel syndrome in the extensor digitorum communis muscle and also found that a substantial portion of the normal range was on the descending limb [42].

In repetitive motions like swimming and locomotion considered above, efficient force generation is of fundamental importance, and lengths near L_O would seem to be highly desirable. Morgan and Lynn have also suggested another important reason for avoiding the descending limb of the F-L function during locomotion [46, 50]: There is likely to be a considerable degree of variability present in the sarcomere lengths along muscle fibers. Any sarcomeres that reach the descending limb are inherently unstable when other sarcomeres are still at L_O or on the ascending limb. That is, the longer sarcomeres will get pulled apart, or "popped," by the shorter sarcomeres. This tendency should be greatly increased when muscle is lengthening, as occurs in antigravity muscles in locomotion. Furthermore, the longer the range of muscle lengths at which an activity takes place, the more likely a larger proportion of sarcomeres will become popped. Morgan and colleagues [46, 50] have hypothesized that this is a major source of muscle damage during eccentric contractions and, thus, avoidance of conditions that tend to cause popping may be one reason why a muscle like the medial gastrocnemius operates at L_O or shorter. In contrast, in single or infrequent movement, efficiency is less important and, thus, a full range of motion may require use of all portions of the F-L function. For the present, however, these conclusions are highly speculative, and considerable further work in this area is needed.

Operating Range on the Force-Velocity Relationship

The F-V relationship of a muscle, and where on this relationship a muscle normally operates, is a key design element. It is intimately linked with locomotor speed, energy use, and fatigue. Muscle velocities during locomotion have been estimated by inverse calculation from video records in numerous species (reviewed in ref. 7) and from direct measurement in cats (see below). Clearly, even at the modest locomotor speeds associated with walking or slow running, the muscle velocities reach peak values that result in substantial modulation of force because of the F-V relationship.

The role of the F-V relationship has been carefully quantified during jumping. Lutz and Rome [45] studied the semimembranosus muscle in frogs during maximal jumps. By studying maximal jumps, they assumed that activation was also maximal and, thus, avoided the problem of measuring motor firing rates. Length of the muscle was estimated from video records and anatomical analysis, and the EMG was used to determine when the muscle was active. An isolated muscle bundle was then driven through the same movement during maximal stimulation over the same interval. They concluded that the muscle operated at the optimal velocity to produce peak power. In addition, they found the timing of EMG allowed for full activation of the muscle before shortening and the muscle operated at L_O. This straightforward result in contrast to the more complex results obtained by Zajac [66, 68] during maximal jumps in cats and humans. These jumps result from a more complex system involving the exact timing of multiple limb segments. Their model indicated that the strength of the muscle was more important than shortening velocity. Zajac believed substantial energy is stored in a stretched tendon just prior to the jump. The tendon can recoil at high speeds independently of muscle shortening velocity. Walmsley et al. [63] measured the force of cat soleus and medial gastrocnemius during jumps, but their results were not directly compared to F-V properties of the muscles. Their results also appear complex, because soleus force is diminished only somewhat during the jump compared to that of slow walking (see Architecture Specializations and Locomotion).

Muscle velocities could be obtained from the chronic data available on muscle length (e.g., see refs. 2, 35, and 63), potentially providing an indication of the role of the F-V function in force generation in normal movements when activation is less than maximal. However, as yet, systematic analyses of these velocities, in comparison to those of specific muscle F-V functions are not available, with one important exception. Gregor et al. [19, 20] measured actual forces and velocities of cat medial gastrocnemius and soleus muscles, using standard chronic techniques in freely moving animals. Their results clearly showed that these muscles underwent a wide range of velocities in normal locomotion. Comparison of these actual locomotor velocities to those of the F-V function of the same muscle, which was measured in the same animals in a terminal experiment under deep anesthesia, indicated the existence of large-velocity dependent modulations of force. In addition, Gregor et al. [19, 20] showed that, during high-speed locomotion in soleus but not medial gastrocnemius, the force during the initial rapid shortening that follows the stretch at the onset of the stance phase was actually greater than that associated with the maximal F-V function at the same speed of shortening. The most likely reason for this was that the stretch stored elastic energy in the tendon and other structures, which was then released during the subsequent shortening.

Uncertainty about the degree to which a tendon is stretched complicates interpretation of F-V data. Is the change in length occurring in the muscle fiber or in the tendon? Gregor et al. [20] measured force during locomotion that exceeds the maximum isometric force, indicating that the muscle fibers were stretched. It is unknown if muscle stretch during locomotion is large enough to break the cross-bridges (short-term elasticity). Eccentric contraction remains a poorly understood area. Recently, Griffiths [22] used sonomicrometers to measure fiber length and demonstrated that fibers can sometimes shorten when the whole muscle-tendon unit is lengthening.

Muscle Stiffness and Tendon Stretch During Locomotion

The storage and recovery of potential energy is an important component in efficient locomotion [3]. A common theme in the locomotor patterns of a wide variety of species is the cyclic transfer of kinetic to potential energy during the step cycle. Potential energy can be stored either in the change in the center of mass of the animal or in the stretch of the muscle tendon units [67]. The stiffness of excised tendons has been measured, and they can store and return up to 80% of the energy used to stretch them [3]. Additional energy storage may reside in the cross-bridges, yet, as mentioned above, uncertainty remains as to exactly where in the muscle tendon unit the elasticity resides.

Griffiths [21] used a buckle force transducer, EMG, and high-speed cinematography to study hopping in wallabies. He found that as speed increased, more energy was stored in the tendon, compared to the amount of storage in the muscle. At high speeds, he believed that muscle force and stretch were high enough to cause cross-bridge recycling (yielding) and energy loss. Lin and Rymer [43] recently studied eccentric contraction in cat soleus. In contrast to previous studies, they found that the muscle could operate in a stable state after yield, so that the muscle could continue to transmit substantial force, even after stretches large enough to forcibly break cross-bridge attachments.

Architecture Specializations and Locomotion

Comparisons between the soleus and medial gastrocnemius are interesting, because they are synergists, yet they have markedly different fiber composition and different architecture [64]. The soleus is composed primarily of rather long, Type S fibers, arranged with moderate angles of pennation and connected to a rather stiff tendon. The medial gastrocnemius, on the other hand, has primarily shorter Type F fibers, with larger angles of pennation and a more compliant tendon. Spector et al. [59] estimated the V_{max} of the sarcomeres in the medial gastrocnemius to be 2.9 times faster than the sarcomeres in the soleus. However, because the fibers in the gastrocnemius are shorter, the whole muscle V_{max} of the medial gastrocnemius is only 1.6 times faster than the soleus. The short fibers and steep pennation angle allow many fibers to be packed into the gastrocnemius, increasing its isometric tension, as compared to its mass, but as a consequence, reducing the width of the F-L curve [64].

This architectural specialization is probably important in locomotion. Walmsley et al. [63] used buckle transducers to measure the force from the soleus and medial gastrocnemius during walking, running, and jumping. They found that the soleus developed the same peak force throughout a range of speeds from slow walk to fast run. Initially, this seems surprising, because one would expect lower force at higher shortening velocities. The explanation lies with the timing of the activation. During the step cycle, activation and peak force occur before the end of the yield phase, when the muscle is lengthening. Force measured from the medial gastrocnemius increased 3-fold as gait speed increased. However, even during fast running, the soleus produced as much or more peak force than the gastrocnemius. During vertical jumping the gastrocnemius produced much larger forces, up to 110% of its maximum isometric tension. The trade-offs in architectural design are intriguing. The quickly fatigued gastrocnemius seems designed to deliver large forces during occasional jumps. The narrow width of its F-L curve may be mitigated by its compliant tendon. Alternately, for jumping, the additional force may be needed only over a portion of its range of motion. Thus, synergistic muscle may have different "gear ratios." The slow intrinsic speed of the soleus is offset by its long fiber lengths. This example was included to demonstrate that while the F-V properties of a muscle are undoubtedly important to the design and use a muscle, the interpretation from force measurements alone is often difficult. Very few basic design principles may as yet be understood.

Possible Roles of Complex Muscle Properties during Locomotion

From the foregoing it is clear that the basic F-L and F-V properties play an essential role in muscle performance, even though there are few quantitative measures of how muscle systems avoid the limitations imposed by these relationships. Knowledge about the role of other muscle properties during normal movement is more uncertain. For example, is the interaction between stimulus rate and the F-L function an important determinate of force in normal posture or movement? Do history-dependent properties, like doublet potentiation and the effects of prior shortening and stretch on subsequent isometric forces, play important roles? Recent studies have shown that the response of muscle to constant velocity stretches is relatively independent of prior mechanical history, in that repeated stretches evoke con-

FIGURE 4.2.

Comparison of experimental force with Hill model predictions during a simulated slow walk. The solid line *depicts the force measured from whole cat soleus muscle when the muscle was stimulated with a pulse train to simulate the firing of a single motor unit and was driven by a servomechanism to impose a length change observed during walking. The* light line *shows the results of the Hill-type model. All parameters (tendon stiffness, F-V, and F-L) used in Hill model were measured from the same muscle. The F-V curve was scaled by length and activation. Activation was determined by inverse calculation, using the same stimulus during an isometric contraction.*

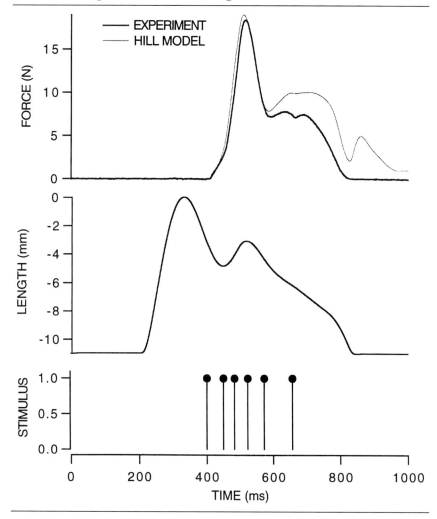

sistent responses [43, 58]. Thus, in a repetitive movement like locomotion, history dependence may not be important—but until a more direct test is available, this question must remain open.

One possible approach to answering these questions is to replicate the conditions of normal movements in isolated preparations, in which the high degree of experimental control is highly advantageous for identifying the effect of each muscle property. Prochazka et al. [35] pioneered this approach in their investigation of the complex firing patterns of muscle spindle afferents during locomotion. After recording spindle afferent discharges and muscle lengths, using chronic techniques in freely moving cats, these researchers turned to the controlled conditions afforded by anesthetized preparations for analysis. By replicating the locomotor length changes with a muscle puller, they were able to identify how the spindle afferent locomotor discharge patterns were generated by the interaction between muscle length and gamma motoneuron activity.

In muscle mechanics, an important step in this same direction is the work-loop technique of Josephson and colleagues [36]. Here, sinusoidal movements at a frequency that resembles locomotion allowed the sustained power output in repetitive tasks to be quantified. Figure 4.2 shows results of a preliminary study in which actual locomotor length changes were used to evaluate the effectiveness of a Hill-type model in predicting locomotor force in the cat soleus muscle. Although every effort was made to construct an accurate Hill-type model of each soleus muscle studied (accurate measurements of the muscle's F-L and F-V functions and its tendon compliance were made, and activation was estimated based on inverse computation from an isometric contraction), the resulting predictions of locomotor force still contained errors on the order of 20–30%. This is probably the best performance that can be obtained with a Hill-type model and suggests that the complex muscle behaviors not included in this model make important contributions to force in locomotor conditions.

Summary of Muscle and Motor Unit Use during Locomotion

In this final section, we will summarize certain basic features that show how locomotor forces arise in the cat triceps surae (medial and lateral gastrocnemius and soleus), perhaps the most thoroughly studied of all muscles in this regard. The first step is to consider use of the heterogeneous motor units in a single muscle. In the previous section, computer simulations were used to estimate the effect of recruitment and rate modulation on F-L and F-V functions for the medial gastrocnemius. To a limited degree, it is possible to compare these simulation results to muscle force outputs actually measured in chronic recording conditions in freely moving animals. The value of this approach is that by matching corresponding simulation and actual force outputs in a given mechanical state, it is then possible to use the simulation to work backwards to define the underlying motor unit use patterns.

FIGURE 4.3.

Computer simulations of the pool input-output relations between synaptic input (y axis) and force (z axis) and velocity outputs (x axis). Surface shading and y-scale at upper left indicate the percent of total force generated by FF units. Single unit I-F, R-F, and F-V functions are based on the cat medial gastrocnemius muscle [25, 27, 53]. Lines labeled with various motor tasks indicate approximate ranges of forces (y axis) and velocities (x axis) measured in medial gastrocnemius with chronically implanted devices. Force ranges are estimated from the peak stance period forces, which occur in near isometric conditions as muscle velocity undergoes the transition between the extension and flexion phases of stance. Force data from ref. 63. Velocity ranges are taken from the peak velocities of shortening during the later portion of the stance phase, when rapid flexion is developing but the muscle is still active. Jump heights ranged from about 0.5–1.2 m. Velocities for slow walking are taken from Weytjens (unpublished data, 1991). For faster speeds and jumping, velocities are estimated from the length records of Walmsley et al. [63]. Bars for running and jumping indicate that fastest velocities probably exceed the range of the figure, which falls well short of the maximum velocity for medial gastrocnemius. Modified from ref. 5.

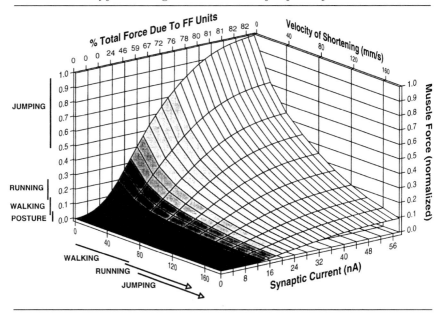

This analysis largely follows that of Walmsley et al. [63], who relied on a motoneuron pool input-output model based solely on recruitment of motor units at their isometric tetanic forces. The simulations reviewed above expand our ability to include realistically the effects of rate modulation, as well as the effects of the F-L and F-V functions. Figure 4.3 summarizes the relation between synaptic input, motor unit recruitment, and F-V function for the cat medial gastrocnemius muscle. The forces and velocities of movement required by various basic locomotor tasks, obtained with the use of chronic techniques, are indicated by the arrows along the *y* and *z* axes. The recruitment scale specifies the percent of total force contributed by FF units (see notation along x axis at the upper left; in addition, the shading of the surface is in proportion to this scale) and thus provides a direct indication of how fatigue resistance varies as a function of neural drive. It should be emphasized that this figure will look different for different muscles—for example, medial gastrocnemius has a relatively small proportion of Type S units.

It is clear that medial gastrocnemius generates only small forces during posture, <10% of maximum. These levels are primarily generated by the fatigue-resistant S and FR units. In addition, velocities during posture are low, so the large proportion force generated by S unit is not a problem. During walking and running, force demands stay modest but are nonetheless sufficiently large as to require substantial recruitment of the fatigable FF units. In addition, peak velocities are very large, far exceeding the capabilities of the Type S units. Jumping in the cat requires the greatest forces and velocities and clearly requires full recruitment of all units, but fatigue resistance dramatically declines. In general, these relations between functional demands and motor unit recruitment are much as they have been envisioned by Henneman and colleagues more than 30 years ago [28, 29].

Actual forces in locomotion are, of course, generated by several synergist muscles, and the relative proportion of the total force within muscle groups varies across different tasks (e.g., see refs. 30 and 63). To a degree, these differences reflect differences in motor unit populations. Among cat ankle extensors, the cat soleus is entirely composed of Type S units and plays the primary role in posture and, in fact, reaches its maximal force generation at low locomotor speeds. Higher forces for faster locomotion and jumping require both medial and lateral gastrocnemius, both of which are composed predominantly of Type FR and FF units. However, separation of function across muscles also allows the architectural specializations discussed above to be used to advantage.

SUMMARY

Over the last century, progress has been made in understanding the basic structure and function of muscle. The emphasis on muscle research has become increasingly focused at the molecular level, and startling advances have been made. Surprisingly, at the whole muscle level significant questions remain unanswered. The details of how muscles are actually used in locomotion are lacking. The foregoing sections have discussed some basic muscle properties and then reviewed instances in which they have been directly measured during locomotor movements. Although most of the basic functional properties of muscle are known, some simple questions such as what the preferred operating point is on the F-L and F-V curves remain unanswered. Design principles of muscle structure and their control by the CNS have yet to be illuminated.

Most in vivo techniques to study muscle function are difficult to use. This precludes their use on all but a small number of specialized muscles. With the exception of photography and electromyography, at best a small number of muscles can be studied at a time. The technique of measuring some muscle properties in vivo and then duplicating the conditions in an isolated muscle for further measurements seems promising. Combinations of mathematical models and careful experimental verification will also be necessary.

ACKNOWLEDGMENTS

Funding for the authors' work on muscle was provided by National Institutes of Health Grant R01 AR41531.

REFERENCES

1. Abbott, B. C., and X. M. Aubert. The force exerted by active striated muscle during and after change in length. *J Physiol.* 117:77–86, 1952.
2. Abrahams, L. D., and G. E. Loeb. The distal musculature of the cat. *Exp. Brain Res.* 58:580–593, 1985.
3. Alexender, R. M. Mechanics of skeleton and tendon. *Handbook of Physiology, Section 1: The Nervous System: Motor Control.* V. B. Brooks. (ed.) Vol. II, Part 1. Bethesda, MD: American Physiological Society, 1981, pp. 17–42.
4. Bagust, J., S. Knott, D. M. Lewis, J. C. Luck, and R. A. Westerman. Isometric contractions of motor units in a fast twitch muscle of the cat. *J. Physiol.* 231:87–104, 1973.
5. Binder, M. D., C. J. Heckman, and R. K. Powers. The physiological control of motoneuron activity. *Handbook of Physiology, Section 12: Integration of Motor, Circulatory, Respiratory and Metabolic Control during Exercise.* L. B. Rowell and J. T. Shephard (eds). Bethesda, MD: American Physiological Society, in press 1995.
6. Binder-Macleod, S. A., and H. P. Clamann. Force output of cat motor units stimulated with trains of linearly varying frequency. *J. Neurophysiol.* 61:208–217, 1989.
7. Bogart, A. J. V. D. Analysis and stimulation of mechanical loads on the human musculoskeletal system: a methodological overview. *Exc. Sport Sci. Rev.* 22:23–51, 1994.
8. Botterman, B. R., G. A. Iwamoto, and W. J. Gonyea. Gradation of isometric tension by different activation rates in motor units of cat flexor carpi radialis muscle. *J. Neurophysiol.* 56:494–506, 1986.
9. Burke, R. E. Motor units: anatomy, physiology, and functional organization. *Handbook of Physiology, Section 1: The Nervous System: Motor Control.* V. B. Brooks. (ed). Vol. II, Part 1. Bethesda, MD: American Physiological Society, 1981, pp. 345–422.
10. Burke, R. E., R. P. Dum, J. W. Fleshman, L. L. Glenn, T. A. Lev, M. J. O'Donovan, and M. J. Pinter. A HRP study of the relation between cell size and motor unit type in cat ankle extensor motoneurons. *J. Comp. Neurol.* 209:17–28, 1982.
11. Burke, R. E., P. Rudomin, and F. E. Zajac. The effect of activation history on tension production by individual muscle units. *Brain Res.* 109:515–529, 1976.
12. Calvert, T. W. and A. E. Chapman. The relationship between the surface EMG and force transients in muscle: simulation and experimental studies. *Proc. IEEE* 65:682–689, 1977.
13. Chanaud, C. M., C. A. Pratt, and G. E. Loeb. Functionally complex muscles of the cat

hindlimb. 2. Mechanical and architectural heterogeneity within the biceps-femoris. *Exp. Brain Res.* 85:257–270, 1991.

14. Devasahayam, S. R., and T. G. Sandercock. Velocity of shortening of single motor units from rat soleus. *J. Neurophysiol.* 67:1133–1145, 1992.

15. Emonet-Denand, F., Y. Laporte, and U. Proske. Summation of tension in motor units of the soleus muscle of the cat. *Neurosci. Lett.* 116:112–117, 1990.

16. Fleshman, J. W., J. B. Munson, G. W. Sypert, and W. A. Friedman. Rheobase, input resistance, and motor-unit type in medial gastrocnemius motoneurons in the cat. *J. Neurophysiol.* 46:1326–38, 1981.

17. Fuglevand, A. J., D. A. Winter, and A. E. Patla. Models of recruitment and rate coding organization in motor-unit pools. *J. Neurophysiol.* 70:2470–2488, 1993.

18. Gans, C., and A. S. Gaunt. Muscle architecture in relation to function. *J. Biomech.* 24(Suppl 1):53–65, 1991.

19. Gregor, R. J., and T. A. Abelew. Tendon force measurements and movement control: a review. *Med. Sci. Sports Exerc.* 26:1359–1372, 1994.

20. Gregor, R. J., R. R. Roy, W. C. Whiting, R. G. Lovely, J. A. Hodgson, and V. R. Edgerton. Mechanical output of the cat soleus during treadmill locomotion: *in vivo* vs. *in situ* characteristics. *J. Biomech.* 21:721–732, 1988.

21. Griffiths, R. I. The mechanics of medial gastrocnemius muscle in the freely hopping wallaby (*Thylogale billardierii*). *J. Exp. Biol.* 147:439–456, 1989.

22. Griffiths, R. I. Shortening of muscle fibres during stretch of the active cat medial gastrocnemius muscle: the role of tendon compliance. *J. Physiol.* (Lond.) 436:219–236, 1991.

23. Gustafsson, B., and M. J. Pinter. An investigation of threshold properties among cat spinal alpha-motoneurones. *J. Physiol.* (Lond.) 357:453–483, 1984.

24. Heckman, C. J. Computer simulations of the effects of different synaptic input systems on the steady-state input-output structure of the motoneuron pool. *J. Neurophysiol.* 71:1717–1739, 1994.

25. Heckman, C. J., and M. D. Binder. Computer simulation of the steady-state input-output function of the cat medial gastrocnemius motoneuron pool. *J. Neurophysiol.* 65:952–967, 1991.

26. Heckman, C. J., J. F. Miller, M. Munson, and W. Z. Rymer. Differences between steady-state and transient post-synaptic potentials elicited by stimulation of the sural nerve. *Exp. Brain Res.* 91:167–170, 1992.

27. Heckman, C. J., J. F. L. Weytjens, and G. F. Loeb. Effect of velocity and mechanical history on the forces of motor units in the cat medial gastrocnemius muscle. *J. Neurophysiol.* 68:1503–1515, 1992.

28. Henneman, E., and L. M. Mendell. Functional organization of motoneuron pool and its inputs. *Handbook of Physiology, Section 1: The Nervous System: Motor Control.* (V. B. Brooks (ed). Vol. II, Part 1. Bethesda, MD: American Physiological Society, 1981, pp. 423–507.

29. Henneman, E., and C. B. Olson. Relations between structure and function in the design of skeletal muscle. *J. Neurophysiol.* 28:581–598, 1965.

30. Herzog, W., T. R. Leonard, and A. C. Guimaraes. Forces in gastrocnemius, soleus, and plantaris tendons of the freely moving cat. *J. Biomech.* 26:945–953, 1993.

31. Herzog, W., T. R. Leonard, J. M. Renaud, J. Wallice, G. Chaki, and S. Bornemisza. Force-length properties and functional demands of cat gastrocnemius, soleus and plantaris muscles. *J. Biomech.* 25:1329–1335, 1992.

32. Hill, A. V. The heat of shortening and the dynamic constants of muscle. *Proc. R. Soc. Lond.* (Biol.) 126:136–195, 1938.

33. Hoffer, J. A., G. E. Loeb, W. B. Marks, M. J. O'Donovan, C. A. Pratt, and N. Sugano. Cat hindlimb motoneurons during locomotion. I. Destination, axonal conduction velocity, and recruitment threshold. *J. Neurophysiol.* 57:510–529, 1987.

34. Hoffer, J. A., N. Sugano, G. E. Loeb, W. B. Marks, M. J. O'Donovan, and C. A. Pratt. Cat hindlimb motoneurons during locomotion. II. Normal activity patterns. *J. Neurophysiol.* 57:530–553, 1987.

35. Hulliger, M., F. Horber, A. Medved, and A. Prochazka. An experimental simulation method for iterative and interactive reconstruction of unknown (fusimotor) inputs contributing to known (spindle afferent) responses. *J. Neurosci.* 21:225–238, 1987.

36. Josephson, R. K. Contraction dynamics and power output of skeletal muscle. *Annu. Rev. Physiol.* 55:527–546, 1993.

37. Joyce, G. C., P. M. H. Rack, and D. R. Westbury. The mechanical properties of cat soleus muscle during controlled lengthening and shortening movements. *J. Physiol.* 204:461–474, 1969.

38. Kernell, D. Rhythmic properties of motoneurones innervating muscle fibres of different speed in m. gastrocnemius medialis of the cat. *Brain Res.* 160:159–162, 1979.

39. Kernell, D., O. Eerbeek, and B. A. Verhey. Relation between isometric force and stimulus rate in cat's hindlimb motor units of different twitch contraction time. *Exp. Brain Res.* 50:220–227, 1983.

40. Kernell, D., and B. Zwaagstra. Input conductance, axonal conduction velocity and cell size among hindlimb motoneurones of the cat. *Brain Res.* 204:311–326, 1980.

41. Lieber, R. L., and J. L. Boakes. Sarcomere length and joint kinematics during torque production in the frog hindlimb. *Am. J. Physiol.* 254:C759–C768, 1988.

42. Lieber, R. L., G. J. Loren, and J. Friden. In vivo measurements of human wrist extensor muscle sarcomere length changes. *J. Neurophysiol.* 71:874–881, 1994.

43. Lin, D. C., and W. Z. Rymer. Mechanical properties of cat soleus muscle elicited by sequential ramp stretches: implications for motor control. *J. Neurophysiol.* 70:997–1008, 1993.

44. Loeb, G. E., and C. Gans. *Electromyography for Experimentalists.* Chicago: University of Chicago Press, 1986.

45. Lutz, G. J., and L. C. Rome. Built for jumping: the design of the frog muscular system. *Science* 263:370–372, 1994.

46. Lynn, R., and D. L. Morgan. Decline running produces more sarcomeres in rat vastus intermedius muscle fibers than does incline running. *J. Appl. Physiol.* 77:1439–1444, 1994.

47. Mashima, H., K. Akazawa, H. Kushima, and K. Fujii. The load-force-velocity relation and the viscous-like force in frog skeletal muscle. *Jap. J. Physiol.* 22:103–120, 1972.

48. McMahon, T. A. *Muscle, Reflexes and Locomotion.* Princeton, NJ: Princeton University Press, 1984.

49. Morgan, D. L. Separation of active and passive components of short-range stiffness of muscle. *Am. J. Physiol.* 232:C45–C49, 1977.

50. Morgan D. L. New insights into the behavior of muscle during active lengthening. *Biophys. J.* 57:209–221, 1990.

51. Otten, E. Concepts and models of functional architecture in skeletal muscle. *Exerc. Sport Sci. Rev.* 16:89–137, 1988.

52. Partridge, L.D. and L. A. Benton. Muscle, the motor. *Handbook of Physiology, Section 1: The Nervous System: Motor Control.* V. B. Brooks (ed). Vol. II, Part 1. Bethesda, MD: American Physiological Society, 1981, pp. 43–106.

53. Petit, J., M. Chua, and C. C. Hunt, Maximum shortening speed of motor units of various types in cat lumbrical muscles. *J. Neurophysiol.* 69:442–448, 1993.

54. Petit, J., G. M. Filippi, F. Emonet-Denand, C. C. Hunt, and Y. Laporte. Changes in muscle stiffness produced by motor units of different types in peroneus longus muscle of cat. *J. Neurophysiol.* 63:190–197, 1990.

55. Powers, R. K. and M. D. Binder. Summation of motor unit tensions in the tibialis posterior muscle of the cat under isometric and nonisometric conditions. *J. Neurophysiol.* 66:1838–1846, 1991.

56. Rack, P. M. H., and D. R. Westbury. The effects of length and stimulus rate on tension in the isometric cat soleus muscle. *J. Physiol.* (Lond.) 204:443–460, 1969.

57. Rome, L.C., R. P. Funke, R. M. Alexander, G. A. Lutz, H. D. Aldridge, F. Scott, and M. Freadman. Why animals have different fiber types. *Nature* 355:824–827, 1988.

58. Scott, S. H., I. E. Brown, and G. Loeb. Mechanics of feline soleus. 1. Effect of fascicle length and velocity on force output. *J. Muscle Res. Cell Motil.*, in press, 1996.
59. Spector, S. A., P. F. Gardiner, R. F. Zernicke, R. R. Roy, and V. R. Edgerton. Muscle architecture and force velocity characteristics of cat soleus and medial gastrocnemius: implications for motor control. *J. Neurophysiol.* 44:951–960, 1980.
60. Stephens, J. A., R. M. Reinking, and D. G. Stuart. The motor units of cat medial gastrocnemius: electrical and mechanical properties as a function of muscle length. *J. Morphol.* 146:495–512, 1975.
61. Trotter, J. A. Functional morphology of force transmission in skeletal muscle. *Acta Anat.* 146:205–222, 1993.
62. Trotter, J. A., F. J. R. Richmond, and P. P. Purslow. Functional morphology and motor control of series-fibered muscle. *Exerc. Sport Sci. Rev.* 23:167–213, 1995.
63. Walmsley, B., J. A. Hodgson, and R. E. Burke. Forces produced by medial gastrocnemius and soleus muscles during locomotion in freely moving cats. *J. Neurophysiol.* 41:1203–1216, 1978.
64. Walmsley, B., and U. Proske. Comparison of stiffness of soleus and medial gastrocnemius muscle in cats. *J. Neurophysiol.* 46:250–259, 1981.
65. Winters, J. M. Hill-based models: a systems engineering perspective. J. M. Winters and S. L.-Y. Woo (eds). *Multiple Muscle Systems: Biomechanics and Movement Organization.* New York: Springer-Verlag, 1990, pp. 69–93.
66. Zajac, F. E. Thigh muscle activity during maximum-height jumps by cats. *J. Neurophysiol.* 53:979–994, 1985.
67. Zajac, F. E. Muscle and tendon: properties, models, scaling, and application to biomechanics and motor control. *Crit. Rev. Biomed. Eng.* 17:359–411, 1989.
68. Zajac, F.E. Muscle coordination of movement: a perspective. *J. Biomech.* 26(Suppl. 1):109–124, 1993.

5
Do Physical Activity and Physical Fitness Avert Premature Mortality?

I-MIN LEE, M.B., B.S., Sc.D.
RALPH S. PAFFENBARGER, Jr., M.D., Dr.P.H.

Over the past 2 decades or so, evidence has been accumulating that indicates that an inverse relation exists between physical activity and risk of chronic diseases, such as coronary heart disease [3, 76], hypertension [20, 106], noninsulin-dependent diabetes mellitus [30, 49, 50], certain site-specific cancers (in particular, colon cancer and, possibly, breast cancer) [4, 42, 101], and osteoporosis [17]. Moreover, the proposed biological mechanisms that enable an individual to benefit from physical activity appear highly plausible and make a case for a causal relation [32, 33]. If physical activity indeed reduces the risk of developing these chronic diseases, it is logical to surmise that premature mortality—from any cause—can be averted or delayed by physical activity. Conversely, we can expect physical activity to enhance longevity.

In this chapter, we will review the epidemiological data on the association between physical activity and longevity to summarize the current state of knowledge. We will examine studies in which investigators specifically have analyzed the endpoint of all-cause mortality. (For studies of physical activity and coronary heart disease, the reader is referred to two comprehensive reviews by Powell et al. [76] and Berlin and Colditz [3]. We will distinguish between physical activity and physical fitness, two interrelated measures [9, 13]. Physical activity is an optional behavior, whereas physiological fitness is an achieved condition. Physical activity modifies physiological fitness over time, whereas physiological fitness limits the amount of physical activity that may be performed. Thus, physical activity and physical fitness each may act independently to favor longevity.

EARLY OBSERVATIONS

The concept that physical activity and physical fitness promote health and longevity certainty is not new. In ancient China, circa 2500 B.C. we find perhaps the earliest records of organized exercise used for health promotion by Hua T'o [48]. The Greek physicians, Hippocrates and Plato (circa 460 to 370 B.C.) and, later, Galen (circa 200 to 129 B.C.) also believed in the importance of a physically active life-style for well-being and its usefulness in treating disease and disability [48]. Hippocrates and Galen, however, eschewed the excess training of the professional athlete in their day, favoring, instead, more moderate physical activity [82]. Later, in 18-century Italy, Ramazzini continued to note the well-being of foot messengers ("runners"), as contrasted to the ill-health of sedentary workers, such as cobblers and tailors [78].

Beginning with the 19th century, investigators attempted to measure the benefits associated with physical activity more objectively, using numerical quantification. In some of the earliest such observations made about occupational physical activity and mortality, Smith noted, in 1864, that the mortality rate among British tailors was much higher than that among agricultural laborers [99]. Meanwhile, across the Atlantic Ocean, in 1923, when Sivertsen and Dahlstrom classified men in Minnesota according to occupational physical activity, they observed that death rates declined with increasing physical activity on the job [96]. Furthermore, investigators noted that the average age at death increased in a gradient fashion with physically more demanding occupations. However, the potential for job selection was not addressed: Men developing chronic diseases might have changed to physically less taxing occupations, thus contributing toward the higher death rates in these occupations.

With respect to nonoccupational forms of physical activity, rowing is one of the oldest sports with formal rules and organization. Thus, early in its history, this sport provided an opportunity for investigators to study mortality associated with vigorous physical activity. During the 19th century, the prevailing belief regarding vigorous exercise had not changed from the time of Hippocrates and Galen namely, that it was harmful [52]. However, 19th- and early 20th-century studies of oarsmen from Cambridge, Oxford, and Harvard Universities showed, in fact, the opposite: The life expectancy of these men tended to exceed that of the general population [28, 77]. Studies of other sportsmen—such as college men excelling in different sporting activities (e.g., track-and-field athletes, cricketers, football players, etc.) and cross-country skiers—also failed to show that these sportsmen died at earlier ages than their less athletically distinguished counterparts [18, 36, 75, 83]. On the contrary, some investigations showed, instead, that these men lived longer [18, 36, 75].

THE ASSOCIATION OF PHYSICAL ACTIVITY OR PHYSICAL FITNESS WITH AVOIDANCE OF PREMATURE MORTALITY

Studies examining the association of physical activity or physical fitness with total mortality generally have been prospective cohort in design. These studies have used two different strategies. First, investigators have classified men according to physical activity or fitness categories and then have examined all-cause mortality rates within each category. Secondly, investigators have analyzed mortality rates according to categories of men who did or did not change their physical activity or fitness profile over time.

We will now proceed to discuss studies belonging to the first category, ordered by date of publication and with related studies grouped together.

Study of U.S. Railroad Industry Employees, 1962

In this study, Taylor et al. [103] wanted to test the hypothesis that men in physically active occupations experience lower rates of coronary heart disease than those in sedentary occupations. In the course of their analyses, they also examined all-cause mortality rates. Investigators chose the U.S. railroad industry for study, because conditions in this industry discouraged men from shifting from one occupation to another, that is, labor contracts prevented the transferring of seniority from one occupation to another. Thus, classifying a railroad worker by his occupation was unlikely to lead to misclassification of physical activity on the job over time. However, because leisure-time physical activity was not measured, misclassification of total physical activity might have occurred. One other advantage of studying railroad employees was that the retirement board of this industry paid out higher disability and retirement benefits than did Social Security; it also paid out death benefits. Thus, morbidity and mortality follow-up among workers was believed to be recorded with high accuracy and completeness.

In this analysis, investigators enrolled white men working as clerks (deemed most sedentary), switchmen or section men (deemed physically most active) in the U.S. railroad industry for study. Additionally, men had to have worked for 10 yr by 1951 and still be employed in 1954. Subjects were followed for mortality from 1955 to 1956. Only deaths occurring at ages 40–64 yr were included in the study. During follow-up, a total of 1978 deaths occurred in 191,609 person-yr.

The age-adjusted death rates per 1,000 were 11.83 for clerks, 10.29 for switchmen, and 7.62 for section men (Table 5.1), with the differences statistically significant. However, the lower mortality rates may have resulted from differences in physical activity, but because of differences in other

TABLE 5.1.
Mortality Rates (1955–1956) among Employees of the U.S. Railroad Industry, according to Occupation in 1954

Occupation	No. of Deaths	Person-Yr	Mortality Rate[a] (/1000)
Clerks (most sedentary)	999	85,112	11.83
Switchmen	638	61,630	10.29
Section men (most active)	341	44,867	7.62

[a]Data are from ref. 103. Age-adjusted.

characteristics predictive of mortality (e.g., cigarette smoking, obesity, diet, etc.). The authors were unable to address potential confounding by these other variables.

The U.S. Railroad Study: Physical Activity and All-Cause Mortality, 1989

This study [98] also enrolled men working in the U.S. railroad industry; here, investigators primarily were interested in leisure-time, rather than occupational, physical activity. The U.S. Railroad Study (n = 3043) comprised one cohort of the Seven-Countries Study, an investigation of the predictors of coronary heart disease among sixteen cohorts in seven countries that was begun in the late 1950s [38]. For the U.S. Railroad Study, data on all-cause mortality also was collected.

In this particular analysis, Slattery et al. [98] investigated 2562 white railroad workers, ages 22–79 yr, who were free of cardiovascular disease, were not retired at baseline, and provided data on leisure-time physical activities. Between 1957 and 1960, these men received a medical examination. During the examination, the men were questioned regarding their frequency and duration of participation in more than fifty different leisure-time activities, using the Minnesota Leisure-Time Physical Activity Questionnaire [102]. Based on these data, an estimate of energy expended on leisure-time physical activities was made for each man (in kilocalories per week). Additionally, this estimated energy expenditure was partitioned into kilocalories per week, derived from light-to-moderate activities and from intense activities (e.g., hunting large game, backpacking, jogging/running, skiing, swimming, shoveling snow, etc.). Investigators then followed the men for mortality until 1977.

Table 5.2 shows that the age-adjusted mortality rates among men declined with increasing leisure-time energy expenditure. After additional adjustment in analysis for differences in cigarette smoking, systolic blood pressure and serum cholesterol, the energy expended in leisure-time physical

TABLE 5.2.
Rates and Relative Risks of All-Cause Mortality (1957–1977) in the U.S. Railroad Study, according to Leisure-Time Physical Activity in 1957–1960

Leisure-Time Physical Activity(kcal/wk)	No. of Men	Mortality Rate[a] (/100)	Relative Risk[b] (95% CI)
≤250	635	29.8	1.21 (1.03–1.42)
251–1000	1015	25.5	1.08 (1.01–1.15)
1001–1999	478	24.7	1.04 (1.01–1.08)
≥2000	434	26.2	1.00 (referent)

[a]Data are from ref. 98. Age-adjusted.
[b]Adjusted for age, cigarette smoking, systolic blood pressure, and serum cholesterol. CI, confidence interval.

activities continued to be significantly and inversely related to all-cause mortality. The least active men had 1.21 times (95% confidence interval, 1.03–1.42) the mortality rate of the most active men, during the 17–20 yr of follow-up. Investigators also examined, separately, men who were occupationally sedentary and those who were active at work. Within each category, all-cause mortality rates tended to decline with increasing leisure-time physical activity; however, this was not statistically significant for either group.

Finally, investigators examined, separately, the association of light-to-moderate leisure-time physical activity and intense leisure-time physical activity with all-cause mortality. In this analysis, they adjusted mutually for both kinds of energy expenditure, as well as for the potential confounding factors listed above. The energy expended in intense leisure-time physical activity significantly predicted lower mortality rates, but the energy expended in light-to-moderate leisure activities did not. For coronary heart disease mortality, the association with intense leisure-time physical activity also was significant; however, the association with light-to-moderate leisure-time physical activity now was of borderline significance.

The U.S. Railroad Study: Physical Fitness and All-Cause Mortality, 1988

In the U.S. Railroad Study [97] at the time of their baseline examination in 1957 to 1960, the men also were examined for physical fitness. As described previously, this cohort originally comprised 3043 men. For this analysis, Slattery et al. [97] studied 2431 men, ages 22–79 yr who were free of cardiovascular disease, were not retired at baseline, and had data available on physical fitness, cigarette smoking, blood pressure, and serum cholesterol. Physical fitness was assessed, using a submaximal treadmill exercise test. Investigators than used heart rate after the exercise test to classify men into four categories of physical fitness, with lower heart rates indicating higher degrees of fitness. As in the study of physical activity, men were followed for mortality after the baseline examination until 1977. Among the 2431 men, 631 deaths occurred.

Table 5.3 shows that the age-adjusted mortality rates were significantly and directly related to exercise test heart rates. That is, higher levels of physical fitness were predictive of lower all-cause mortality rates. Findings remained significant after additional adjustment for differences in cigarette smoking, blood pressure and serum cholesterol. After adjustment for these variables, the least fit men had 1.23 times (95% confidence interval, 1.17–1.30) the mortality rate of those most fit, during the 17–20 years of follow-up.

Investigators then tried to determine the independent associations of physical activity and physical fitness with reduction of all-cause mortality. In multivariate analysis, with simultaneous adjustment for physical activity and physical fitness, only physical fitness, but not physical activity, was significantly predictive of lower all-cause mortality rates. The authors thus concluded that the inverse relation between physical activity and all-cause mortality was likely mediated by favorable changes in physical fitness.

TABLE 5.3.
Rates and Relative Risks of All-Cause Mortality (1957–1977) in the U.S. Railroad Study, according to Exercise Test Heart Rate in 1957–1960

Exercise Test Heart Rate (beats/min)	No. of Men	Mortality Rate[a] (/100)	Relative Risk[b] (95% CI)
≤105 (most fit)	548	22.8	1.00 (referent)
106–115	665	22.3	1.07 (1.02–1.13)
116–127	692	27.8	1.15 (1.10–1.21)
>127 (least fit)	526	31.4	1.23 (1.17–1.30)

[a]Data are from ref. 97. Age-adjusted.
[b]Adjusted for age, cigarette smoking, systolic blood pressure, and serum cholesterol. CI, confidence interval.

Study of British Civil Servants, 1978

Morris and co-workers [14, 56] have pioneered research on the relation between physical activity and risk of developing coronary heart disease, laying the ground work for much of what we know today. Their findings, with observations dating as far back as the 1940s, were derived from the study of London bus drivers and conductors, postal service workers and civil servants [14, 53–58]. These data indicated that physical activity, whether occupational or leisure-time, was inversely associated with coronary heart disease risk. Furthermore, no benefit was found for total energy expenditure; only energy expended in vigorous sporting activities (those apt to require peaks of energy expenditure of 7.5 kcal/min) was associated with reduced incidence of coronary heart disease. Men engaging in such vigorous sporting activities experienced less than half the coronary heart disease rates of those who did not take part in such activities. This held true within categories of men without and with other risk factors for coronary heart disease (cigarette smoking, hypertension, high body mass, short stature, and parental history of premature cardiovascular mortality).

In the above investigators' study of British civil servants, observations also were made for all-cause mortality. This particular analysis involved 17,944 male, executive-grade civil servants, ages 40–65 years. Between 1968 and 1970, these men were asked on a Monday morning to fill out a 5-min-by-5-min diary of their physical activities on the preceding Friday and Saturday. Men were not forewarned, so they presumably reported on their usual pattern of physical activities for a typical weekday and a typical weekend day. Coding of these 7-page physical activity diaries was a very time-consuming process, carefully done without knowledge of the medical history of the civil servants. In their report on all-cause mortality, the investigators based their findings on a 20% random sample of men (n = 3591). Men were classified as not having or having engaged in vigorous exercise (activities apt to require peaks of energy expenditure of 7.5 kcal/min, e.g., vigorous sports and recreation). The men were followed until 1977; during follow-up, 268 deaths occurred. Because subjects were civil servants, their morbidity and mortality experience could be traced with a high degree of completeness through the National Health Service Central Register and the Civil Service Medical Advisory Service.

For men reporting no vigorous exercise, 8.4% died during follow-up, as compared with 4.2% of men who reported vigorous exercise (Table 5.4). Men who reported vigorous exercise tended to smoke less; of those who did, fewer cigarettes were smoked. For coronary heart disease mortality, at least, when nonsmokers and smokers were examined separately, vigorous exercise was associated with lower such mortality in each group. Furthermore, there was no evidence that the increased coronary heart disease mortality among men not reporting vigorous exercise was because of disability or ill health. Were this the case, as these unhealthy men died over time, the inverse association would disappear with the passage of time. When investigators divided the follow-up period into the first 3 yr, the next 3 yr, and subsequent years, the same inverse association was noted for all three periods. Because dietary data were unavailable, investigators could not address the potential for dietary factors to confound the association between physical inactivity and mortality.

Study of Men and Women in Eastern Finland, 1982

This is one of the few studies in this review that has included women [86]. Study subjects were a random sample of the population living in two counties of Eastern Finland, an area with extremely high morbidity and mortality from cardiovascular disease. A total of 3978 men (ages 30–59 yr) and 3688 women (ages 35–59 yr), who were free of cardiovascular disease in the 12 mo preceding the baseline survey and had data on the variables of interest, were included in this study. Baseline information on risk factors was collected via a self-administered questionnaire in 1972. At the same time, blood pressure and serum cholesterol also were measured. Investigators assessed physical activity at work and during leisure, using two multiple-choice type questions. For the purpose of this analysis, subjects were dichotomized into those hav-

TABLE 5.4.
Mortality Rates (1968–1977) among British Civil Servants, according to Physical Activity in 1968–1970

Physical Activity	No. of Deaths	No. of Men	Mortality Rate (/100)
No vigorous exercise	235	2814	8.4
Vigorous exercise	33	777	4.2
			P < .001

Data are from refs. 14 and 56.

ing low or high physical activity at work and during leisure. Subjects were followed after baseline through 1978, during which 172 men and 75 women died. Mortality follow-up presumably was complete, as deaths were traced from the national death certificate data register.

Low physical activity at work predicted increased mortality during follow-up among both men and women (Table 5.5). The relative risks for dying, adjusted for age, cigarette smoking, diastolic blood pressure, serum cholesterol, and body mass index, were 1.9 (90% confidence interval, 1.5–2.5) for men with low physical activity, 2.2 (1.5–3.3) for women with low physical activity. Low physical activity during leisure-time also predicted increased mortality. The corresponding relative risks were 1.5 (1.2–2.0) for men and 1.6 (1.0–2.3).Although the study's investigators calculated 90%, rather than 95%, confidence intervals, all relative risks were reported as statistically significant at P < .05.

Investigators next divided the follow-up period into the first 2 years and the next 5 years, in order to examine potential bias arising from unhealthy men who decreased their physical activity at baseline. (Because of the small number of deaths, this analysis would not have been meaningful for the women studied). There was some evidence of such an artifactual association, although it did not completely explain the inverse relation between physical activity and mortality. For work, low physical activity increased mortality risk among men by 2.7 times (90% confidence interval, 1.4–5.2) during Years 1–2 and 1.7 times (1.2–2.3) during Years 3–7, after adjustment for the variables listed above. For leisure-time, the corresponding figures were 3.5 (1.8–6.8) and 1.1 (0.8–1.5), respectively.

TALE 5.5
Relative Risks for All-Cause Mortality (1972–1978) among Men and Women in Eastern Finland, according to Physical Activity at Work and during Leisure in 1972

Physical Activity	Relative Risk[a] (90% CI)
Men, work	
High physical activity	1.0 (referent)
Low physical activity	1.9 (1.5–2.5)
Men, leisure-time:	
High physical activity	1.0 (referent)
Low physical activity	1.5 (1.2–2.0)
Women, work	
High physical activity	1.0 (referent)
Low physical activity	2.2 (1.5–3.3)
Women, leisure-time	
High physical activity	1.0 (referent)
Low physical activity	1.6 (1.0–2.3)

[a]Data are from ref. 86. Adjusted for age, cigarette smoking, diastolic blood pressure, serum cholesterol, and body mass index. CI, confidence interval.

Finally, investigators classified subjects into three categories of work and leisure-time physical activity: low physical activity, both at work and during leisure; high physical activity at work or during leisure; or high physical activity both at work and during leisure. In age-adjusted analyses, comparing the third with the first category yielded relative risks for mortality of 3.9 (95% confidence interval, 2.7–5.5) in men and 3.5 (1.9–6.3) in women.

The Harvard Alumni Health Study, 1986, 1993, and 1995

Morris in England and Paffenbarger in the United States, with their colleagues, beginning in the 1950s, conducted some of the earliest epidemiological studies on the health benefits associated with physical activity, studying coronary heart disease in particular [43, 62, 64]. Like Morris, Paffenbarger noted that physical activity was inversely related to the risk for this disease. Such observations have been based on data from the College Alumni Health Study (comprising alumni from Harvard University and the University of Pennsylvania) and from studies of occupational physical activity among San Francisco longshoremen [11, 43, 61–65, 67–71, 105].

In 1986, Paffenbarger et al. made one of the first rigorous attempts to quantify added years of life from being physically active. Investigators used data from the Harvard Alumni Health Study. This is an ongoing, prospective cohort study of the predictors of chronic disease in men matriculating as undergraduates at Harvard University between 1916 and 1950. The men provided information on their sociodemographic characteristics, personal and family medical history, and health habits via mailed questionnaires that were returned. The initial or baseline questionnaire was mailed to alumni in 1962 or 1966 (referred to as 1962/1966); since then, data have been updated periodically by means of further mailed questionnaires. Additionally, information on the medical history and health habits of these men during their youth, obtained from a standardized medical examination at the time of college entry, also was available from college archives. Deaths in this cohort have been traced, using information from the Harvard Alumni Office, with mortality follow-up that is more than 99% complete.

In this particular study of added years of life, investigators enrolled 16,936 men, ages 35–74 years, who were free of self-reported, physician-diagnosed coronary heart disease at baseline (1962/1966). On the baseline questionnaire, men were asked about the number of flights of stairs climbed daily, the number of city blocks walked daily, the types of sports or recreational activities engaged in, and the time spent on each of these sports and recreational activities. Although investigators did not inquire specifically about occupational activity, alumni were unlikely to have expended much energy on the job, apart from walking and climbing stairs. Investigators quantified physical activity thus: Walking seven city blocks rated 56 kcal, whereas climbing seven flights of stairs rated 28 kcal. Sports and recreational activities were classified as light (requiring 5 kcal/min of energy expenditure), vigorous (10 kcal/min), or mixed (7.5 kcal/min). Investigators then summed kilocalories per week from blocks walked, flights climbed, and sports or recreational activities carried out, to obtain an index of weekly energy expenditure. Physical activity then was related to all-cause mortality between 1962/1966 and 1978. A total of 1413 men died during the 12–16 years of follow-up, encompassing 213,716 person-yr.

Table 5.6 shows that the age-adjusted mortality rates among alumni generally declined with increasing physical activity, although this benefit appeared to taper off after 3500 kcal/wk. Men expending 3000–3499 kcal/wk experienced only 0.46 times the mortality of those expending <500 kcal/wk. When investigators examined men of ages 35–49, 50–59, 60–69 and 70–84 years separately, the inverse association held within each age stratum. Furthermore, the inverse relation was significant, regardless of the absence or presence of other factors predictive of mortality: cigarette smoking, hypertension, weight-for-height, weight change since college, early parental death, and college athleticism.

Next, investigators estimated the proportion of deaths in the cohort that might have been averted between 1962/1966 and 1978, had all alumni expended ≥2000 kcal/wk. This figure stood at 16.1%, ranking second in importance after avoidance of cigarette smoking (22.5%); it was more important than avoiding hypertension (6.4%) or having no early parental death (4.8%). Finally, investigators estimated the number of years that might be gained, up to age 80, from an active life-style. In their most contrasted comparison, they compared men who expended ≥2000 kcal/wk with those who expended only <500 kcal/wk (Table 5.7). After taking into account differences in cigarette smoking, hypertension, weight change since college, and early parental death, it was shown that active alumni, on average, might be expected to live more than 2 years longer than those who were inactive.

TABLE 5.6.
Rates and Relative Risks of All-Cause Mortality (1962/1966–1978) in the Harvard Alumni Health Study, according to Physical Activity in 1962/1966

Physical Activity (kcal/wk)	No. of Deaths[a]	Mortality Rate[b] (/10,000)	Relative Risk[b]
<500	308	93.7	1.00 (referent)
500–999	322	73.5	0.78
1000–1499	202	68.2	0.73
1500–1999	121	59.3	0.63
2000–2499	89	57.7	0.62
2500–2999	62	48.5	0.52
3000–3499	42	42.7	0.46
≥3500	203	58.4	0.62
			P, trend < .0001

[a]Data are from ref. 62. Total deaths do not add up to 1413 because of missing data.
[b]Age-adjusted.

TABLE 5.7.
Estimated Years of Added Life, up to Age 80, Comparing Men Expending ≥ 2000 kcal/wk with Men Expending <500 kcal/wk in Physical Activity in the Harvard Alumni Health Study

Age at Entry (yr)	Estimated Added Life (yr), up to Age 80[a]
35–39	2.51
40–44	2.34
45–49	2.10
50–54	2.11
55–59	2.02
60–64	1.75
65–69	1.35
70–74	0.72
75–79	0.42
35–79	2.15

[a]Data are from ref. 62. Adjusted for cigarette smoking, hypertension, weight change since college, and early parental death.

Subsequent analyses of Harvard alumni examined all-cause mortality in relation to physical activity in 1977. The eligible men for this study were 10,269 individuals, ages 45–84 years in 1977, who were free of self-reported, physician-diagnosed cardiovascular disease, diabetes, cancer, and chronic obstructive pulmonary disease at that time. Men were followed from 1977–1985, with 476 dying in 90,650 person-years. Findings were congruent with those from earlier analyses; however, a benefit continued to be observed with energy expenditure of ≥3500 kcal/wk (Table 5.8). In addition, men were classified according to the intensity of their sports or recreational activities, being categorized as engaging in light (<4.5 METs, or multiples of resting metabolic rate) or moderately vigorous (≥4.5 METs) activities. Table 5.8 shows that in age-adjusted analyses, light activities were not significantly related to all-cause mortality rates, but moderately vigorous activities were. Investigators also examined the influence of change in physical activity on all-cause mortality; these findings will be discussed later in the chapter.

In a further attempt to clarify the role of intensity in averting premature mortality, investigators launched a more detailed scrutiny of the intensity of physical activities carried out by these Harvard men. Specifically, they sought to answer the question: Is a set amount of energy expended in vigorous activities associated with benefit equivalent to that of the same amount of energy expended in nonvigorous activities? This study involved 17,321 men, ages 30–79 years, who were free of self-reported, physician-diagnosed cardiovascular disease, cancer and chronic obstructive pulmonary disease at baseline (1962/1966). Additionally, subjects had to provide data on physical activity and other potential confounding factors of interest.

TABLE 5.8.
Rates and Relative Risks of All-Cause Mortality (1977–1985) in the Harvard Alumni Health Study, according to Physical Activity in 1977

Physical Activity (kcal/wk)	No. of Deaths[a]	Mortality Rate[b] (/10,000)	Relative Risk[b] (95% CI)
<500	101	74.0	1.00 (referent)
500–999	92	53.8	0.73 (0.54–0.95)
1000–1499	75	52.3	0.71 (0.53–0.96)
1500–1999	50	47.3	0.64 (0.46–0.92)
2000–2499	37	42.3	0.57 (0.40–0.87)
2500–2999	34	54.7	0.74 (0.50–1.12)
3000–3499	27	59.8	0.81 (0.52–1.32)
≥3500	59	38.6	0.52 (0.39–0.75) P, trend < .001
Sports or recreational activity[c]			
None	81	58.6	1.00 (referent)
Light only	103	77.7	1.33 (0.98–1.75)
Light and moderately vigorous	149	48.0	0.82 (0.62–1.08)
Moderately vigorous only	123	42.6	0.73 (0.52–0.95) P, trend < .001

[a]Data are from ref. 64. Total deaths do not add up to 476 because of missing data.
[b]Age-adjusted. CI, confidence interval.
[c]Light, requiring <4.5 METs; moderately vigorous, requiring ≥4.5 METs.

Investigators assessed physical activity at baseline, 1962/1966, and again in 1977. The energy expended on walking and stair climbing was estimated as described earlier. For sports and recreational activities, investigators assigned a multiple of resting metabolic rate (MET score) to every activity [1]. The energy expended on each activity was estimated by multiplying its MET score with body weight (in kilograms) and hours per week of participation. Investigators then summed kilocalories per week from blocks walked, flights climbed, and activities carried out, to provide an index of total energy expenditure per week. The investigators further divided total energy expenditure into two components: that derived from vigorous activities—apt to require ≥6 METs—and that derived from nonvigorous (i.e., light and moderate) activities—requiring <6 METs. (Because walking speed was not ascertained in 1962/1966 and 1977, all walking was deemed nonvigorous, whereas stair climbing was considered vigorous.) Men then were classified into five categories each of vigorous and nonvigorous energy expenditure, using the same cutpoints: <150, 150–399, 400–749, 750–1499, and ≥1500 kcal/wk. The investigators followed men for mortality after return of the 1962/1966 questionnaire through 1988. A total of 3728 men died in 384,681 person-years of observation.

In relating vigorous and nonvigorous energy expenditure estimated in 1962/1966 to all-cause mortality from 1962/1966 through 1988, investigators found that vigorous expenditure, but not nonvigorous, significantly predicted decreased mortality. The relative risks, adjusted for age, cigarette smoking, hypertension, diabetes mellitus, body mass index, and early parental death, for all-cause mortality associated with the five categories of vigorous energy expenditure were 1.00 (referent), .88, .95, .87, and .87, respectively; P, trend = .007. For nonvigorous energy expenditure, the corresponding relative risks were 1.00 (referent), .89, 1.00, .98 and .92, respectively; P, trend = .36. Analyses of the two kinds of energy expenditure were mutually adjusted.

Because physical activity was likely to have changed over the 26 years of follow-up, this misclassification may have attenuated the relation between physical activity and all-cause mortality. A further potential for bias might have arisen from men with illnesses, other than the exclusionary diseases, who decreased their activity levels. Such men would likely die early in follow-up. Thus, to minimize these potential limitations, investigators conducted additional analyses, first, allowing physical activity (and potential confounding variables) to be assessed in 1962/1966 and updated in 1977 and, second, excluding an arbitrarily chosen 5 years of follow-up after each assessment of physical activity. Table 5.9 and Figure 5.1 show the findings from this analysis, covering 1702 deaths. Vigorous energy expenditure was even more strongly related to decreased all-cause mortality (adjusted rela-

TABLE 5.9.
Relative Risks of All-Cause Mortality (1967/1971–1977 and 1983–1988)[a] in the Harvard Alumni Health Study, by Vigorous and Nonvigorous Physical Activity[b] Assessed in 1962/1966 and Updated in 1977

Physical Activity (kcal/wk)	No. of Deaths	Relative Risk[c] (95% CI)
Vigorous activity		
<150	637	1.00 (referent)
150–399	526	0.89 (0.79–1.00)
400–749	215	0.83 (0.71–0.97)
750–1,499	143	0.76 (0.63–0.91)
≥1500	181	0.75 (0.64–0.89)
		P, trend < .001
Nonvigorous activity		
<150	222	1.00 (referent)
150–399	292	0.94 (0.79–1.12)
400–749	343	0.97 (0.82–1.15)
750–1,499	387	0.96 (0.81–1.14)
≥1,500	458	0.89 (0.75–1.04)
		P, trend = .18

[a]Data are from ref. 43. That is, excluding the first 5 yr after each physical activity assessment.
[b]Vigorous, requiring ≥6 METs; nonvigorous, requiring <6 METs.
[c]Adjusted for age, cigarette smoking, hypertension, diabetes mellitus, body mass index, and early parental death. Vigorous and nonvigorous energy expenditure were mutually adjusted. CI, confidence interval.

FIGURE 5.1

Graph of relative risks of all-cause mortality (1967/1971–1977 and 1983–1988, that is, excluding first 5 yr after each physical activity assessment) in the Harvard Alumni Health Study, according to vigorous and nonvigorous physical activity assessed in 1962/1966, and updated in 1977. Vigorous, requiring ≥6 METs; nonvigorous, requiring <6 METs. Data were adjusted for age, cigarette smoking, hypertension, diabetes mellitus, body mass index, and early parental death. Vigorous and nonvigorous energy expenditure were mutually adjusted. Data are from ref. 43.

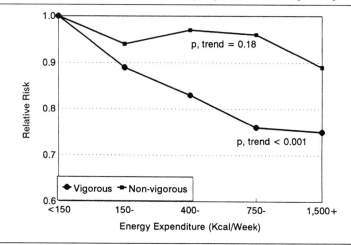

tive risks, 1.00, .89, .83, .76, and .75, respectively; P, trend < .001), while nonvigorous energy expenditure continued to be nonsignificantly related (1.00, .94, .97, .96, and .89, respectively; P, trend = .18).

In a final effort to disentangle the independent associations of the two kinds of energy expenditure with mortality, investigators examined alumni who reported only one kind of activity in 1962/1966. Of the 919 alumni who engaged only in vigorous activities (and no nonvigorous exercise), 259 died between 1962/1966 and 1988. Although numbers for certain categories were small, Table 5.10 shows a marginally significant trend of decreasing age-standardized mortality rates with increasing vigorous energy expenditure (P = .05). Of the 1195 alumni who reported only nonvigorous activity (and no vigorous exercise) in 1962/1966, 380 died during follow-up.Table 5.10 shows nonvigorous energy expenditure and mortality to be not significantly related (P = .99).

Investigators hypothesized that the most likely alternate explanation for the lack of association between nonvigorous energy expenditure and all-cause mortality was less precise accounting of these activities on questionnaire. The resulting misclassification could have obscured a true inverse relation. Dietary differences were unlike to account for findings. Investigators

TABLE 5.10.
Relative Risks of All-Cause Mortality (1962/1966–1988) in the Harvard Alumni Health Study among Men Who Engaged Only in Vigorous or Only in Nonvigorous Physical Activities in 1962/1966

Physical Activity (kcal/wk)	No. of Deaths	Mortality Rate[a] (/10,000)	Relative Risk[a]
Vigorous activity[b]			
<500	197	143.01	1.00 (referent)
500–999	23	134.08	0.94
1000–1499	10	136.08	0.95
1500–1999	6	111.40	0.78
2000–2499	6	66.39	0.46
2500–2999	3	79.70	0.56
3000–3499	5	128.16	0.90
≥3500	9	109.53	0.77
			P,trend = .05
Nonvigorous activity[c]			
<500	156	149.05	1.00 (referent)
500–999	70	155.03	1.04
1000–1499	53	165.72	1.11
1500–1999	25	132.36	0.89
2000–2499	23	176.47	1.18
2500–2999	13	125.36	0.84
3000–3499	10	199.53	1.34
≥3500	30	142.50	0.94

[a]From ref. 43. Age-adjusted.
[b]Requiring ≥6 METs. Among these men, nonvigorous energy expenditure = 0.
[c]Requiring <6 METs. Among these men, vigorous energy expenditure = 0.

did not collect detailed dietary data at baseline or 1977, but did so in 1988. For the subset of alumni who provided dietary information in 1988, estimated total calories consumed increased with increasing total, vigorous, and nonvigorous energy expenditure in 1962/1966. However, the proportion of total calories consumed as fat or saturated fat did not vary across activity categories. Thus, confounding by fat intake was unlikely, assuming that later diet was indicative of earlier habits.

The Alameda County, California, Study (Human Population Laboratory), 1987

In this study, Kaplan et al. [35] were interested in whether factors associated with increased mortality risk among older men and women were the same as those for younger individuals. Investigators used data from the Alameda County Study, a prospective cohort study of the predictors of mortality among a random sample of 6928 adult residents of Alameda County, California.

In this analysis, the investigators restricted the study population to 4174 men and women who were age 38 years or older at baseline, 1965, so that these individuals would be at least age 55 at the end of the 17-year follow-up.

Study subjects completed a questionnaire on demographic, behavioral, social, and psychological characteristics in 1965. Physical activity was assessed, based on frequency and presumed intensity of leisure-time participation in active sports, swimming, long walks, physical exercise, gardening, and hunting and fishing. Based on these data, investigators classified men and women as inactive or active. Subjects were followed for 17 years, until 1982. By that time, 1219 men and women had died. Investigators estimated that the completeness of mortality follow-up among study participants was 90%.

Table 5.11 shows that after adjusting for age, self-reported health status and factors predictive of mortality in this cohort (cigarette smoking, alcohol intake, weight-for-height, hours of sleep, regular breakfast, and snacking), physical inactivity was a significant predictor of mortality among those in the age groups 38–49, 50–59, 60–69, and ≥70 yr. Indeed, when crude survival curves were plotted by age group over the 17 years, the differential in mortality between inactive and active subjects was more marked in the oldest than in the youngest age group.

The Multiple-Risk Factor Intervention Trial (MRFIT), 1987

The MRFIT was a randomized, multicenter primary prevention trial designed to test whether multifactor intervention could reduce coronary heart disease mortality in men, ages 35–57 years, who were at high risk for this disease based on their cigarette habit, diastolic blood pressure, and serum cholesterol [45]. Of the 12,866 men enrolled in the MRFIT cohort, all were free of clinical coronary heart disease at baseline, 1973–1976.

For this study of physical activity and its association with all-cause mortality, investigators enrolled 12,138 men with acceptable data on physical activity. Physical activity was assessed in 1973–1976 using the Minnesota Leisure-Time Physical Activity Questionnaire (a later version of the questionnaire used in the US Railroad Study) [102]. Men were queried regard-

TABLE 5.11.
Relative Risks of All-Cause Mortality (1965–1982) in the Alameda County Study, according to Physical Activity in 1965

Age Group (yr)	Relative Risk,[a] Comparing Inactive with Active Men and Women (95% CI)
38–49	1.48 (1.08–2.02)
50–59	1.27 (0.97–1.66)
60–69	1.38 (1.09–1.75)
≥70	1.37 (1.09–1.72)

[a]Data are from ref. 35. Adjusted for age, self-reported health status, cigarette smoking, alcohol intake, weight for height, hours of sleep, regular breakfast and snacking. CI, confidence interval.

ing the frequency and duration of participation in 62 individual physical activities, per month, over the past year. These activities were considered light (requiring 2–4 kcal/min of energy expenditure), moderate (4.5–5.5 kcal/min) or heavy (≥6.0 kcal/min). Investigators estimated leisure-time physical activity for each person, in minutes per day, as well as in kilocalories expended per day. Based on these data, men were classified into tertiles: Tertile 1 having a mean of 15 min of leisure-time physical activity per day at a cost of 74 kcal; Tertile 2, 47 min and 224 kcal/day; Tertile 3, 134 min and 638 kcal/day. However, investigators did not separate out the energy expended on light-to-moderate activities from that expended on heavy activities. They then followed men for mortality for 6–8 yr, with a mean follow-up period of 7 yr during which 488 men died.

Table 5.12 presents the relative risks for all-cause mortality, adjusted for age, treatment assignment, cigarette smoking, diastolic blood pressure, and blood cholesterol, associated with leisure-time physical activity. The greatest benefit was experienced by men in Tertile 2, with a 27% reduction in mortality risk, when they were compared with subjects in Tertile 1. Meanwhile, the most active men in Tertile 3 had a nonsignificant 13% reduction in mortality. These findings from the MRFIT contrast with the U.S. Railroad Study and the Harvard Alumni Health Study, with respect to the importance of high-intensity physical activity. In the MRFIT, a benefit was observed among men in Tertile 2, who expended energy mainly on light and moderate activities (on average, only 19% of the total daily energy expenditure was spent on heavy activities). In the other two studies, investigators found only intense or vigorous (but not nonintense or nonvigorous) physical activity to be significantly related to decreased mortality.

In an updated analysis of data from the MRFIT, with an average follow-up of 10.5 yr, investigators observed generally similar trends regarding leisure-time physical activity and all-cause mortality [44].

TABLE 5.12.
Rates and Relative Risks of All-Cause Mortality, in a 7-Yr Follow-up of Men in the Multiple-Risk Factor Intervention Trial, according to Leisure-Time Physical Activity in 1973–1976

Leisure-Time Physical Activity	No. of Deaths	Mortality Rate[a] (/1000)	Relative Risk[b] (95% CI)
Tertile 1 (least active)	190	47.7	1.00 (referent)
Tertile 2	138	33.7	0.73 (0.59–0.91)
Tertile 3 (most active)	160	39.5	0.87 (0.70–1.07)

[a]Data are from ref. 45. Age-adjusted.
[b]Adjusted for age, treatment assignment, cigarette smoking, diastolic blood pressure, and blood cholesterol. CI, confidence interval.

Study of Finnish Men, 1987

This group of Finnish men represents yet another cohort belonging to the Seven Countries Study [38]. For the present analysis [74], investigators restricted the study population to 636 healthy Finnish men, ages 45–64 yr at baseline in 1964. Physical activity was assessed at baseline, with men being interviewed regarding their leisure-time and occupational habits. Leisure-time physical activity covered habitual walking, bicycling, and cross-country skiing. Occupational physical activity was classified as sedentary and light (mainly sitting), moderate (e.g., shopkeeping or truck driving), heavy (mainly farming), or very heavy (mainly lumberjacking). Investigators then classified men into two categories of overall physical activity: low (n = 386, 60.7%) or high (n = 250, 39.3%), with the latter category consisting of men whose work involved heavy or very heavy activity and who also walked ≥5 km daily on a regular basis, cycled ≥150 km/mo for ≥6 mo of the year, or cross-country-skied ≥200 km every winter. Men were followed for 20 yr until 1984, with 287 deaths observed. Mortality follow-up was 100% complete.

Investigators first compared men with low and high physical activity, according to cigarette habit, in the first and second 10 yr of follow-up (Table 5.13). (It is unclear as to why they did not provide findings for the subgroup of men who were smokers with low physical activity.) Smoking as expected, increased mortality risk. Physical inactivity was found to predict increased mortality, but only in the first 10 yr of follow-up, with the benefit disappearing in the second 10 yr. This was confirmed when investigators plotted crude survival curves over 20 years for the two physical activity groups. There was a distinct advantage of the high physical activity group for perhaps the first 16 yr, with the two survival curves merging after that. This led investigators to hypothesize that physical activity can reduce premature mortality but cannot extend life span (at the end of the 20-yr follow-up, the oldest of these Finnish men was 85, perhaps close to the life span).

TABLE 5.13.
Relative Risks of All-Cause Mortality (1964–1984) among Finnish Men, according to Physical Activity in 1964

Physical Activity/ Cigarette Habit	Relative Risk[a]	
	1964–1974	*1975–1984*
High activity/nonsmoker	1.00 (referent)	1.00 (referent)
Low activity/nonsmoker	1.35	0.82
High activity/smoker	1.31	1.31

[a]Data are from ref. 74. Adjusted for age, systolic blood pressure, serum cholesterol, and body mass index. Comparing high vs. low physical activity, P = .92; comparing nonsmokers vs. smokers, P = .03.

Investigators also estimated, for men who had died, the additional years lived by men with high physical activity. At baseline, the mean age of men in the low and high physical activity groups was 54.9 and 55.2 yr, respectively. At the end of the 20-yr follow-up, 44.6 and 46.0%, respectively, of men in the low and high physical activity groups had died. Their mean ages at death were 67.4 and 69.1 yr, respectively. After adjustment for differences in age, cigarette smoking, systolic blood pressure, serum cholesterol, and body mass index, the more active men had survived for an additional 2.1 (95% confidence interval, 0.8–3.4) yr.

The Lipid Research Clinics Mortality Follow-up Study, 1988

The original purpose of the Lipid Research Clinics Prevalence Study, conducted between 1972 and 1976, was to describe the lipid profile of men and women from 10 different centers in North America [19]. Participating subjects were examined up to two times (Visit 1, n = 33,800; Visit 2, n = 8,200). Subsequently, investigators started the Lipid Research Clinics Mortality Follow-up Study, examining the relation between factors ascertained at the second visit and later mortality among participants, aged ≥30 yr, who were examined at this visit.

In this study of physical fitness, investigators were interested primarily in cardiovascular disease mortality, but they also provided data on all-cause mortality. They enrolled 3755 white men, 3106 healthy and 649 with cardiovascular disease, ages 30–69 yr at baseline, with valid exercise test data. (Women were excluded because the small number of deaths precluded meaningful analyses.) Physical fitness was assessed at Visit 2, using a submaximal treadmill exercise test, according to a modified Bruce protocol. Men then were classified as unfit or fit, according to the amount of time they spent on the treadmill. Additionally, they were categorized into quartiles of fitness, by heart rate at Stage 2 of the exercise test. Investigators followed men for mortality until 1983 or 1984, an average of 8.5 yr. During this time, 45 fatalities from cardiovascular disease occurred among 3106 healthy men and 46 among 649 men with cardiovascular disease. Number of total deaths was not provided. Mortality follow-up was 99% complete.

Among healthy men, physically unfit men experienced 1.8 times (95% confidence interval, 1.2–2.6) the mortality of fit men during follow-up, after taking into account differences in age, cigarette smoking, systolic blood pressure, and high-density and low-density lipoprotein cholesterol (Table 5.14). For men with preexisting cardiovascular disease, the corresponding relative risk was 2.9 (1.7–4.9). The difference in time on treadmill between unfit and fit men was 4.4 min for the former group, 5.5 min for the latter. For cardiovascular mortality in healthy men, investigators also examined plots of cumulative mortality, adjusted for the variables listed above, according to quartiles of Stage 2 exercise test heart rate. Over the 8.5 yr of follow-up, the curves for the least and most fit men continued to diverge, suggesting that the ben-

TABLE 5.14.
Relative Risks for All-Cause Mortality (1972–1984) in the Lipid Research Clinics Mortality Follow-up Study, according to Physical Fitness in 1972–1976

Physical Fitness	Relative Risk[a] (95% CI)
Healthy men	
High physical fitness	1.0 (referent)
Low physical fitness	1.8 (1.2–2.6)
Men with cardiovascular disease	
High physical fitness	1.0 (referent)
Low physical fitness	2.9 (1.7–4.9)

[a]Data are from ref. 19. Adjusted for age, cigarette smoking, systolic blood pressure, and high-density and low-density lipoprotein cholesterol. CI, confidence interval.

efit of physical fitness was unlikely to be artifactual, resulting from early mortality among men with subclinical illness who were unfit.

The Aerobics Center Longitudinal Study, 1989

This study represents the largest one to date of physical fitness and all-cause mortality [7]. Additionally, it is one of the few studies in this review that included women. For this analysis, investigators enrolled 10,244 men and 3,210 women, ages 20–60 plus yr, who received a preventive medical examination between 1970 and 1981 at the Cooper Institute for Aerobics Research in Dallas, Texas. Subjects were predominantly white and of middle to upper socioeconomic status. As part of their medical examination, men and women underwent a maximal treadmill exercise test. Investigators used total treadmill test time, specific for each sex and age group, to classify subjects into quintiles of physical fitness; then they followed subjects through 1985, or for an average of more than 8 yr, during which 240 men and 43 women died in 110,482 person-yr. Mortality follow-up was 95% complete.

Table 5.15 presents the age-adjusted mortality rates for men and women according to their physical fitness category. There was a strong inverse association between fitness level and all-cause mortality in men. Although the number of deaths was small, the pattern appeared similar in women. The least fit men had more than 3-fold increased risk of mortality than the most fit men, the least fit women more than a 4-fold increase than the least fit women. The largest mortality differential occurred between Quintiles 1 and 2, the two lowest fitness categories. The inverse associations persisted after additional adjustment for cigarette smoking, systolic blood pressure, serum cholesterol, serum glucose, body mass index, and parental history of coronary heart disease. Furthermore, investigators noted the inverse association between physical fitness and mortality to hold within categories of each of these risk factors.

Investigators next estimated the proportion of deaths among study sub-

TABLE 5.15.
Relative Risks of All-Cause Mortality (1970 to 1985) in the Aerobics Center Longitudinal Study, according to Physical Fitness Assessed in 1970 to 1981

Physical Fitness	No. of Deaths	Mortality Rate[a] (/10,000)	Relative Risk[a] (95% CI)
Men			
Quintile 1 (least fit)	75	64.0	3.44 (2.05–5.77)
Quintile 2	40	25.5	1.37 (0.76–2.50)
Quintile 3	47	27.1	1.46 (0.81–2.63)
Quintile 4	43	21.7	1.17 (0.63–2.17)
Quintile 5 (most fit)	35	18.6	1.00 (referent)
Women			
Quintile 1 (least fit)	18	39.5	4.65 (2.22–9.75)
Quintile 2	11	20.5	2.42 (1.09–5.37)
Quintile 3	6	12.2	1.43 (0.60–3.44)
Quintile 4	4	6.5	0.76 (0.27–2.11)
Quintile 5 (most fit)	4	8.5	1.00 (referent)

[a]Data are from ref. 7. Age-adjusted. CI, confidence interval.

jects that might have been averted had all subjects been fit (i.e., belonging to Quintiles 2 to 4, instead of Quintile 1). This figure was 9.0% in men, ranking third after avoidance of high serum cholesterol (11.2%) and having neither parent die from coronary heart disease (10.1%). For women, being physically fit was the most important characteristic, potentially helping to avoid 15.3% of deaths during follow-up.

The Seventh-Day Adventist Mortality Study, 1991

Subjects of the Seventh-Day Adventist Mortality Study [47] comprised 27,530 members of the Seventh-Day Adventist Church in California, who filled out a questionnaire on demographic, medical, and life-style characteristics in 1960. For this analysis of physical activity and all-cause mortality, investigators limited the study population to 9484 men, ages ≥30 yr at baseline. Physical activity at work and during leisure was assessed using a single, multiple-choice question on the baseline questionnaire. Men then were classified as inactive, moderately active, or highly active. Investigators followed men for mortality through 1985, observing 3799 deaths in the 26 yr. Mortality follow-up was more than 93% complete.

Between 1960 and 1985, 798 (38.5%) of 2072 inactive men died, as did 2495 (43.0%) of 5803 moderately active men and 506 (31.4%) of 1609 highly active men. Mean ages at baseline of men in the three groups were 51.6, 54.7, and 49.9 yr, respectively. Table 5.16 shows the association between physical activity and all-cause mortality according to categories of attained age at the end of follow-up or age at death if this occurred. Like men in the MRFIT, moderate physical activity was associated with greater bene-

TABLE 5.16.
Relative Risks of All-Cause Mortality (1960–1985) in the Seventh-Day Adventist Mortality Study, according to Physical Activity Assessed in 1960 and Attained Age

Attained Age[a] (yr)	Relative Risk[b] (95% CI)		
	Inactive	Moderately Active	Highly Active
50	1.00 (referent)	0.61 (0.50–0.74)	0.66 (0.50–0.87)
60	1.00 (referent)	0.68 (0.59–0.78)	0.76 (0.63–0.92)
70	1.00 (referent)	0.76 (0.69–0.83)	0.89 (0.78–1.01)
80	1.00 (referent)	0.85 (0.78–0.92)	1.03 (0.91–1.16)
90	1.00 (referent)	0.94 (0.84–1.06)	1.19 (0.99–1.43)

[a]Data are from ref. 47. Age at the end of follow-up or at death.
[b]Adjusted for race, education, marital status, medical history, cigarette smoking, body mass index, and diet. CI, confidence interval.

fit among Seventh-Day Adventist men than were high levels. Moreover, at higher attained ages, the impact of physical activity on decreased mortality began to disappear. Investigators hypothesized, as did Pekkanen et al. in their study of Finnish men [74], that physical activity served to postpone mortality of Seventh-Day Adventist men but could not extend life span.

Study of Norwegian Men, 1993

Subjects for this study [88] of physical fitness and all-cause mortality were recruited from five companies in Oslo, Norway. A total of 2014 healthy men, ages 40–59 yr, received a medical examination between 1972 and 1975; 54 were excluded because of cardiovascular disease, leaving 1960 men in this analysis. As part of their medical examination, men performed a symptom-limited exercise tolerance test on a bicycle ergometer. Depending on the total work performed, investigators then divided men into quartiles of physical fitness. Men also were questioned about their physical activity. Investigators classified men as inactive or active, with the latter group being those who exercised at least twice per week at an intensity sufficient to produce sweating and shortness of breath or participated in sports competitions (or both). Men were followed until 1989, or for an average of 16 years, during which 271 died. Mortality follow-up was 100% complete.

After adjusting for differences in age, cigarette smoking, systolic blood pressure, blood cholesterol, blood triglyceride, glucose tolerance, vital capacity, resting heart rate, body mass index, and physical activity, men in the most fit quartile had 0.54 times the mortality risk of those in the least fit quartile (Table 5.17). Mortality risks among men in Quartiles 1, 2, and 3, meanwhile, were similar, in contrast to findings from the Aerobics Center Longitudinal Study [7]. Investigators also plotted age-adjusted cumulative mortality over the 16 yr of follow-up. The mortality curves for the least and

TABLE 5.17.
Relative Risks of All-Cause Mortality (1972–1989) among Norwegian Men,
according to Physical Fitness in 1972–1975

Physical Fitness	No. of Deaths	Relative Risk [a] (95% CI)
Quartile 1 (least fit)	106	1.00 (referent)
Quartile 2	77	0.92 (0.66–1.28)
Quartile 3	64	1.00 (0.71–1.41)
Quartile 4 (most fit)	24	0.54 (0.32–0.89)

[a]Data are from ref. 88. Adjusted for age, cigarette smoking, systolic blood pressure, blood cholesterol, blood triglyceride, glucose tolerance, vital capacity, resting heart rate, body mass index, and physical activity. CI, confidence interval.

most fit quartiles continued to diverge over time. Interestingly, for cardiovascular disease mortality, active men did not differ in risk from inactive men, after adjustment for the variables listed above and for physical fitness.

THE ASSOCIATION OF CHANGES IN PHYSICAL ACTIVITY OR PHYSICAL FITNESS WITH AVOIDANCE OF PREMATURE MORTALITY

To date, only two studies have investigated all-cause mortality in relation to changes in physical activity or fitness. With regard to coronary heart disease, Paffenbarger et al. had examined, in an earlier study, the risk of heart attack associated with continuities and changes in physical activity during college and in middle life [71]. Investigators reported on the importance of contemporary physical activity: Only men who continued to be active during their middle years experienced lower risk, regardless of their physical activity status during college years.

The Harvard Alumni Health Study, 1993

The population for this study previously has been described. Briefly, this analysis [64] involved 10,629 Harvard alumni, ages 45–84 yr in 1977, who were free of self-reported, physician-diagnosed cardiovascular disease, diabetes, cancer, and chronic obstructive pulmonary disease then. Men provided information via questionnaires on their physical activities in either 1962 or 1966 (1962/1966) and again in 1977. Based on these data, investigators estimated an index of total energy expenditure for each man, during each of the two times. Furthermore, each reported activity was classified according to intensity [1]. Men were followed from 1977 to 1985, with 476 dying in 90,650 person-yr. Mortality follow-up in this cohort was more than 99% complete.

Table 5.18 examines the association between changes in physical activity

TABLE 5.18.
Rates and Relative Risks of All-Cause Mortality (1977–1985) in the Harvard Alumni Health Study, according to Changes in Physical Activity between 1962/1966 and 1977

Physical Activity	1962/ 1966	1977	No. of Deaths[a]	Mortality Rate[b] (/10,000)	Relative Risk[b] (95% CI)
Energy expenditure	No	No	221	54.6	1.00 (referent)
≥2000 kcal/week	Yes	No	85	60.3	1.10 (0.78–1.50)
	No	Yes	69	46.6	0.85 (0.65–1.13)
	Yes	Yes	83	44.8	0.82 (0.63–1.08)
Activities at	No	No	139	61.7	1.00 (referent)
≥4.5 METs	Yes	No	26	70.7	1.15 (0.73–1.71)
	No	Yes	131	47.4	0.77 (0.58–0.96)
	Yes	Yes	116	43.8	0.71 (0.55–0.96)

[a]Data are from ref. 64. Total number of deaths do not add up to 476 because of missing data.
[b]Adjusted for age, cigarette smoking, hypertension and body mass index. CI, confidence interval.

and all-cause mortality. With respect to energy expenditure, men who changed from being inactive (<2000 kcal/wk) to active (≥2,000 kcal/wk) had about the same mortality rate as men who were active at both time points, with these two rates somewhat lower than that among men who were inactive at both times. Turning to intensity of physical activity, men who did not engage in any moderately vigorous activities (requiring ≥4.5 METs) in 1962/1966 but did so in 1977 had a 23% lower mortality than those who never reported such activities, the difference being statistically significant. Meanwhile, men who habitually engaged in moderately vigorous activities had a 29% lower mortality, which was also statistically significant. These analyses were adjusted for differences in age, cigarette smoking, hypertension, and body mass index. When men of ages 45–54, 55–64, 65–74, and 75–84 yr were examined separately, similar risk reductions for each age group were observed among men taking up moderately vigorous activities, although the reductions were no longer significant because of the smaller number of deaths.

Investigators further estimated added years of life from change in physical activity. For these alumni, ages 45–84 yr in 1977, added years of life to age 85, associated with increasing energy expenditure, was 0.37 yr, amounting to a nonstatistically significant increase. However, taking up moderately vigorous activities added a significant 0.78 yr. To put this into perspective with other predictors of mortality, quitting cigarette smoking added 1.46 yr of life.

Investigators also conducted parallel analyses for the larger group of 14,786 men, that included those with self-reported, physician-diagnosed chronic diseases in 1977 [66]. They then adjusted for the presence of these diseases in analyses. Trends similar to those described here were observed.

The Aerobics Center Longitudinal Study, 1995

The population for the Aerobics Center Longitudinal Study also has been described previously. Extended follow-up of this population [6] has enabled investigators to examine changes in physical fitness in relation to all-cause mortality rates. The present analysis involved 9777 men, ages 20–82 yr, who received two preventive medical examinations between 1970 and 1989. Of these men, 6819 were healthy, whereas 2958 had a variety of chronic conditions (referred to from here on as "unhealthy"). The interval between examinations ranged from 1 to 18 yr, with a mean of 4.9 yr. As described previously, physical fitness was assessed with a maximal treadmill exercise test. Investigators used total treadmill test time from the first examination, specific for each age group, to classify men into quintiles of physical fitness. Because previous findings had shown that mortality among the least fit men was substantially higher than that among men in the second quintile, in this analysis, unfit men were those belonging to Quintile 1; all others were considered fit. Follow-up for mortality occurred after the second examination through 1989, with mean follow-up of 5.1 years. Among healthy men, 103 men died, among those unhealthy, 120 died in a total of 47,561 person yr.

Among all men, the lowest age-adjusted mortality rates occurred among men who were fit at both examinations, whereas the highest rates occurred among those who were unfit at both examinations (Table 5.19). Men who changed in fitness, whether from unfit to fit, or vice versa, experienced intermediate mortality rates that were similar for the two changed groups. Investigators next examined men, ages 20–39, 30–49, 50–69, and ≥60 yr, separately, and observed the same pattern in each age group. They then examined healthy and unhealthy men, separately, and adjusted additionally for baseline fitness level, cigarette smoking, systolic blood pressure, blood cholesterol, glucose tolerance, weight, family history of coronary heart disease, and interval between examinations. For healthy men, each

TABLE 5.19.
Rates and Relative Risks of All-Cause Mortality (1970–1989) in the Aerobics Center Longitudinal Study, according to Changes in Physical Fitness between 1970 and 1989

Physical Fitness		No. of Deaths	Mortality Rate[a] (/10,000)	Relative Risk[a] (95% CI)
1st exam	2nd exam			
Unfit	Unfit	32	122.0	1.00 (referent)
Unfit	Fit	25	67.7	0.56 (0.41–0.75)
Fit	Unfit	9	63.3	0.52 (0.38–0.70)
Fit	Fit	157	39.6	0.33 (0.23–0.47)

[a]Data are from ref. 6. Age-adjusted. CI, confidence interval.

one minute improvement in treadmill test time from the first to the second examination was associated with approximately 10% reduction in mortality, statistically significant, over follow-up. For unhealthy men, the corresponding risk reduction was about 6%; however, that reduction only achieved borderline significance.

Finally, investigators compared the magnitude of benefit associated with favorable changes in various predictors of mortality. After adjusting for the variables listed above, as well as for health status, this magnitude was largest for favorable change in physical fitness (approximately 60% risk reduction), followed by quitting cigarette smoking (approximately 50% risk reduction). Favorable changes in systolic blood pressure, blood cholesterol, or body mass index were not associated with appreciable reductions in risk of dying during follow-up.

DISCUSSION

All of the studies reviewed above describe significant inverse associations between physical activity or physical fitness and all-cause mortality, suggesting that physical activity or fitness may avert premature mortality and enhance longevity. However, because all studies were observational in nature, rather than experimental, cause and effect cannot be assumed [100]. First, we need to ask, are these observations valid? One concern is that a selective process—perhaps genetic—might operate, rendering an individual capable of achieving high levels of physical activity or fitness, as well as favoring him or her with longevity. This argument has been made less cogent by the findings of Paffenbarger et al. and Blair et al. in their studies of changes in physical activity or physical fitness [6, 64, 66, 71]. Paffenbarger et al. [64] found that men who took up moderately vigorous physical activities in midlife experienced mortality rates (47.4/10,000) similar to those of men who consistently engaged in such activities (43.8/10,000). Even more encouraging, this trend was seen even among older men, ages 75–84 yr, who took up moderately vigorous activities in the previous 11–15 yr. Meanwhile, men who stopped these activities fared as badly (70.7/10,000) as those who never undertook such activities (61.7/10,000). Similarly, Blair et al. [6] reported that men who changed, over an average of 4.9 yr, from being physically unfit to fit experienced lower mortality rates (67.7/10,000) than those who remained unfit (122.0/10,000). Men who were consistently fit over that period experienced the lowest mortality rates (39.6/10,000). In light of these data, the argument for a selection process is weakened but not entirely negated, as in the study of Blair et al., the men who changed from being physically fit to unfit experienced mortality rates (63.3/10,000) similar to those of men who changed from being unfit to fit. One could argue, thus, that those consistently unfit were those selected out to be unfit and to suffer premature mortality.

A second bias to consider is that subjects might self-select themselves into the lower spectrum of physical activity because of disability or occult disease, which would result in an artifactual observation of higher mortality among those with little physical activity (and, hence, low physical fitness). With longer follow-up, however, the impact of this bias would be diluted as the force of mortality removes those unhealthy individuals, leaving a cohort of healthy survivors. Most investigators have tried to minimize this bias by studying ostensibly healthy subjects (e.g., those free of cardiovascular disease, the most prevalent chronic condition). Moreover, follow-up typically has been long; apart from the 2-yr follow-up of railroad employees [103], other investigators have followed subjects from 6 [45] to 26 yr [43, 47] for mortality. In the study of changes in physical activity, men were followed for up to 9 yr [64], whereas in the study of changes in fitness, mean follow-up among men was 5 yr [6]. To further circumvent the effect of occult antecedent disease, some investigators have allowed a lag period after physical activity assessment [43] or have examined the association between physical activity and mortality according to segments of follow-up [14, 66, 74, 86].

In prospective cohort studies, findings may be rendered invalid when subjects are lost to follow-up, because this loss may be related to their physical activity or fitness levels. Of the studies reviewed, despite the long follow-up, loss has been minimal, with the lowest rate of follow-up at 90% [35].

Whereas physical fitness may be measured more precisely, it is difficult to assess physical activity with a high degree of precision [41]. Moreover, physical activity patterns are likely to change over time. However, because investigators of the studies discussed above measured physical activity prospectively, any misclassification would have been random (i.e., unrelated to mortality). Thus, this would tend to attenuate the true relation between physical activity and all-cause mortality; that is, the observed reductions in mortality rates associated with physical activity are likely underestimates.

Individuals who exercise, or are physically fit also may differ with respect to other of their health habits [12, 94]. Investigators have attempted to control, in analyses, for confounding by various other predictors of mortality, among them age, cigarette habit, alcohol consumption, body mass index, and family medical history. However, few reports have assessed the impact of dietary habits [35, 43, 47]; in these studies, investigators have continued to note an inverse association between physical activity and all-cause mortality. Other investigators have attempted to account for dietary differences indirectly by adjusting for serum cholesterol levels in analyses [6, 7, 19, 45, 74, 86, 88, 97, 98]. Again, the inverse association between physical activity or fitness and all-cause mortality has persisted in these studies. However, some have argued that a favorable change in lipid profile [27, 111] represents one of the mechanisms through which exercise imparts a beneficial effect towards longevity; thus, serum cholesterol and other lipid parameters should not be controlled for in analyses, because they represent events in the causal pathway [85]. The same argument has been made to explain nonadjustments for blood pressure and glucose tolerance.

After consideration of the issues discussed above, we conclude that the finding of an inverse relation between physical activity or fitness and all-cause mortality is valid. We then need to ask: Is this association one of cause and effect? Several criteria have been suggested to make this evaluation [32, 33]. Certainly, the data appear consistent. The temporal sequence also appears correct: Physical activity or fitness precedes the occurrence of mortality. Issues regarding the strength of the association and dose-response will be discussed later. Perhaps the most important criteria to consider are the coherence and biological plausibility of the association. Available data show that exercise training benefits the cardiovascular system. In rats, physical training induced lower heart rates and increased the resistance of heart muscle to ventricular fibrillation [60, 109]. Monkeys fed an atherogenic diet and exercised fared better than sedentary controls fed the same diet: Their heart rates were lowered, favorable changes in lipid profile occurred, and atherogenic changes in the aorta and other arteries were less severe [39]. Similar benefits are seen in humans: Physical activity increases oxygen supply to the heart, decreases oxygen demand, and improves electrical stability [8, 15, 87]. It also increases collateral coronary artery formation, increases the diameter and dilating capacity of coronary arteries, and reduces the rate of atherosclerotic progression in these arteries [22, 26, 81]. Moreover, physical activity reduces the tendency for platelet aggregation and increases fibrinolytic activity [10, 37, 80]. Physical activity further induces favorable changes in lipid profile, decreases blood pressure, increases insulin sensitivity, and improves glucose tolerance [16, 24, 27, 29, 46, 79, 106, 111].

Whereas the above mechanisms represent favorable events that can stave off mortality from atherosclerotic, hypertensive, and metabolic diseases, physical activity also appears capable of inducing changes in the immune and endocrine systems that can prevent cancer. Data from both animal and human studies consistently show that moderate amounts of physical activity enhance various components of the immune system, including natural killer cells, cytotoxic T lymphocytes, and cells of the monocyte-macrophage system [34, 59, 73, 91, 92, 112, 113]. Because the immune system is responsible for eliminating tumor cells from the body, it is plausible for physical activity to reduce mortality from cancer. Additionally, various hormones are necessary for the development of male and female reproductive cancers [23, 31, 84]. In females, physical activity can delay the onset of menarche, reduce the number of ovulatory cycles, and lower estrogen and progesterone levels, potentially reducing breast cancer incidence and premature mortality from this disease [5, 89, 107]. Similarly, in males, physical training can lower testosterone levels, potentially reducing prostate cancer incidence and mortality [25, 108].

Therefore, we conclude that the inverse relation between physical activity and all-cause mortality is likely to be causal, with the underlying physiological processes appearing highly coherent and plausible. What, then, is the role of physical fitness? As discussed previously, physical activity can modify physical fitness over time. Thus, the biological mechanisms discussed above also should apply for physical fitness. In fact, Slattery and Jacobs found no independent effect of physical activity on all-cause mortality after accounting for physical fitness, leading these investigators to conclude that the benefit of physical activity was mediated entirely by changes in physical fitness [97]. Similarly, for cardiovascular mortality, Sandvik et al. observed no independent effect of physical activity after consideration of physical fitness [88]. However, because physical activity was assessed rather simply in this latter study, the resulting misclassification may have obscured a true inverse association. Not all investigators have concurred: A dissenting result was noted by Lakka et al., when studying acute myocardial infarction [40]. In this study of Finnish men, physical activity was assessed, using the Minnesota Leisure-Time Physical Activity Questionnaire [102]; physical fitness was assessed, using a maximal, symptom-limited exercise tolerance test on a bicycle ergometer. Investigators found both physical activity and physical fitness to predict lower risk of this disease independently.

What is the magnitude of benefit conferred by physical activity or fitness on all-cause mortality? Comparing those most active or fit with those least so, mortality rates have been found to be 17 [98] to 78% lower [7] among most active or fit individuals, with most investigators observing death rates that were, perhaps, between a quarter and one-half lower. This magnitude translates to a benefit that is on par with other established predictors of mortality. The difference in mortality rates is comparable, approximately, to that between nonsmokers and smokers and between persons of ideal weight and those 20% heavier [7, 43, 62]. Looked at from another perspective, middle-aged individuals might expect to gain, on average, some 2 yr of life from being physically active [62, 74]. However, physical activity does not appear to extend life span; its benefit appears to come from postponing mortality (i.e., from making the survival curve more rectangular) [47, 74]. It is encouraging to note that even older individuals do benefit from a physically active life [35, 62]. Among men and women of ages ≥70 yr who were followed for 17 yr, physical activity was associated with a 27% decreased risk of dying [35], whereas among men of ages 75–79 yr, Paffenbarger et al. estimated that an additional 0.42 yr might be gained, to age 80, from being active [62].

Most studies indicate a dose-response relation: The higher the level of physical activity or fitness, the lower the mortality rate. However, data from the MRFIT and the Seventh-Day Adventist Study suggest a threshold effect for physical activity [45, 47], whereas the findings of Blair et al. and Sandvik et al. suggest a threshold effect for physical fitness [7, 88]. In the first two studies, moderate levels of physical activity were associated with the lowest mortality rates; men with higher activity levels did not benefit as much.

Meanwhile, Blair et al. observed mortality rates to decline sharply from the least fit quintile to the second quintile of men, with little additional benefit seen thereafter. Among women, based on small numbers, a dose-response was more evident. In contrast, Sandvik et al. noted that only the most fit quartile of men experienced lower mortality rates than the least fit quartile; little benefit was seen among men in the second and third quartiles. Is there a limit beyond which physical activity proves hazardous? Paffenbarger et al. found mortality rates to climb beyond 3000 kcal/wk [62]; however, in an updated analysis of this same cohort of men, mortality rates continued to decline at ≥3500 kcal/wk [64]. In a study of British men, Shaper and Wannamethee observed that for healthy men, heart attack risk among the most active men was significantly higher than that among men with moderate physical activity [90]. Thus, the question of whether an upper threshold for benefit from physical activity exists remains unresolved.

Only three of the studies reviewed included women as subjects [7, 35, 86]. Based on these limited data, it appears that, qualitatively, there are no marked differences between the sexes. Further research focusing on women is needed. Moreover, available data have been collected almost exclusively in white populations. This shortcoming urgently needs to be rectified.

Of public health significance is this question: What physical activity regimen should we recommend in order to enhance longevity? Unfortunately, the answer evades us for the present. Few studies have investigated which kinds (intensities) of physical activity may be best. We know even less regarding the optimum frequency and duration of physical activity. With respect to exercise intensity, Slattery et al. found that only intense physical activities significantly decreased mortality rates among railroad workers [98]. Light-to-moderate physical activities were not significantly predictive of lower mortality. Similarly, Lee et al. observed that only vigorous activities apt to require ≥6 METs were associated with decreased all-cause mortality in Harvard alumni [43]. Nonvigorous activities requiring >6 METs were not significantly related to mortality. For coronary heart disease, Morris et al. also noted that only vigorous sporting activities, but not other kinds of activities, decreased risk in British civil servants [54, 56]. Meanwhile, Lakka et al. [40] reported decreased risk of myocardial infarction only among Finnish men engaging in conditioning types of physical activity (with mean intensity of 6 METs). Nonconditioning physical activity (mean intensity, 3.6 METs) and walking or bicycling to work (mean intensity, 4.0 METs) were not significantly associated with reduced risk. A dissenting view was offered by Leon et al. [45]: In the MRFIT, an inverse relation was seen between physical activity and all-cause mortality, even though men engaged primarily in light-to-moderate physical activities only. However, in this latter study, investigators did not separate the energy expended on light-to-moderate activities from that expended on heavy activities.

In view of the many sedentary adults living in the United States today [93], it seems sensible, as an initial step, to adopt this recommendation from the Centers for Disease Control and Prevention and the American College of Sports Medicine [72]: "Every U.S. adult should accumulate 30 minutes or more of moderate-intensity physical activity on most, preferably all, days of the week." Because available data indicate a dose-response relation and because several studies suggest that intense or vigorous activities are more beneficial, we further propose, as the next step, that healthy persons should proceed to engage in more intense activities. Of course, we recognize that there are those—for example, the infirm and the old—for whom that next step is ill advised, and the guidelines for exercise prescription drawn up by the American College of Sports Medicine and the American Heart Association should be followed [2, 21]. We emphasize the importance of gradually increasing the amount (intensity and duration) of physical activity, because high-intensity activities can precipitate acute myocardial infarction, with the risk especially severe among those habitually sedentary [51, 95, 104,110].

CONCLUSION

Physical activity, as well as physical fitness, is inversely related to all-cause mortality in men and women. This association is likely to be causal; moreover, there appears to be a dose-response relation. The most active or fit individuals experience mortality rates that are, perhaps, one-quarter to one-half lower than the rates among those least active or fit. Expressed differently, among middle-aged persons, approximately 2 yr of life, on average, may be gained from being physically active. The benefit of physical activity appears to be from averting premature mortality, rather than extending life span. It remains unclear what kinds of physical activity may be most beneficial, although several studies suggest it to be intense or vigorous physical activity, rather than light-to-moderate or nonvigorous activity. Further research is needed to determine optimum frequency and duration of physical activity and to ascertain whether an upper limit to the benefit of physical activity exists. Also, data on women and minority populations need to be expanded.

ACKNOWLEDGMENTS

Dr. Lee was supported in part by National Institutes of Health Grants CA47988, HL43851 and HL 34174. Dr. Paffenbarger was supported in part by National Institutes of Health Grant HL 34174.

REFERENCES

1. Ainsworth, B. E., W. L. Haskell, A. S. Leon, et al. Compendium of physical activities: Classification of energy costs of human physical activities. *Med. Sci. Sports Exerc.* 25:71–80, 1993.

2. American College of Sports Medicine. *Guidelines for Exercise Testing and Prescription*, 4th Ed. Philadelphia: Lea & Febiger, 1991.
3. Berlin, J. A., and G. A. Colditz. A meta-analysis of physical activity in the prevention of coronary heart disease. *Am. J. Epidemiol.* 132:612–628, 1990.
4. Bernstein, L., B. E. Henderson, R. Hanisch, J. Sullivan-Halley, and R. K. Ross. Physical exercise and reduced risk of breast cancer in young women. *J. Natl. Cancer Inst.* 86:1403–1408, 1994.
5. Bernstein, L., R. K. Ross, R. A. Lobo, R. Hanisch, M. D. Krailo, and B. E. Henderson. The effects of moderate physical activity on menstrual cycle patterns in adolescence: implications for breast cancer prevention. *Br. J. Cancer.* 55:681–685, 1987.
6. Blair, S. N., H. W. Kohl III, C. E. Barlow, R. S. Paffenbarger, Jr., L. W. Gibbons, and C. E. Macera. Changes in physical fitness and all-cause mortality: a prospective study of healthy and unhealthy men. *J.A.M.A.* 273:1093–1098, 1995.
7. Blair, S. N., H. W. Kohl III, R. S. Paffenbarger, Jr., D. G. Clark, K. H. Cooper, and L. W. Gibbons. Physical fitness and all-cause mortality: a prospective study of healthy men and women. *J.A.M.A.* 262:2395–2401, 1989.
8. Blomqvist, C. G., and B. Saltin. Cardiovascular adaptations to physical training. *Annu. Rev. Physiol.* 45:169–189, 1983.
9. Bouchard, C., and R. J. Shephard. Physical activity, fitness, and health: the model and key concepts. C. Bouchard, R. J. Shephard, and T. Stephens (eds). *Physical Activity, Fitness, and Health: International Proceedings and Consensus Statement.* Champaign, IL: Human Kinetics, 1994, pp. 77–88.
10. Bourey, R.E., and S. A. Santoro. Interactions of exercise, coagulation, platelets, and fibrinolysis: a brief review. *Med. Sci. Sports Exerc.* 20:439–446, 1988.
11. Brand, R. J., R. S. Paffenbarger, Jr., R. I. Sholtz, and J. B. Kampert. Work activity and fatal heart attacks studied by multiple logistic risk analysis. *Am. J. Epidemiol.* 110:52–62, 1979.
12. Buring, J. E., and I-M. Lee. Confounding in epidemiologic research. *Am. J. Public Health* 82:164–165, 1995.
13. Caspersen, C. J., K. E. Powell, and G. M. Christenson. Physical activity, exercise, and physical fitness: definitions and distinctions for health-related research. *Public Health Rep.* 100:126–131, 1985.
14. Chave, S. P. W., J. N. Morris, S. Moss, and A. M. Semmence. Vigorous exercise in leisure time and the death rate: a study of male civil servants. *J. Epidemiol. Community Health* 32:239–243, 1978.
15. Clausen, J. P. Effect of physical training on cardiovascular adjustments to exercise in man. *Physiol. Rev.* 57:779–815, 1977.
16. Deprés, J. P., and B. Lamarche. Low-intensity endurance exercise training, plasma lipoproteins and the risk of coronary heart disease. *J. Intern. Med.* 236:7–22, 1994.
17. Drinkwater, B. L. Physical activity, fitness, and osteoporosis. C. Bouchard, R. J. Shephard, and T. Stephens (eds). *Physical Activity, Fitness, and Health: International Proceedings and Consensus Statement.* Champaign, IL: Human Kinetics, 1994, pp. 724–736.
18. Dublin, L. I. *Statistical Bulletin.* NY: Metropolitan Life Insurance, August 1932, pp. 5–7.
19. Ekelund, L.-G.,W. L. Haskell, J. L. Johnson, F. S. Whaley, M. H. Criqui, and D. S. Sheps. Physical fitness as a predictor of cardiovascular mortality in asymptomatic North American men: The Lipid Research Clinics Mortality Follow-up Study. *N. Engl. J. Med.* 319:1379–1384, 1988.
20. Fagard, R. H., and C. M. Tipton. Physical activity, fitness, and hypertension. C. Bouchard, R. J. Shephard, and T. Stephens (eds). *Physical Activity, Fitness, and Health: International Proceedings and Consensus Statement.* Champaign, IL: Human Kinetics, 1994, pp. 633–655.
21. Fletcher, G. F., S. N. Blair, J. Blumenthal, et al. Statement on exercise. Benefits and recommendations for physical activity programs for all Americans: A statement for health professionals by the Committee on Exercise and Cardiac Rehabilitation of the Council on Clinical Cardiology, American Heart Association. *Circulation* 86:340–344, 1992.

22. Fuster, V., L. Badimon, J. J. Badimon, and J. H. Chesebro. The pathogenesis of coronary artery disease and the acute coronary syndromes. *N. Engl. J. Med.* 326:242–250, 310–318, 1992.

23. Gittes, R. F. Carcinoma of the prostate. *N. Engl. J. Med.* 324:236–245, 1991.

24. Gordon, D. J., and B. M. Rifkind. High-density lipoprotein—The clinical implications of recent studies. *N. Engl. J. Med.* 321:1311–1316, 1989.

25. Hackney, A.C., W. E. Sinning, and B. C. Bruot. Reproductive hormonal profiles of endurance-trained and untrained males. *Med. Sci. Sports Exerc.* 20:60–65, 1988.

26. Hambrecht, R., J. Niebauer, C. Marburger, et al. Various intensities of leisure time physical activity in patients with coronary artery disease: effects on cardiorespiratory fitness and progression of coronary atherosclerotic lesions. *J. Am. Coll. Cardiol.* 22:468–477, 1993.

27. Hardman, A. E., A. Hudson, P. R. M. Jones, and N. G. Norgan. Brisk walking and plasma high-density lipoprotein cholesterol concentration in previously sedentary women. *Br. Med. J.* 299:1204–1205, 1989.

28. Hartley, P. H. S., and G. F. Llewellyn. The longevity of oarsmen: a study of those who rowed in the Oxford and Cambridge boat race from 1829–1928. *Br. Med. J.* 1:657–662, 1939.

29. Haskell, W. L. Exercise-induced changes in plasma lipids and lipoproteins. *Prev. Med.* 13:23–36, 1984.

30. Helmrich, S. P., D. R. Ragland, R. W. Leung, and R. S. Paffenbarger, Jr. Physical activity and reduced occurrence of non-insulin-dependent diabetes mellitus. *N. Engl. J. Med.* 325:147–152, 1991.

31. Henderson, B. E., R. K. Ross, and M. C. Pike. Hormonal chemoprevention of cancer in women. *Science* 259:633–638, 1993.

32. Hennekens, C. H., and J. E. Buring. *Epidemiology in Medicine*. Boston: Little, Brown, 1987, pp. 30–53.

33. Hill, A. B. The environment and disease: association or causation? *Proc. R. Soc. Med.* 58:295–300, 1965.

34. Hoffman-Goetz, L. Exercise, natural immunity, and tumor metastasis. *Med. Sci. Sports Exerc.* 26:157–163, 1994.

35. Kaplan, G. A., T. E. Seeman, R. D. Cohen, L. P. Knudsen, and J. Guralnik. Mortality among the elderly in the Alameda County Study: Behavioral and demographic risk factors. *Am. J. Public Health* 77:307–312, 1987.

36. Karvonen, M. J. Endurance sports, longevity, and health. *Ann. N.Y. Acad. Sci.* 301:653–655, 1977.

37. Kestin, A. S., P. A. Ellis, M. R. Barnard, A. Errichetti, B. A. Rosner, and A. D. Michelson. Effect of strenuous exercise on platelet activation state and reactivity. *Circulation* 88:1502–1511, 1993.

38. Keys, A. *Seven Countries: A Multivariate Analysis of Death and Coronary Heart Disease*. Cambridge, MA: Harvard University Press, 1980.

39. Kramsch, D. M., A. J. Aspen, B. M. Abramowitz, T. Kreimendahl, and W. B. Hood, Jr. Reduction of coronary atherosclerosis by moderate conditioning exercise in monkeys on an atherogenic diet. *N. Engl. J. Med.* 305:1483–1489, 1981.

40. Lakka, T. A., J. M. Venalainen, R. Rauramaa, R. Salonen, J. Tuomilehto, and J. T. Salonen. Relation of leisure-time physical activity and cardiorespiratory fitness to the risk of acute myocardial infarction in men. *N. Engl. J. Med.* 330:1549–1554, 1994.

41. LaPorte, R. E., H. J. Montoye, and C. J. Caspersen. Assessment of physical activity in epidemiologic research: Problems and prospects. *Public Health Rep.* 100:131–145, 1985.

42. Lee, I-M. Physical activity, fitness, and cancer. C. Bouchard, R. J. Shephard, and T. Stephens (eds). *Physical Activity, Fitness, and Health: International Proceedings and Consensus Statement*. Champaign, IL: Human Kinetics, 1994, pp. 814–831.

43. Lee, I-M, C.-c. Hsieh, and R. S. Paffenbarger, Jr. Exercise intensity and longevity in men: The Harvard Alumni Health Study. *J.A.M.A.* 273:1179–1184, 1995.

44. Leon, A. S., and J. Connett, for the MRFIT Research Group. Physical activity and 10.5 year mortality in the Multiple Risk Factor Intervention Trial (MRFIT). *Int. J. Epidemiol.* 20:690–697, 1991.

45. Leon, A. S., J. Connett, D. R. Jacobs, Jr., and R. Rauramaa. Leisure-time physical activity levels and risk of coronary heart disease and death: The Multiple Risk Factor Intervention Trial. *J.A.M.A.* 258:2388–2395, 1987.

46. Lie, H., R. Mundal, and J. Erikssen. Coronary risk factors and incidence of coronary death in relation to physical fitness: Seven-year follow-up study of middle-aged and elderly men. *Eur. Heart J.* 6:147–157, 1985.

47. Lindsted, K. D., S. Tonstad, and J. W. Kuzma. Self-report of physical activity and patterns of mortality in Seventh-Day Adventist men. *J. Clin. Epidemiol.* 44:355–364, 1991.

48. Lyons, A. S., and R. J. Petrucelli. *Medicine: An Illustrated History.* New York: Harry N. Abrams, pp. 130, 195–203, 1978.

49. Manson, J. E., and D. M. Nathan, A. S. Krolewski, M. J. Stampfer, W. C. Willett, and C. H. Hennekens. A prospective study of exercise and incidence of diabetes among U.S. male physicians. *J.A.M.A.* 268:63–67, 1992.

50. Manson, J. E., E. B. Rimm, M. J. Stampfer, et al. Physical activity and incidence of non-insulin-dependent diabetes mellitus in women. *Lancet* 338:774–778, 1991.

51. Mittleman, M. A., M. Maclure, G. H. Tofler, J. B. Sherwood, R. J. Goldberg, and J. E. Muller. Triggering of acute myocardial infarction by heavy physical exertion: protection against triggering by regular exertion. *N. Engl. J. Med.* 329:1677–1683, 1993.

52. Morgan, J. E. *University Oars.* London: MacMillan and Co., pp 1–126, 1873.

53. Morris, J. N., S. P. W. Chave, C. Adam, C. Sirey, L. Epstein, and D. J. Sheehan. Vigorous exercise in leisure-time and the incidence of coronary heart-disease. *Lancet* 1:333–339, 1973.

54. Morris, J. N., D. G. Clayton, M. G. Everitt, A. M. Semmence, and E. H. Burgess. Exercise in leisure-time: coronary attack and death rates. *Br. Heart J.* 63:325–334, 1990.

55. Morris, J. N., and M. D. Crawford. Coronary heart disease and physical activity of work: evidence of a national necropsy survey. *Br. Med. J.* 2:1485–1496, 1958.

56. Morris, J. N., M. G. Everitt, R. Pollard, S. P. W. Chave, and A. M. Semmence. Vigorous exercise in leisure-time: protection against coronary heart disease. *Lancet* 2:1207–1210, 1980.

57. Morris, J. N., J. A. Heady, P. A. B. Raffle, C. G. Roberts, and J. W. Parks. Coronary heart-disease and physical activity of work. I. Coronary heart-disease in different occupations. *Lancet* 2:1053–1057, 1953.

58. Morris, J. N., J. A. Heady, P. A. B. Raffle, C. G. Roberts, and J. W. Parks. Coronary heart-disease and physical activity of work. II. Statement and testing of provisional hypothesis. *Lancet* 2:1111–1120, 1953.

59. Nieman, D. C. Exercise, upper respiratory tract infection, and the immune system. *Med. Sci. Sports Exerc.* 26:128–139, 1994.

60. Noakes, T. D., L. Higginson, and L. H. Opie. Physical training increases ventricular fibrillation thresholds of isolated rat hearts during normoxia, hypoxia, and regional ischemia. *Circulation* 67:24–30, 1983.

61. Paffenbarger, R. S., Jr., and W. E. Hale. Work activity and coronary heart mortality. *N. Engl. J. Med.* 292:545–550, 1975.

62. Paffenbarger, R. S., Jr., R. T. Hyde, A. L. Wing, and C.-c. Hsieh. Physical activity, all-cause mortality, and longevity of college alumni. *N. Engl. J. Med.* 314:605–613, 1986.

63. Paffenbarger, R. S., Jr., R. T. Hyde, A. L. Wing, and C.-c. Hsieh. Physical activity and longevity of college alumni. *N. Engl. J. Med.* 315:400–401, 1986.

64. Paffenbarger, R. S., Jr., R. T. Hyde, A. L. Wing, I-M. Lee, D. L. Jung, and J. B. Kampert. The association of changes in physical activity level and other lifestyle characteristics with mortality among men. *N. Engl. J. Med.* 328:538–545, 1993.

65. Paffenbarger, R. S., Jr., R. T. Hyde, A. L. Wing, and C. H. Steinmetz. A natural history of athleticism and cardiovascular health. *J.A.M.A.* 252:491–495, 1984.

66. Paffenbarger, R. S., Jr., J. B. Kampert, I-M. Lee, R. T. Hyde, R. W. Leung, and A. L. Wing. Changes in physical activity and other lifeway patterns influencing longevity. *Med. Sci. Sports. Exerc.* 26:857–865, 1994.

67. Paffenbarger, R. S., Jr., M. E. Laughlin, A. S. Gima, and R. A. Black. Work activity of longshoremen as related to death from coronary heart disease and stroke. *N. Engl. J. Med.* 282:1109–1114, 1970.

68. Paffenbarger, R. S., Jr., J. Notkin, D. E. Krueger, et al. Chronic disease in former college students. II. Methods of study and observations on mortality from coronary heart disease. *Am. J. Public Health* 56:962–971; 1966.

69. Paffenbarger, R. S., Jr., and A. L. Wing. Chronic disease in former college students. X. The effects of single and multiple characteristics on risk of fatal coronary heart disease. *Am. J. Epidemiol.* 90:527–535, 1969.

70. Paffenbarger, R. S., Jr., P. A. Wolf, J. Notkin, and M. C. Thorne. Chronic disease in former college students. I. Early precursors of fatal coronary heart disease. *Am. J. Epidemiol.* 83:314–328, 1966.

71. Paffenbarger, R. S., Jr., A. L. Wing, and R. T. Hyde. Physical activity as an index of heart attack risk in college alumni. *Am. J. Epidemiol.* 108:161–175, 1978.

72. Pate, R. R., M. Pratt, S. N. Blair, et al. Physical activity and public health: A recommendation from the Centers for Disease Control and Prevention and the American College of Sports Medicine. *J.A.M.A.* 273:402–407, 1995.

73. Pedersen, B. K., and H. Ullum. NK cell response to physical activity: possible mechanisms of action. *Med. Sci. Sports. Exerc.* 26:140–146, 1994.

74. Pekkanen, J., B. Marti, A. Nissinen, J. Tuomilehto, S. Punsar, and M. Karvonen. Reduction of premature mortality by high physical activity: a 20-year follow-up of middle-aged Finnish men. *Lancet* 1:1473–1477, 1987.

75. Pomeroy, W. C., and P. D. White. Coronary heart disease in former football players. *J.A.M.A.* 167:711–714, 1958.

76. Powell, K. E., P. D.Thompson, C. J. Caspersen, and J. S. Kendrick. Physical activity and the incidence of coronary heart disease. *Annu. Rev. Public Health* 8:253–287, 1987.

77. Prout C. Life expectancy of college oarsmen. *J.A.M.A.* 220:1709–1711, 1972.

78. Ramazzini, B. *DeMorbis Artificum Diatriba.* (The Latin text of 1713, revised with translation and notes by Wright, W. C.) *Diseases of Workers.* Chicago: University of Chicago Press, 1940, pp. 281–285, 295–301.

79. Rauramaa, R. Relationship of physical activity, glucose tolerance and weight management. *Prev. Med.* 13:37–46, 1984.

80. Rauramaa, R., J. T. Salonen, K. Kukkonen-Harjula, et al. Effects of mild physical exercise on serum lipoproteins and metabolites of arachidonic acid: a controlled randomized trial in middle-aged men. *Br. Med. J.* 288:603–606, 1984.

81. Richardson, P. D., M. J. Davies, and G. V. R. Born. Influence of plaque configuration and stress distribution on fissuring of coronary atherosclerotic plaques. *Lancet* 2:941–944, 1989.

82. Robinson, R. S. *Sources for the History of Greek Athletics.* Chicago, IL: Area Publishers Inc., pp 191–197, 1955.

83. Rook, A. An investigation into the longevity of Cambridge sportsmen. *Br. Med. J.* 1:773–777, 1954.

84. Ross, R., L. Bernstein, H. Judd, R. Hanisch, M. Pike, and B. Henderson. Serum testosterone levels in healthy and young black and white men. *J. Natl. Cancer Inst.* 76:45–48, 1986.

85. Rothman, K. J. *Modern Epidemiology.* Boston: Little, Brown, 1986, pp. 77–97.

86. Salonen, J. T., P. Puska, and J. Tuomilehto. Physical activity and risk of myocardial infarction, cerebral stroke and death: a longitudinal study in Eastern Finland. *Am. J. Epidemiol.* 115:526–537, 1982.

87. Saltin, B. Cardiovascular and pulmonary adaptation of physical activity. C. Bouchard, R. J. Shephard, T. Stephens, J. R. Sutton, and B. D. McPherson (eds). *Exercise, Fitness, and Health: A Consensus of Current Knowledge.* Champaign, IL: Human Kinetics, 1990, pp. 187–203.

88. Sandvik, L., J. Erikssen, E. Thaulow, G. Erikssen, R. Mundal, and K. Rodahl. Physical fitness as a predictor of mortality among healthy, middle-aged Norwegian men. *N. Engl. J. Med.* 328:533–537, 1993.

89. Shangold, M. M. Exercise and the adult female: hormonal and endocrine effects. *Exerc. Sport Sci. Rev.* 12:53–79, 1984.

90. Shaper, A. G., G. Wannamethee, and R. Weatherall. Physical activity and ischaemic heart disease in middle-aged British men. *Br. Heart. J.* 66:384–394, 1991.

91. Shephard, R. J., T. J. Verde, S. G. Thomas, and P. Shek. Physical activity and the immune system. *Can. J. Sport Sci.* 16:169–185, 1991.

92. Shephard, R. J., S. Rhind, and P. N. Shek. The impact of exercise on the immune system: NK cells, interleukins 1 and 2, and related responses. *Exerc. Sport Sci. Rev.* 23:215–241, 1995.

93. Siegel, P. Z., R. M. Brackbill, E. L. Frazier, P. Mariolis, L. M. Sanderson and M. N. Waller. Behavioral Risk Factor Surveillance, 1986–1990. *M.M.W.R. Morb. Mortal. Wkly. Rep.* 40(SS–4):1–23, 1991.

94. Simoes, E. J., T. Byers, R. J. Coates, M. J. Serdula, A. H. Mokdad, and G. W. Heath. The association between leisure-time physical activity and dietary fat in American adults. *Am. J. Public Health* 85:240–244, 1995.

95. Siscovick, D. S., N. S. Weiss, R. H. Fletcher, and T. Lasky. The incidence of primary cardiac arrest during vigorous exercise. *N. Engl. J. Med.* 311:874–877, 1984.

96. Sivertsen, I., and A. W. Dahlstrom. The relation of muscular activity to carcinoma: a preliminary report. *J. Cancer. Res.* 6:365–378, 1922.

97. Slattery, M. L., and D. R. Jacobs, Jr. Physical fitness and cardiovascular disease mortality: the US Railroad Study. *Am. J. Epidemiol.* 127:571–580, 1988.

98. Slattery, M. L., D. R. Jacobs, Jr., and M. Z. Nichaman. Leisure time physical activity and coronary heart disease death: The US Railroad Study. *Circulation* 79:304–311, 1989.

99. Smith, E. Report on the sanitary conditions of tailors in London. *Report of the Medical Officer.* London: The Privy Council, 1864, pp. 416–430.

100. Smith, G. D., A. N. Phillips, and J. D. Neaton. Smoking as "independent" risk factor for suicide: illustration of an artifact from observational epidemiology? *Lancet* 340:709–712, 1992.

101. Sternfeld, B. Cancer and the protective effect of physical activity: the epidemiological evidence. *Med. Sci. Sports Exerc.* 24:1195–1209, 1992.

102. Taylor, H. L., D. R. Jacobs, B. Schucker, J. Knudsen, A. S. Leon, and G. DeBacker. A questionnaire for the assessment of leisure-time physical activities. *J. Chronic Dis.* 31:741–755, 1978.

103. Taylor, H. L., E. Klepetar, A. Keys, W. Parlin, H. Blackburn, and T. Puchner. Death rates among physically active and sedentary employees of the railroad industry. *Am. J. Public Health* 52:1697–1707, 1962.

104. Thompson, P. D., E. J. Funk, R. A. Carleton, and W. Q. Sturner. Incidence of death during jogging in Rhode Island from 1975 through 1980. *J.A.M.A.* 247:2535–2538, 1982.

105. Thorne, M. C., A. L. Wing, and R. S. Paffenbarger, Jr. Chronic disease in former college students. VII. Early precursors of nonfatal coronary heart disease. *Am. J. Epidemiol.* 87:520–529, 1968.

106. Tipton, C. M. Exercise, training, and hypertension: an update. *Exerc. Sport Sci. Rev.* 19:447–505, 1991.

107. Warren, M. P. The effects of exercise on pubertal progression and reproductive function in girls. *J. Clin. Endocrinol. Metab.* 51:1150–1157, 1980.

108. Wheeler, G. D., S. R. Wall, A. N. Belcastro, and D. C. Cumming. Reduced serum testosterone and prolactin levels in male distance runners. *J.A.M.A.* 252:514–516, 1984.

109. Williams, R. S., T. F. Schaible, T. Bishop, and M. Morey. Effects of endurance training on cholinergic and adrenergic receptors of the rat heart. *J. Mol. Cell Cardiol.* 16:395–403, 1984.

110. Willich, S. N., M. Lewis, H. Löwel, H.-R. Arntz, F. Schubert, and R. Schröder. Physical exertion as a trigger of acute myocardial infarction. *N. Engl. J. Med.* 329:1684–1690, 1993.
111. Wood, P. D., M. L. Stefanick, P. T. Williams, and W. L. Haskell. The effects on plasma lipoproteins of a prudent weight-reducing diet, with or without exercise, in overweight men and women. *N. Engl. J. Med.* 325:461–466, 1991.
112. Woods, J. A., and J. M. Davis. Exercise, monocyte/macrophage function, and cancer. *Med. Sci. Sports Exerc.* 26:147–156, 1994.
113. Woods, J. A., J. M. Davis, M. L. Kohut, A. Ghaffar, E. P. Mayer, and R. P. Pate. Effects of exercise on the immune response to cancer. *Med. Sci. Sports Exerc.* 26:1109–1115, 1994.

6
Force-Sharing Among Synergistic Muscles: Theoretical Considerations and Experimental Approaches

W. HERZOG

The determination of the forces generated by individual muscles during voluntary movements has become one of the primary research topics in biomechanics since the pioneering works of Seireg and Arvikar [97, 98] and Penrod et al. [87, 88] in the early 1970s. From an engineering or biomedical engineering point of view, knowledge of the forces exerted by muscles is important, because muscles are believed to contribute more to the loading of skeletal structures, particularly joints, than other forces, such as inertial forces or forces transmitted by ligaments. Also, muscles are the primary producers of moments about joints and, therefore, are the primary creators of movement. Knowledge of the force-time histories of muscles crossing a joint is not only of interest from the point of view of mechanics but also from the point of view of physiology and movement control. Knowing the forces in muscles at any instant in time during a specific movement is like having a window to the central nervous system and its organization and control of movement.

Individual muscle forces may be determined theoretically or experimentally. Theoretically, most force predictions have been performed using optimization theory [15, 17, 18, 25, 26, 48, 86, 88, 98], except for cases in which muscles were grouped into functional units [78, 79, 84] and/or cases in which only a select number of muscles (for example, the prime movers of a system) were considered. Experimentally, individual muscle forces have been determined in many animal models, either by fixing force transducers to the target tendon [9, 63, 109] or within the target tendon [19, 114], or to the bone at or near the attachment site of the target muscle [23]. Also, muscle forces have been estimated experimentally, using a variety of approaches other than direct-force measurements, with estimation of muscle forces from electromyogram (EMG) signals probably the most popular method [40, 65, 83, 107].

Crowninshield and Brand [17] summarized the research on individual muscle force estimates nearly 15 years ago. Although their work was motivated by predicting the forces in joint structures (muscles/tendons, ligaments, and bones), their discussion was centered almost exclusively around the determination of muscle forces, because they, like many others, recognized that joint moments are produced primarily by muscle forces; the possible contributions of ligament and bony contact forces to the resultant joint moments were assumed to be small and were essentially ignored in their considerations. At the end of their comprehensive review, Crowninshield and Brand [17] summarized the present shortcomings (as of 1981) of the techniques used to predict forces in joint structures, particularly in muscles. These shortcomings included: 1) a lack of quantitative measures of the anatomy of the musculoskeletal system; 2) the neglect of physiological knowledge for the prediction of muscle forces; 3) an insufficient effort to validate the theoretical predictions of (muscle) forces; 4) the neglect of EMGs as quantitative tools for estimating muscle forces; and 5) the lack of inquiry into methods of validating the predicted (muscle) forces.

This chapter will address the shortcomings mentioned by Crowninshield and Brand [17]; its aim is to assess the progress in research on individual muscle force predictions since 1981 and to evaluate critically the present state of knowledge in this area.

THEORETICAL CONSIDERATIONS

Force-sharing among synergistic muscles is defined here as the distribution of forces among synergistic muscles at any given instant in time. For a movement extending over a finite time period, force-sharing refers to the force-time histories of the individual muscles over the time period of the movement of interest. Therefore, the force sharing between two muscles may be expressed as $f_1 = (g(f_2)$, where f_1 and f_2 are the force magnitudes of Muscles 1 and 2, respectively, and g is a variable (possibly of a functional nature) relating f_1 and f_2.

In this part of the chapter, I will concentrate on the theoretical aspects of force sharing among muscles. For many of the parts of this chapter, such as "The General Distribution Problem" or "Optimization Approaches before 1981," theory clearly dominates the experiment, although experimental aspects may have to be considered in specific cases. Later in this chapter, we will discuss the validation of the theoretical force predictions and the estimation of individual muscle forces from EMG, topics in which the theoretical work is tightly interwoven with experimental research and, for the sake of clarity, were not separated artificially. Therefore, the title of this chapter, "Theoretical Considerations," should be considered in the broadest sense, i.e., the theory was of primary interest but experimental information was required. Similarly, the part of this chapter entitled "Experimental Considerations" will not be completely free of theoretical analysis.

The General Distribution Problem

In order to calculate the forces exerted by individual muscles and, thus, to determine the force sharing among muscles, the so-called "distribution problem" is typically solved first [17]. The distribution problem relates the forces and moments produced by structures in and around a joint to the in-

tersegmental resultant force and moment, and it is based on the idea that
any distributed force/moment system may be replaced by a single force and
moment that are equipollent to the distributed force/moment system. The
joint equipollence relationship may be expressed as follows (note, bold
characters designate vectors) [17]:

$$\boldsymbol{F}^0 = \sum_{i=1}^{m} (\boldsymbol{f}_i^m + \sum_{j=1}^{l} (\boldsymbol{f}_j^l) + \sum_{k=1}^{c} (\boldsymbol{f}_k^c) \qquad 1$$

$$\boldsymbol{M}^0 = \sum_{i=1}^{m} (\boldsymbol{r}_i^m \times \boldsymbol{f}_i^m) + \sum_{j=1}^{l} (\boldsymbol{r}_j^l \times \boldsymbol{f}_j^l) + \sum_{k=1}^{c} (\boldsymbol{r}_k^c \times \boldsymbol{f}_k^c) \qquad 2$$

where $\boldsymbol{F}$ and $\boldsymbol{M}$ are the intersegmental resultant force and moment, respectively, and the superscript "0" designates the joint center 0 (which, from
a mathematical point of view, may be defined arbitrarily within the joint);
$f_i^m, f_j^l,$ and f_k^c are the forces in the ith muscle, jth ligament, and kth bony contact, respectively; $r_i^m, r_j^l,$ and r_k^c are location vectors from the joint center to
any point on the line of action of the corresponding force; "x" denotes the
vector (cross) product; and $m, l,$ and c designate the number of muscles/
tendons, ligaments crossing the joints, and individual articular contact
areas within the joint, respectively.

When solving the distribution problem (i.e., Eq. 1 and 2), the purpose is
to determine the ligamentous, muscular, and bony contact forces from the
intersegmental resultant moment and force. The intersegmental resultants
may be determined by using the inverse dynamics approach [6], when the
kinematics (obtained, for example, by filming the movement of interest, using high-speed video or film) and the external forces acting on the system
of interest (except for the intersegmental resultants, which are to be determined) are known. It is important to note here that the intersegmental
resultant force and moment are conceptual kinetic quantities; they cannot
be measured, and they are not present in an identifiable structure.

Equations 1 and 2 represent the general distribution problem. When
solving these two equations in practical situations, simplifying assumptions
are typically made. Particularly when calculating the forces in muscles for
the normal range of everyday movements, it is commonly assumed that ligaments do not transmit appreciable forces. Also, the joint center is usually
assumed to fall on the line of action of the resultant joint contact force;
therefore, the distributed joint contact forces do not contribute to the resultant intersegmental moments. When these two assumptions are made,
Equations 1 and 2 are reduced to:

$$\boldsymbol{F}^0 = \sum_{i=1}^{m} (\boldsymbol{f}_i^m) + \sum_{k=1}^{c} (\boldsymbol{f}_k^c) \qquad 3$$

$$\boldsymbol{M}^0 = \sum_{i=1}^{m} (\boldsymbol{r}_i^m \times \boldsymbol{f}_i^m) \qquad 4$$

Equations 3 and 4 are two-vector equations in three-dimensional space; they give six independent scalar equations. For calculating individual muscle forces, it is preferable to use Equation 4 only, because Equation 3, although adding one vector (or three scalar) equation(s) to the description of the system of interest, also introduces at least one additional vector (or three scalar) unknown(s) in the form of the resultant(s) of the distributed forces of the joint contact(s), f_k^c.

Assuming that the resultant intersegmental moment, M^0, has been determined using the inverse dynamics approach, Equation 4 contains $2 \cdot m$ vector unknowns, m unknown location vectors, r_i^m, and m unknown muscle forces, f_i^m. The location vectors, r_i^m (or the corresponding scalar moment arms) can be determined experimentally, using cadaveric specimens [35, 58, 104] or imaging techniques [94, 104]. Although the experimental determination of moment arms is by no means trivial (nor is it a problem that has been solved conclusively), it is usually assumed that moment arms are known. Also, the lines of action of the muscles are often determined experimentally; therefore, the only remaining unknowns in Equation 4 are the magnitudes of the muscle forces, f_i^m. Because Equation 4 gives three independent scalar equations, but the number of muscles crossing a given joint in humans (or in animals) typically exceeds three, Equation 4 represents a mathematically indeterminate system (i.e., a system that contains more unknowns than equations).

Mathematically indeterminate systems generally have an infinite number of possible solutions. For example, the equation x + y = 12 (which contains two unknowns, x and y) has an infinite number of possible solutions (e.g., x = 6, y = 6; x = 1, y = 11; x = −17, y = 29, etc.). An indeterminate system may be made determinate and, so, give a unique solution to a problem, by 1) adding equations to the system, or 2) eliminating unknowns until the number of unknowns and the number of equations match. For example, adding the equation x − y = 4 to equation x + y =12 will result in a unique solution for x and y (i.e., x = 8, y = 4). Unknowns may be eliminated by grouping them or by relating them in some fashion. For example, when we assume that x is the same as y, equation x + y = 12 becomes 2x = 12, and we have a unique solution for x (x = 6).

Similarly, in biomechanics, the prediction of forces in individual muscles crossing a joint (often, an indeterminate mathematical problem) has been solved by adding system equations or by eliminating unknowns. System equations may be added not only by considering the mechanical relation between muscular forces and joint moments but also by incorporating other known mechanical or neurophysiological relations between muscular forces and joint moments [89, 91]. Reducing the number of unknown muscular forces when solving the distribution problem has been done by grouping individual muscles into functional units [79, 84]. Neither the addition of system equations nor the reduction of system unknowns is a satisfactory solution, because additional system equations are normally based on assumptions about system behavior, and grouping muscles into functional units introduces a series of new problems (e.g., What is the line of action of a group of muscles or the moment arm about a given joint?), and it does not solve the problem of interest (i.e., What is the amount of force sharing among individual muscles during movements?).

The most common approach to solving for individual muscle forces during movement has been mathematical optimization. This elegant way of solving the distribution problem is simple enough that analytical solutions for many realistic musculoskeletal models can be obtained, and the idea that human (or animal) movements obey some law of optimal control has both a strong appeal and a long history [110].

OPTIMIZATION APPROACHES BEFORE 1981

In their review article, Crowninshield and Brand [17] summarized the work on individual muscle force predictions that used optimization up to that time. They criticized the fact that "most researchers who have advanced methods to solve the distribution problem have overemphasized the mathematical possibility of solutions and underemphasized the physiologic basis of the method." Furthermore, they advised that "more attention should be directed toward investigating the physiologic significance of many numerical optimization procedures."

Up to 1981, most optimization approaches that were used to determine individual muscle forces were linear [87, 88]. The most severe limitation of linear optimization is that the number of predicted active muscles will, in general, be restricted to the number of degrees of freedom of the system [17, 43]. This limitation has sometimes been overcome by imposing upper limit constraints on the forces or stresses of muscles [16]; however, the solution of such a case is dominated by the constraint equations, rather than by the "chosen" objective function of the optimization algorithm.

Pedotti et al. [86] were the first to use nonlinear optimization to predict the forces in lower limb muscles during walking. Their research was followed by one other nonlinear optimization approach by 1981, the work of Crowninshield and Brand [18]. In their work, Crowninshield and Brand [18] emphasize the physiological derivation of their objective function (i.e., the minimization of muscle stresses). They further justify their choice of a nonlinear objective function with the known nonlinear relation between endurance time (the time during which a muscle can maintain a given amount of stress) and muscular stress. They suggested that when a criterion for selecting muscles to contribute to walking is the maximization of the time that the movement can be performed, then maximization of this endurance time is equivalent to minimizing the sum of the muscular stresses.

Although this line of reasoning is correct for a single muscle, it is not quite correct when one is considering systems of multiple synergistic muscles [22]. Nevertheless, the work of Crowninshield and Brand [18] stimulated the notion of deriving objective functions for individual muscle force predictions, based on physiological criteria.

One of the best attempts at relating the physiology of a system to an optimization approach aimed at predicting individual muscle forces was made by Hardt [42] in an unpublished doctoral dissertation. Hardt [42] derived a function relating the energy requirements of a muscle to its contractile speed and then used this energy function to calculate individual muscle forces based on the idea that total energy requirements should be minimized during movement. Although some aspects of the doctoral dissertation were published [43], the critical ideas of Hardt's work did not become public (to my knowledge), and thus, this promising attempt at individual muscle force predictions was not pursued further. For a detailed review of all optimization works up to 1981, the reader is referred to Crowninshield and Brand [17].

Optimization after 1981

Although there are dozens of published manuscripts that attempt to use optimization mathematics to predict individual muscle forces, only a few selected examples are mentioned here. These examples were chosen because they either contained a physiologically derived optimization model (rather than a purely mathematical model), or they aimed to validate theoretical predictions, using experimentally measured muscle forces.

Dul et al. [26] evaluated a series of published optimization algorithms and proposed an objective function for individual muscle force predictions, which was an attempt to maximize the amount of time that a movement (or isometric contraction) could be maintained [25]. The objective function of Dul et al. [25] was the first to require input about the fiber-type distribution of the studied muscles. Dul et al. [25] evaluated their optimization algorithm by first comparing the predicted contraction times to contraction times measured experimentally in lower limb muscles of humans during isometric tasks. They then attempted to validate their proposed optimization scheme by deriving the force-sharing relationship for cat soleus and gastrocnemius muscles theoretically, based on their proposed model, and then comparing the predicted force sharing between these two muscles to the maximal forces measured in cat soleus and gastrocnemius for standing, walking, trotting, galloping, and jumping. The theoretically predicted results were said to fit the experimental results well (and, clearly, fitted the experimental results better than any of the predictions from previously published works). Nevertheless, the comparisons made by Dul et al. [25] had several limitations: 1) the musculoskeletal input required for the theoretical model and the muscle force measurements were obtained from different animals; 2) the maximal forces in soleus and gastrocnemius during cat locomotion do not occur at the same instant in time [55, 56], whereas the force-sharing equation required (implicitly) that comparisons of force values between muscles be made at the same instant in time; 3) only maximal values, rather than the force-time histories throughout the movements, were used for comparisons.

Furthermore, the force-sharing predictions of Dul et al. [25] had the following conceptual shortcomings: 1) the force sharing between muscles was dependent only on the maximal isometric force and the fiber-type distribution (two constants) of the muscles; therefore, all force-sharing relations derived from their algorithm had a unique functional relation, which means that a given force in Muscle 1 will always be associated with a given force in Muscle 2 (Fig. 6.1). Direct muscle force measurements at a variety of speeds of locomotion in the cat, however, demonstrate that a given force in the soleus, for example, can be associated with a large range of forces in a synergistic muscle (i.e., the gastrocnemius, Fig. 6.2); 2) the force-sharing relations derived from the model by Dul et al. [25] are steadily increasing; that is, if the force in Muscle 1 increases, the force in Muscle 2 has to increase as well. Again, experimental data from cat soleus and gastrocnemius demonstrate convincingly that gastrocnemius forces increase steadily from stand-

FIGURE 6.1.
Theoretical prediction of the force sharing between cat soleus and medial gastrocnemius muscles for a variety of activities (solid line) and the corresponding peak forces in soleus and medial gastrocnemius (MG), obtained experimentally (triangles, static; dots, dynamic). Adapted from ref. 25.

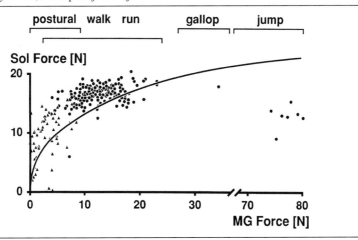

FIGURE 6.2.

Force sharing between cat soleus and gastrocnemius muscles obtained experimentally for nominal speeds of locomotion of 0.4, 0.7, 1.2, and 2.4 m/s. All force-sharing loops represent the average of a minimum of 10 consecutive step cycles. For a force of 10 N in the soleus, forces as low as 4 N (0.4 m/s) and as high as 47 N (2.4 m/s) could be observed in the gastrocnemius. Adapted from ref. 50.

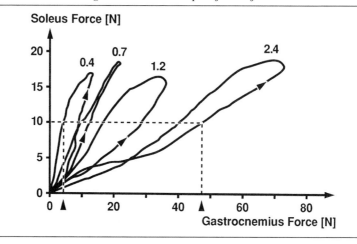

ing to walking to running to jumping; whereas soleus forces tend to increase slightly from standing to walking, they remain constant for a large range of speeds of locomotion, and they tend to decrease for jumping (Fig. 6.1).

Herzog [47, 48] presented an optimization algorithm for the solution of individual muscle forces that had an objective function that contained explicitly the instantaneous contractile conditions (length and rate of change in length) and the force-length-velocity properties of the muscles of interest. This algorithm allowed for the prediction of a wide range of muscle forces for one muscle while the other muscle's force remained constant. Therefore, the force-sharing "loops" measured experimentally between two muscles. (Fig. 6.2) could, at least conceptually, be accommodated. Furthermore, the algorithm predicted smooth force transitions in muscles, whereas previous (strictly static) algorithms predicted large instantaneous force changes. The drawbacks of the algorithm proposed by Herzog [47, 48] were associated with its difficult implementation. For example, the force-length-velocity properties of most muscles are unknown, and their behavior under submaximal levels of contraction can at best be approximated.

Davy and Audu [21] introduced dynamic optimization for predicting the forces of nine lower limb muscle groups during the swing phase of walking. The dynamic algorithm was motivated by the fact that force-time histories of muscles, using static optimization, often showed unrealistic discontinuities. The results of the dynamic optimization proposed by Davy and Audu [21] were compared to those of the static optimization algorithm of Crowninshield and Brand [18] and to those of the EMG envelopes during the swing phase of walking [86]. Lacking a rigorous validation, it is difficult to assess the appropriateness of the dynamic algorithm proposed by Davy and Audu [21]. Furthermore, their results of the comparison of the static and dynamic algorithms must be considered with caution, because the results shown for the static algorithm contained cocontraction of two single-joint antagonistic muscles in a planar model, which represents an impossible solution for the algorithm of Crowninshield and Brand [18, 51, 52].

The first validation of optimization algorithms predicting the force sharing among synergistic muscles was performed by Herzog and Leonard [55]. In this study, the force-sharing among the cat soleus, gastrocnemius, and plantaris muscles was predicted theoretically, based on the most common optimization algorithms proposed up to that time. The required input parameters for the optimization algorithms were largely determined directly from working with the experimental animals. The predicted force-sharing behavior was then compared to the actual force measurements obtained from the target muscles for a variety of speeds of locomotion. It was found that the tested theoretical algorithms were conceptually not able to predict actual force-sharing behavior among the muscles of a synergistic group. In the study of Herzog and Leonard [55], static linear and nonlinear optimization algorithms were evaluated, whereas dynamic algorithms or algorithms requiring instantaneous contractile conditions were ignored. An evaluation of the algorithm proposed by Herzog [48], containing the instantaneous contractile conditions of the muscles, was performed in the form of a pilot study [54], and although the initial comparisons between the theoretical and experimental force-sharing behavior of cat soleus and gastrocnemius were encouraging, a thorough analysis revealed that the predictions based on Herzog's [48] work did not predict experimental findings well (W. Herzog, unpublished results). The question as to whether optimization-based muscle force predictions are useful in predicting the actual muscle forces remains unresolved; further research aimed at developing good theoretical predictions of individual muscle forces is required. Experimental data on the force-sharing among synergistic muscles are now available for comparison from a variety of laboratories, which was not the case in 1981. It is hoped that researchers will take advantage of this situation in the coming decade.

Muscle Force Predictions from Electromyographical Signals

In their 1981 review article, Crowninshield and Brand [17] recommended that "the correlation of predicted muscle forces to measured EMG activity has been useful in validation and should be more intensively applied." EMG signals have been used frequently to correlate times of activity of muscles with the times of predicted muscle forces [16, 17, 71, 85, 86, 98]. Good temporal agreement between the EMG activity and theoretically predicted muscle forces was taken as a temporal validation of the theoretical algorithms. The results of these studies must be interpreted with some caution, because it can be shown that nonlinear objective functions predict muscle forces to occur during fixed time periods for a given activity and that nonphysiological (or even arbitrary mathematical objective functions) can predict reasonable temporal patterns of muscle activity [16]. For an (adequate) nonlinear objective function, the period of force production of a one-joint muscle will largely coincide with the resultant joint moment; that is, when the resultant moment is in the same direction as the moment produced by the muscle upon contraction, the muscle will typically be predicted to be active; when the resultant joint moment is in the opposite direction of he moment produced by the muscle, the muscle will normally (but not always) be silent [51, 52].

Attempts to predict muscle forces from the corresponding EMG signals have been performed (see Basmajian and de Luca [7] for a review). The relation between some processed form of the EMG signal and muscle force has been found to be linear [65, 75, 76, 99] or nonlinear [74, 108] for isometric contractions. Differences in the EMG-force relationship have been found for the same muscle (e.g., the human biceps brachii: linear [75] and nonlinear [117]); therefore, the qualitative relation between these two parameters is largely unknown, even for the relatively "simple" cases involving isometric contractions.

Despite the difficulties in trying to relate EMG to force during isometric contractions, a few attempts have been made to predict dynamic muscle forces from electromyographical signals. The first attempts were made, using well-controlled isokinetic contractions [10, 11, 14, 45, 72, 73], followed more recently by investigations of unrestrained movement tasks [24, 64, 83, 100, 107].

Van den Bogert et al. [107] predicted the in vivo forces of the deep digital flexor of the horse, based on a four-component model of the muscle of interest and the measured EMG signals. The force of the contractile component of the model was assumed to be proportional to the "active state," which was represented by the rectified and low-pass filtered (30 Hz) EMG signal. The remaining three components of the muscle model consisted of an elastic element in parallel with the contractile element, an elastic element in series with the contractile and the first-mentioned elastic element, and a linear damper. Therefore, the model was length- and velocity-dependent. Van den Bogert et al. [107] derived the necessary input for their model using "irregular" walking and then predicted the forces for "normal'" walking in the deep digital flexor. The theoretically predicted forces were compared to the experimentally measured forces, which were obtained using a mercury-in-silastic strain gauge. The predicted forces were similar to the measured forces, and the RMS prediction error was given as 143 N for actual forces ranging from 0 N to about 1200 N (estimated based on Fig. 5c in ref. 107). Most notably, the predicted forces always deviated substantially from the actual forces at the end of the stance phase, when the actual forces were close to zero, and the predicted forces became negative (up to about −400 N, estimated from Fig. 5c).

A further attempt to predict dynamic muscle forces from EMG signals was made by Norman et al. [82]. These researchers measured the soleus forces in a cat walking on a treadmill, using a "buckle" tendon force transducer [109]. EMG signals were obtained from the same muscle, using indwelling fine-wire electrodes. The EMG signals were digitized (2000 Hz), rectified and filtered (double-pass Butterworth filter, 2–10 Hz) to produce "linear envelopes" [7]. Force magnitudes of the soleus were predicted as follows:

$$f_p = f_{iso} \, (EMG/EMG_{iso}) \qquad\qquad 5$$

where f_p is the instantaneous predicted force, f_{iso} is the measured tendon force when the cat is standing still, *EMG* is the instantaneous value of the linear envelope when the cat is walking, and EMG_{iso} is the average of the linear envelope signal over 2 s while the cat is standing still.

The root mean square (RMS) difference between the actual and the predicted force curves, normalized with respect to the actual forces, was 23% over four consecutive step cycles. Despite the fact that the electromechanical delay was not accounted for in the model, there appeared to be little shift in the temporal aspects between the actual and predicted forces. The limitation of this particular approach is that an experimentally measured force (the measured tendon force when the cat is standing still) and the corresponding EMG were required as input into the prediction model.

Guimaraes et al. [39–41] performed a series of studies aimed at evaluating the relation between dynamic force and EMG in the cat soleus muscle. In the first two of their experiments, they attempted to determine quantitatively the relation between force and EMG in acute preparations and under isometric contractions. Forces were measured using a calibrated strain gauge attached to the end of a linear motor; EMGs were recorded, using indwelling wire electrodes [59] and a patch-type surface electrode [77], sutured to the epimysium of the soleus muscle. Stimulation of the soleus was produced through 10 independent channels hooked up to 10 bundles of ventral root filaments on the L7/S1 levels. Stimulation frequencies in each stimulation channel could be controlled independently, as could the pseudorandom interpulse interval statistics [116]. This setup allowed for a realistic production of EMG signals, and a smooth development of force, even at low levels of stimulation frequency. Guimaraes et al. [40] found an S-shaped relation between the integrated EMG signals and the mean force, which was highly linear in the region of physiological stimulation frequencies and normally occurring forces. These results were extended to different soleus lengths, covering the normal physiological range [41]. The dynamic relation between the soleus force and EMG for cats walking and running at various speeds turned out to be highly nonlinear (as expected), and could be explained partly by the instantaneous contractile properties of the muscle [39]. Nevertheless, many detailed aspects of the relation remain unknown.

In an attempt to determine whether the EMG signal alone contained enough information to predict dynamic muscle forces, Herzog et al. [50] predicted the experimentally measured forces in the cat plantaris from the corresponding EMG signals, using an adaptive filtering approach. Forces in this experiment were measured using an "E"-shaped tendon force transducer, and EMG signals were obtained using bipolar, indwelling fine-wire electrodes [50]. The EMG signals were used as input for the adaptive filter, and the predicted forces were directly compared and adjusted using the known actual forces. The agreement between predicted and actual forces was excellent after the first step cycle, indicating that the EMG signal should contain sufficient information to predict individual muscle forces adequately. However, such predictions (in which the actual forces were not used as reference input) have not been successful to date (W. Herzog, unpublished observations).

Motivated by the partially successful results derived from using adaptive filters to predict muscle forces from EMG, Savelberg and Herzog [96] attempted to predict experimentally measured forces from cat gastrocnemius muscles, using EMG alone or EMG and hindlimb kinematics, as input into an artificial neural network with a back propagation algorithm. Excellent preliminary predictions of gastrocnemius forces were obtained for one animal (at a given speed of walking) when the artificial neural network was trained, using steps of two other animals (at the same speed of walking) (Fig. 6.3). Although adaptive filtering techniques or artificial neural networks may not help to further the understanding of the relation between EMG and force, they appear (at a first glance, at least, and based on pilot experiments only) to be powerful predictors of individual muscle forces from EMG. It must be kept in mind, though, that although the predictions of muscle forces, using the artificial neural network approach, were extremely good, the actual muscle forces (albeit from different animals than those for which the predictions were made) needed to be known for training the network.

EXPERIMENTAL CONSIDERATIONS

By definition, experimental work on force-sharing among muscles requires that a minimum of two individual muscle forces is measured simultaneously. Although direct muscle force measurements have been done in a variety of animals (e.g., in horses [107], kangaroos [37], pigeons [23] and

FIGURE 6.3.

Experimentally measured (solid line) and theoretically predicted (dashed line) gastrocnemius forces for cat walking at a nominal speed of 0.8 m/s. The predictions were made using an artificial neural network approach with a back propagation algorithm, with which EMG, ankle angle, and ankle angular speed as input were used. The artificial neural network was trained using the measured forces and the measured input parameters of two cats, and the predictions were made for a third cat.

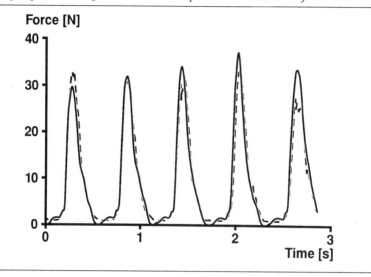

kangaroo rats [9]), multiple force recordings from individual muscles have been performed primarily in the cat hindlimb.

Walmsley et al. [109] pioneered multiple-force measurements in the freely moving cat. These researchers recorded the forces of soleus and medial gastrocnemius for a variety of activities (walking, trotting, galloping, and jumping). They found that the peak forces in the soleus muscle remained nearly constant, independent of the speed of locomotion, whereas the peak forces in the gastrocnemius increased with increasing speeds of locomotion. Walmsley et al. [109] explained that peak soleus forces were constant, because soleus was fully (or nearly fully) activated at low force requirements and, therefore, its activation could not be increased with increasing demands on force or moment production; its peak force was determined by the contractile conditions. Primarily, it was suggested that soleus forces would tend to increase with increasing speeds of locomotion because of the increased speed in stretch of the muscle just before reaching peak forces. However, they suggested that this effect was offset by the decreasing time available from the onset of activation of the muscle to peak force attainment with increasing speeds.

Other researchers repeated the experiments performed by Walmsley et al. [109] with similar results [63, 112]. Interestingly enough, however, Hodgson [63] interpreted the force sharing between cat soleus and medial gastrocnemius quite differently than Walmsley et al. [109]. Hodgson [63] believed that the instantaneous contractile conditions of soleus and medial gastrocnemius are about the same during locomotion; therefore, the contractile conditions were assumed to have a negligible effect on the force sharing between the two muscles. The increasing peak medial gastrocnemius forces were associated with the increasing activation of this muscle for increasing speeds of locomotion; the constant peak soleus forces were associated with a lack of increase in activation of the soleus. Hodgson [63] believed that the constant activation of the soleus muscle at increasing speeds of locomotion was the result of two competing factors: an increase in the activation from descending pathways and a decrease in the activation through rubrospinal and cutaneous pathways [13].

At present, it is not known whether the explanation given by Walmsley et al. [109] or that offered by Hodgson [63] is correct; however, some comments about their conclusions can be made. The observations made by Walmsley et al. [109] that the speed of stretch of the soleus increases and the time available to build up peak forces decreases with increasing speeds of locomotion appear to be correct [31, 32, 34] and, therefore, may be accepted in principle. The conclusions suggested by Hodgson may be criticized on various accounts. For example, the idea that the instantaneous contractile conditions (length and rate of change in length) of soleus and medial gastrocnemius are about the same during locomotion appears to be correct [32]; however, the contractile conditions normalized with respect to the contractile properties (maximal force, maximal speed of shortening, optimal length) are different in the two muscles [5, 57, 92, 102] and must be considered in an analysis of force sharing between these muscles. Furthermore, Hodgson [63] argued that the activation of the soleus was constant across speeds. Activation was quantified as the integrated EMG signal over 50-ms periods, which is a questionable method to use. Our own unpublished observations appear to suggest that the root mean square values [7] of EMG signals from the soleus increase to a similar extent as the corresponding signals of the gastrocnemius (and plantaris) for increasing speeds of locomotion ranging, from 0.4 to about 2.0 m/s.

Abraham and Loeb [3] recorded individual muscle forces from the cat hindlimb of five animals. One or maximally two muscle forces were measured in a given animal for standing, walking, trotting, dropping, paw shaking, and scratching. Forces were obtained from the flexor digitorum longus, tibialis posterior, plantaris, flexor digitorum brevis, and the total Achilles tendon. The results shown were primarily used to describe the patterns of normal use. Little attempt was made to explain the patterns of use or the force-sharing patterns between muscles.

About 5 yr ago, we started to perform systematic measurements of the forces and EMG signals of four cat ankle muscles (soleus, gastrocnemius, plantaris,and tibialis anterior) during locomotion at a variety of speeds [40, 55–57, 61, 92]. A typical pattern of force sharing between the three plantar flexor muscles is shown in Figure 6.4. Comparison of the experimentally measured forces with theoretically predicted forces obtained from the primary force-sharing algorithms available at the time revealed the following limitations of the theoretical algorithms: 1) the algorithms predicted a unique relation between the forces in synergistic muscles, whereas the experimental evidence shows clearly that a given force in one muscle (e.g., 10 N in soleus) can be associated with a large range of forces in another muscle (e.g., 4–47 N in the gastrocnemius; see Fig. 6.2); 2) the algorithms predicted a continuously increasing force-sharing function, with increasing demands on the resultant joint moment, whereas experimental evidence from the cat plantar flexors suggests that gastrocnemius forces may increase from one activity to another (e.g., from walking to jumping), whereas soleus forces decrease [101, 109].

Using a model of the three primary cat plantar flexors, based on anatomical measurements of experimental animals, the force-length and force-velocity properties from the literature [57, 102], as well as sinusoid muscle length changes coupled with sinusoid changes in activation, it is possible to recover the basic force-sharing patterns of the cat soleus, gastrocnemius, and plantaris for a movement cycle (Fig. 6.5). Once the basic mechanical properties of the model were chosen, subtle changes in the shape or magnitude of the force-sharing patterns could be produced by small changes in the magnitude or timing of the activation patterns. Although the results shown in Figure 6.5 cannot be considered predictions of force-sharing patterns, they illustrate how acceptable force-sharing patterns can be produced by incorporating basic properties of the muscles studied.

At this point, we might reconsider Crowninshield and Brand's [17] statement that insufficient effort at validating theoretically predicted muscle forces has been made. At present, the situation is much the same. Although Dul et al. [25] used peak force measurements of soleus and medial gastrocnemius and compared them to theoretically predicted forces, the study was flawed in several ways, as discussed earlier. Similarly, Herzog and Leonard [55] compared direct muscle force recordings from soleus, gastrocnemius, and plantaris in the freely moving cat with the predictions of the most prominent theoretical algorithms. Their work was limited by the number of experimental observations made and the theoretical algorithms chosen for comparison, algorithms that were static in nature and did not contain the instantaneous contractile conditions of the muscles. Theoretical algorithms, based on dynamic optimization [21] or based on knowledge of the instantaneous contractile conditions [47, 49], were ignored for validation, because it is virtually impossible to obtain the required input for

FIGURE 6.4.

Force sharing among cat soleus, gastrocnemius, and plantaris muscles, obtained experimentally for nominal speeds of locomotion of 0.4, 0.7, 1.2, and 2.4 m/s. All force-sharing loops represent the average of a minimum of 10 consecutive step cycles. Reproduced from ref. 50.

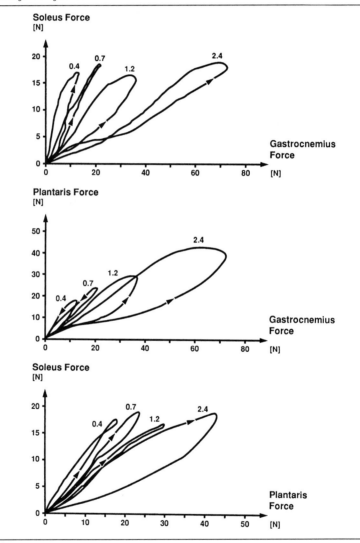

FIGURE 6.5.

Theoretically predicted force sharing among cat soleus, gastrocnemius, and plantaris muscles for simulated speeds of locomotion of 0.4, 0.7, 1.2, and 2.4 m/s. The muscles were given experimentally determined force-length-velocity properties. Activation was modeled on a one-half period of a sinusoidal wave, and activation was linearly related to force.

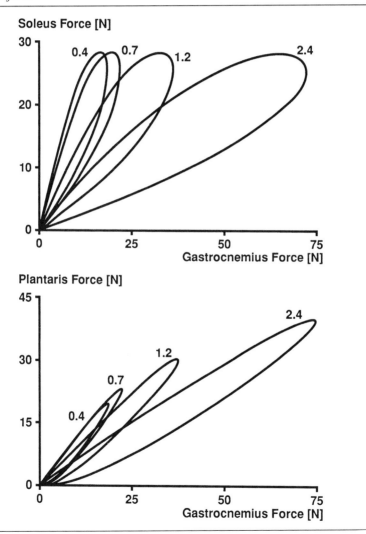

these algorithms accurately (i.e., the instantaneous length, rate of change in length, angles of pinnation, stiffness, etc.). Some of these problems will be addressed in Chapter 7.

Quantitative Musculoskeletal Anatomy

The force a muscle can exert depends on, among other things, its size and structure, its active state, its instantaneous contractile conditions, and its contractile history. Furthermore, the moment produced by the force of a muscle about a joint depends on its moment arm, determined by the muscle's line of action and the point used to represent an anatomical joint. Many of these anatomical and structural parameters are required as input into theoretical models aimed at predicting the force sharing between muscles. Here, a short summary is given of some selected attempts to quantify the musculoskeletal anatomy, the morphology of muscles, and the instantaneous contractile conditions of dynamically working muscles.

SIZE OF MUSCLES. The size of a muscle is generally quantified using the physiological cross-sectional area (PCSA). It has been suggested that the maximal isometric force that a muscle can exert is proportional to PCSA, and a typical value for the proportionality factor is about 25–40 N/cm^2, although values ranging from 9.8 N/cm^2 [110] to 147 N/cm^2 [86] have been used in the literature. Typically, *PCSA* is defined by:

$$PCSA = \left[\frac{\text{Muscle volume}}{\text{Fiber (fascicle) length}} \right] \cos(\alpha) \qquad 6$$

where α represents the angle of pinnation [20, 95]. The problem with the above definition is that *PCSA* of a muscle is not constant, because the angle of pinnation, α, changes during contractions [118] and is different for steady-state, isometric contractions at different muscle lengths [12]. Therefore, the preferred definition for *PCSA* is yielded by:

$$PCSA = \frac{\text{Muscle volume}}{\text{Fiber (fascicle) length}} \qquad 7$$

where fiber (fascicle) length refers to some defined reference length, normally, the optimal length. This definition has the advantage over the previous one in that the *PCSA* of a muscle is constant, and two muscles of equal volume and fiber length have the same *PCSA* and, consequently, the same potential to produce force. The component of the force coinciding with the muscle's line of action can then be calculated, when the variable of pinnation is known.

The PCSAs of human skeletal muscles have been determined quantitatively in a variety of studies. For example, values for most lower limb muscles are available in the literature [4, 29, 113]; however, these PCSAs were determined from cadaveric specimens and, therefore, are not subject specific. Cutts and Seedhom [20] performed one of the rare studies in which

PCSAs were determined in vivo in four active males (19–32 yr of age), using radiographic techniques. As one might expect, the PCSAs of the knee extensor and flexor muscles in the active young subjects were substantially larger than in the corresponding muscles of cadaveric specimens. Interestingly enough, however, Cutts and Seedhom [20] found that the relative PCSAs of the knee extensors and the knee flexors in their subjects were similar to the corresponding values found in previous studies, using cadaveric specimens. Consequently, in models of force sharing between muscles requiring only ratios of PCSAs, rather than absolute values, cadaveric information of PCSAs may be adequate. This result is encouraging, as it has been shown that in many models of force sharing among muscles, only the ratios, and not the absolute values of the PCSAs, are required [25, 49].

MUSCLE LINES OF ACTION AND MOMENT ARMS. Muscles produce movements of the skeletal system, primarily because they create a moment about the joints they cross. When considering the force-sharing between, for example, two agonistic muscles, the force in the two muscles may be the same at a specific instant in time, but the moment these muscles produce about a joint axis may be different because of differences in the moment arms. Most theoretical models aimed at predicting the absolute forces generated by muscles require information about moment arms as input, and most models of force sharing among muscles require at least the ratio of the moment arms, with the (possibly lone) exception of the force-sharing model proposed by Dul et al. [25], in which the force-sharing equation between two muscles does not contain (or require) the moment arms (or their ratio).

In order to define a moment arm of a muscle, the joint center and the line of action of the muscle must be defined. Joint centers are typically defined as fixed points, often coinciding with palpable or visible bony landmarks, for example, the femoral condyles for the knee or the malleoli for the ankle.

More recently, joint centers have been defined as moving points, for example, the instantaneous contact point of the lateral femoral condyle and the lateral tibial plateau in the human knee [81], or the instantaneous center of rotation [94]. However, defining the joint center as a moving point has two disadvantages: 1) the joint center is hard to determine and 2) the moment produced by the distributed joint contact force cannot generally be neglected. Using the instantaneous center of rotation as the joint center, moment arms of muscles can be determined with the tendon travel approach [103, 104]. This approach is probably the preferred method of quantifying moment arms of muscles accurately, because it incorporates the notion of the moving joint center (and a moving joint axis) and does not require that the muscle's line of action be known. Determining the line of action of a muscle is a specific problem that will not be dealt with here: an excellent review of the relevant literature in this area of research has just been published [90].

INSTANTANEOUS CONTRACTILE CONDITIONS AND CONTRAC-
TILE PROPERTIES OF SKELETAL MUSCLES. The contractile properties
of skeletal muscles are typically described by the force-length and and the
force-velocity relationships. The force-length property describes the maximal isometric force a muscle can exert as a function of its length. When incorporating the force-length relationship into a model aimed at predicting
individual muscle forces, the following problems arise: 1) The force-length
relationship of most human skeletal muscles is unknown; therefore, an estimate of the relationship must be provided [60]. 2) The force-length relationship is plastic and may adapt to the requirements of everyday life, for
example, to the chronic training of high-performance athletes [53]. 3) The
force-length relationship for submaximal levels of contraction differs vastly
from those obtained during maximal levels of contraction [41, 46, 93]. 4)
Obviously, the force-length properties will differ, depending on the
"length" that is being measured and the "length" that is held isometric during an experiment. The two extreme choices are the sarcomere length [30]
and the muscle-tendon length [33, 93]. The resulting properties depend
strongly on this choice and, 5) to determine the force-length properties of
in vivo human skeletal muscles, artificial or voluntary stimulation may be
used. Artificial stimulation is painful but will demonstrate the muscular
properties independent of length-dependent activation. Maximal voluntary contractions by subjects are easy to perform but may contain the effects
of a variable activation as a function of muscle length [7, 8, 28, 44].

The force-velocity property describes the maximal force a muscle can exert as a function of its speed of contraction. Typically, this property is evaluated at optimal muscle length [62], and the force is determined once the
muscle reaches a steady-state value (i.e., the initial transient behavior,
which may be of importance in many movement situations, is ignored).
When one is attempting to incorporate the force-velocity property into a
model of individual muscle force prediction, the following problems arise:
1) The force-velocity properties of individual human skeletal muscles are
virtually unknown, and, therefore, must be estimated in most cases. 2)
Stretch-related phenomena, for example, "yielding," i.e., the abrupt decrease in force when a muscle is stretched at a constant speed [70, 80, 105],
are not well understood. 3) the force-velocity relation is not unique and appears to depend on whether the experiment is performed using force or
speed control [69]. 4) the force-velocity relation for submaximal activation
differs substantially from that obtained at maximal activation.

Aside from the multitude of problems associated with defining and describing the force-length and force-velocity properties of muscles, a further
difficulty arises when these two properties are combined. Hill [62] suggested that his force-velocity equation, which was derived for optimal muscle fiber lengths (Eq. 8), would also hold at lengths other than the optimal

length when F_0 (Eq. 8) was replaced by the maximal isometric force at the fiber length of interest

$$F = (F_0 b - av) / (b + v) \qquad\qquad 8$$

where F is the variable force produced by the muscle, F_0 is the maximal isometric force at optimal fiber length, v is the speed of shortening, and a and b are thermodynamic constants with the units of force and speed, respectively. Although Abbott and Wilkie [2] provided experimental evidence that substituting F_0 in Equation 8 with the maximal isometric force of the appropriate length was correct; performing this substitution results in the speed of unloaded shortening being highest at optimal length and scaled linearly with the maximal force as a function of length. However, measurements on single frog skeletal fibers showed that the speed of unloaded shortening was not affected within a large range of fiber length [27]. The precise combination of the force-length and the force-velocity relationship, therefore, is not known and remains a matter of controversy.

Finally, it has been known for a long time now that the isometric force production of a muscle depends not only on muscle length but also on the history of its contractile conditions. Abbott and Aubert [1] showed that, for muscles from frogs, toads, and dogfish, the isometric force after a stretch or release was higher or lower, respectively, then the corresponding force obtained under strictly isometric conditions. Figure 6.6 illustrates this phenomenon for cat soleus. Furthermore, Abbott and Aubert [1] also found that the steady-state force reached after a stretch (or release) depended on the speed of the stretch (release). Slow stretches yielded a higher steady-state force, and slow releases yielded a lower steady-state force than the corresponding (i.e., the same magnitude of stretch or release) fast stretches. This speed-dependence of the final steady-state force was also observed in experiments on cat soleus (Fig. 6.6). Such history-dependent force enhancements after stretch and force depressions after release are not completely understood and, as a result, are rarely considered in descriptions of the contractile properties of skeletal muscles.

DETERMINATION OF INSTANTANEOUS CONTRACTILE CONDITIONS IN VIVO. Assuming that appropriate force-length and force-velocity properties have been described for a muscle, forces can be calculated only when the instantaneous contractile conditions (i.e., the instantaneous length and rate of change in length of the contractile elements) are known. (For the sake of argument, we will ignore other factors that influence force production at this time.) The contractile elements or a muscle are the sarcomeres. Sarcomere lengths behave nonuniformly in a contracting muscle [106] and, at present, it is impossible to track the length and length changes of each sarcomere; even when such measurements were possible, it is not clear what the force properties of such a nonuniform arrangement of sarcomeres are or how they could be modeled.

FIGURE 6.6.

Releases of cat soleus muscle from a fully active state (top panel) using speeds of 5, 10, and 20 mm/s; the subsequent recovery is also shown (top panel). Note that the recovery to the corresponding isometric force value (dashed horizontal line) is very slow and incomplete for the slowest speed of release. Stretching of cat soleus muscle from a fully active state is shown (bottom panel), using speeds of 5, 10, and 20 mm/s; the subsequent force decay is also shown. Note that the decay to the corresponding isometric force value (dashed line) is very slow and incomplete for all speeds of stretching shown here.

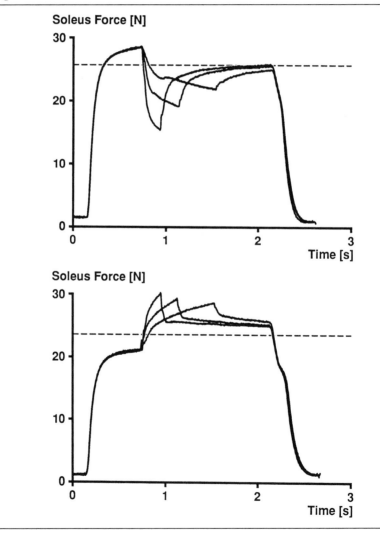

Representing the force-length and force-velocity properties, using muscle-tendon length (and rate of change of the muscle-tendon length) as input for the contractile properties of sarcomeres, is also not possible, because the sarcomere lengths do not depend solely on the muscle-tendon length but also on the muscle force [115]. A reasonable middle ground is the representation of the instantaneous contractile conditions, using fiber (-bundle) lengths and the corresponding first-time derivatives. However, there are few reports in which fiber (-bundle) lengths have been measured in vivo.

In vivo measurements of fiber (bundle) lengths were typically performed in the cat medial gastrocnemius, using pulsing ultrasound, the transit times of which were recorded with piezoelectric crystals at the ends of fiber bundles [36]. For the medial gastrocnemius, there is agreement that, at the instant of paw contact, the muscle-tendon unit is stretched while the corresponding fiber bundles continue to shorten [38, 66, 67, 110]. However, such methods are not without limitations [36, 67], and although it appears that different investigators found similar results, there are some noteworthy discrepancies among those findings. For example, the muscle-tendon length measurements performed by Hoffer et al. [67] (using saline-filled silicone tubing) are significantly different from the corresponding records of Goslow et al. [31], which were obtained from the knee and ankle joint angles and geometrical consideration. In particular, at the instant of paw-off, Hoffer et al. [67] recorded a sharp local maximum of the muscle-tendon length, compared to a local minimum for Goslow et al. [31]. Other researchers have also found a local minimum for medial gastrocnemius lengths at paw-off in the walking cat [92, 111], thereby bringing into question the results of Hoffer et al. [67].

Also, the fiber-bundle length changes occurring at paw contact in the cat medial gastrocnemius muscles appear to differ slightly in the literature. Griffiths showed a smooth continuous shortening of the fiber-bundles at that instant in time ([38], Griffiths' Fig. 2); Hoffer et al. [67] showed a distinct discontinuity of the fiber length traces (although they continuously shorten, their Fig. 2); and finally, Weytjens [111] showed some increase in the fiber-bundle length (although not as large an increase as for the muscle-tendon length, Weytjen's Fig. 4.1B).

Measurements of the angles of pinnation of the cat medial gastrocnemius muscle in vivo (using the same ultrasound technique) have also yielded different results. For example, Weytjens [111] reports a consistent 5–10° decrease in the angle of pinnation immediately after paw contact, whereas these changes do not appear in results presented by Hoffer et al. ([66], their Fig. 1). Thus, although attempts at in vivo measurements of the instantaneous contractile conditions have been made, the results are inconsistent among researchers (for the same muscle in the same animal), and, therefore, further investigation and improvement of the methods used are required before such information may be used with confidence.

CONSIDERATIONS FOR THE FUTURE

Probably the biggest contribution one can make to an area of research is the formulation of a paradigm that can be used to formulate specific hypotheses, which, in turn, can be tested experimentally. Huxley [68] made such a contribution for the force production of skeletal muscles when formulating the cross-bridge theory. In the area of "force sharing among synergistic muscles," such as paradigm is presently not available; therefore, a strict testing of hypotheses is not possible, and there is no framework for orientation. Paradigms have been suggested; for example, Hardt [43] proposed that "force-sharing among synergistic muscles occurs in such a way that the metabolic cost of the movement is minimized." Hardt [43], Crowninshield and Brand [18], and Dul et al. [25] proposed that the endurance time of a movement is maximized. However, the effects made to convert these ideas into detailed paradigms were insufficient. Therefore, this author believes that the biggest contribution (and also, possibly, the biggest challenge) lies in the formulation of a detailed paradigm of force sharing among synergistic muscles during normal movements.

Experimentally, a series of paths have opened in the past decade that may be followed to describe the force-sharing among synergistic muscles more comprehensively. At present, the maximal number of individual force measurements that can be made for a given limb is four [50]. In the future, measurements of all muscle forces crossing (at least) a single joint would be helpful, so that the precise control of joint movement, stiffness, and force transmission could be studied. Performing such an experiment appears quite feasible in the near future.

As Crowninshield and Brand pointed out in 1981, there is tremendous potential for adequately predicting muscle forces through the corresponding EMG signals [17]. Interestingly, this area of research was more prominent 10 or 20 years ago, before such promising techniques as adaptive filtering and artificial neural networks were introduced to biomechanics.

Another area of experimental focus should be the determination of force-length and force-velocity properties of in vivo human skeletal muscles for maximal and submaximal activation. Also, more accurate and reliable methods than those presently available for the description of the instantaneous contractile condition of muscles are required.

Crowninshield and Brand [17], in their review of force predictions in skeletal muscles, emphasized the need for validation. Although this appeal was followed to a certain extent [25, 55], systematic validations of the theoretically predicted forces of individual muscles have not been performed. Finally, there appears to be some reluctance on the part of theoreticians to predict force sharing among synergistic muscles. This area of research was blooming in the 1970s and up to the mid-1980s; however, there were relatively few reports on this issue in the past decade [15]. The establishment of a testable paradigm of force sharing among muscles requires a theoretical framework, and the testing of hypotheses cannot stop at the experimental level. At present, the timing is right. The theory preceded the experiment in the 1970s; it is unfortunate that now, when the measurement of multiple individual muscle forces (at least in animal models) has become quite standard, the theoreticians should remain silent.

REFERENCES

1. Abbott, B. C., and X. M. Aubert. The force exerted by active striated muscle during and after change of length. *J. Physiol. (Lond.)* 117:77–86, 1952.
2. Abbott, B. C., and D. R. Wilkie. The relation between velocity of shortening and the tension-length curve of skeletal muscle. *J. Physiol. (Lond.)* 120:214–223, 1953.
3. Abraham, L. D., and G. E. Loeb. The distal hindlimb musculature of the cat. *Exp. Brain Res.* 58:580–593, 1985.
4. Alexander, R. M., and A. Vernon. The dimensions of knee and ankle muscles and the forces they exert. *J. Hum. Movement. Stud.* 1:115–123, 1975.
5. Allinger, T., and W. Herzog. Calculated fiber lengths in cat gastrocnemius muscle during walking (Abstract). *Proc. North Am. Cong. Biomech.* 81–82, 1992.
6. Andrews, J. G. Biomechanical analysis of human motion. *Kinesiology* 4:32–42, 1974.
7. Basmajian, J. V., and C. J. de Luca. *Muscles Alive.* Baltimore: Williams & Wilkins, 1985.
8. Basmajian, J. V., T. P. Harder, and E. M. Regenos. Integrated actions of the four heads of quadriceps femoris: an EMG study. *Anat. Rec.* 172:15–20, 1972.
9. Biewener, A. A., R. Blickhan, A. K. Perry, N. C. Heglund, and C. R. Taylor. Muscle forces during locomotion in kangaroo rats: force platform and tendon buckle measurements compared. *J. Exp. Biol.* 137:191–205, 1988.
10. Bigland, B., and O. C. J. Lippold. The relation between force, velocity and integrated electrical activity in human muscles. *J. Physiol. (Lond.)* 123:214–224, 1954.
11. Bigland-Ritchie, B., and J. J. Woods. Integrated EMG and oxygen uptake during dynamic contractions of human muscles. *J. Appl. Physiol.* 36:475–479, 1974.
12. Brooks, J. G., W. Herzog, and T. R. Leonard. Fiber dynamics of unipennate cat medial gastrocnemius during active shortening (Abstract). Proceedings of the 8th Conference of the Canadian Society for Biomechanics, Calgary, 1994, pp. 72–73.
13. Burke, R. E., G. Ten Bruggencate, and E. Jankowska. A comparison of peripheral and rubrospinal input to slow and fast twitch motor units of triceps surae. *J. Physiol. (Lond.)* 207:709–732, 1970.
14. Close, J. R., E. D. Nickel, and F. N. Todd. Motor-unit action potential counts. *J. Bone Joint Surg. Am.* 42:1207–1222, 1960.
15. Collins, J. J. The redundant nature of locomotor optimization laws. *J. Biomech.* 28: 251–267, 1995.
16. Crowninshield, R. D. Use of optimization techniques to predict muscle forces. *J. Biomech. Eng.* 100:88–92, 1978.
17. Crowninshield, R. D., and R. A. Brand. The prediction of forces in joint structures: distribution of intersegmental resultants. *Exerc. Sport Sci. Rev.* 9:159–181, 1981.
18. Crowninshield, R. D., and R. A. Brand. A physiologically based criterion of muscle force prediction in locomotion. *J. Biomech.* 14:793–801, 1981.
19. Cummings, J. F., J. P. Holden, E. S. Grood, R. R. Wroble, D. L. Butler, and J. A. Schafer. In-vivo measurements of patellar tendon forces and joint position in the goat model. (Abstract). *Trans. Orthop. Res. Soc.* 16:601, 1991.
20. Cutts, A., and B. B. Seedhom. Validity of cadaveric data for muscle physiological cross-sec-

tional area ratios: a comparative study of cadaveric and *in-vivo* data in human thigh muscles. *Clin. Biomech.* 8:156–162, 1993.

21. Davy, D. T., and M. L. Audu. A dynamic optimization technique for predicting muscle forces in the swing phase of gait. *J. Biomech.* 20:187–201, 1987.

22. Denoth, J. Methodological problems in prediction of muscle forces. *Biomechanics 11A*:82–87, 1988.

23. Dial, K. P., and A. A. Biewener. Pectoralis muscle force and power output during different modes of flight in pigeons (Columba livia). *J. Exp. Biol.* 176:31–54, 1993.

24. Dowling, J. J. The prediction of force in individual muscles crossing the human elbow joint. University of Waterloo, 1987. *Ph. D Thesis.*

25. Dul, J., G. E. Johnson, R. Shiavi, and M. A. Townsend. Muscular synergism—II. A minimum-fatigue criterion for load sharing between synergistic muscles. *J. Biomech.* 17:675–684, 1984.

26. Dul, J., M. A. Townsend, R. Shiavi, and G. E. Johnson. Muscular synergism—I. On criteria for load sharing between synergistic muscles. *J. Biomech.* 17:663–673, 1984.

27. Edman, K. A. P. The velocity of unloaded shortening and its relation to sarcomere length and isometric force in vertebrate muscle fibres. *J. Physiol. (Lond.)* 291:143–159, 1979.

28. Eloranta, V. Patterning of muscle activity in static knee extension. *Electromyogr. Clin. Neurophysiol.* 29:369–375, 1989.

29. Friedrich, J. A., and R. A. Brand. Muscle fibre architecture in the lower limb. *J. Biomech.* 23:91–95, 1990.

30. Gordon, A. M., A. F. Huxley, and F. J. Julian. Tension development in highly stretched vertebrate muscle fibres. *J. Physiol. (Lond.)* 184:143–169, 1966.

31. Goslow, G. E., Jr., R. M. Reinking, and D. G. Stuart. The cat step cycle: hind limb joint angles and muscle lengths during unrestrained locomotion. *J. Morphol.* 141:1–42, 1973.

32. Goslow, G. E., Jr., R. M. Reinking, and D. G. Stuart. Physiological extent, range and rate of muscle stretch for soleus, medial gastrocnemius and tibialis anterior in the cat. *Eur. J. Physiol.* 341:77–86, 1973.

33. Goslow, G. E., Jr., and K. M. Van DeGraaff. Hindlimb joint angle changes and action of the primary ankle extensor muscles during posture and locomotion in the striped skunk (*Mephitis mephitis*). *J. Zool. Lond.* 197:405–419, 1982.

34. Gregor, R. J., R. R. Roy, W. C. Whiting, R. G. Lovely, J. A. Hodgson, and V. R. Edgerton. Mechanical output of the cat soleus during treadmill locomotion: *in vivo* vs *in situ* characteristics. *J. Biomech.* 21:721–732, 1988.

35. Grieve, D. W., S. Pheasant, and P. R. Cavanagh. Prediction of gastrocnemius length from knee and ankle joint posture. *Biomechanics 6A:*405–412, 1978.

36. Griffiths, R. I. Ultrasound transit times gives direct measurement of muscle fiber length in vivo. *J. Neurosci. Meth.* 21:159–165, 1987.

37. Griffiths, R. I. The mechanics of the medial gastrocnemius muscle in the freely hopping wallaby (Thylogale billardierii). *J. Exp. Biol.* 147:439–456, 1989.

38. Griffiths, R. I. Shortening of muscle fibres during stretch of the active cat medial gastrocnemius muscle: The role of tendon compliance. *J. Physiol. (Lond.)* 436:219–236, 1991.

39. Guimaraes, A. C., W. Herzog, T. L. Allinger, and Y. T. Zhang. EMG-force relation of the cat soleus muscle during locomotion, and its association with contractile conditions. *J. Exp. Biol.* 198:975–987, 1995.

40. Guimaraes, A. C., W. Herzog, M. Hulliger, Y. T. Zhang, and S. Day. EMG-force relation of the cat soleus muscle: Experimental simulation of recruitment and rate modulation using stimulation of ventral root filaments. *J. Exp. Biol.* 186:75–93, 1994.

41. Guimaraes, A. C., W. Herzog, M. Hulliger, Y. T. Zhang, and S. Day. Effects of muscle length on the EMG-force relation of the cat soleus muscle using non-periodic stimulation of ventral root filaments. *J. Exp. Biol.* 193:49–64, 1994.

42. Hardt, D. E. A minimum energy solution for muscle force control during walking [*Ph. D Thesis*]. Cambridge, MA: MIT, 1978.

43. Hardt, D. E. Determining muscle forces in the leg during normal human walking—an application and evaluation of optimization methods. *J. Biomech. Eng.* 100:72–78, 1978.

44. Hasler, E. M., J. Denoth, A. Stacoff, and W. Herzog. Influence of hip and knee joint angles on excitation of knee extensor muscles. *Electromyogr. Clin. Neurophysiol.* 34:355–361, 1994.

45. Heckathorne, C. W., and D. S. Childress. Relationships of the surface electromyogram to the force, length, velocity, and contraction rate of the cineplastic human biceps. *Am. J. Physical Med.* 60:1–19, 1981.

46. Heckman, C. J., J. L. F. Weytjens, and G. E. Loeb. Effect of velocity and mechanical history on the forces of motor units in the cat medial gastrocnemius muscle. *J. Neurophysiol.* 68:1503–1515, 1992.

47. Herzog, W. Considerations for predicting individual muscle forces in athletic movements. *Int. J. Sports Biomech.* 3:128–141, 1987.

48. Herzog, W. Individual muscle force estimation using a non-linear optimal design. *J. Neurosci. Methods* 21:167–179, 1987.

49. Herzog, W. Sensitivity of muscle force estimations to changes in muscle input parameters using nonlinear optimization approaches. *J. Biomech. Eng.* 114:267–268, 1992.

50. Herzog, W. Muscle. B. M. Nigg and W. Herzog (eds). *Biomechanics of the Musculo-Skeletal System.* New York: John Wiley, 1994, pp. 154–190.

51. Herzog, W., and P. Binding. Predictions of antagonistic muscular activity using nonlinear optimization. *Math. Biosci.* 111:217–229, 1992.

52. Herzog, W., and P. Binding. Cocontraction of pairs of antagonistic muscles: analytical solution for planar static nonlinear optimization approaches. *Math. Biosci.* 118:83–95, 1993.

53. Herzog, W., A. C. S. Guimaraes, M. G. Anton, and K. A. Carter-Erdman. Moment-length relations of rectus femoris muscles of speed skaters/cyclists and runners. *Med. Sci. Sports Exerc.* 23:1289–1296, 1991.

54. Herzog, W., J. A. Hoffer, and S. K. Abrahamse. Synergistic load sharing in cat skeletal muscles. *Proceedings of the 5th Biennial Conference of the Canadian Society for Biomechanics, Ottawa, Ontario, Spodym Publishers, London, Ontario, Canada, Ottawa* 1988, pp. 78–79.

55. Herzog, W., and T. R. Leonard. Validation of optimization models that estimate the forces exerted by synergistic muscles. *J. Biomech.* 24(Suppl. 1):31–39, 1991.

56. Herzog, W., T. R. Leonard, and A. C. S. Guimaraes. Forces in gastrocnemius, soleus, and plantaris tendons of the freely moving cat. *J. Biomech.* 26(8):945–953, 1993.

57. Herzog, W., T. R. Leonard, J. M. Renaud, J. Wallace, G. Chaki, and S. Bornemisza. Force-length properties and functional demands of cat gastrocnemius, soleus and plantaris muscles. *J. Biomech.* 25(11):1329–1335,1992.

58. Herzog, W., and L. J. Read. Lines of action and moment arms of the major force-carrying structures crossing the human knee joint. *J. Anat.* 182:213–230, 1993.

59. Herzog, W., A. Stano, and T. R. Leonard. Telemetry system to record force and EMG from cat ankle extensor and tibialis anterior muscles. *J. Biomech.* 26:1463–1471, 1993.

60. Herzog, W., and H. E. D. J. ter Keurs. A method for the determination of the force-length relation of selected in-vivo human skeletal muscles. *Eur. J. Physiol.* 411:637–641, 1988.

61. Herzog, W., V. Zatsiorsky, B. I. Prilutsky, and T. R. Leonard. Variations in force-time histories of cat gastrocnemius, soleus and plantaris muscles for consecutive walking steps. *J. Exp. Biol.* 191:19–36, 1994.

62. Hill, A. V. The heat of shortening and the dynamic constants of muscle. *Proc. R. Soc. Lond.*:136–195, 1938.

63. Hodgson, J. A. The relationship between soleus and gastrocnemius muscle activity in conscious cats—a model for motor unit recruitment? *J. Physiol. (Lond.)* 337:553–562, 1983.

64. Hof, A. L., C. N. A. Pronk, and J. A. van Best. Comparison between EMG to force processing and kinetic analysis for the calf muscle moment in walking and stepping. *J. Biomech.* 20:167–178, 1987.

65. Hof, A. L., and J. Van den Berg. Linearity between the weighted sum of the EMGs of the human triceps surae and the total torque. *J. Biomech.* 10:529–539, 1977.

66. Hoffer, J. A., A. A. Caputi, and I. E. Pose. Activity of muscle proprioceptors in cat posture and locomotion: relation to EMG, tendon force, and the movement of fibres and aponeurotic segments. L. Jami, E. Pierrot-Deseilligny, and D. Zytnicki (eds). *Muscle Afferents and Spinal Control of Movement.* Oxford, England: Pergamon Press, 1992, pp. 113–121.

67. Hoffer, J. A., A. A. Caputi, I. E. Pose, and R. I. Griffiths. Roles of muscle activity and load on the relationship between muscle spindle length and whole muscle length in the freely walking cat. *Prog. Brain Res.*:75–85, 1989.

68. Huxley, A. F. Muscle structure and theories of contraction. *Prog. Biophys. biophys. Chem.* 7:255–318, 1957.

69. Joyce, G. C., and P. M. H. Rack. Isotonic lengthening and shortening movements of cat soleus muscle. *J. Physiol. (Lond.)* 204:475–491, 1969.

70. Joyce, G. C., and P. M. H. Rack, and D. R. Westbury. The mechanical properties of cat soleus muscle during controlled lengthening and shortening movements. *J. Physiol. (Lond.)* 204:461–474, 1969.

71. Kaufman, K. R., K. N. An, W. J. Litchy, and E. Y. S. Chao. Physiological prediction of muscle forces—II. Application to isokinetic exercise. *Neuroscience* 40:793–804, 1991.

72. Knowlton, G.C., F. T. Hines, K. W. Keever, and R. L. Bennet. Relation between EMG voltage and load. *J. Appl. Physiol.* 9:473–476, 1956.

73. Komi, P. V. Relationship between muscle tension, EMG and velocity of contraction under concentric and eccentric work. J. E. Desmedt (ed). *New Developments in Electromyography and Clinical Neurophysiology.* Basel, Switzerland: Karger, 1973, pp. 596–606.

74. Komi, P. V., and J. H. T. Viitasalo. Signal characteristics of EMG at different levels of muscle tension. *Acta Physiol. Scand.* 96:267–276, 1976.

75. Liberson, W. T., M. Dondey, and M. M. Asa. Brief repeated isometric maximal exercises. *Am. J. Physical Med.* 41:3–14, 1962.

76. Lippold, O. C. J. The relation between integrated action potential in human muscle and its isometric tension. *J. Physiol. (Lond.)* 117:492–499, 1952.

77. Loeb, G. E., and C. Gans. *Electromyography of Experimentalists.* Chicago: University of Chicago Press, 1986.

78. Morrison, J. B. Bioengineering analysis of force actions transmitted by the knee joint. *Biomed. Eng.* 3:164–170, 1968.

79. Morrison, J. B. The mechanics of muscle function in locomotion. *J. Biomech.* 3:431–451, 1970.

80. Nichols, T. R., and J. C. Houck. Improvement in linearity and regulation of stiffness that results from actions of stretch reflex. *J. Neurophysiol.* 39:119–142, 1976.

81. Nissel, R., G. Nemeth, and H. Ohlsen. Joint forces in extension of the knee. *Acta. Orthop. Scand.* 57:41–46, 1986.

82. Norman, R. W., R. J. Gregor, and J. J. Dowling. The prediction of cat tendon force from EMG in dynamic muscular contractions. *Proceedings of the 5th Biennial Conference of the Canadian Society for Biomechanics, Ottawa, Ontario, Spodyin Publishers, London, Ontario, Canada* 1988, pp. 120–121.

83. Olney, S. J., and D. A. Winter. Predictions of knee and ankle moments of force in walking from EMG and kinematic data. *J. Biomech.* 18:9–20, 1985.

84. Paul, J. P. Bioengineering studies of the forces transmitted by joints. II. R. M. Kenedi (ed). *Biomechanics and Related Bioengineering Topics.* London: Pergamon Press, 1965.

85. Pedersen, D. R., R. A. Brand, C. Cheng, and J. S. Arora. Direct comparison of muscle force predictions using linear and nonlinear programming. *J.Biomech. Eng.* 109:192–199, 1987.

86. Pedotti, A., V. V. Krishnan, and L. Stark, Optimization of muscle-force sequencing in human locomotion. *Math. Biosci.* 38:57–76, 1978.

87. Penrod, D. D., D. T. Davy, and D. P. Singh. An optimization approach to tendon force analysis. *Proceedings of the 25th Conference on Engineering and Medical Biology.* 1972, p. 247.

88. Penrod, D. D., D. T. Davy, and D. P. Singh. An optimization approach to tendon force analysis. *J. Biomech.* 7:123–129, 1974.

89. Pierrynowski, M. R. A physiological model for the solution of individual muscle forces during normal human walking. [*Ph.D. Thesis*] Simon Fraser University, Burnaby, British Columbia, Canada. 1982.
90. Pierrynowski, M. R. Analytic representation of muscle line of action and geometry. P. Allard, I. A. F. Stokes, and J.-P. Blanchi (eds). *Three-Dimensional Analysis of Human Movement.* Champaign, IL: Human Kinetics, 1995, pp. 215–256.
91. Pierrynowski, M.R., and J. B. Morrison. A physiological model for the evaluation of muscular forces in human locomotion: theoretical aspects. *Math. Biosci.* 75:69–101, 1985.
92. Prilutsky, B. I., W. Herzog, and T. L. Allinger. Force-sharing between cat soleus and gastrocnemius muscles during walking: explanations based on electrical activity, properties, and kinematics. *J. Biomech.* 27:1223–1235, 1994.
93. Rack, P. M. H., and D. R. Westbury. The effects of length and stimulus rate on tension in the isometric cat soleus muscle. *J. Physiol. (Lond.)* 204:443–460, 1969.
94. Rugg, S. G., R. J. Gregor, B. R. Mandelbaum, and L. Chin. In vivo moment arm calculations at the ankle using magnetic resonance imaging (MRI). *J. Biomech.* 23:495–501, 1990.
95. Sacks, R. D., and R. R. Roy. Architecture of the hind limb muscles of cats: functional significance. *J. Morphol.* 173:185–195, 1982.
96. Savelberg, H. C. M., and W. Herzog. Artificial neural networks used for the prediction of muscle forces from EMG patterns. *Proceedings of the International Society of Biomechanics Jyväskylä,* 1995.
97. Seireg, A., and R. J. Arvikar. A mathematical model for evaluation of force in lower extremities of the musculoskeletal system. *J. Biomech.* 6:313–326, 1973.
98. Seireg, A., and R. J. Arvikar. The prediction of muscular load sharing and joint forces in the lower extremities during walking. *J. Biomech.* 8:89–102, 1975.
99. Seyfert, S., and H. Kunkel. Analysis of muscular activity during voluntary contraction of different strengths. *Electromyogr. Clin Neurophysiol.* 14:323–330, 1974.
100. Sherif, M. H., R. J. Gregor, L. M. Liu, R. R. Roy, and C. L. Hager. Correlation of myoelectric activity and muscle force during selected cat treadmill locomotion. *J. Biomech.* 16:691–701, 1983.
101. Smith, J. L., V. R. Edgerton, B. Betts, and T. C. Collatos. EMG of slow and fast ankle extensors of cat during posture, locomotion, and jumping. *J. Neurophysiol.* 40:503–513, 1977.
102. Spector, S. A., P. F. Gardiner, R. F. Zernicke, R. R. Roy, and V. R. Edgerton. Muscle architecture and force-velocity characteristics of cat soleus and medial gastrocnemius: implications for motor control. *J. Neurophysiol.* 44:951–960, 1980.
103. Spoor, C. W., and J. L. van Leeuwen. Knee muscle moment arms from MRI and from tendon travel. *J. Biomech.* 25:201–206, 1992.
104. Spoor, C. W, J. L. van Leeuwen, C. G. M. Meskers, A. F. Titulaer, and A. Huson. Estimation of instantaneous moment arms of lower-leg muscles. *J. Biomech.* 23:1247–1259, 1990.
105. Sugi, H. Tension changes during and after stretch in frog muscle fibers. *J. Physiol. (Lond.)* 225:237–253, 1972.
106. Sugi, H., and T. Tsuchiya. Stiffness changes during enhancement and deficit of isometric force by slow length changes in frog skeletal muscle fibres. *J. Physiol. (Lond.)* 407:215–229, 1988.
107. van den Bogert, A. J., W. Hartman, H. C. Schamhardt, and A. A. H. J. Sauren. In-vivo relationship between force, EMG and length change in deep digital flexor muscle of the horse. A. P. Hollander, P. A. Huijing, and G. J. van Ingen Schenau (eds). *Biomechanics XI-A.* Amsterdam: Free University, 1988, pp. 68–74.
108. Vredenbregt, J., and G. Rau. Surface electromyography in relation to force, muscle length and endurance. J. E.Desmedt (ed). *New Developments in Electromyography and Clinical Neurophysiology.* Basel, Switzerland: Karger, 1973, pp. 607–622.
109. Walmsley, B., J. A. Hodgson, and R. E. Burke. Forces produced by medial gastrocnemius and soleus muscles during locomotion in freely moving cats. *J. Neurophysiol.* 41:1203–1215, 1978.

110. Weber, W., and E. Weber. *Mechanik der menschlichen Gehwerkzeuge.* Göttingen: West Germany, W. Fischer-Verlag, 1836.
111. Weytjens, J. L. F. Determinants of cat medial gastrocnemius muscle force during simulated locomotion. *Ph. D. Thesis.* University of Calgary, Calgary Canada. 1992.
112. Whiting, W. C., R. J. Gregor, and V. R. Edgerton. A technique for estimating mechanical work of individual muscles in the cat during treadmill locomotion. *J. Biomech.* 17:685–694, 1984.
113. Wickiewicz, T. L., R. R. Roy, P. L. Powell, and V. R. Edgerton. Muscle architecture of the human lower limb. *Clin. Orthop. Related Res.* 179:275–283, 1983.
114. Xu, W. S., D. L. Butler, D. C. Stouffer, E. S. Grood, and D. L. Glos. Theoretical analysis of an implantable force transducer for tendon and ligament structures. *J. Biomech. Eng.* 114:170–177, 1992.
115. Zajac, F. E., and M. E. Gordon. Determining muscle's force and action in multi-articular movement. *Exer. Sport Sci. Rev.* 17:187–230, 1989.
116. Zhang, Y. T., W. Herzog, P. A. Parker, M. Hulliger, and A. C. S. Guimaraes. Distributed random electrical neuromuscular stimulation: dependence of EMG median frequency on stimulation statistics and motor unit action potentials. L. Draganich, R. Wells, and J. Bechtold (eds). *Proceedings of the Second North American Congress on Biomechanics.* Chicago: American Society of Biomechanics, 1992, pp. 185–186.
117. Zuniga, E. N., X. T. Truong, and D. G. Simons. Effects of skin electrodes on averaged electromyographic potentials. *Arch. Phys. Med. Rehabil.* 50:264–272, 1970.
118. Zuurbier, C. J., and P. A. Huijing. Changes in geometry of actively shortening unipennate rat gastrocnemius muscle. *J. Morphol.* 218:167–180, 1993.

7
Effects of Acute and Chronic Exercise on Fat Metabolism

WADE H. MARTIN, III, M.D.

It has been well recognized for many years that fat is an important substrate for skeletal muscle contraction [14, 36, 84]. However, the proportion of energy derived from fatty acid oxidation during exercise is highly variable; it is influenced by a number of factors, including dietary and nutritional status [4, 13]; hormonal milieu [25]; exercise mode, intensity, and duration [46, 67]; and state of training [38, 81]. Less well appreciated are the effects of these physiological variables on the source of fatty acids metabolized and the mechanisms that regulate mobilization from each of the available sources. Thus, the major purpose of this communication is to summarize current knowledge regarding the contributions of various triglyceride pools in supplying fatty acids to skeletal muscle under differing exercise and training conditions. This information will be discussed in the context of mechanisms that regulate fatty acid release from each of these pools. The first part of the chapter will provide a brief general review of the different triglyceride pools, their regulatory control, and their relative importance as sources of fatty acids for skeletal muscle metabolism in both experimental animals and humans under differing exercise conditions. The focus of the second part will be on adaptations to endurance training that modify the sources of fatty acids oxidized during exercise.

SOURCES OF FATTY ACIDS

Of the triglyceride pools that have been implicated in supplying fatty acids to skeletal muscle, only two are of major importance during exercise. The first of these is adipose tissue, which releases fatty acids into the plasma after the action of lipolytic hormones such as the catecholamines [35]. Because of their insolubility in aqueous medium, these plasma free fatty acids (FFA) are complexed with albumin to permit dissolution during intravascular transport to their site of uptake in peripheral tissues such as skeletal muscle, which are likely to be anatomically remote from the site of triglyceride hydrolysis [22, 30, 38]. The second important source of fatty acids for contracting skeletal muscle is locally available in the form of triglycerides stored within the muscle fibers themselves [19, 28]. Use of these intramuscular triglycerides occurs primarily in fast-twitch oxidative (Type 2A) fibers, to a lesser extent in slow-twitch (Type 1) myocytes, and is negligible in fast-twitch glycolytic (Type 2B) fibers [68, 74]. Although a major role for this fuel source is not universally accepted [5, 70], it is the only triglyceride pool that is likely to provide sufficient fatty acids to account for the large discrepancy between the rates of total fat and plasma FFA oxidation during moderate-strenuous exercise of large muscle groups [34]. Other potential fat substrates include plasma triglycerides bound to lipoproteins, fat deposits interspersed among skeletal muscle fibers, and plasma ketones and ketoacids.

The skeletal muscle uptake of fatty acids from plasma lipoproteins increases slightly with contractile work, especially in the fasting state, but plasma triglycerides are thought to contribute only ~5–15% of the energy derived from fatty acid oxidation during exercise [37, 40, 44, 53, 76]. However, accurate measurement of the rate of skeletal muscle uptake of fatty acids released exclusively from plasma triglycerides is complicated by several factors. During exercise, the rate of hydrolysis of plasma triglycerides appears to be relatively low, in comparison with hydrolysis of triglycerides in adipose tissue and skeletal muscle [12, 37]. After hydrolysis, fatty acids released from plasma triglycerides intermingle in the vascular space with FFA originating from adipose tissue stores. In addition to this diluent effect and the modest fractional extraction of fatty acids by skeletal muscle, particularly during exercise [37], fatty acids from both plasma triglyceride and adipose tissue sources may be oxidized shortly after they are taken up, precluding their detection in tissue specimens analyzed for retention of radioactive label previously administered as exogenous triglyceride [75, 76]. In part because of these difficulties, definitive data are lacking, and it is conceivable that the role of plasma triglycerides as a fuel source for skeletal muscle contraction is somewhat greater than is generally appreciated. Nevertheless, investigations in both experimental animals and humans suggest that plasma triglycerides contribute less than 10% of the total energy derived from fatty acid metabolism during exercise.

Skeletal muscle uptake and oxidation of fatty acids released directly into the interstitial space from adipocytes interspersed among muscle fibers, without entrance of these fatty acids into the plasma compartment, has never been demonstrated. However, this process is unlikely to occur at a physiologically meaningful rate, given the low interstitial concentration of albumin, which is necessary for binding fatty acids in an aqueous environment.

Ketones and ketacids are not produced or metabolized to a significant degree in healthy, well-nourished individuals [25]. Thus, the only non-plasma FFA source of fat that is likely to supply a physiologically important proportion of substrate to skeletal muscle during exercise is the intermuscular triglycerides.

LIPOLYSIS AND PLASMA FFA METABOLISM

Evidence that fat is a major fuel for muscular work was obtained more than 50 years ago from measurements of the respiratory exchange ratio [14]. In the 1950s and 1960s, it became apparent that plasma FFA contributed an appreciable amount of this fat both at rest and during mild-to-moderate exercise [22, 23, 36, 37, 84]. For humans who ingest a typical Western diet, plasma FFA are comprised of ~40% oleate, 25% palmitate, 15% stearate, and 10% linoleate, and the remainder are a mixture of saturated and unsaturated fatty acids, having chain lengths of 12–20 carbon atoms [33]. The three most abundant fatty acids are oxidized approximately in proportion to their relative fraction of the total plasma FFA pool [33]. Thus, total plasma FFA kinetics can be estimated reliably from radioactive or stable isotope tracer studies of palmitate kinetics when the palmitate and total FFA concentrations are known.

Classical investigations of plasma FFA kinetics performed more than 30 years ago indicated that the rates of whole body FFA uptake and oxidation generally were limited by the rate of lipolysis in adipose tissue [1, 33]. The latter is influenced by a number of factors, the most important being the level of neurohumoral stimulation or inhibition and the rate of adipose tissue blood flow [2, 11]. Although it is meaningful in a physiological sense to consider the total proportion of energy derived from plasma FFA, there are large differences in lipolytic responses to hormonal action among adipocytes isolated from separate anatomical sites [78]. For example, there is good evidence that the lipolytic action of catecholamines is at least 10-fold greater in fat cells obtained from visceral abdominal adipose tissue than in those from the subcutaneous fat of the extremities [62, 78]. Intermediate responses are found in subcutaneous abdominal adipocytes [62, 78], and the action of insulin on adipocytes from different locations may vary in an analogous fashion [8]. However, the extent to which these in vitro observations are applicable under in vivo conditions is unknown and is likely to be a very fruitful subject for future investigation. The regulation of blood flow and sympathetic and neural outflow to different adipose tissue regions is also poorly understood.

Under resting conditions, the rate of whole body plasma FFA turnover is highly dependent on nutritional state and recent dietary intake [47]. After an overnight fast, fat supplies most of the resting caloric needs in healthy subjects, and a plasma FFA turnover rate of ~4–5 μmol/kg/min is sufficient to meet this substrate requirement [45, 47]. The onset of dynamic large muscle mass exercise, such as walking or running, is associated with an immediate increase in skeletal muscle uptake of FFA that exceeds the more slowly rising rate of lipolysis, resulting in a decrease in plasma FFA concentration during the initial 10–15 min of work [23, 36, 37]. Subsequently, the rate of lipolysis and FFA influx into plasma surpasses the rate of efflux and FFA concentration increases gradually for the remainder of the exercise bout [82]. During mild cycle ergometer work at ~40% $\dot{V}O_{2max}$, plasma FFA turnover after 15–20 min of exercise is about three to four times the resting rate and rises progressively to about six times the resting rate after 4 hr [84]. For low exercise intensities in the range of 25–40% $\dot{V}O_{2max}$, the turnover rate of plasma FFA is rapid enough that the substrate requirements of skeletal muscle can be met entirely from this source. However, during more strenuous work at ~65% $\dot{V}O_{2max}$, fat still supplies 40–60% of total substrate requirements, and the absolute rate of fat oxidation is ~40% higher than at 25% $\dot{V}O_{2max}$. Under these conditions, the plasma FFA turnover rate was found by Romijn et al. [67] to be similar to that at 25% $\dot{V}O_{2max}$ and well below the total rate of fat oxidation, as shown in Figure 7.1. Thus, the supply of plasma FFA is only adequate to account for 50–60% of the total fatty acids metabolized in the first 60 min of exercise at 65% $\dot{V}O_{2max}$. On the other hand, during very prolonged moderate-intensity exercise lasting for more than 1–2 hr, the continually increasing rate of lipolysis enhances the availability of FFA such that the latter substrate may become the dominant one [67], particularly in the fasting state [4]. These changes in substrate use with increasing duration of exercise are illustrated in Figure 7.2, also from studies of Romijn

FIGURE 7.1.

Whole body plasma-free fatty acid uptake (hatched bars) and total fat oxidation (open bars) after 30 min of cycle ergometer exercise at 25, 65, and 85% $\dot{V}O_{2max}$. Data are means ± SE. *, $P < .05$ vs. 25% $\dot{V}O_{2max}$; + $P < .05$ vs 25 and 85% $\dot{V}O_{2max}$; #, $P < .05$ vs. 65% $\dot{V}O_{2max}$. Adapted from ref. 67.

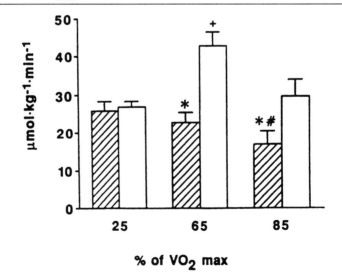

FIGURE 7.2.

Effect of exercise duration on the relative contribution of plasma FFA and glucose and muscle triglycerides (Tg) and glycogen to energy production during 120 min of cycle ergometer exercise at 65% $\dot{V}O_{2max}$ (A) and 25% $\dot{V}O_{2max}$ (B). Adapted from ref. 67.

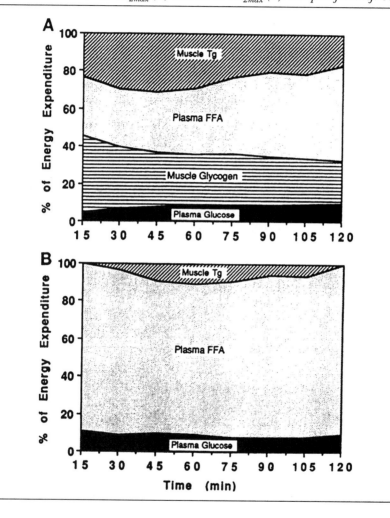

et al. [67]. At still higher work intensities (e.g., 85% $\dot{V}O_{2max}$) that usually cannot be maintained for 60 min, most of the substrate needs of skeletal muscle are provided by carbohydrate fuel sources, that ~25–30% of the total energy expenditure is still derived from fat oxidation [69]. Because the turnover rate of plasma FFA is ~25% lower at 85% than at 65% $\dot{V}O_{2max}$, a substantial proportion (>40%) of the fatty acids oxidized during high-intensity work originates from a nonplasma FFA source.

Hormonal Regulation

The rate of whole body lipolysis is well-known to be highly dependent on the action of several hormones, the most potent of which in humans are the catecholamines and insulin [2]. During exercise, plasma catecholamines and sympathetic neural activity rise exponentially with increasing exercise intensity, especially at work rates above ~70% $\dot{V}O_{2max}$ [49, 71], as shown in Figure 7.3. At or near maximal effort, plasma epinephrine and norepinephrine concentrations may attain levels more than 20-fold above those at rest [49], values that are equivalent to those seen under other conditions of extreme physiological stress, such as shock, myocardial infarction, diabetic ketoacidosis, or hypoglycemia [18]. In addition, the plasma epinephrine concentration increases with duration of exercise, particularly during very prolonged work that results in hypoglycemia [25]. As illustrated in Figure 7.3, the level of sympathoadrenal stimulation during physical activity of a given relative intensity is also dependent on exercise mode [49], being greatest for work involving a large muscle mass, such as running or two-leg cycling, and least for work requiring a small muscle mass, such as single-arm flexion

FIGURE 7.3.

Plasma catecholamine concentrations during one-arm, one-leg, and two-leg cycle ergometer exercise at various submaximal and maximal intensities. Data are means ± SE. Adapted and reproduced with permission from Circulation Research. Copyright 1981 American Heart Association.

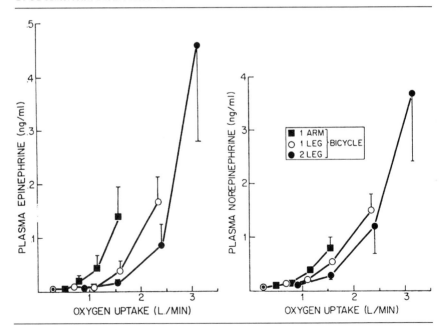

(curl). Despite the major role of the sympathoadrenal system in promoting lipolysis during physical activity and the close relationship between work intensity and level of sympathoadrenal stimulation, the effect of exercise intensity on the rate of lipolysis is much less predictable. As discussed above, plasma FFA turnover after 30 min of exercise is reported to be most rapid (about four to five times the resting rate) during mild exertion (e.g., 25% $\dot{V}O_{2max}$), when plasma catecholamine concentrations are only 50–60% above those at rest. In contrast, during exercise at 65 and 85% $\dot{V}O_{2max}$, plasma FFA turnover is ~10 and 35%, respectively, below that at 25% $\dot{V}O_{2max}$, yet plasma catecholamine concentrations at these higher work rates are 3–6 and 17–19 times, respectively, those at rest [67]. These findings illustrate that, despite the fact that the rate of lipolysis at rest is directly related to the level of catecholamine stimulation [26], during exercise the situation is more complex, and a variety of other factors, such as blood flow to adipose tissue [11] and the plasma lactic acid concentration [9, 42] also may be of considerable importance. The other hormone of major significance in regulation of lipolysis is insulin. In contrast to the effects of catecholamines, the action of insulin is antilipolytic at plasma concentrations occurring under most conditions in healthy subjects. The plasma insulin concentration generally decreases during mild-to-moderate intensity exercise, and the magnitude of the decline is related to work intensity, possibly because of sympathoadrenally mediated α-adrenergic inhibition of insulin release [26]. The antilipolytic action of insulin is evident at a lower plasma hormone concentration than is required for stimulation of glucose transport [61]. Thus, an exercise-induced decline in insulin concentration to a value below the previous baseline level may contribute to enhanced plasma FFA turnover in the first 10–30 min of physical activity. However, for more prolonged bouts of exercise, the progressive increase in lipolysis is accompanied by only modest or no further decreases in insulin concentration [81], casting doubt on the role of this mechanism in directly augmenting lipolysis under these conditions. During a 2-hr bout of cycle ergometer work performed at 64% peak $\dot{V}O_2$, the plasma insulin concentration of subjects studied in our laboratory declined 25–30% in the first 30 min of exercise, as shown in Figure 7.4 with only minor changes over the remaining 90 min of the cycling protocol [39]. The plasma concentration of glycerol, which is more closely related to the rate of lipolysis than the FFA concentration because of the relative absence of glycerol metabolism in adipose tissue and skeletal muscle, rose 20–30% over the same time interval as the decrease in insulin concentration in the initial 30 min of exercise (see Fig. 7.4). On the other hand, the glycerol level rose nearly fourfold in the 90 min thereafter when the plasma insulin concentration was stable or decreasing slowly from a level ~25% below that at baseline. Nevertheless, the early decrease in insulin concentration during exercise is likely to have a permissive effect that facilitates amplification of the rate of lipolysis in the later stages of prolonged work.

FIGURE 7.4.

Plasma insulin and blood glycerol concentrations at rest and at various time points during cycle ergometer exercise at 64% peak $\dot{V}O_2$ for 120 min. Data are means $\pm$ SD. Adapted from ref. 39.

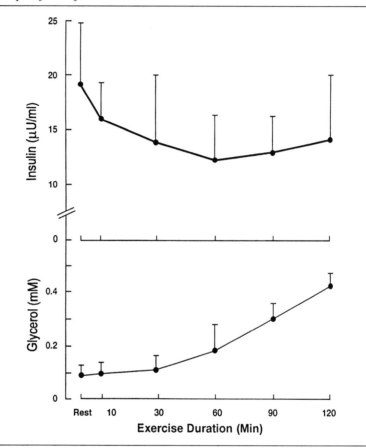

Several other hormones may stimulate lipolysis directly or enhance the lipolytic response to catecholamines, but their role in mediating the increase in FFA turnover during exercise is more doubtful. Plasma growth hormone concentration is directly related to exercise intensity and duration [7, 31, 32], but the time course of its rise is too slow to account for the prompt stimulation of lipolysis at the onset of exercise. In addition, growth hormone concentration may decline with very prolonged or exhausting work that elicits the most pronounced increase in FFA turnover [32]. Hypophysectomy plus β-adrenergic blockade with propranolol completely inhibited adipose tissue lipolysis in rats in which propranolol alone reduced this process by only 45% [29]. These results suggest that adrenocorticotrophic hormone (ACTH), thyroid-stimulating hormone (TSH), or other pituitary polypeptides could stimulate lipolysis in some species of animals during exercise, but it is unclear as to whether this is true in humans. Glucagon also is a potent stimulant of lipolysis in experimental animals, such as rats, but its importance in regulating this process in people under physiological conditions has recently been questioned [59]. Hormones such as estrogen and testosterone may modulate lipolysis directly or via alteration of lipolytic sensitivity to catecholamines in some adipose tissue regions of humans [63, 83]. However, a role for sex hormones in mediating exercise-induced lipolysis has not been established. Thus, much remains to be learned about hormonal and other aspects of regulation of lipolysis during exercise.

Limitations to the Role of Plasma FFA as a Substrate Source

Although early radioisotopic studies in dogs and humans demonstrated that plasma FFA could supply all or most of the substrate requirements of skeletal muscle under resting conditions or during mild exercise, these investigations also revealed that only about half of the infused FFA label was immediately oxidized [34, 36, 42]. Recent findings from stable isotope investigations indicate that a significant portion of the administered label of an FFA tracer can be accounted for in products of exchange reactions that result in label fixation into nonfatty acids moieties, such as glutamate and lactate, during the first or later revolutions through the tricarboxylic acid cycle [73]. However, the amount of label metabolized in this fashion becomes progressively less with increasing exercise intensity because of more rapid flux through the tricarboxylic acid cycle, relative to the rates of these exchange reactions, which do not increase and may even decrease with exercise. Nevertheless, during moderate-intensity work, when 20% or less of the FFA label appears in exchange reaction products, plasma FFA provide only about 50–70% of the total energy derived from fat metabolism, based on simultaneous isotopic tracer and indirect calorimetric measurements of FFA turnover and total fat oxidation [34, 36, 67]. Indeed, one recent report suggests that even if all FFA extracted from the plasma were immediately oxidized, FFA could provide no more than 25–30% of the total energy derived from fat during moderate or strenuous exercise [45]. Thus, several lines of evidence support the concept that a significant, and under some circumstances, major proportion of fatty acids oxidized during exercise originate from sources other than FFA released from adipose tissue.

MUSCLE TRIGLYCERIDE METABOLISM

The most important nonplasma FFA source of fatty acids for oxidation during moderate-strenuous exercise involving large muscle groups is the triglycerides stored within skeletal muscle fibers. Investigations conducted more than 40 yr ago indicated that during prolonged exercise, these triglycerides may be the preferred substrate in highly oxidative muscle fibers of pigeons [28]. This also appears to be true for a variety of other species of birds and fish [19, 27], suggesting that the processes of intramuscular triglyceride storage and use evolved in ancient times. A number of migratory fish and birds accumulate vast quantities of triglycerides within locomotor (fin or flight) muscle fibers in preparation for their journey, and these are severely depleted in muscle specimens obtained from such animals after arrival at their destination [27].

Evidence consistent with a physiologically important role of intramuscular triglycerides as a fuel source in nonmigratory species such as mammals became available about 20 yr ago. A single bout of exhausting physical activity lasting several hours was found to result in disappearance of 30–70% of preexercise triglyceride stores from the active musculature of rats [64, 74]. Plasma FFA oxidation accounted for only ~50% of total fat oxidation during moderate-intensity exercise in normal dogs [40], and the percentage was considerably lower in animals with pancreatectomy-induced diabetes or after treatment with nicotinic acid [41], which inhibits lipolysis in adipose tissue. Subsequent studies in rats performing exhausting aquatic exercise demonstrated that the magnitude of muscle triglyceride depletion was dependent on fiber type, being ~70% in fast-twitch red muscle of the deep quadriceps, ~25% in slow-twitch fibers of the soleus, and minimal in fast-twitch white muscle of the superficial quadriceps [64]. This contrasted with the pattern of glycogen depletion, which was 70–75% in all skeletal muscles examined and nearly complete in the liver. At about the same time, it was reported that the triglyceride concentration in homogenates of human vastus lateralis muscle decreased ~25% after 90 min of strenuous cycle ergometry [12] and ~50% after several hours of cross-country skiing [24]. In the latter investigation, up to two-thirds of the total fatty acids oxidized were estimated to be supplied by muscle triglyceride stores. However, it was unclear from such studies whether the triglycerides used were originally contained within skeletal muscle fibers or were released from adipose tissue deposits interspersed among the fibers.

More recent information on the contribution of muscle triglycerides to total energy expenditure during cycle ergometry suggests that the role of this fuel source is highly dependent on exercise intensity, duration, and mode. In the cycle ergometer studies of Romijn et al. [67], estimated muscle triglyceride use ranged from 0 to 10% of total fat oxidation during cycling at 25% $\dot{V}O_{2max}$ to ~50% of total fat oxidation for the first hour of ergometry at 65% $\dot{V}O_{2max}$ (see Fig. 7.2). With increasing duration of work at the latter intensity, the role of muscle triglycerides gradually declined and represented only ~30% of the total fat being oxidized at 2 hr. On the other hand, at 85% $\dot{V}O_{2max}$, muscle triglycerides were estimated to supply 40–

50% of the fat but only ~10–15% of the total substrate metabolized. However, no muscle biopsies were performed in this investigation, and muscle triglyceride use was estimated as the difference between total fat oxidation determined by indirect calorimetry and the rate of plasma FFA uptake evaluated with stable isotope techniques. In contrast to these findings, muscle triglyceride use, quantified directly in skeletal muscle biopsies, was found to be negligible during 3 hr of single leg thigh extension exercise at ~60% peak thigh extension capacity but only ~25% peak $\dot{V}O_2$[77]. These contrasting results illustrate the metabolic flexibility of mechanisms regulating the supply of fatty acids from separate substrate sources under differing exercise and metabolic conditions.

Regulation of Muscle Triglyceride Use

The regulation of triglyceride hydrolysis in skeletal muscle is less well-studied than is control of lipolysis in adipose tissue. Nevertheless, β-adrenergic stimulation appears to be essential for exercise-induced muscle triglyceride use, in contrast to adipose tissue lipolysis, which is only partially inhibited by β-adrenergic blockade. Nearly 20 yr ago, it was first reported that the nonselective β-adrenergic antagonist, propranolol, completely prevented the disappearance of triglycerides from fast-twitch red and intermediate skeletal muscles of rats performing exhausting aquatic exercise [74]. In the same animals, the increase in plasma FFA levels after 3 hr of exercise was only reduced ~50% by propranolol. Thus, hydrolysis of muscle triglycerides may be even more sensitive to catecholamine stimulation than lipolysis in adipose tissue. More recently, nonselective β-adrenergic blockade with nadolol also was found by Cleroux et al. [15] to result in total inhibition of triglyceride use in the vastus lateralis muscle of human subjects during strenuous cycle ergometer work to an end point of exhaustion (Fig. 7.5). In contrast, muscle triglyceride use was greater after treatment with the β_1-selective blocking agent, atenolol, than with placebo. Exercise time to exhaustion was reduced 33% by nadolol in the same individuals but only 14% by β_1-selective blockade. Muscle glycogen depletion and the plasma FFA concentration at exhaustion were not significantly different among treatments (see Fig. 1.5). These results suggest that the inability to mobilize muscle triglycerides may have been a critical factor in the earlier onset of fatigue after nonselective β-blockade. Despite the absence of any statistically apparent effect of β-blockade on the serum FFA concentration at exhaustion, the rise in serum glycerol with exercise was blunted with the β_1-selective antagonist, atenolol and, to an even greater degree, with the nonselective β-blocker, nadolol. The latter findings and normal use of muscle triglycerides during atenolol treatment are consistent with inhibition of skeletal muscle lipolysis by nonselective but not β_1-selective adrenergic blockade. Radioligand binding analyses indicate that skeletal muscle β-adrenergic receptors are of the β_2-subtype [50, 80], in contrast to those in adipose tissue which,

FIGURE 7.5.

Effects of β_1-selective and nonselective β-adrenergic blockade on vastus lateralis muscle triglyceride and glycogen and serum FFA and glycerol concentrations at rest and during or immediately after cycle ergometer exercise at 189 W to an end point of exhaustion. Data are means ± SE. *, P < .05;**, P < .01 vs. placebo. Adapted from ref. 15.

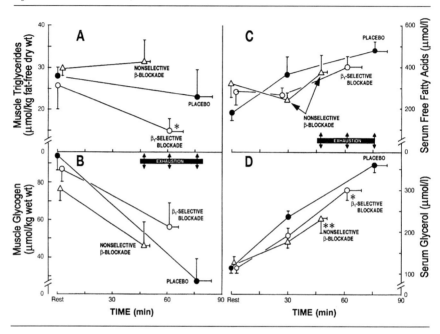

until recently, were considered to be β_1 in nature [6, 48] but may be of a distinct subtype (i.e., the recently cloned β_3-adrenergic receptor) [20].

THE ROLE OF PLASMA TRIGLYCERIDES

Although plasma lipoproteins appear to play a minor role in supplying fatty acids to skeletal muscle during exercise, they are likely to be of considerable importance in replenishing muscle triglyceride stores in the postexercise resting state. Fatty acid release from chylomicrons and very low-density lipoproteins is mediated by the action of lipoprotein lipase in the capillary endothelium [66]. Moreover, the rate of fatty acid uptake from chylomicrons was found by Mackie et al. [53] to be closely correlated with lipoprotein lipase activity in skeletal muscles of differing fiber type, as shown in Figure 7.6. In these studies, lipoprotein lipase activity and the rate of uptake of fatty acids from plasma chylomicrons was more than fivefold greater in

FIGURE 7.6.

Relative uptake of chylomicron [14C]-triglyceride (TG) in slow-twitch (soleus), fast-twitch red (deep lateral gastrocnemius), and fast-twitch white (superficial medial gastrocnemius) muscle sections as a function of tissue lipoprotein lipase (LPL) activity as reported by Borensztajn et al. Am J Physiol 229:394–397, 1975) and Linder et al. (Am J Physiol 231:860–864, 1976). Filled symbols are fasting data. Adapted from ref. 53.

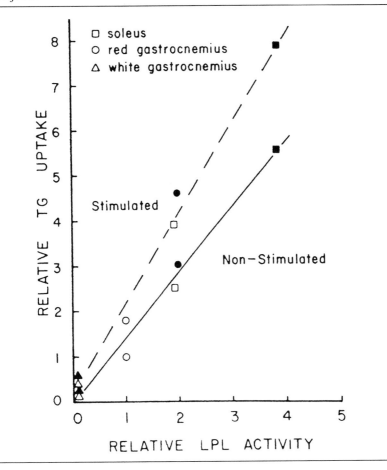

slow-twitch and fast-twitch red fibers than in fast-twitch white muscle fibers of the rat [53]. Under resting conditions,most of the fatty acids taken up by skeletal muscle from plasma chylomicrons are subsequently detected in acylglycerides, rather than in nonesterified fatty acids of analyzed tissue samples [75]. These findings and the fact that muscle fibers that metabolize triglycerides during exercise (i.e., fast-twitch red fibers of the deep vas-

TABLE 7.1.
Fatty Acid Turnover from Circulating Triglycerides and Plasma FFA at Indicated Concentrations in the Resting-Fed Condition for Human, Dog, and Rats

		Plasma Concentration (μmol/ml)	Fatty Acid Turnover (μmol/kg/min)
Human	TG[a]	1.25	~13
	FFA	0.3	10
Dog	TG	1.4	57
	FFA	0.4	12
Rat	TG	2.0	21
	FFA	0.4	12

Adapted from ref 76.
[a]TG, triglycerides.

tus and slow-twitch fibers of the soleus) take up fatty acids from plasma chylomicrons much more avidly than fast-twitch white fibers, from which little or no triglycerides are used during muscle contraction, provide further evidence that intramuscular triglycerides are an important fuel for contractile activity.

Both plasma triglycerides and nonesterified FFA are important sources of fatty acids for repletion of intramuscular triglycerides stores after prolonged exercise. However, for this process the role of chylomicrons and very low-density lipoproteins may be greater than that of plasma FFA in both humans and experimental animals, as suggested by Terjung et al. (Table 7.1; see ref 76). At rest in the postprandial state, higher insulin and low plasma catecholamine concentrations (in comparison with exercise) minimize the rate of lipolysis in adipose tissue while enhancing its lipoprotein lipase activity [69]. The concentration of FFA is low relative to that of plasma triglycerides under these conditions (Table 7.1). In the fasting state, both insulin and catecholamine levels are low at rest, but after one or more preceding bouts of prolonged exercise, lipoprotein lipase activity and gene expression in skeletal muscle are enhanced relative to those in adipose tissue [52, 68]. Although the rate of uptake of plasma triglyceride-derived fatty acids in skeletal muscle is slower at rest than during exercise, over the course of several hours it appears sufficient to restore muscle triglyceride concentrations to the pre-exercise state in slow-twitch and fast-twitch red fibers that preferentially use fat as a substrate for contractile work [75].

EFFECTS OF ENDURANCE TRAINING ON FAT METABOLISM

One of the most important adaptations to endurance exercise training is the enhanced capacity of skeletal muscle to oxidize long-chain fatty acids

[60]. This biochemical adaptation is accompanied by an increase in the proportion of energy derived from fat oxidation and a corresponding decrease in carbohydrate use during submaximal exercise [14, 38]. The magnitude of training-induced alterations in substrate use may be 30–50%, based on measurements of the respiratory exchange ratio and other metabolic parameters. Studies were conducted in our laboratory to quantify changes in the proportion and source of substrates oxidized during a 120-min bout of two-leg cycle ergometry performed at the same absolute work intensity (64% pretraining peak $\dot{V}O_2$) before and after 3 mo of training [39]. The training program consisted of ~45 min of running or cycle ergometry on alternate days 6 days/wk. Included in these sessions were six 5-min bouts of cycle ergometer interval training at peak $\dot{V}O_2$ 1–3-days/wk. Biopsy samples obtained from the vastus lateralis of these individuals demonstrated that the activity of skeletal muscle β-hydroxy CoA dehydogenase, a marker of fatty acid oxidative capacity, increased ~90% after completion of the training program. The magnitude of this effect is very similar to the doubling of fatty acid oxidative capacity observed in skeletal muscle of rats after an equivalent duration of training [60]. In the human subjects, the cumulative proportion of energy derived from fat oxidation during the 120-min bout of cycle ergometry at 64% $\dot{V}O_{2max}$ rose from ~40% before training to ~60% afterward (Fig. 7.7). There was a corresponding decrease in carbohydrate oxidation that was partially accounted for by a 40% decline in glycogen depletion from the vastus lateralis muscle. Subsequent studies by Coggan et al. [16] showed that plasma glucose oxidation also is reduced by 30% during moderate-intensity exercise in the trained state. Thus, multiple independent metabolic observations support the conclusion that one of the salient adaptations to endurance exercise training is a diminished dependence on carbohydrate energy sources and an increase in total fat oxidation during mild-moderate intensity exercise.

Adaptations of Lipolytic Hormones to Training

Early cross-sectional studies in trained and untrained human subjects performing different modes of exercise were interpreted to indicate that plasma FFA transported from remote adipose tissue stores are the source of the additional fat oxidized by physically conditioned individuals during submaximal exercise [33,36]. However, this view is difficult to reconcile with the markedly decreased lipolytic hormone response to exercise elicited by even a few weeks of training. Winder et al. [81] demonstrated that the plasma concentrations of glucagon and of epinephrine and norepinephrine, the most potent stimulants of lipolysis, are reduced by 30–70% at the same absolute work intensity (~60% pretraining peak $\dot{V}O_2$) in the trained state, as shown in Figure 7.8. This adaptation is virtually complete within 3 wk of initiation of the same alternate-day running and cycle ergometry program as that which markedly enhances fat oxidation during

FIGURE 7.7.

Cumulative energy derived from oxidation of carbohydrates, fatty acids, and all substrate sources during 120 min of cycle ergometer exercise at 64% pretraining peak $\dot{V}O_2$. Open circles, before training; closed circles, afterward. Data are means ± SD. **, P < .01 after vs. before. Adapted from ref. 39.

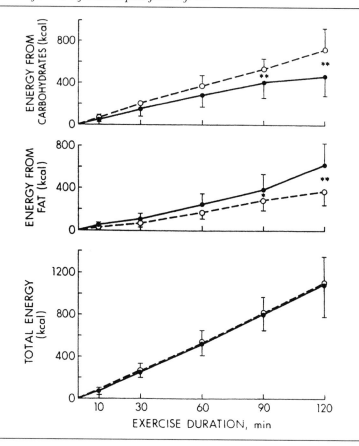

moderate-intensity exercise. A somewhat smaller but still significant decrease in the plasma catecholamine response to exercise was also reported previously by Hartley et al. in young healthy subjects who engaged in seven weeks of vigorous sports activities conducted three hours/day three days/week [32]. In the same study, the effect of training on plasma catecholamines was statistically significant, even for exercise bouts performed at equivalent relative work rates (i.e., higher absolute work rates in the trained state). However, the plasma growth hormone response to exercise was not consistently altered by physical conditioning in this investigation.

In addition to observing lower catecholamine levels, several investigators

FIGURE 7.8.

Effect of duration of endurance training on plasma norepinephrine (NE) and epinephrine (E) concentrations at the end of 90 min of cycle ergometer work at 58% initial $\dot{V}O_{2max}$. Data are means ± SE. Adapted from ref. 81.

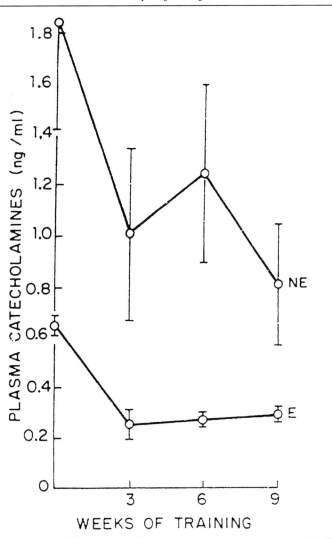

have also reported a higher plasma insulin concentration or less pronounced decline in insulin during prolonged exercise in the trained state [7, 25, 31, 81]. Although a lower insulin level is usually observed in trained subjects at rest, the antilipolytic action of a higher insulin concentration during exercise is likely to exacerbate the blunted sympathoadrenal response to exercise in trained individuals, further reducing adipose tissue lipolysis under such conditions. These hormonal changes are associated with lower plasma FFA and glycerol levels at the same absolute work rate in the trained state [7, 43, 65, 81]. The decrease is particularly noteworthy for glycerol, a more reliable indicator of the rate of whole body lipolysis than the plasma FFA concentration, because the relative absence of glycerokinase activity in adipocytes and skeletal myocytes precludes glycerol reesterification in these tissues after triglyceride hydrolysis [51]. Glycerol may be reesterified or metabolized in the liver but the lower blood flow to this organ during moderate-strenuous exercise versus rest [68] is likely to limit any exercise-induced increase in glycerol clearance. In contrast, plasma FFA are metabolized in many tissues, and FFA uptake briefly may exceed the rate of lipolysis under some non-steady-state conditions, such as the onset of exercise when plasma FFA turnover increases and concentration decreases [23, 36, 37]. In any case, both plasma glycerol and FFA levels during exercise are lower after training than beforehand, suggesting that the rate of adipose tissue lipolysis is decreased and that plasma FFA are unlikely to be the source of the additional fat oxidized in physically conditioned subjects.

Adaptations of Adipose Tissue to Training

The effect of training-induced neurohumoral adaptations on lipolysis during exercise probably would be even greater without the concurrent increase in the lipolytic response of adipose tissue to catecholamines, which also occurs. Glycerol and fatty acid release from isolated fat cells during catecholamine exposure is enhanced by chronic exercise in both experimental animals and humans [3, 17]. This effect is not explained by differences or changes in body weight or adipocyte size and number [3]. It is mediated by augmentation of the β-adrenergic action of catecholamines, rather than by diminution of their α-adrenergic antagonism of lipolysis [17]. The adaptation appears to be a postreceptor effect, because adipose tissue β-adrenergic receptor density is not altered by training, at least in rats [79]. Studies conducted in our laboratory in highly conditioned human subjects indicate that plasma glycerol and FFA responses to intravenous epinephrine infusion are 50–80% greater in the trained state than after the same subjects stop exercising for only four days (Fig. 7.9; see ref 55). No further decrease in epinephrine-induced lipolysis occurred after 3 and 8 wk of reduced physical activity. The rapid change in lipolytic response to epinephrine with cessation of training was observed at equivalent plasma cate-

FIGURE 7.9.

*Effect of duration of detraining on serum FFA and blood glycerol responses to constant-rate epinephrine infusion. Data are means ± SE. *, P < .01 vs. trained. Adapted from ref. 55.*

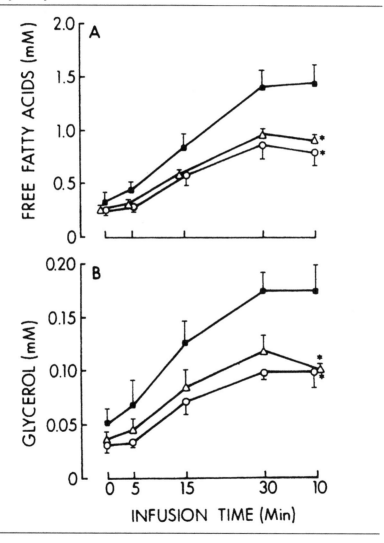

cholamine levels, and the epinephrine concentrations were in the range elicited by strenuous exercise. The diminished lipolytic response also before any changes in body weight, skinfold adiposity, or the plasma insulin concentration became evident. Thus, in humans, enhanced epinephrine-induced lipolysis may be primarily an effect of recent bout(s) of exercise, rather than of training per se. On the other hand, Askew et al. reported in rats that epinephrine-sensitive lipolysis is not altered in sedentary animals by a single preceding bout of exhausting exercise [3]. Additional studies will be necessary to clarify the relative roles of acute vs. chronic exercise in modulating catecholamine-induced lipolysis.

Effect of Training on Plasma FFA Kinetics

Plasma FFA turnover is too slow to account for more than about half of all fatty acids oxidized during exercise of more than mild intensity [34, 36, 40, 45, 67]. As noted above, physical conditioning decreases plasma FFA and glycerol concentrations while simultaneously increasing the rate of total fat oxidation under these conditions [7, 38, 43, 65, 81]. There is considerable evidence that plasma FFA uptake and oxidation are directly related to the plasma FFA concentration [1, 40]. In the context of these findings, it is not logical that the greater amount of fat oxidized in physically conditioned subjects during exercise would be supplied by plasma FFA transported from adipose tissue, unless training also increases skeletal muscle FFA uptake at the same or a lower plasma concentration of this substrate.

To investigate this possibility, studies were conducted in our laboratory to quantify the effect of training on the rates of plasma FFA turnover and oxidation [56] and the use of the most likely alternative source of fatty acids, the intramuscular triglycerides [39], in young healthy human subjects during prolonged exercise. These investigations were carried out before and after 12 wk of the strenuous endurance training program described earlier. $\dot{V}O_{2max}$ increased ~25% after completion of the program. The respiratory exchange ratio during the final 30–60 min of a 90 to 120 min bout of cycle ergometer work performed at the same absolute work rate (64% pretraining peak $\dot{V}O_2$) decreased from 0.88 ± 0.01 before training to 0.82 ± 0.01 afterward (P < .01). Based on these data, the proportion of energy derived from fat oxidation during this time interval increased from 41% initially to 62% after physical conditioning. Plasma palmitate and FFA kinetics were characterized for the same time intervals. These results were calculated from gas chromatography-mass spectrometry analysis of ^{13}C isotopic enrichment and the concentrations of palmitate and total FFA in plasma samples drawn during a constant-rate intravenous infusion of the stable isotope tracer [1-^{13}C]palmitate [26]. Palmitate is a saturated 16-carbon fatty acid that comprises ~25% of the total plasma (and adipose tissue) fatty acid mass, and its kinetics resemble those of most other long-chain plasma FFA [33]. Thus, total plasma FFA kinetics can be estimated reliably

TABLE 7.2.
Effect of 12 Wk of Endurance Training on Plasma Palmitate Kinetics and Substrate Concentrations during Prolonged Cycle Ergometer Exercise[a]

	Before Training	After Training
Plasma palmitate R_a (μmol/kg/min)	5.27 ± 0.66	$3.55 \pm 0.24^*$
Plasma palmitate R_d (μmol/kg/min)	5.15 ± 0.67	$3.45 \pm 0.24^*$
Plasma palmitate concentration (μM)	261 ± 28	$184 \pm 21^*$
Plasma FFA concentration (μM)	1010 ± 120	$690 \pm 70^*$
Plasma glycerol concentration (μM)	400 ± 50	$320 \pm 60^\dagger$
Plasma palmitate oxidation rate (μmol/kg/min)	2.52 ± 0.23	$1.92 \pm 0.21^*$

[a]Adapted from ref. 56. Data are means $\pm$ SE. R_a, = rate of appearance into plasma; R_d, = rate of disappearance from plasma. Values given are averages for the final 30–60 min of cycle ergometer exercise at 64% pretraining peak $\dot{V}_{O_2}$. $^*P < .05$; †, $P < .01$ vs. before training.

from the palmitate data. The plasma palmitate kinetics and substrate concentration data in our subjects for the final 30–60 min of cycle ergometry are shown in Table 7.2. Despite the large training-induced increase in total fat oxidation in these individuals, the rates of inflow and outflow of palmitate to and from the plasma, respectively, declined by about one-third after training. This effect was accompanied by 20–32% decreases in the plasma concentrations of palmitate, total FFA, and glycerol, providing further evidence of a substantial reduction in the rate of adipose tissue lipolysis in the trained state. Because the concentration ratio of palmitate to total plasma FFA (~26%) did not change, the estimated decrease in FFA turnover after physical conditioning was nearly identical in magnitude to the decrement in palmitate turnover. The rate of plasma palmitate oxidation, evaluated by isotope ratio mass spectrometric analyses of $^{13}CO_2$ isotopic enrichment in expired air samples [57], was 24% lower during cycle ergometry after completion of the endurance training program. There was a very high correlation between the plasma palmitate concentration and its rate of oxidation both before and after training (R = .90–.92), consistent with several studies from various laboratories, indicating that the rate of FFA oxidation is dependent on the FFA plasma concentration under steady-state conditions [1, 33, 36]. The FFA kinetics data also provide evidence that physical conditioning does not enhance skeletal muscle uptake of plasma FFA during moderately strenuous exercise involving a large muscle mass.

Effect of Training on Intramuscular Triglyceride Use

In the investigations discussed above, oxidation of plasma FFA accounted for ~44% of energy derived from fat metabolism before training and ~23% afterward, as illustrated in Figure 7.10. Thus, in highly conditioned subjects, more than three-fourths of fatty acids oxidized during moderate-intensity exercise may originate from a source other than plasma FFA. Ad-

FIGURE 7.10.

Percentage of total energy derived from carbohydrate (CHO), nonplasma fatty acid (FA), and plasma FA fuel sources during prolonged cycle ergometer exercise before and after training. Adapted from ref. 56.

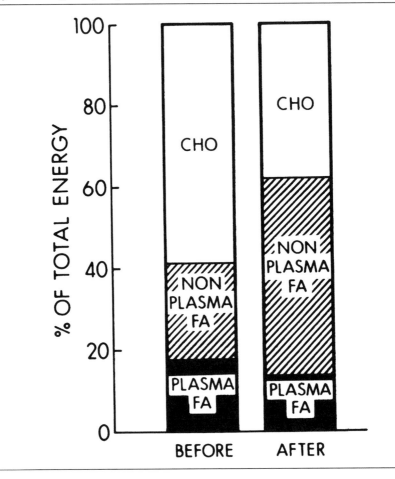

ditional studies of skeletal muscle biopsy samples obtained from the same individuals were conducted to quantify the effect of training on use of intramuscular triglycerides [39]. The biopsy samples were taken from the vastus lateralis muscle before and immediately after completion of the 90 to 120-min bout of cycle ergometer exercise at 64% pretraining peak $\dot{V}O_2$. Histochemical staining of tissue sections revealed no visible evidence of fat deposits interspersed among muscle fibers, even in the sedentary state. Nevertheless, to prevent commingling of fat from intramyocytic and extramyocytic stores and selectively quantify triglyceride use from the intramuscular compartment alone, triglyceride content was assayed in freeze-dried fibers that had been individually separated from all extraneous nonmyocytic material. Several hundred fibers were isolated from each specimen and were combined subsequently for the triglyceride analyses. There was a difference in the pre-exercise muscle fiber triglyceride content after as opposed to before training. The measured content of ~60 mmol/kg dry weight is similar to that reported by other investigators in pre-exercise skeletal muscle samples [12, 21, 24] if results are adjusted for a tissue water content of 75% [64].

Depletion of intramuscular triglycerides during cycle ergometry nearly doubled in the trained state, rising from ~21% of the preexercise triglyceride content on the baseline evaluation to ~41% of the corresponding value of the follow-up study. The mass of triglycerides metabolized was 12.7 mmol/kg dry weight before training and 26.1 mmol/kg dry weight afterward. If triglycerides are assumed to have an average molecular weight of 860 g/mol [82], which yields 9.46 kcal of energy/g of triglycerides [58] when the latter are fully metabolized, and the active muscle mass is ~8 kg (2 kg dry weight) for cycle ergometry at a $\dot{V}O_2$ of 1.7 L/min (8.3 kcal/min), then the energy derived from use of intramuscular triglycerides was 207 kcal in the untrained state and 425 kcal after physical conditioning. This accounts for ~20% of the total energy expenditure on the first study and more than 40% after training. Of the energy derived from fat, about 90% of that unaccounted for by plasma FFA oxidation is explained by use of intramuscular triglycerides.

POSSIBLE MECHANISMS

Given that muscle triglyceride use appears to be entirely dependent on β_2-adrenergic stimulation [15, 74], it is somewhat surprising that intramuscular triglyceride metabolism is increased in trained subjects in whom sympathoadrenal activity during exercise is much lower than it is in sedentary individuals [31, 32, 81]. However, as previously discussed, there is good evidence that catecholamine-induced lipolysis is markedly enhanced in isolated adipocytes from physically conditioned humans and experimental animals [3, 17]. Williams et al. concluded that this was a postreceptor effect [79] because, in contrast to skeletal muscle [80], β-adrenergic receptor density of isolated adipocytes was not altered in trained rats, despite a marked increase in the lipolytic response of these cells to catecholamines in the same animals. On the other hand, Buckenmeyer et al. reported that β-adrenergic receptor density is increased in slow- and fast-twitch oxidative but not fast-twitch glycolytic skeletal muscle fibers of rats after a 12-wk exercise program [10]. This adaptation may be specific to certain species, however, because we did not observe such an effect in any skeletal muscle fiber type of human subjects after a training regimen of similar duration [54]. These differences notwithstanding, it seems conceivable that enhanced β-adrenergic receptor-adenylate cyclase coupling or other molecular adaptations could mediate the augmented triglyceride hydrolysis despite reduced sympathoadrenal stimulation during exercise in physically conditioned human skeletal muscle. Little information is available on this topic, and further studies will be necessary to determine which, if any, metabolic responses to catecholamines are altered by training in human skeletal muscle and to elucidate the molecular mechanism(s) by which increased intramuscular triglyceride hydrolysis is achieved.

Caveats during Exercise of Small Muscle Groups

Despite our observations on the effect of large muscle group training on muscle triglyceride use during the same type of exercise, there are some circumstances under which these results may not be applicable. In a cross-sectional investigation by Turcotte et al. [77], plasma FFA uptake was greater in trained than in untrained subjects during the third hour of a single-leg thigh extension exercise protocol. However, plasma FFA uptake was not different in the two groups during the first 2 hr of this protocol. The increase in plasma catecholamine concentrations during single-leg thigh extension exercise was only one- or twofold above the resting level in this study, slightly greater than the 70% rise observed with two-leg cycling at 25% $\dot{V}O_{2max}$, in which plasma FFA were found by Romijn et al [67] to supply more than 80% of total substrate requirements. A longitudinal study by Kiens et al. [46] reported little or no triglyceride use by the quadriceps muscle during 3 hr of single-leg thigh extension exercise, either before or after training. In this investigation, plasma catecholamine concentrations during exercise did not rise above the resting level on either occasion. Studies discussed earlier in this chapter demonstrating that muscle triglyceride use may be completely inhibited by β-adrenergic blockade, while adipose tissue lipolysis during exercise is only partially prevented by this treatment [15, 74], suggest that a certain threshold of β-adrenergic stimulation may be necessary for intramuscular triglyceride hydrolysis to occur. In any case, results of these single-leg thigh extension investigations emphasize the extent to which the relative roles of plasma FFA and muscle triglycerides as energy sources are highly dependent on exercise mode, intensity, and duration.

SUMMARY

Fatty acids are an important source of energy for skeletal muscle contraction, particularly during exercise of mild-moderate intensity, prolonged duration, and in the fasting state. Plasma FFA transported from remote adipose tissue stores and triglycerides contained within skeletal muscle fibers are the major sources of these fatty acids. The relative contribution of each source is dependent on the mode, intensity, and duration of exercise and on training status. Plasma FFA oxidation is directly related to the rate of lipolysis in adipose tissue. The most potent stimulants of the latter are the catecholamines, but a lower plasma insulin concentration during exercise also plays a contributory role. In contrast, intramuscular triglyceride hydrolysis appears to be mediated entirely by β^2-adrenergic stimulation. Endurance training substantially enhances fatty acid oxidative capacity in skeletal muscle and increases the proportion of energy derived from fatty acid oxidation during exercise. In addition, the sympathoadrenal response to exercise is markedly blunted in the trained state. Studies conducted in our laboratory indicate that plasma FFA and glycerol concentrations and whole body FFA uptake and oxidation are all decreased during moderate-intensity exercise at the same absolute work rate after physical conditioning, probably because of the reduction of sympathoadrenal activity. However, the lipolytic response to catecholamines also is enhanced in trained subjects. Perhaps as a consequence, the magnitude of the decrease in lipolysis and plasma FFA oxidation is less than the decrement in sympathoadrenal activity in the same individuals during exercise in the trained state.

Other investigations were conducted in our laboratory to determine the source of the additional fatty acids oxidized in physically conditioned subjects. These studies demonstrated that during moderate-intensity exercise at the same absolute work rate, depletion of triglycerides from within skeletal muscle fibers was twice as great after, as opposed to, before training. Regardless of training status, intramuscular triglyceride use accounted for about 90% of the oxidized fatty acids that were not supplied from adipose tissue via the plasma. Intramuscular triglycerides were the source of virtually all of the additional fatty acids oxidized in the trained state. Both before and after physical conditioning they explained the discrepancy between the rates of plasma FFA and total fat oxidation during moderate-intensity exercise of up to 2 hr in duration.

ACKNOWLEDGMENTS

The contributions of current and former faculty members, postdoctoral fellows, the technical staff of the Division of Applied Physiology and the Department of Medicine of Washington University School of Medicine, and the many research subjects who participated in these investigations are recognized with deep appreciation. The author was supported by National Heart, Lung, and Blood Institute (NHLBI) Grant HL-41290 and by National Institute on Aging Institutional National Research Service Award AG-00078. The research conducted by our group at Washington University was supported by National Institutes of Health (NIH) Resource for Biomedical

Mass Spectrometry Grant RR-00954, General Clinical Research Center Grant RR-00036, Diabetes Research and Training Center Grant AM-20579, and NIH Grants AM-18986 and NS-18387.

REFERENCES

1. Armstrong, D. T., R. Steele, N. Altszuler, A. Dunn, J. S. Bishop, and R. C. DeBodo. Regulation of plasma free fatty acid turnover. *Am. J. Physiol.* 201:9–15, 1961.
2. Arner, P. Control of lipolysis and its relevance to development of obesity in man. *Diabetes Metab. Rev.* 4:507–515, 1988.
3. Askew, E. W., R. L. Huston, C. G. Plopper, and A. L. Hecker. Adipose tissue cellularity and lipolysis. Response to exercise and cortisol treatment. *J. Clin. Invest.* 56:521–529, 1975.
4. Astrand, P.-O. Diet and athletic performance. *Fed. Proc.* 26:1772–1777, 1967.
5. Astrand, P.-O., and K. Rodahl. *Textbook of Work Physiology. Physiological Bases of Exercise.* New York: McGraw-Hill, 1986, p. 460.
6. Bahouth, S. W., and C. C. Malbon. Subclassification of β-adrenergic receptors of rat fat cells: a re-evaluation. *Mol. Pharmacol* 34:318–326, 1988.
7. Bloom, S. R., R. H. Johnson, D. M. Park, M. J. Rennie, and W. R. Sulaiman. Differences in the metabolism and hormonal response to exercise between racing cyclists and untrained individuals. *J. Physiol. Lond.* 258:1–18, 1976.
8. Bolinder, J., L. Kager, J. Ostman, and P. Arner. Differences at the receptor and postreceptor levels between human omental and subcutaneous adipose tissue in the action of insulin on lipolysis. *Diabetes* 32:117–123, 1983.
9. Boyd, A. E., S. R. Giamber, M. Mager, and H. E. Lebovitz. Lactate inhibition of lipolysis in exercising man. *Metabolism* 23:531–542, 1974.
10. Buckenmeyer, P. J., A. H. Goldfarb, J. S. Partilla, M. A. Pineyro, and E. M. Dax. Endurance training, not acute exercise, differentially alters β-receptors and cyclase in skeletal fiber types. *Am. J. Physiol* 258 (*Endocrinol. Metab.* 21):E71–E77, 1990.
11. Bulow, J. Subcutaneous adipose tissue blood flow and triacylglycerol mobilization during prolonged exercise in dogs. *Pflugers. Arch.* 392:230–234, 1981.
12. Carlson, L. A., L.-G. Ekelund, and S. O. Froberg. Concentration of triglycerides, phospholipids and glycogen in skeletal muscle and of free fatty acids and β-hydroxybutyric acid in blood in man in response to exercise. *Eur. J. Clin. Invest.* 1:248–254, 1971.
13. Christensen, E. H., and O. Hansen. Arbeitsf ahigkeit und Ernahrung. *Skand. Arch. Physiol.* 81:160–171, 1939.
14. Christensen, E. H., and O. Hansen. Respiratorischer Quotient and O_2-Aufnahme. *Skand. Arch. Physiol.* 81:180–189, 1939.
15. Cleroux, J. P. Van Nguyen, A. W. Taylor, and F. H. H. Leenen. Effects of β_1-vs. $\beta_1 + \beta_2$-blockade on exercise endurance and muscle metabolism in humans. *J. Appl. Physiol.* 66:548–554, 1989.
16. Coggan, A. R., W. M. Kohrt, R. J. Spina, D. M. Bier, and J. O. Holloszy. Endurance training decreases plasma glucose turnover and oxidation during moderate-intensity exercise in men. *J. Appl. Physiol.* 68:990–996, 1990.
17. Crampes, F., M. Beauville, D. Riviere, and M. Garrigues. Effect of physical training in humans on the response of isolated fat cells to epinephrine. *J. Appl. Physiol.* 61:25–29, 1986.
18. Cryer, P. E. Physiology and pathophysiology of the human sympathoadrenal neuroendocrine system. *N. Engl. J. Med.* 303:436–444, 1980.
19. Drummond, G. I. and E. C. Black. Comparative physiology:fuel of muscle metabolism. *Annu. Rev. Physiol* 22:169–190, 1960.
20. Emorine, L. J., S. Marullo, M. M. Briend-Sutren, et al. Molecular characterization of the human β_3-adrenergic receptor. *Science* 245:1118–1121, 1989.

21. Essen, B. L. Hagenfeldt, and L. Kaijser. Utilization of blood-borne and intramuscular substrates during continuous and intermittent exercise in man. *J. Physiol. Lond.* 265:489–506, 1977.

22. Fredrickson, D. S., and R. S. Gordon, Jr. The metabolism of albumin-bound C^{14}-labeled unesterified fatty acids in normal human subjects. *J. Clin. Invest.* 37:1504–1515, 1958.

23. Friedberg, S. J., W. R. Harlan, and E. H. Estes, Jr. The effect of exercise on the concentration and turnover of plasma nonesterified fatty acids. *J. Clin. Invest.* 39:215–220, 1960.

24. Froberg, S. O., and F. Mossfeldt. Effect of prolonged strenuous exercise on the concentration of triglycerides, phospholipids and glycogen in muscle of man. *Acta Physiol. Scand.* 82:167–171, 1971.

25. Galbo, H. *Hormonal and Metabolic Adaptations to Exercise.* New York: Thieme-Stratton, 1983, pp 5–7, 30–35, 64–69.

26. Galster, A. D., W. E. Clutter, P. E. Cryer, J. A. Collins, and D. M. Bier. Epinephrine plasma thresholds for lipolytic effects in man. *J. Clin. Invest.* 67:1729–1738, 1981.

27. George, J. C., and D. Jyoti. The lipid content and its reduction in the muscle and liver during long and sustained muscular activity. *J. Anim. Morphol. Physiol.* 2:31–37, 1955.

28. George, J. C., and R. M. Naik. Relative distribution and chemical nature of the fuel store of the two types of fibres in the pectoralis major muscle of the pigeon. *Nature* 181:709–711, 1958.

29. Gollnick, P. D., R. G. Soule, A. W. Taylor, C. Williams, and C. D. Ianuzzo. Exercise-induced glycogenolysis and lipolysis in the rat:hormonal influence. *Am. J. Physiol.* 219:729–733, 1970.

30. Gordon, R. S., Jr. and A. Cherkes. Unesterified fatty acids in human blood plasma. *J. Clin. Invest.* 35:206–212, 1956.

31. Hartley, L. H., J. W. Mason, R. P. Hogan, et al. Multiple hormonal responses to graded exercise in relation to physical training. *J. Appl. Physiol.* 33:602–606, 1972.

32. Hartley, L. H., J. W. Mason, R. P. Hogan, et al. Multiple hormone responses to prolonged exercise in relation to physical training. *J. Appl. Physiol.* 33:607–610, 1972.

33. Havel, R. J., L. A. Carlson, L.-G. Ekelund, and A. Holmgren. Turnover rate and oxidation of different fatty acids in man during exercise. *J. Appl. Physiol.* 19:613–619, 1964.

34. Havel R. J., L.-G. Ekelund, and A. Holmgren. Kinetic analysis of the oxidation of palmitate-1-^{14}C in man during prolonged heavy muscular exercise. *J. Lipid Res.* 8:366–373, 1967.

35. Havel, R. J., and A. Goldfein. The role of the sympathetic nervous system in the metabolism of free fatty acids. *J. Lipid Res.* 1:102–108, 1959.

36. Havel R. J., A. Naimark, and C. F. Borchgrevink. Turnover rate and oxidation of free fatty acids of blood plasma in man during exercise:studies during continuous infusion of palmitate-1-C^{14}. *J. Clin. Invest.* 42:1054–1063, 1963.

37. Havel R. J., B. Pernow, and N. L. Jones. Uptake and release of fatty acids and other substrates in the legs of exercising men. *J. Appl. Physiol.* 23:90–99, 1967.

38. Henriksson, J. Training-induced adaptations of skeletal muscle and metabolism during submaximal exercise. *J. Physiol. (Lond.)* 270:661–665, 1977.

39. Hurley, B. F., P. M. Nemeth, W. H. Martin, III, J. M. Hagberg, G. P. Dalsky, and J. O. Holloszy. Muscle triglyceride utilization during exercise: effect of training. *J. Appl. Physiol.* 60:562–567, 1986.

40. Issekutz, B., H. I. Miller, P. Paul, and K. Rodahl. Source of fat oxidation in exercising dogs. *Am. J. Physiol.* 207:583–589, 1964.

41. Issekutz, B., Jr., and P. Paul. Intramuscular energy sources in exercising normal and pancreatectomized dogs. *Am. J. Physiol.* 215:197–204, 1968.

42. Issekutz, B., Jr, B. A. S. Shaw, and T. B. Issekutz. Effect of lactate on FFA and glycerol turnover in resting and exercising dogs. *J. Appl. Physiol.* 39:349–353, 1975.

43. Johnson, R. H., J. L. Walton, H. A. Krebs, and D. H. Williamson. Metabolic fuels during and after severe exercise in athletes and nonathletes. *Lancet* ii:452–455, 1969.

44. Jones, N. L., and R. J. Havel. Metabolism of free fatty acids and chylomicron triglycerides during exercise in rats. *Am. J. Physiol.* 213:824–828, 1967.

45. Kanaley, J. A., C. D. Mottram, P. D. Scanlon, and M. D. Jensen. Fatty acid kinetic responses to running above and below the lactate threshold. *J. Appl. Physiol.* 79:439–447, 1995.

46. Kiens, B., B. Essen-Gustavsson, N. J. Christensen, and B. Saltin. Skeletal muscle substrate utilization during submaximal exercise in man: effect of endurance training. *J. Physiol. (Lond.)* 469:459–478, 1993.

47. Klein, S., V. R. Young, G. L. Blackburn, B. R. Bistrian, and R. R. Wolfe. Palmitate and glycerol kinetics during brief starvation in normal weight young adult and elderly subjects. *J. Clin. Invest.* 78:928–933, 1986.

48. Lands, A. M., A. Arnold, J. P. McAuliff, F. P. Luduena, and T. G. Brown. Differentiation of receptor systems activated by sympathomimetic amines. *Nature* 214:597–598, 1967.

49. Lewis S. F., W. F. Taylor, R. M. Graham, W. A. Pettinger, J. E. Schutte, and C. G. Blomqvist. Cardiovascular responses to exercise as functions of absolute and relative work load. *J. Appl. Physiol.* 54:1314–1323, 1983.

50. Liggett, S. B., S. D. Shah, and P. E. Cryer. Characterization of β-adrenergic receptors of human skeletal muscle obtained by needle biopsy. *Am. J. Physiol.* 254 (*Endocrinol. Metab.* 17):E795–E798, 1988.

51. Lin, E. C. C. Glycerol utilization and its regulation in mammals. *Annu. Rev. Biochem.* 46:765–795, 1977.

52. Lithel, H., J. Orlander, R. Schele, B. Sjodin, and J. Karlsson. Changes in lipoprotein-lipase activity and lipid stores in human skeletal muscle with prolonged heavy exercise. *Acta Physiol. Scand.* 107:257–261, 1979.

53. Mackie, B. G., G. A. Dudley, H. Kaciuba-Uscilko, and R. L. Terjung. Uptake of chylomicron triglycerides by contracting skeletal muscle in rats. *J. Appl. Physiol.* 49:851–855, 1980.

54. Martin, W. H., III, A. R. Coggan, R. J. Spina, and J. E. Saffitz. Effects of fiber type and training on β-adrenoceptor density in human skeletal muscle. *Am. J. Physiol.* 257(*Endrocrinol Metab* 20):E736–E742, 1989.

55. Martin, W. H., E. F. Coyle, M. Joyner, D. Santeusanio, A. A. Ehsani, and J. O. Holloszy. Effects of stopping exercise training on epinephrine-induced lipolysis in humans. *J. Appl. Physiol.* 56:845–848, 1984.

56. Martin, W. H., G. P. Dalsky, B. F. Hurley, et al. Effect of endurance training on plasma free fatty acid turnover and oxidation during exercise. *Am. J. Physiol.* 265(*Endocrinol. Metab.* 28):E708–E714, 1993.

57. Mathews, D. E., K. J. Motil, D. K. Rohrbaugh, J. F. Burke, V. R. Young, and D. M. Bier. Measurement of leucine metabolism in man from a primed continuous infusion of L-[1-^{13}C]leucine. *Am. J. Physiol.* 238(*Endocrinol. Metab.* 1):E473–E479, 1980.

58. McGilvery, R. W. *Biochemistry. A Functional Approach.* Philadelphia: W. B. Saunders, 1970, p. 516.

59. Miles, J. M., and M. D. Jensen. Editorial:Does glucagon regulate adipose tissue lipolysis? *J. Clin. Endocrinol. Metab.* 77:5A–6A, 1993.

60. Mole, P.A., L. B. Oscai, and J. O. Holloszy. Adaptation of muscle to exercise. Increase in levels of palmityl CoA synthetase, carnitine palmityltransferase, and palmityl CoA dehydrogenase, and in the capacity to oxidize fatty acids. *J. Clin. Invest.* 50:2323–2330, 1971.

61. Nurjhan, N., P. J. Campbell, F. P. Kennedy, J. M. Miles, and J. E. Gerich. Insulin dose-response characteristics for suppression of glycerol release and conversion to glucose in humans. *Diabetes* 35:1326–1331, 1986.

62. Rebuffe-Scrive, M., B. Andersson, L. Olbe, et al. Metabolism of adipose tissue in intraabdominal depots of nonobese men and women. *Metabolism* 38:453–458, 1989.

63. Rebuffe-Scrive, M., J. Fidh, L.-O. Hafstrom, and P. O. Bjorntorp. Metabolism of mammary, abdominal, and femoral adipocytes in women before and after menopause. *Metabolism* 35:792–797, 1986.

64. Reitman, J., K. M. Baldwin, and J. O. Holloszy. Intramuscular triglyceride utilization by red, white, and intermediate skeletal muscle and heart during exhausting exercise. *Proc. Soc. Exp. Biol. Med.* 142:628–631, 1973.

65. Rennie, M. J., and R. H. Johnson. Alteration of metabolic and hormonal responses to exercise by physical training. *Eur. J. Appl. Physiol. Occup. Physiol.* 33:215–226, 1974.
66. Robinson, D. S. The function of the plasma triglycerides in fatty acid transport. M. Florkin and E. H. Stotz (eds). *Comprehensive Biochemistry, Lipid Metabolism,* Vol. 18. Amsterdam: Elsevier, 1970, pp. 51–116.
67. Romijn, J.A., E. F. Coyle, L. S. Sidossis, et al. Regulation of endogenous fat and carbohydrate metabolism in relation to exercise intensity and duration. *Am. J. Physiol.* 265(*Endocrinol. Metab.* 28):E380–E391, 1993.
68. Rowell, L. B., J. R. Blackmon, and R. A. Bruce. Indocyanine green clearance and estimated hepatic blood flow during mild to maximal exercise in upright man. *J. Clin. Invest.* 43:1677–1690, 1964.
69. Sadur, C. N., and R. H. Eckel. Insulin stimulation of adipose tissue lipoprotein lipase activity. *J. Clin. Invest.* 69:1119–1125, 1982.
70. Saltin, B., and P.-O. Astrand. Free fatty acids and exercise. *Am. J. Clin Nutr.* 57(Suppl.): 752S–758S, 1993.
71. Seals, D. R., R. G. Victor, and A. L. Mark. Plasma norepinephrine and muscle sympathetic discharge during rhythmic exercise in humans. *J. Appl. Physiol.* 65:940–944, 1988.
72. Seip, R. J., T. J. Angelopoulos, and C. F. Semenkovich. Exercise induces human lipoprotein lipase gene expression in skeletal muscle but not adipose tissue. *Am. J. Physiol.* 268(*Endocrinol. Metab.* 31):E229–E236, 1995.
73. Sidossis, L. S., A. R.Coggan, A. Gastaldelli, and R. R. Wolfe. Pathway of free fatty acid oxidation in human subjects. Implications for tracer studies. *J. Clin. Invest.* 95:278–284, 1995.
74. Stankiewicz-Choroszucha, B., and J. Gorski. Effect of beta-adrenergic blockade on intramuscular triglyceride mobilization during exercise. *Experientia* 34:357–358, 1978.
75. Terjung, R. L., L. Budohoski, K. Nazar, A. Kobryn, and H. Kaciuba-Uscilko. Chylomicron triglyceride metabolism in resting and exercising fed dogs. *J. Appl. Physiol.* 52:815–820, 1982.
76. Terjung, R., B. G. Mackie, G. A. Dudley, and H. Kaciuba-Uscilko. Influence of exercise on chylomicron triacylglycerol metabolism: plasma turnover and muscle uptake. *Med. Sci. Sports Exerc.* 15:340–347, 1983.
77. Turcotte, L. P., E. A. Richter, and B. Kiens. Increased plasma FFA uptake and oxidation during exercise in trained vs. untrained humans. *Am. J. Physiol.* 262(*Endocrinol. Metab.* 25):E791–E799, 1992.
78. Wahrenberg, H., F. Lonnqvist, and P. Arner. Mechanisms underlying regional differences in lipolysis in human adipose tissue. *J. Clin. Invest.* 84:458–467, 1989.
79. Williams, R. S., and T. Bishop. Enhanced receptor-cyclase coupling and augmented catecholamine-stimulated lipolysis in exercising rats. *Am. J. Physiol.* 243(*Endocrinol. Metab.* 6):E345–E351, 1982.
80. Williams, R. S., M. G. Caron, and K. Daniel. Skeletal muscle β-adrenergic receptors: variations due to fiber type and training. *Am. J. Physiol.* 246(*Endocrinol. Metab.* 9):E160–E167, 1984.
81. Winder, W. W., R. C. Hickson, J. M. Hagberg, et al. Training-induced changes in hormonal and metabolic responses to submaximal exercise. *J. Appl. Physiol.* 46:766–771, 1979.
82. Wolfe, R. R., S. Klein, F. Carraro, and J.-M. Weber. Role of triglyceride-fatty acid cycle in controlling fat metabolism during and after exercise. *Am. J. Physiol.* 258(*Endocrinol. Metab.* 21):E382–E389, 1990.
83. Xu, X., G. DePergola, and P. Bjorntorp. Testosterone increases lipolysis and the number of β-adrenoceptors in male rat adipocytes. *Endocrinology* 128:379–382, 1991.
84. Zierler, K. L. Fatty acids as substrates for heart and skeletal muscle. *Circ. Res.* 38:459–463, 1976.

8
Growth, Physical Activity, and Bone Mineral Acquisition

DONALD A. BAILEY, P.E.D.
ROBERT A. FAULKNER, Ph.D.
HEATHER A. McKAY, Ph.D

Skeletal fragility leading to fractures represents a public health problem of major importance, both socially and economically [35, 60]. The size of this problem is certain to grow as the population ages. The percentage of the total population over age 55 (those at highest risk) is growing rapidly in North America and Europe [134]. Although osteoporosis is primarily a disease of the elderly, attainment of a strong, dense skeleton during the growing years may be the best way to prevent osteoporosis in the older population [9, 113].

Our lack of knowledge concerning the determinants of bone mineral accretion during the years of growth limits our understanding of osteoporosis in the elderly. Adult bone mineral status is a reflection of bone mineral accrual during growth and subsequent loss with advancing years. The establishment of an optimum level of bone mineral in childhood and adolescence is of crucial concern in terms of lifelong skeletal adequacy. Because bone mineral loss is a normal consequence of aging, those who acquire a greater bone mineral balance during the first two decades of life should be at reduced risk for the health problems associated with skeletal fragility later in life.

The impact of exercise and physical activity on skeletal integrity is an area of considerable interest and extensive study, especially in view of the well-documented relationship between adult bone mineral density status and fracture risk in the elderly. Fracture frequency increases as bone mineral density decreases [137]; thus, a major risk factor for fracture is a low bone mineral density [59]. Heredity is the major determinant of bone mineral status, which has been demonstrated in studies on twins and studies of familial patterning [59, 73, 86, 115, 133]. A recent study, however, indicates that nearly half the variance in bone mineral density is attributable to nonhereditary factors [64], and there is evidence that physical activity may be an important contributor. It is well established that immobilization results in bone mineral loss. Thus, the potential of weight-bearing physical activity to reduce the age-related decrease in bone mineralization in older adults has been widely studied, and there are a number of excellent reviews covering this topic [13, 19, 33, 51]. In growing children, however, our knowl-

233

edge about the long-term effects of physical activity on bone mineral accretion is incomplete. Only recently have studies on healthy pediatric populations been undertaken.

The purpose of this chapter is to review the principles of skeletal development and adaptation, with an emphasis on the preeminent role of mechanical loading factors. Data from current developmental studies on bone mineral accrual in growing children are reviewed, and studies investigating the role of physical activity in the regulation of bone mineral accretion during growth are summarized.

THE HUMAN SKELETON

The human skeleton is comprised of 206 individual bones that function as a framework for the body providing, among other things, support against gravity, protection for vital organs and tissues, and a lever system for muscle action. Bones also play an essential role in terms of a number of vital body processes related to calcium and phosphate homeostasis, immune system function, and hematopoiesis. The composition of skeletal tissue is primarily a combination of collagen fibers and other proteins, as well as minerals in the form of hydroxyapatite. Close to 30% of the mass of a mature skeleton is mineral; protein, fat, and water make up the remainder. Calcium accounts for approximately 37% of the total mineral content in bone with phosphorous, sodium, potassium, zinc, magnesium, and other trace minerals making up the rest [114]. The compression-resisting hydroxyapatite crystals have a high-strength component and account for 80–90% of the variance in bone compression strength [81]. The tension-resisting collagen fibers provide flexibility, thereby allowing the composite material to respond to strong forces by bending, rather than breaking. Bone remains elastic for up to about three-quarters of its breaking stress [3].

Bone tissue is mineralized in an ordered fashion into two basic forms: cortical or compact bone and trabecular or cancellous bone. Total skeletal mass is made up of 75–80% cortical bone and 20–25% trabecular bone. Cortical bone is the densely compacted tissue that forms the outer surface of all bones, including the shafts of the long bones. Trabecular bone consists of a meshwork of thin, bony horizontal and vertical plates, occurring inside the cortical shell in some of the flat bones, the vertebral bodies, and the distal ends of the long bones. The proportion of each component will vary for different parts of the body (axial vs. appendicular), from bone to bone and within the same bone at different sites and ages. Trabecular bone, which has a relatively greater surface area: volume ratio than cortical bone, is thought to be more susceptible to changes in hormonal milieu [39], whereas cortical and trabecular bone are responsive to mechanical loading factors [89].

Measurement of the Mineral Component of Bone

Over the years, many methods have been used to describe skeletal development and assess changes in bone mineralization with age. Early assessments, using postmortem anatomical specimens, included skeletal weighing and direct bone morphometry. Radiographs were also used for morphometric analysis, and photo densitometry was used to estimate bone mineralization. Over the last 25 years, newer noninvasive techniques have been developed that have provided more precise, sensitive, and accurate estimates of bone mineralization. These methods include photon absorption techniques, which have progressed from single-photon (SPA), to dual-photon (DPA), to dual energy X-ray absorptiometry (DXA). Quantitative computed tomography (QCT) and broadband ultrasound attenuation have also been applied to the study of bone mineralization. DXA and QCT have been used to assess bone mineral in various regions of the body, including the distal and midradius, the lumbar spine, the proximal femur, the calcaneus, and the total body, and excellent reviews deal with the scientific basis, strengths, and weaknesses of the various techniques [81, 129]. For the purposes of this chapter, bone mineral content (BMC) will be defined as the absolute amount of mineral present in a bone or regions of a bone and bone mineral density (BMD) as the relative amount of bone mineral per measured area or volume of bone.

It is important to understand the distinction between BMC and BMD. Quantitative information about skeletal development is provided by BMC, whereas BMD provides a qualitative assessment that attempts to control for size differences. For instance, women in general have a lower BMC than men, because their skeletons are anatomically smaller, but sexual dimorphism in BMD is still controversial and may vary according to the skeletal site measured. The merits of expressing the mineral component of bone as BMC or as BMD have been reviewed elsewhere [22]. Another important semantic distinction needs to be made. The literature is full of references to bone mass and peak bone mass. The problem with this terminology is that current measurement techniques do not measure bone mass per se; they measure the mineral content of bone. Numerous studies have used BMC and, in some cases, BMD as a measure of bone mass. In this chapter, unless otherwise stated, peak bone mineral content will be used as a surrogate measure for peak bone mass.

Skeletal Adaptation Processes

Contrary to early thought, bone tissue is in a constant state of flux throughout life. Three processes are involved in this dynamic condition: growth, modeling, and remodeling. During the life span, a single process may dominate at certain times, or the three processes may function concurrently at other times. In the immature skeleton all three processes are active simultaneously; each has a different function [19].

GROWTH. Growth is the expression of the genetically programmed process of enlargement of the entire skeleton without regard to concurrent changes in shape that may be occurring regionally in response to local loading factors. In humans, maturity is marked by the cessation of skeletal growth. Growth is primarily under the control of the endocrine system, a topic too large to be covered in this review but thoroughly reviewed elsewhere [93, 100].

MODELING. Modeling is the process that alters the shape and mass of bones in response to mechanical loading factors. Modeling occurs primarily during the growing years and represents a regional response to current loading conditions. Bone strength is increased by adding mass and improving internal architecture at high-load locations. Modeling involves the addition of bone, without prior resorption, to surfaces for which bone deformation through loading is greatest, resulting in a net gain of bone over time. The modeling response to regular involvement in weight-bearing physical activity in the young may result in a reserve of bone beyond that needed for normal activity [37]. The ability of bone to adapt to loading factors is much greater during growth than after maturity [33, 96]. Although modeling occurs primarily during the growing years, recent evidence suggests that under certain metabolic or loading conditions, limited modeling can occur following skeletal maturation [20].

REMODELING. Remodeling, although present in the young, is the dominant bone process modifying shape and mass in adults. The principal purpose of remodeling is to replace fatigue-damaged bone tissue with new bone; thus, remodeling serves a maintenance function. The remodeling cycle begins with an activation phase, followed in sequence by a resorption phase, then a formation phase. This sequence of events allows the skeleton to maintain its mechanical integrity through the renewal of bone and provides a mechanism for the maintenance of calcium homeostasis. Over time, however, remodeling results in a net loss of bone, as new bone never completely replaces the bone that has been resorbed, particularly on the endosteal surface, where bone is in contact with marrow. This is responsible for the decrease in bone mineral that accompanies aging. Thus, the processes of modeling and remodeling have opposite long-term effects, even though they are both initiated by mechanical loading stimuli.

BONE MINERALIZATION: DEVELOPMENTAL CONSIDERATIONS

The establishment of an optimum level of bone mineral during the growing years, when modeling is superimposed on growth, is an important consideration in terms of lifelong skeletal adequacy. Two determinants have been advanced to explain the cause of dangerously low bone mineral density in some older members of the population: excessive bone loss during aging and failure to attain a sufficiently high bone mineral content during the years of growth. Thus, the antecedents of low bone mineral and skeletal fragility in the elderly may begin during the first two decades of life [113], which has led to developmental studies of bone mineral accrual in children and adolescents.

In evaluating the results of such developmental studies, it should be kept in mind that the skeleton is not a single entity: There are regional differences in bone mineralization, just as there are regional differences in overall growth. The age of onset, the rate of bone mineral accrual, and the age of attainment of peak bone mineral content vary, according to gender and the bone region being studied [41, 48, 113]. For example, as shown in data from a study of Canadian children (Fig. 8.1), with advancing age, BMC of the skull decreased as a percentage of total body BMC whereas, in other regions, particularly the legs, BMC increased. In boys, the legs accounted for nearly half the total increase in BMC (600–700 g) between 8 and 15 years of age, whereas the other sties increased by 100–200 g. In females, there was

FIGURE 8.1.
Regional BMC at the skull, lower limbs, trunk, and upper limbs, expressed as a percentage of total body BMC. Adapted from ref. 113.

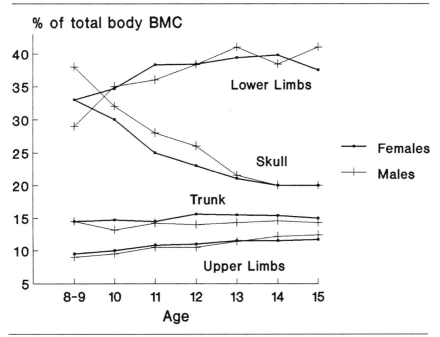

a relatively greater increase in trunk BMC with increasing age, whereas in boys the legs showed a relatively greater increase. In terms of regional differences in BMD accrual, McKay et al. [85] compared premenarcheal adolescent girls (mean age, 11.1 yr) to their premenopausal mothers (mean age, 40 yr). They found that although the girls had attained 78% of the mothers' total body BMD, they had attained 81% of the mothers' BMD at the femoral neck and only 68% at the lumbar spine. These trends are in agreement with previous values for the femoral neck and lumbar spine, as reported by others [16].

Considering the fact that the calcium component of bone mineral increases from about 25 g at birth to about 1000 g by 15–20 yr of age; this gain is more than double the age-associated loss of calcium during adult years [40, 80], which suggests that any interruption in mineral accrual during the growing years that results in a deficit in peak bone mineral content may be more detrimental to skeletal health than later loss [96, 113].

Bone Mineral Accrual during Growth

Although there is a rapid increase in bone mineral accrual (BMC) accompanying linear growth, interpretation of BMD values across the growing years is complex and difficult, particularly when bone density is measured by currently favored projectional methods, including the photon absorption techniques (DPA and DXA). These methods scan in only two directions (length and width) and yield an area density (BMD is expressed as grams per square centimeter), which is obtained by dividing the BMC by the bone area under the scan. This provides an incomplete correction for size, because it fails to take into account the depth of bone being scanned. Thus, larger bones resulting from growth will yield higher BMD values than previously smaller bones, even when there is no difference in true mineral density [21]. This has led to confusion as to the magnitude of change in BMD during the first two decades of life and has prompted attempts to provide an "apparently" true density by estimating bone volume based on geometric assumptions [21, 61, 67]. Using this approach, Katzman et al. estimated that across adolescence, 99% of the change in total body and femoral neck BMC and 50% of the change in lumbar spine BMC was attributable to bone expansion, rather than to an increase in bone mineral per unit volume [61]. Clearly, volumetric density (BMD is expressed as grams per cubic centimeter) as provided by QCT, is the preferred bone density measure in developmental studies of growing children, in whom bone size is changing, but ethical considerations usually mitigate against the exposure to ionizing radiation involved in this procedure.

The gains in BMC at adolescence are more a function of pubertal stage than chronological age [49, 66, 104, 123], which is supported by biochemical bone marker studies. In girls, markers of bone turnover are at a maximum during midpuberty (Tanner Stages 2 and 3), then decrease toward adult values after menarche [15]; markers of bone formation clearly rise during puberty [57]. In terms of chronological age, bone turnover markers peak at an approximate age of 12 in girls and 14 in boys, with each representing the average age of peak linear growth in children [11, 46].

SITE SPECIFIC AND GENDER DIFFERENCES IN BMC ACQUISITION. There are small or nonexistent gender differences in BMC at axial or appendicular skeletal sites during childhood, but during the pubertal growth period, the gender differences observed in adults become apparent [16, 17, 24, 29, 41, 46, 55, 63, 104, 124]. The most comprehensive longitudinal data set on children is from our own laboratory, where more than 100 boys and 100 girls, ranging from 8 to 19 yr old, have been measured annually over the past 4 yr. Figures 8.2–8.4 represent cross-sectional distance and velocity bone mineral accrual curves for the total body, femoral neck, and lumbar spine (L1/L4) for subjects in this study. As indicated in Figure 8.2, total body BMC is similar in boys and girls until about age 13, but after that age, BMC gains are greater in boys. These data are consistent with those of others, who have reported no differences in radial or total body BMC values in prepubertal boys and girls but show boys to have a more pronounced increase in BMC during puberty and at skeletal maturity [17, 42, 47, 55, 104, 110, 145]. Based on the current literature, it is difficult to reach consensus on other site-specific gender variations in BMC during growth. The difficulty arises because some investigators use BMD and BMC synonymously when defining bone mass, and others use inappropriate statistical analyses (for example, univariate approaches, when data clearly are multivariate), and many studies have small sample sizes, resulting in low statistical power. Nevertheless, there are some gender variations apparent. For example, several studies have shown greater BMC or BMD values in males at the femoral neck at some stage in growth or certainly by late adolescence [16, 66, 67, 72, 127, 145]. Others, although reporting no statistically significant gender differences for femoral neck BMC or BMD, have found a trend toward greater values in males [49, 88, 128]. Our data (Fig. 8.3) suggest that boys have greater femoral neck BMC at all ages but that the differences between them and girls are clearly accentuated after age 13.

There are also some inconsistencies in the data comparing gender differences at the lumbar spine. Although some studies report small or no gender differences in BMC or BMD during childhood or adolescence [25, 49, 88, 123], others report greater values in females [67, 72], while still others have reported greater values in females until about ages 15–18 yr, when males' values surpass those of females [41, 46, 82, 110, 145]. As presented in Figure 8.4, our values show that girls have slightly greater BMC values at the lumbar spine until about age 15, when the boys' values surpass those of the girls. These data are in agreement with previous studies (which controlled for maturity status), reporting no significant gender differences at the lumbar spine prior to puberty, but by late puberty showing males to

FIGURE 8.2.

Total body BMC distance (a) and velocity (b) curves for males and females, derived from cross-sectional data, using a least-squares curve fitting model [100]. PHV indicates where peak height velocity occurs for boys and girls in this cross-sectional sample.

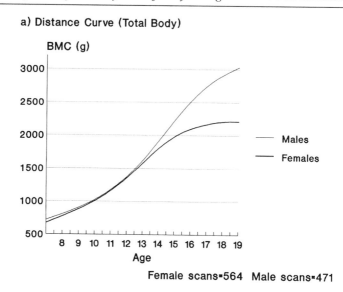

a) Distance Curve (Total Body)

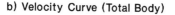

Female scans■564   Male scans■471

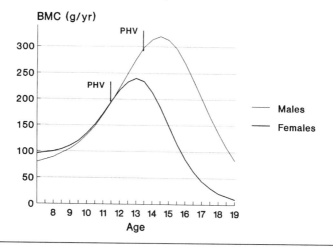

b) Velocity Curve (Total Body)

FIGURE 8.3.

Femoral neck BMC distance (a) and velocity (b) curves for males and females, derived from cross-sectional data, using a least-squares curve fitting model [100]. PHV indicates where peak height velocity occurs for boys and girls in this cross-sectional sample.

a) Distance Curve (Lumbar Spine)

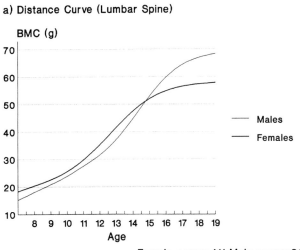

Female scans=411 Male scans=312

b) Velocity Curve (Lumbar Spine)

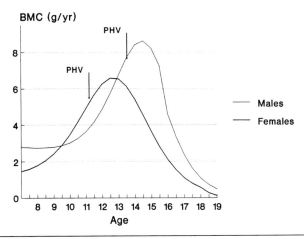

FIGURE 8.4.

Lumbar spine (L1-L4) BMC distance (a) and velocity (b) curves for males and fe-males, derived from cross-sectional data, using a least-squares curve fitting model [100]. PHV indicates where peak height velocity occurs for boys and girls in this cross-sectional sample.

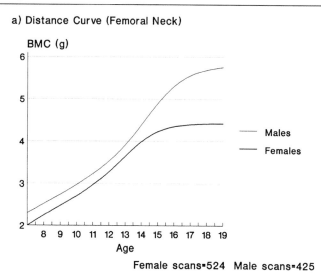

a) Distance Curve (Femoral Neck)

Female scans=524   Male scans=425

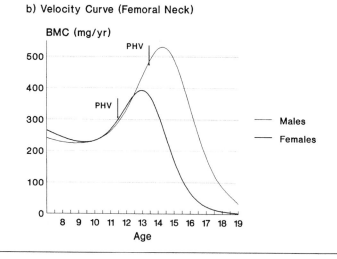

b) Velocity Curve (Femoral Neck)

have greater BMC values [16, 127]. Others, using QCT, have demonstrated that the greater lumbar spine BMC found in postpubertal males is a function of their larger vertebral bodies [43].

In general, at skeletal maturation, males have greater BMC than females. This postpubertal gender difference at skeletal sites containing relatively greater amounts of cortical bone is a result of a greater skeletal size and cortical shell in males [1, 41, 72, 87]. There are smaller gender differences, however, at sites containing relatively more cancellous bone [42, 43, 45].

The timing of the peak gains in bone accrual, reported as BMC or BMD, showing earlier peaks in girls (Fig. 8.2–8.4), is consistent with the earlier onset of sexual maturation in girls [24, 25, 44, 66, 103, 127]. In our data, for the lumbar spine, femoral neck, and total body, peak gains in BMC occurred at an approximate age of 13.0 for girls and 14.4 yr for boys. For comparative purposes, the age of peak linear growth (peak height velocity, PHV) for this cross-sectional sample of children occurred over 1 yr earlier than peak gain in BMC, in both boys and girls. At a similar developmental age (the age of peak height velocity), girls and boys had attained 90% of their adult height, 70% of adult BMC at the femoral neck, and 57% of adult lumbar spine and total body BMC. These values are in agreement with the findings of Lloyd et al. [70], who reported that premenarcheal girls (age 11.9 yr) had reached 90% of adult reference height and 53% of adult reference total body BMC.

Regardless of site, at the time of peak BMC velocity, boys were acquiring bone mineral at an approximate rate of 5:4 over girls (320 g/yr in boys, 247 g/yr in girls, for total body BMC). The more advanced mineralization of the femoral neck, in comparison to that of the lumbar spine, suggests that there may be different rates of mineralization between cortical and trabecular bone. Mora et al. [89], using QCT at the lumbar spine, found that cortical bone increased linearly during childhood and adolescence, whereas trabecular bone stayed constant before puberty, then increased rapidly during late adolescence.

BONE MINERAL ACCRUAL DURING ADOLESCENCE. The period between 9 and 20 yr of age is critical in attaining an optimum peak bone mineral content [77]. For example, depending on site, at least 90%, and probably more, of the adult bone mineral content is deposited by the end of adolescence [17, 46, 78, 118, 126, 133]. Total body BMC more than doubles in children between 8 and 15 yr of age [29]. In our data (Figs. 8.2–8.4), in the 3 yr around a similar developmental age during adolescence (the age of peak height velocity), about 30% of BMC in the total body and lumbar spine is laid down, and about 20% of femoral neck BMC is accumulated. These values are similar for both girls and boys, and they are in agreement with those of others, who have reported that in the 3 yr around the onset of puberty, almost one-third of the total bone mineral in the lumbar spine of an adult woman is accumulated [118]. As depicted in Figures 8.2–8.4, there is a steady increase in BMC at all sites, until about age 12 or 13, when there is an acceleration of bone mineral accrual. The data are consistent with previous studies showing that bone mineralization increases progressively in early childhood [29, 46, 72, 98] and then accelerates during adolescence [16, 45, 46, 82, 127]. Recent data on younger children suggest that there is a critical bone mineralization period between birth and 3 yr of age [24, 123], but it is clearly during adolescence when the largest gains occur.

LINEAR GROWTH AND BMC. Height is closely correlated with BMC in children up to 15 yr of age [16, 46, 110] but is dissociated after linear growth ceases; that is, bone mineral accumulation continues after the cessation of longitudinal growth [24, 63]. In girls, by age 14 long bone growth declines, and by age 16 all epiphyses are closed in most girls, but skeletal consolidation continues as shoulders and hips continue to broaden [76]. Matkovic et al. [78] showed that, in girls, skeletal height reached a maximum 1–7 yr earlier than maximum values in BMC and BMD (depending on site). In our data (Fig. 8.2), both girls and boys achieved about 90% of their final adult height at PHV but had only achieved about 57% of their adult total body BMC values, clearly illustrating that bone mineral accrual continues after the cessation of longitudinal growth. For all sites, PHV in BMC occurred more than a year later than PHV in both girls and boys. Thus, there is a transient period of relative bone weakness during adolescence, resulting in increased fracture risk during the adolescent growth spurt [2, 10, 14, 96].

The adolescent dissociation of BMC from height and subsequent skeletal consolidation is explained by changes in calcium requirements during this period of rapid gain in bone length. The need for calcium during peak growth is extensive, and even optimum intake and absorption may be insufficient to meet the demands for calcium [75, 97]. Additional calcium needed for growth in bone length is thought to come from the cortical shell; that is, calcium is "borrowed" from cortical bone to meet the demands of the growing metaphyses in the long bones. Once growth in length ceases, consolidation of cortical bone occurs, provided that sufficient calcium is available from dietary sources [96].

PEAK BONE MASS. There is still some controversy as to the age when peak bone mineral content is attained. For example, some earlier studies suggested that peak bone mass did not occur in subjects until their mid-30s [105, 108, 111], but more recent data indicates that peak BMD may occur before the third decade [72]. Most studies show no significant differences in BMC or BMD in most sites from the third to the fifth decades [42, 54, 55, 80, 94], whereas several have demonstrated a decrease in area BMD at the proximal femur from the early 20s to mid- to late 30s [55, 79, 108].

Recker et al. [102], in a prospective study of young adult women, found that BMC and BMD at the forearm, lumbar spine, and total body continued to increase between 18 and 30 yr of age but was stable by age 30, which suggests that the end point for BMC and BMD had been reached. Matkovic et al. [78], however, demonstrated that rapid cessation of bone mineral accumulation occurred at most bone sites by age 18. The exceptions were at the distal radius and an estimated volumetric spine site, where gains continued until ages 22 and 27 yr, respectively. Total body BMC and BMD showed very small gains in subjects up to age 50, but these gains were not statistically significant after age 18 yr. Teegarden et al. reported that females reach 90% of their total body BMC by age 17 yr and 99% by age 26 yr [126]. Lu et al. [72], in a sample of 4–27 yr olds, found no significant changes in BMD at the femoral neck, lumbar spine, or total body after about age 17.5 yr in boys, and age 15.8 yr in girls, suggesting that peak BMD values were attained before the end of the second decade. As shown in Figures 8.2–8.4, the BMC accrual curves for females in our sample of children are beginning to level off by age 19 yr for all sites. This suggests that little bone mineral acquisition occurs in females after age 19 yr. Others also have shown that peak levels of bone mineral occur in the second or third decade. Gilsanz et al. [44] reported that maximal volumetric BMD (measured by QCT) of the lumbar spine was achieved soon after menarche; there were no differences in BMD between 16- and 30-yr-old women. Ortolani et al. [95] found that peak BMD at the lumbar spine was reached by 20–25 yr of age in females, and the BMD value stayed fairly constant until menopause; they also reported that the age of peak BMD at the proximal femur occurred around 30 yr of age, although the estimate was less reliable because of the smaller number of young subjects studied.

Although there are some discrepancies, it is apparent that peak bone mass, whether measured in terms of BMC or BMD, occurs before age 30. The variation may be attributable to measurement technique differences and sample bias. Also, as indicated previously, BMD and BMC are not synonymous terms, yet both have been used as an index of bone mass, which has led to some confusion. In addition there is a paucity of longitudinal data; thus, conclusions reached must be treated with some caution because of the inherent biases in cross-sectional data. Based on available evidence, however, it appears that the indicators of peak bone mass, whether BMD or BMC, reach maximal values before the end of the third decade of life. There is certainly no evidence to suggest that there are any significant gains in BMD or BMC at any site or in either sex beyond age 30 yr [17, 92].

Hormonal Status and Bone Mineralization

The endocrine involvement in bone mineral accrual is too extensive a topic to be covered in detail in this chapter. The relative contributions of growth hormone, insulin like growth factor (IGF-1), the thyroid hormones, and the sex steroids differ during the growth process. The prepubertal increase in BMC appears to be largely growth hormone dependent, whereas the pubertal increase is dependent on sex hormones as well [42, 70]. Estrogen and testosterone are critical hormones affecting bone mineralization during adolescence. Androgens and estrogens are thought to have similar effects on trabecular bone, with androgens having a relatively greater impact on cortical bone [41, 42, 58]. There are also differences in bone mineralization between the axial and appendicular skeleton. The axial skeleton is relatively more dependent on sex hormones, whereas the appendicular skeleton is relatively more dependent on growth hormone [101].

The importance of sex hormones in bone mineral acquisition during adolescence is of particular concern for some adolescent girls. A well-documented consequence of a long-term energy deficit profile (whether caused by reduced caloric intake, as in anorexia or by an extremely high energy expenditure from chronic intense exercise, or by a combination of the two) is an alteration in the normal menstrual cycle leading, in some cases, to amenorrhea and markedly reduced estrogen levels [71, 143]. The skeletal hazard of chronic menstrual dysfunction in young women has been well documented [4, 26, 141]. Estimates as to the extent of compromised reproductive function and irregular menses in athletic women range from 2 to 51%, depending on the activity engaged in, as compared to 2–5% in nonathletes [120]. The reduction in bone mineral accrual rate or bone mineral loss may have irreversible consequences. For example, Bachrach et al. [5] found that values for BMD at four skeletal sites were 56–82% below normal in recovered anorectics 2 yr after the resumption of normal menses and the restoration of normal body weight.

The effect of caloric restriction or intense long-term exercise on hormonal status in boys has not been thoroughly investigated, but delayed puberty has been shown to result with reduced BMD values in young adults, suggesting that the timing of puberty, with associated increases in testosterone levels, is a determinant of bone mineralization in men [32].

Developmental Summary

The attainment of an optimum peak BMC is a critical factor in the prevention of osteoporosis; the adolescent growth period is the critical time for bone mineral accretion. During the adolescent growth spurt, there is dissociation between linear growth and bone acquisition, resulting in a brief period of relative skeletal fragility. After growth ceases, there is consolidation of the skeleton, as calcium borrowed from cortical bone for metaphyseal growth is rapidly reinstated in the cortical shell [96]. Girls experience a rapid gain in bone mineralization about 2 yr before boys (coincident with earlier maturation in girls). At skeletal maturation, males have greater overall skeletal mass, which is primarily a function of having a greater cortical shell; there are small or nonexistent gender differences in cancellous bone. Bone mineral acquisition during adolescence is largely sex steroid dependent. Sufficient concentrations of estrogen are clearly important for bone mineralization in females. Peak values for both BMC and BMD are attained as early as the end of the second decade of life and certainly before age 30.

The observation that adolescence is the critical time for bone mineral accretion and that peak bone mineral levels are reached shortly after cessation of growth should not be surprising: As noted by Parfitt [96], by the time growth ceases, the skeleton must be as strong as it will ever need to be, and any mechanism that significantly increases bone mass and strength after cessation of growth would be of little purpose.

BONE MINERALIZATION: MECHANICAL LOADING AND PHYSICAL ACTIVITY CONSIDERATIONS DURING GROWTH

The effects of a changed mechanical loading environment, particularly disuse, on the skeleton have been recognized for more than a century, but it is only within the last 20 yr that investigators have demonstrated that the key intermediate variable between mechanical loading and bone adaptation is induced mechanical strain [68]. Increased loading results in a minute change in the surface curvature of bones that induces a strain gradient signal that activates bone cell response. Recently, it has been suggested that the induced mechanical strain signal is amplified by interstitial fluid flow forced from more compressed to less compressed regions during bending [19, 34].

The Adaptive Response of Bone to Mechanical Loading

Most researchers suggest that bone adaptation is error driven [19], which means that bone will not respond unless it perceives that it is not adapted to the new mechanical load. The implication of this is that bone will only respond within certain ranges of loading. Induced strains must be above or below threshold levels for bone to have an adaptive response. This concept has been called the "mechanostat theory," of Frost [36], and it maintains that bone adaptation is dependent on the mechanical environment described by four mechanical usage windows. Each window is defined by minimum effective strain (MES) thresholds (Fig. 8.5). The window within which a less than adequate mechanical stimulus is provided is called the trivial loading zone, in which remodeling will be the predominant process, with a resultant loss of bone. The physiological loading zone is defined by a lower threshold called the remodeling MES and an upper threshold called the modeling MES. Within this window the mechanical loading stimulus is sufficient to control the remodeling process such that bone remodeling remains in a steady state, and there is little or no effect on bone turnover. The overload zone is entered when loads exceed the upper set point of the physiological loading zone and elicit a modeling response. In this situation, bone is added and structurally ordered to respond to a new level of mechanical demand. Extremely high loads that induce very high strains push bone into a repair zone, whereby disorganized (woven) bone

FIGURE 8.5.

Mechanical usage windows, as defined by Frost's mechanostat theory [36]. In the trivial loading zone, strains are low, resulting in increased remodeling, with subsequent loss of bone, as in immobilization or disuse. In the physiological loading zone, strains are sufficient to maintain bone, remodeling is in a steady state, and bone is neither gained nor lost. In the overload zone, modeling is stimulated to add more bone and to organize it to respond to high strains. At very high strains, bone enters a repair mode, in which unorganized bone is added to meet a severe and immediate need. $\mu\epsilon$ = microstain, MES = minimum effective strain. Adapted from refs. 19 and 34.

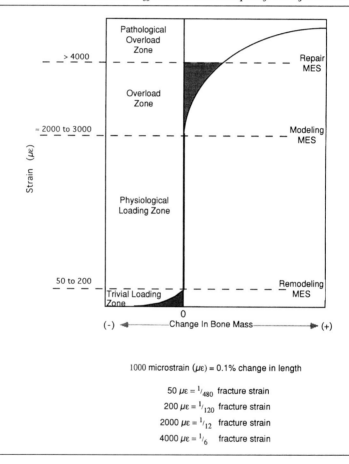

1000 microstrain ($\mu\epsilon$) = 0.1% change in length

$$50\ \mu\epsilon = {}^1/_{480}\ \text{fracture strain}$$
$$200\ \mu\epsilon = {}^1/_{120}\ \text{fracture strain}$$
$$2000\ \mu\epsilon = {}^1/_{12}\ \text{fracture strain}$$
$$4000\ \mu\epsilon = {}^1/_{6}\ \text{fracture strain}$$

of poor quality is added to meet an acute need. The resulting bone is subsequently replaced by better organized bone [109, 130].

The mechanostat theory rests on the premise that bone adaptation is dependent on mechanical stimuli; however, it should be noted that, with no change in mechanical loading, a change in the set point thresholds would elicit a similar adaptive response [38]. Thus, the altered hormonal milieu in girls experiencing menstrual dysfunction could result in the skeleton initiating remodeling, even though normal mechanical usage has not changed. It should also be emphasized that the control of bone mass is localized, because mechanical strains differ greatly in different parts of the skeleton, so that there may be net bone loss and net bone gain occurring simultaneously, even in different regions of the same bone.

Physical Activity Studies of Children and Adolescents

The potential of weight-bearing physical activity to positively influence bone mineral acquisition in children and adolescents is a topic of increasing interest. As described in the mechanostat model, strains on bone above the modeling MES threshold will induce a modeling response to increase bone mass to meet the increasing load requirements. Because this modeling response occurs mainly during the years of growth, the importance of investigating the effects of weight-bearing physical activity on bone mineralization during the growing years becomes apparent.

Although there are gaps in our understanding about the precise role of physical activity in bone mineral accretion in children and adolescents, there have been a number of studies that have investigated the relationship between activity and bone mineralization. A summary of these studies is presented in Table 8.1; in addition, studies on adolescents in which the effects of physical activity have been modulated by hormonal status have also been reviewed. The activity studies have been categorized according to the experimental design followed, which includes controlled or prospective trials; unilateral control studies in which one limb has been preferentially stressed; observational and correlative studies of athletic and nonathletic groups; and retrospective activity assessment studies, in which historical activity as a child is related to adult bone status.

CONTROLLED OR PROSPECTIVE TRIALS. Of six prospective studies, only two have included data on prepubertal children. One study reported a significant effect of physical activity on BMD accrual over 3 yr at the lumbar spine, proximal femur, and distal radius in prepubertal children but not in peripubertal children [118]. The other study found no significant relationship between BMD accrual rate over a 1-yr period and physical activity in a group of children 7–20 yr of age, although there was a trend for greater BMD in the more active children [66].

Studies in older adolescents show mixed results. In males, age 18–21 yr, 14 wk of intense daily military training resulted in significant BMC gains in the lower limbs for those subjects who completed the training course [74]. That 40% of the subjects dropped out of the course because of stress fractures demonstrates the severity of this training regime. In females, activities such as resistance training, running, and gymnastics have been shown to significantly increase BMD at the lumbar spine by a modest amount but not at

TABLE 8.1
Studies of Physical Activity and Bone Mineralization in Children and Adolescents

Study and Design[a]	Subjects n (Age in yr)	Measurement[b]	Physical Activity Type, Measure	Effects Description	Effects Summary[c]
Kroger et al. [66]: I (Finland)	65 (7–20) 37F 28 M	BMC/BMD (DXA), FN, LS	I. (FN) little or no PA II. (LS) 3 hr/wk III. Regular athletes 5 hr/wk	No relationship between PA and any bone measure	FN ⇒ LS ⇒
Margulies et al. [74]: I (Israel)	286 M (18–21)	BMC (SPA), tibia, fibula	Demanding basic training 8 hr/day, 7 day/wk, 14 wk	L leg, +11.1% R leg, +5.2%	Tib/Fib ⇑
Nichols et al. [90]: I (Texas)	22F 11 gymnasts 11 controls	BMD, (DXA), PF, LS, TB	5 mo gymnastic program	Gymnasts initially higher on all BMD measures after 5 mo reg, menstruating gymnasts signif + 2.1% at LS	PF ⇔ LS ⇑ TB ⇔
Rice et al. [103]: I (Ontario)	35 F (14–18) 17 wt trained 18 controls	BMD (DPA), LS, TB	26 wk of wt training on hydrogym 3x/wk circuit of 13 exer/4 sets	No SD BMD between groups Signif. increase in strength in training group	LS ⇔ TB ⇔
Slemenda et al. [118]: I (Indiana)	45 (6–14) 32 F 13 M	BMD (SPA), radius; BMD (DPA), PF, LS	Normally active (questionnaire)	PA was a signif. predictor of prepubertal BMD at all sites, M and F	PF ⇑ LS ⇔
Snow-Harter et al. [121]:I (California, Oregon)	30 F (x = 19.9) 1) 12 wt. trained 2) 10 runners 3) 8 controls	BMD (DXA), PF, LS	(1) 8 mo: progressive wt training 3x/wk or (2) run 3x/wk (up to 10 mi/wk)	(PF, LS)—no diff wt trained +1.2% Runners +1.3%, controls 0.8%	PF ⇔ LS ⇑
Bailey et al. [7]: II (Saskatchewan)	17 (7–14) 3 F 14 M	BMD (DXA), PF	Compromised wt bearing in children with unilateral LCPD (Legg-Calvé-Perthes disease)	x diff between PF = 5.6% Involved regions < baseline Noninvolved > baseline	PF ⇑
Faulkner et al. [30]: II (Saskatchewan)	234 (8–16) 124 F 110 M	BMD (DXA), TB, arms, legs	Normal childhood activity range	BMD dominant arm > nondominant arm all ages, M & F No diff in legs	TB (arm) ⇑ TB (leg) ⇒
Haapasalo et al. [52]:	38 F (18–32) 19 athletes	BMC (DXA), radius;	75 min, 4x/wk for 5.7 ± 8.5 yr	Dominant > nondominant (all sites)	Radius ⇑ Humerus ⇑

Study (Location)	Subjects	Measurement	Activity	Findings	Site
II (Finland)	19 controls	BMD, humerus ulna, os calcis			Ulna ⇑ Os calcis ⇑
Robinson et al. [107]: III (Oregon)	60 F (17–27) 1) 21 gymnasts 2) 20 runners 3) 19 nonathletes	BMD (DXA), FN, LS, TB	1) competitive collegiate athletes (47% menstrual dysfunction) 2) 30 mi/wk min (30% menst/dys)	(FN) gymnasts > controls > runners (LS) controls > gymnasts > runners (TB) controls > runners > gymnasts	FN ⇑
Slemenda and, Johnston [116]: III (Indiana)	44 F (10–23) 22 fig. skaters 22 controls	BMD (DPX), TB (regions)	Questionnaire designed for skaters Skating: regional, 12/20 hr/wk; nat'l/int'l, 25–40 hr/wk	Skater (5.5–11%) > cont for lower body regions No signif effect of skating on upper body sites	TB ⇑
Virvidakis et al. [136]: III (14 countries)	59 M (15–20) wt lifters	BMC (SPA), distal radius, prox radius	Nat'l wt lifting champions from 14 countries Not screened for steroid use	BMC at distal and proximal radius > 2 SD's above age-matched controls	Distal radius ⇑ Prox Radius ⇑
Young et al. [144]: III (Australia)	85 F (x̄=17) 1) 44 dancers 2) 18 anorexics 3) 23 controls	BMD (DXA), PF, LS, TB	1) 32 hr/wk	(PF) ballet dancers > controls, anorexics (LS) controls, ballet dancers > anorexics	PF ⇑ LS ⇒
Katzman et al. [61]: IV (California)	45 F 9–21	BMC (SPA), radius; BMD, (DXA), TB, LS, PF; BMD (DPA), TB, LS	Low active, <2x/wk Moderate active, 2–3x/wk High active, >3x/wk for 30 min	No relationship between PA and any bone mineral measure	Radius ⇔ PF ⇔ LS, TB ⇔
Kroger, et al [67]: IV (Finland)	84 (6–19) 44 F 40 M	BMD (DXA), PF, LS	Normal activity evaluated by questionnaire (outside school activities) No/≥3 hr/wk/>5 hr/wk	(PF) high active > low active (LS) no diff (controlled for age, ht, wt)	PF ⇑
Rubin et al. [110]: IV (Connecticut)	299 (6–18) 163 F 136 M	BMC (SPA), radius; BMD (DPA), LS	Questionnaire	(LS) small exercise effect (controlled for wt and pubertal stage)	Radius ⇔ LS ⇑
Ruiz et al. [112]: IV (France)	151 (7–15) 81 F 70 M	BMD (DXA), PF, LS	1–3 hr/wk/3–12 hr/wk	Multiple regression (PF, LS) PA had a signif. effect (F) No diff (M)	PF - ⇑(F) ⇔(M) LS - ⇑(F) ⇔(M)

TABLE 8.1—*continued*

Study and Design[a]	Subjects n (Age in yr)	Measurement[b]	Physical Activity Type, Measure	Effects Description	Summary[c]
Slemenda et al. [117]: IV (Indiana)	118 (5.3–14)	BMC (SPA), radius; BMD, (DPA), PF, LS	Normal activity evaluated by questionnaire (total hr wt bearing)	(PF, radius) signif correlation between BMD and PA (LS) no relationship	Radius ⇑ PF and PA ⇑ LS ⇔
Southard et al. [123]: IV (Ohio)	218 (1–19) 134 F 84 M	BMD (DXA), LS	Low active <2x/wk	No relationship between BMD and PA	LS ⇔
Turner et al. [131]: IV (N Zealand)	138 F (x = 18.4)	BMD (DXA), PF, LS	High school activity assessment	(controlled for wt and maturity) (PF) PA signif + effect (LS) no effect	PF ⇑ LS ⇔
Valimaki et al. [135]: IV (Finland)	264 (9–29) 153 F 111 M	BMD (DXA) (different models), FN, LS	by questionnaire >30 min/wk	(FN) PA signif predictor of BMD in F and M and (LS) BMD in M	FN ⇑ LS ⇑ M ⇒ F
Webber et al. [139]: IV (Ontario)	36 F (14–18)	BMC (DPA), LS; BMD, TB	Questionnaires past yearly, past monthly and current PA Measured strength	(LS) PA signif predictor of BMC (TB) PA signif predictor of BMC and BMD	LS ⇑ TB ⇑
Welten et al. [140]: III (Netherlands)	182 (13–28) 98 F 84 M	BMD (DXA), LS	By questionnaire 4–6x/yr from 13–28 yr BMD measured once at age 28	PA signif predictor of BMC in M Wt signif predictor of BMD in F	LS ⇑ (M) ⇔ (F)
White et al. [141]: IV (Texas)	36 F (15–21) 8 amenorrheics 28 eumenorrheics	BMD (DXA), LS, FN	Leisure activity by questionnaire	(FN) signif relationship in eumen subjects (LS) no effect (controlling for wt—no diff)	FN ⇑ LS ⇔
Fehily et al. [31]: V (Wales)	371 (20–23) 182 F 189 M	BMC (SPA), radius	Sport participation at age 12 evaluated by recall questionnaire	pos. correlation between PA (12 yr) and BMC for F but not M	Radius ⇑
Kriska et al. [65]: V (Pennsylvania)	223 F (x = 57.6)	BMD (QCT) 1/3, radius	Past PA by questionnaire at 14–21 yr (one time period)	Signif diff in BM area but not BMD according to PA levels Age periods 22–24, 35–50, 50+ NS	Radius ⇔

Study	Sample	Measurement	Activity	Results	Findings
Henderson et al. [53]: II (N. Carolina)	38 (2–15) 14 F 24 M	BMD (DXA), PF	Restricted activity due to casting of tibia or femur	x diff between PF = 3.3% Immobilization >8 wk = 4.3%	PF ⇑
Jacobson et al. [56]: II (N. Carolina)	11 F (18–22)	BMC (SPA), radius	Elite tennis performance	Dominant radius signif > non-dominant radius	Radius ⇑
Watson [138]: II (Wisconsin)	203 M (8–19)	BMC (SPA), humerus and radius	Throwing a baseball	Dominant humerus signif > non-dominant humerus, all ages	Humerus ⇑
Conroy et al. [23]: III (USA)	36 M (x = 16.9) 25 wt lifters 11 controls	BMD (DXA), PF, LS	Wt lifters trained for an avg of 2.7 ± 1.4 yr None of the controls had previously wt trained	(PF, LS) SD between wt training and controls: wt training > male ref values LS, 13%; PF, 31%	PF ⇑ LS ⇑
Grimston et al. [50]: III (Alberta)	34 (10–16) 18 F, 16 M 1) 17 runners, gymnasts, dancers 2) 17 swimmers	BMD (DPA), FN, LS	60 min, 3x/wk provincial level competitors	(FN) 1) >swimmers (M, F) (LS) 1) >swimmers (M) (LS) 1) no diff than swimmers (F)	FN ⇑ LS ⇔
Kirchner et al. [62]: III (Georgia)	52 F (18–22) 26 gymnasts 26 controls	BMD (DXA), PF, LS, TB	7 day recall questionnaire 2.6 hr/day hard or very hard 0.5 hr/day hard or very hard	gymnasts > controls, all sites	PF ⇑ LS ⇑ TB ⇑
McCulloch et al. [84]: III (Sask)	68 M/F (13–17) 11/12 soccer pl. 10/10 swimmers 12/13 controls	BMC (SPA), radius; BMD (QCT), os calcis	Elite age class soccer and swim training: swimmers, higher training intensity, and energy expenditure	(Os calcis) soccer pl > controls or swimmers (Radius) no diff between groups	Radius ⇔ Os calcis ⇑
Nichols et al. [91]: III (Texas)	58 F (x = 19.9) 1) 46 athletes 2) 12 nonathletes	BMD (DPX), FN, LS, TB	1) 9.7 ± 3.4 yr wt training (except tennis) 2) <3 hr/wk	athletes BMD signif >at all sites compared to norms (Lunar) Regional lean mass best predictor of BMD	FN ⇑ LS ⇑ TB ⇑
Risser et al. [106]: III (Texas)	44 F (x = 19 yr) 12 vball. 9 bball. 10 swim. 13 controls	BMC (SPA), os calcis; BMD (DPA), LS	Competitive intercollegiate athlete	(LS) volleyball >controls, swimmers controls >swimmers (Os calcis) volleyball, bball > swimmers, controls	LS ⇑ Os calcis ⇑

TABLE 8.1—*continued*

Study and Design[a]	Subjects n (Age in yr)	Measurement[b]	Physical Activity Type, Measure	Effects Description	Summary[c]
McCulloch et al. [83]: V (Saskatchewan)	101 F (20–35)	BMC (SPA), radius; BMD (QCT), os calcis	Adolescent and childhood activity evaluated by recall questionnaire	BMD high activity signif > other groups	Os calcis ⇑
Talmage and Anderson [125]: V (N. Carolina)	1200 F (19–98) Subset >25 yr old	BMC (SPA), radius	Adolescent activity evaluated by recall questionnaire	Secondary school athletics and/or did heavy farm labor higher BMC at 25 yr	Radius ⇑
Tylavsky et al. [132]: V (N. Carolina)	705 F (17–23)	BMC (SPA), radius, midradius	Self-administered activity questionnaire during high school and college	(Distal radius) signif diff high > moderate > low; Long-term PA—greater effect than long-term Ca	Radius ⇑
Zhang et al. [146]: V (N. Carolina)	352 F (40–54)	BMD (DPA), LS; BMD, (SPA), distal, midradius	Adolescent activity evaluated by recall questionnaire	Modest dose-response relationship but not signif at any site	LS ⇔ Distal and mid radius ⇔

Adapted from ref 9.

[a]Study design: Level I, controlled prospective trials. Level IIA, unilateral control; Level III, observational and correlative (activity assessment); Level IV, observational and correlative (athletic groups); Level V, retrospective activity assessment.

[b]Abbreviations used are: BMD, bone mineral density (g/cm²); BMC, bone mineral content (g); PA, physical activity; TB, total body; PF, proximal femur; FN, femoral neck; LS, lumbar spine; SPA, single photon absorptiometry; DPA, dual photon absorptiometry; DXA, dual energy x-ray absorptiometry; QCT, quantitative computerized tomography; x diff, mean difference.

[c]Direction of association: ⇓, negative effects; ⇒, no apparent evidence of PA related to outcome; ⇑, some apparent evidence of beneficial trend of PA related to outcome; ⇑⇑, apparent evidence of beneficial trend of PA related to outcome.

the proximal femur [90, 121]. Others, however, have reported no effect of resistance training on lumbar spine or total body BMD in postmenarcheal girls 14–18 yr of age [103]. A major problem in most of these studies is the limited duration of the intervention and small subject numbers.

UNILATERAL CONTROL STUDIES. Childhood activities that preferentially stress one side of the body over the other provide a unique model for studying the effect of mechanical loading on the growing skeleton. Because genetic, nutritional, and endocrine factors are shared by both limbs, differences in bone mineralization can be attributed to the altered loading pattern of the specific sport activity. Significantly greater BMD or BMC has been reported in the dominant arms of Little League baseball players from 8 to 19 yr old [138], elite female tennis players from 18–22 yr old [56], and elite female squash players [52]. In the study of squash players, the number of years of training was correlated with the BMD and BMC in the humerus of the playing arm. Significantly larger side-to-side differences (22%) were found in players who had started playing before or around menarche than in those who began their playing careers one or more years after menarche (9%). In a study of normal healthy children, from 8–16 yr old, who were involved in nothing more than routine daily activities, the BMC and BMD were significantly higher in the dominant arm, as compared to their level in the nondominant arm [30]. Consistent with the hypothesis that there is a relationship between physical activity and bone accrual are the results of a study by Miller et al. [88]. These investigators studied the relationship between muscularity and BMD in children and report a relationship between girth measures close to the corresponding BMD site (e.g., thigh girth and proximal femoral BMD).

The effects of altered loading patterns on bone mineralization attributable to injury or disease have not been extensively studied in children, but two recent studies are worthy of note. Femoral BMD was measured in children who had experienced an uncomplicated fracture of the tibia or femur, on average, some 2.3 yr earlier [53]. There was a residual deficit in BMD on the injured side, with the side-to-side difference greater in children who had been immobilized for a longer period of time. Similarly, significant differences in BMD of the proximal femur have been reported in children afflicted with unilateral Legg-Calvé-Perthes disease, with BMD on the involved side significantly below normal values and BMD on the noninvolved side significantly above baseline norms. [7].

On the whole, these unilateral control studies provide the strongest evidence for the contribution of physical activity to bone mineral accrual in growing children.

OBSERVATIONAL STUDIES OF ATHLETIC GROUPS. There are no studies comparing BMD among athletic groups in young children, but in adolescents and young adults, physical activities involving relatively high impact loads are associated with higher BMD. For example, several studies have reported BMD at the femoral neck, lumbar spine, or total body to be greater in gymnasts, as compared to that of controls [50, 52, 91, 107]. Competitive adolescent male weight lifters (at 17 yr old) had significantly greater BMD at the femoral neck and lumbar spine, as compared to that of age-matched controls and adult males [23]. These data are in agreement with another study of elite adolescent weight lifters, in which BMC of the radius was more than 2 SDs above the age-matched control value and was highly correlated with strength [136]. Others have found adolescent soccer, basketball, or volleyball players to have a greater BMD than controls at weight-bearing sites, such as the proximal femur and os calcis [50, 84, 106]. The importance of weight-bearing is demonstrated by the fact that swimmers have lower BMD values at such sites than other athletic groups or controls [50, 84, 106].

High-impact loading activities may offset, at least to some degree, the deleterious skeletal effects of menstrual disturbances in young female athletes. For example, gymnasts had greater BMD at the proximal femur, lumbar spine, and total body than eumenorrheic controls, despite the fact that 30% of the gymnasts had menstrual disturbances [62]. Robinson et al. [107] found that gymnasts (47% of whom were oligo- or amenorrheic) had greater BMD at the proximal femur than either runners or eumenorrheic controls. Young figure skaters (40% of whom had menstrual disorders) were found to have significantly greater total body BMD than controls, but the differences were attributable to greater BMD in the lower body of skaters—there were no differences in BMD at upper body sites [117]. Young et al. [144] reported amenorrheic ballet dancers to have greater BMD at the proximal femur than controls but not at the lumbar spine. These results suggest that high-impact loading activities in athletes with abnormal menstrual function have a sparing effect at weight-bearing sites but not to the same extent at nonweight-bearing sites. Activities involving lower impact loads, such as running, do not appear to offset bone loss resulting from menstrual disorders [6, 107].

OBSERVATIONAL ACTIVITY ASSESSMENT OF NONATHLETIC GROUPS. Observational studies investigating the relationship of physical activity (usually assessed by questionnaire) to BMD in nonathletic groups show mixed results. Several studies have reported a significant relationship between physical activity and BMD at the proximal femur or femoral neck in children and/or adolescent males and females [67, 112, 117, 131]; however, others have reported no significant association in females [61, 141].

Although some studies have reported a significant positive relationship between physical activity and BMD at the lumbar spine in males or females [110, 112, 117, 139], others report no relationship [61, 67, 123, 131]. One study reported a positive relationship between physical activity and total body BMD in males and females [139], but others reported no such relationship in females [61].

The inconsistencies in these observational studies probably stem from several factors. As discussed by others, accurate, valid, and reliable measurement of physical activity in children and adolescents is extremely difficult [117]. There is little consistency in the measurement of this parameter across studies, and there is often little information on the reliability and validity of the instrument. Many studies also have small sample sizes and low statistical power. Despite these difficulties, however, it appears that physical activity is more consistently related to BMD at the proximal femur or femoral neck than at the lumbar spine and more consistently so in males than in females.

RETROSPECTIVE ACTIVITY ASSESSMENT STUDIES. The effect of childhood physical activity on BMD status as an adult has been assessed through the use of retrospective questionnaires in a number of studies. The skeletal site evaluated in five of these investigations was a nonweight-bearing site, the distal or midradius. Of these studies, two reported a significant relationship between childhood activity and adult BMD [125, 132]; two reported no significant relationship [65, 146]; and one reported a relationship in women but not in men [31]. In a study that measured BMD at a weight-bearing site, physical activity during childhood was positively related to BMD of the os calcis in young women [83]. In another study, BMD of the lumbar spine was measured in men and women (age 27) whose activity had been assessed six times during and since their teenage years [140]. Using a multiple linear regression analysis, regular weight-bearing activity in adolescence and youth was a significant predictor of adult BMD at the lumbar spine. In a similar study, physical activity measured during childhood and adolescence was a significant predictor of adult BMD at the femoral neck and lumbar spine in males but only at the femoral neck in females [135].

Physical Activity Summary and Recommendations

There have been too few prospective studies on young children to either confirm or reject a biologically important effect of physical activity on bone mineral accrual during growth, although the most rigorous of these studies, by Slemenda et al. [118], is certainly supportive. The unilateral control studies, which look at childhood activities that preferentially stress one side of the body over the other, provide the strongest evidence that local mechanical factors modulate bone mineralization during the growing years, over and above genetic considerations. Studies comparing elite young athletes with control groups also suggest that bone mineral acquisition can be enhanced by weight-bearing activity, but these studies have the problem of self-selection. Questionnaire and activity assessment studies in normal children are equivocal in terms of the relationship between physical activity and bone mineralization. Like the retrospective questionnaire studies, which have investigated the relationship between adult bone status and self-reported childhood activity patterns, these studies suffer from all of the difficulties associated with the valid, reliable, and objective determination of physical activity in children.

Studies that have investigated the response of growing bone in young animals to moderate and intense physical activity have recently been reviewed by Forwood and Burr [33]. These investigators conclude that "animal studies are incontrovertible in showing that growing bone has a greater capacity to add new bone to the skeleton than the bone of adults." The consistency of the evidence suggests that the animal data do have relevance for humans. Considered as a whole, the studies noted above highly suggest that bone mineral in children can be enhanced by loading factors associated with physical activity; however, there are still more questions than answers when it comes to exercise prescription issues, such as frequency, intensity, duration, and type of activity.

Although there remain many questions about the complicated mechanisms controlling bone mineral accretion during the growing years, it is still possible to offer some prudent advice to young people, based on the preceding review of bone-related research in children and adolescents. Suggestions for optimizing bone mineral acquisition during the growing years include the following:

1. A person should make a lifelong commitment to physical activity at an early age. Growing bones respond to weight-bearing activity by the addition of new bone. The ability to adapt to increases in mechanical loading is much greater in the growing, than in the nongrowing, skeleton [96].
2. A variety of vigorous daily activities of short duration is better than prolonged repetitive activity. Activities should be diverse to ensure a varied strain distribution on bone, and they should be vigorous to ensure high strain rates.
3. Weight-bearing activities are better than weight-supported activities, such as swimming or cycling.
4. Activities that increase muscle strength and work all large muscle groups should be encouraged, as these can enhance bone acquisition.
5. As much as possible, periods of immobility and immobilization should be avoided; when this is not achievable because of sickness or injury, even brief daily weight-bearing movements can help to conserve bone mineral.

The responsiveness of the growing skeleton to physical activity is dependent on the sensitivity of bone to circulating hormones [33] and the synergistic relationship between activity and proper nutrition [8]. Therefore, the hormonal milieu during growth and adequate nutrition that is related to calcium absorption are important considerations when normal or enhanced rates of bone mineral accretion are to be maintained, which leads to a number of other important suggestions:

1. In girls, abnormal delay of menarche and chronic menstrual dysfunction represent a potential skeletal hazard in terms of bone mineral acquisition and maintenance. Natural means of restoring an energy balance should be advocated.
2. Disordered eating habits are destructive to the skeleton at any age; when they occur during the growing years, there may develop a permanent deficit in bone mineral status that lasts throughout one's life.
3. Children and adolescents should eat a well-balanced diet that meets the recommended dietary allowance for calcium.
4. Cigarettes should be avoided; they are antiestrogenic and may interfere with the attainment of an optimal level of bone mineral after skeletal maturation.

CONCLUSIONS

Heavy and prolonged physical activity has always been a major determinant of human structure and function [18]. The genetic makeup of humans remains adapted for circumstances as they existed 10,000 yr ago, before the domestication of plants and animals and the rise of agriculture [28]. Humans evolved as active animals designed for an environment demanding high levels of activity. Thus, our present relatively sedentary lives may be out of step with our genetic makeup, which remains adapted to the conditions of another time [27].

Human energy expenditure requirements have declined over the past 10,000 yr, and the decline has been most marked during the twentieth century [12]. Taking this life-style difference into consideration, one would expect early humans to have a relatively greater skeletal mass and denser skeletons than present-day people, and anthropological studies have confirmed this [69, 111, 119, 142]. Although this genetic argument does not prove that physical activity is necessary for skeletal health, it does suggest that we may be playing a dangerous game with our heritage and that we should not forget the preeminent role played by mechanical loading through physical activity, as it applies to bone mineral acquisition during growth.

ACKNOWLEDGMENTS

The authors thank the National Health Research and Development Fund (NHRDP) of Canada and the Health Services Utilization and Research Commission of Saskatchewan (HSURC) for their support of the work carried out in our laboratory. Also, the authors thank Mark Forwood and Stuart Houston for their comments and suggestions in the preparation of this manuscript.

REFERENCES

1. Aharinejad, S., R. Bertagnoli, K. Wicke, W. Firbas, and B. Schneider. Morphometric analysis of vertebrae and intervertebral discs as a basis of disc replacement. *Am. J. Anat.* 189:69–76, 1990.
2. Alffram, P. A., and G. C. H. Bauer. Epidemiology of fractures of the forearm. *J. Bone Joint Surg. Am.* 44:105–114, 1962.
3. Ascenzi, A., and G. Bell. Bone as a mechanical engineering problem. G. Bourne (ed). *The Biochemistry and Physiology of Bone.* New York: Academic Press, 1971,pp. 311–346.
4. Bachrach, L. K., D. Guido, D. K. Katzman, I. F. Litt, and R. Marcus. Decreased bone density in adolescent girls with anorexia nervosa. *Pediatrics* 86:440–447, 1990.
5. Bachrach, L. K., D. K. Katzman, and I. F. Litt. Recovery from osteopenia in adolescent girls with anorexia nervosa. *J. Clin. Endocrinol. Metab.* 72:602–606, 1991.
6. Baer, J. T., L. J. Taper, F. G. Gwazdauskas, et al. Diet, hormonal and metabolic factors affecting bone mineral density in adolescent amenorrheic and eumenorrheic runners. *J. Sports Med. Phys. Fitness* 32:51–58, 1992.
7. Bailey, D. A., R. A. Faulkner, K. Kimber, A. Dzus, and K. Yong-Hing. Altered loading patterns and femoral bone mineral acquisition in children with Legg-Calvé-Perthes disease. In press, 1996.
8. Bailey, D.A., and A. D. Martin. Physical activity and skeletal health in adolescents. *Pediatr. Exerc. Sci.* 6:330–347, 1994.
9. Bailey, D. A., and R. G. McCulloch. Osteoporosis: Are there childhood antecedents for an adult health problem? *Can. J. Pediatr.* 5:130–134, 1992.
10. Bailey, D. A., J. H. Wedge, R. G. McCulloch, A. D. Martin, and S. C. Bernhardson. Epidemiology of fractures of the distal end of the radius in children as associated with growth. *J. Bone Joint Surg. Am.* 71:1225–1231, 1989.
11. Beardsworth, L. J., D. R. Eyre, and I. R. Dickson. Changes with age in the urinary excretion of lysyl- and hydroxylysylpyridinoline, two new markers of bone collagen turnover. *J. Bone Miner. Res.* 5:671–676, 1990.
12. Blair, S. N., H. W. Kohl, and N. F. Gordon. How much physical activity is good for health? *Annu. Rev. Public Health* 11:99–126, 1992.
13. Blimkie, C. J. R., P. Chilibeck, and S. Davison. Bone mineralization: endocrine, nutrition, and physical activity influences during the lifespan. O. Bar-or, D. Lamb, and P. Clarkson (eds). *Perspectives in Exercise and Sports Medicine, Exercise and the Female—A Lifespan Perspective,* Vol. 9. Cooper, in press, 1995.
14. Blimkie, C. J. R., J. Levevre, G. P. Beunen, R. Renson, J. Dequeker, and P. Van Damme. Fractures, physical activity, and growth velocity in adolescent Belgian boys. *Med. Sci. Sports Exerc.* 25:801–808, 1993.
15. Blumsohn, A., R. A. Hannon, R. Wrate, et al. Biochemical markers of bone turnover in girls during puberty. *Clin. Endocrinol.* 40:663–670, 1994.
16. Bonjour, J. P., G. Theintz, B. Buchs, D. Slosman, and R. Rizzoli. Critical years and stages of puberty for spinal and femoral bone mass accumulation during adolescence. *J. Clin. Endocrinol. Metab.* 73:1330–1333, 1991.
17. Bonjour, J. P. G. Theintz, F. Law, D. Slosman, and R. Rizzoli. Peak bone mass. *Osteoporos. Int.* 4(Suppl. 1):S7–S13, 1994.
18. Bortz, W. M. Physical exercise as an evolutionary force. *J. Hum. Evol.* 14:145–155, 1985.
19. Burr, D. Orthopedic principles of skeletal growth, modeling and remodeling. D. Carlson and S. Goldstein (eds). *Bone Dynamics in Orthodontic and Orthopedic Treatment, Craniofacial Growth Series,* Vol. 27. Ann Arbor, MI: Center for Human Growth and Development, 1992, pp. 15–49.
20. Burr, D., M. Schaffler, K. Yang, et al.Skeletal change in response to altered strain environments: Is woven bone a response to elevated strain? *Bone* 10:223–233, 1989.

21. Carter, D. R., M. L. Bouxsein, and R. Marcus. New approaches for interpreting projected bone mineral density data. *J. Bone Miner. Res.* 7:137–145, 1992.
22. Compston, J. Bone density: BMC, BMD, or corrected BMD? *Bone* 16:5–7, 1995.
23. Conroy, B. P.,W. J. Kraemer, C. M. Maresh, S. J. Fleck, M. H. Stone, A. C. Fry, P. D. Miller,and G. P. Dalsky. Bone mineral density in elite junior Olympic weightlifters. *Med. Sci. Sports Exerc.* 25:1103–1109, 1993.
24. del Rio, L., A. Carrascosa, F. Pons, M. Gusinye, D. Yeste, and F. M. Domenech. Bone mineral density of the lumbar spine in white Mediterranean Spanish children and adolescents: changes related to age, sex, and puberty. *Pediatr. Res.* 35:362–366, 1994.
25. De Schepper, J., M. P. Derde, M. Van den Broeck, A. Piepsz, and M. H. Jonckheer. Normative data for lumbar spine bone mineral content in children: influence of age, height, weight, and pubertal stage. *J. Nucl. Med.* 32:216–220, 1991.
26. Dhuper, S., M. Warren, J. Brooks-Gunn, and R. Fox. Effects of hormonal status on bone density in adolescent girls. *J. Clin. Endocrinol. Metab.* 71:1083–1088, 1990.
27. Eaton, S. B., M. J. Konner, and M. Shostak. Stone agers in the fast lane: chronic degenerative diseases in evolutionary perspective. *Am. J. Med.* 84:739–749, 1988.
28. Eaton, S. B., and D. A. Nelson. Calcium in evolutionary perspective. *Am. J. Clin. Nutr.* 54:281S–287S, 1991.
29. Faulkner, R. A., D. A. Bailey, D. T. Drinkwater, A. A. Wilkinson, C. S. Houston, and H. A. McKay. Regional and total body bone mineral content, bone mineral density and total body tissue composition in children 8–16 years of age. *Calcif. Tissue Int.* 53:7–12, 1993.
30. Faulkner, R. A., C. S. Houston, D. A. Bailey, D. T. Drinkwater, H. A. McKay, and A. A. Wilkinson. Comparison of bone mineral content and bone mineral density between dominant and non-dominant limbs in children 8–16 years of age. *Am. J. Hum. Biol.* 5:491–499, 1993.
31. Fehily, A., R. Coles, W. Evans, and P. Elwood. Factors affecting bone density in young adults. *Am. J. Clin. Nutr.* 56:579–586, 1992.
32. Finkelstein, J. S., R. M. Neer, B. M. K. Biller, J. D. Crawford, and A. Kilbanski. Osteopenia in men with a history of delayed puberty. *N. Engl. J. Med.* 325:600–604, 1992.
33. Forwood, M., and D. Burr. Physical activity and bone mass: exercise in futility? *Bone Miner.* 21:89–112, 1993.
34. Forwood, M., and C. Turner. Skeletal adaptations to mechanical usage: results from tibial loading studies in rats. *Bone* in press, 1995.
35. Fox, N., J. Jacobs, W. Wright, and S. Philips. The direct medical costs of osteoporosis for American women aged forty five and older. *Bone* 9:271–279, 1988.
36. Frost, H. Bone mass and the mechanostat: a proposal. *Anat. Rec.* 219:1–9, 1987.
37. Frost, H. Mechanical usage, bone mass, bone fragility: a brief overview. M. Kleerekoper and S. Krane (eds). *Clinical Disorders of Bone and Mineral Metabolism.* New York: Liebert, 1989, pp. 15–40.
38. Frost, H. Perspectives: on a "paradigm shift" developing in skeletal science. *Calcif. Tissue Int.* 56:1–4, 1995.
39. Gallagher, J. The pathogenesis of osteoporosis. *Bone Miner.* 9:215–227, 1990.
40. Garn, S. M., and B. Wagner. The adolescent growth of the skeletal mass and its implications to mineral requirements. F. P. Heald (ed). *Adolescent Nutrition and Growth.* New York: Appleton-Century-Crofts, 1969, pp. 139–161.
41. Geusens, P., F. Cantatore, J. Nijs, W. Proesmans, F. Emma, and J. Dequeker. Heterogeneity of growth of bone in children at the spine, radius and total skeleton. *Growth Dev. Aging* 55:249–256, 1991.
42. Geusens, P., J. Dequeker, A. Verstraeten, and J. Nijs. Age, sex, and menopause-related changes of vertebral and peripheral bone: population study using dual and single photon absorptiometry and radiogrammetry. *J. Nucl. Med.* 27:1540–1549, 1986.

43. Gilsanz, V., M. I. Boechat, T. F. Roe, M. L. Loro, J. W. Sayre, and W.G. Goodman. Gender differences in vertebral body sizes in children and adolescents. *Radiology* 190:673–677, 1994.

44. Gilsanz, V., D. T. Gibbens, M. Carlson, I. Boechat, C. E. Cann, and E. S. Schulz. Peak trabecular bone density: a comparison of adolescent and adult females. *Calcif. Tissue Int.* 43:260–262, 1988.

45. Gilsanz, V., D. T. Gibbens, T. F. Roe, et al. Vertebral bone density in children: effect of puberty. *Radiology* 166:847–850, 1988.

46. Glastre, C., P. Braillon, L. David, P. Cochat, P. J. Meunier, and P. D. Delmas. Measurement of bone mineral content of the lumbar spine by dual energy x-ray absorptiometry in normal children: correlations with growth parameters. *J. Clin. Endocrinol. Metab.* 70:1330–1333, 1990.

47. Gordon, C. L., J. M. Halton, S. A. Atkinson, and C. E. Webber. The contributions of growth and puberty to peak bone mass. *Growth Dev. Aging* 55:257–262, 1991.

48. Gordon, C. L., and C. E. Webber. Body composition and bone mineral distribution during growth in females. *Can. Assoc. Radiol. J.* 44:112–116, 1993.

49. Grimston, S. K., K. Morrison, J. A. Harder, and D. A. Hanley. Bone mineral density during puberty in Western Candian children. *Bone Miner.* 19:85–96, 1992.

50. Grimston, S. K., N. D. Willows, and D. A. Hanley. Mechanical loading regime and its relationship to bone mineral density in children. *Med. Sci. Sports Exerc.* 25(11):1203–1210, 1993.

51. Gutin B., and M. Kasper. Can vigorous exercise play a role in osteoporosis prevention? *Osteoporos. Int.* 2:55–69, 1992.

52. Haapasalo, H., P. Kannus, H. Sievnen, A. Heinonen, P. Oja, and I. Vuori. Long-term unilateral loading and bone mineral density and content in female squash players. *Calcif. Tissue Int.* 54:249–255, 1994.

53. Henderson, R., G. Kemp, and H. Campion. Residual bone mineral density and muscle strength after fractures of the tibia or femur in children. *J. Bone Joint Surg. Am.* 74:211–218, 1992.

54. Hedlund, L. R., and J. C. Gallagher. The effect of age and menopause on bone mineral density of the proximal femur. *J. Bone Miner. Res.* 4:639–642, 1989.

55. Hui, S. L., C. C. Johnston, and R. B. Mazess. Bone mass in normal children and young adults. *Growth* 49:34–43, 1985.

56. Jacobson, P., W. Bevier, S. Grubb, T. Taft, and R. Talmage. Bone density in women: college athletes and older athletic women. *J. Orthop. Res.* 2:328–332, 1984.

57. Johansen, J. S., A. Giwercman, and D. Hartwell. Serum bone GLa protein as a mark of bone growth in children and adolescents: correlation with age, height, serum insulin-like growth factor I and serum testosterone. *J. Clin. Endocrinol. Metab.* 67:273–278, 1988.

58. Johansen, J. S., C. Hassager, J. Podenphant, et al. Treatment of postmenopausal osteoporosis: Is the anabolic steroid nandrolone decanoate a candidate? *Bone Miner.* 6:77–86, 1989.

59. Johnston, C., and C. Slemanda. Risk assessment: theoretical considerations. *Am. J. Med.* 95 (5A): 2S–5S, 1993.

60. Kanis, J., and F. Pitt. Epidemiology of osteoporosis. *Bone* 13:S7–S15, 1992.

61. Katzman, D. K., L. K. Bachrach, D. R. Carter, and R. Marcus. Clinical and anthropometric correlates of bone mineral acquisition in healthy adolescent girls. *J. Clin. Endocrinol. Metab.* 73:1332–1339, 1991.

62. Kirchner, E. M., R. D. Lewis, and P. J. O'Connor. Bone mineral density and dietary intake of female college gymnasts. *Med. Sci. Sports Exerc.* 27:543–549, 1995.

63. Krabbe, S., C. Christiansen, P. Rodbro, and I. Transbol. Effect of puberty on rates of bone growth and mineralisation. *Arch. Dis. Child.* 54:950–953, 1979.

64. Krall, E., and B. Dawson-Hughes. Heritable and lifestyle determinants of bone mineral density. *J. Bone Miner. Res.* 8:1–9, 1993.

65. Kriska, A., R. Sandler, J. Cauley, R. LaPorte, D. Hom, and G. Pambianco. The assessment of historical physical activity and its relation to adult bone parameters. *Am. J. Epidemiol.* 127:53–63, 1988.
66. Kroger, H., A. Kotaniemi, L. Kroger, and E. Alhava. Development of bone mass and bone density of the spine and femoral neck—a prospective study of 65 children and adolescents. *Bone Miner.* 23:171–182, 1993.
67. Kroger, H., A. Kotaniemi, P. Vainio, and E. Alhava. Bone densitometry of the spine and femur in children by dual-energy x-ray absorptiometry. *Bone Miner.* 17:75–85, 1992.
68. Lanyon, L. E. Analysis of surface bone strain in the calcaneous of sheep during normal locomotion. *J. Biomech.* 6:41–49, 1973.
69. Larsen, C. S. Bioarchaeological interpretations of subsistence economy and behavior from human skeletal remains. *Adv. Archaeol. Method Theory* 10:339–445, 1987.
70. Lloyd, T., N. Rollings, M. B. Andon, et al. Determinants of bone density in young women. I. Relationships among pubertal development, total body bone mass, and total body bone density in premenarchal females. *J. Clin. Endocrinol. Metab.* 75:383–387, 1992.
71. Loucks, A., and S. Horvath. Athletic amenorrhea—a review. *Med. Sci. Sports Exerc.* 17:56–72, 1985.
72. Lu, P. W., J. N. Brody, G. D. Ogle, et al. Bone mineral density of total body, spine and femoral neck in children and young adults: a cross-sectional and longitudinal study. *J. Bone Miner. Res.* 9:1451–1458, 1994.
73. Lutz, J., and R. Tesar. Mother-daughter pairs: spinal and femoral bone densities and dietary intakes. *Am. J. Clin. Nutr.* 52:872–877, 1990.
74. Margulies, J. Y., A. Simkin, I. Leichter, et al. Effect of intense physical activity on the bone-mineral content in the lower limbs of young adults. *J. Bone Joint Surg. Am.* 68:1090–1093, 1989.
75. Matkovic, V. Calcium metabolism and calcium requirements during skeletal modeling and consolidation of bone mass. *Am. J. Clin. Nutr.* 54:S245–S260, 1991.
76. Matkovic, V., D. Fontana, C. Tominac, P. Goel, and C. H. Chesnut. Factors which influence peak bone mass formations: A study of calcium balance and the inheritance of bone mass in adolescent females. *Am. J. Clin. Nutr.* 52:878–888, 1991.
77. Matkovic, V., J. Ilich, and L. Hsieh. Influence of age, sex and diet on bone mass and fracture rate. *Osteoporos. Int.* 4:(Suppl. 1):S20–22, 1993.
78. Matkovic, V., T. Jelic, G. M. Wardlaw, et al. Timing of peak bone mass in caucasian females and its implication for the prevention of osteoporosis. *J. Clin. Invest.* 93:799–808, 1994.
79. Mazess, R. B., H. S. Barden, M. Ettinger, et al. Spine and femur density using dual-photon absorptiometry in U.S. white women. *Bone Miner.* 2:211–219, 1987.
80. Mazess, R. B., and J. R. Cameron. Skeletal growth in school children: maturation and bone mass. *Am. J. Phys. Anthropol.* 35:399–408, 1971.
81. Mazess, R., and H. Wahner. Nuclear medicine and densitometry. L. Riggs and L. Melton (eds). *Osteoporosis: Etiology, Diagnosis, and Management.* New York: Raven Press, 1988, pp. 251–295.
82. McCormick, D. P., S. W. Ponder, H. D. Fawcett, and J. L. Palmer. Spinal bone mineral density in 335 normal and obese children: evidence for ethnic and sex differences. *J. Bone Miner. Res.* 6:507–513, 1991.
83. McCulloch, R. G., D. A. Bailey, C. S. Houston, and B. L. Dodd. Effects of physical activity, dietary calcium intake and selected lifestyle factors on bone density in young women. *Can. Med. Assoc. J.* 142:221–227, 1990.
84. McCulloch, R.G., D. A. Bailey, R. Whalen, C. C. Houston, R. A. Faulkner, and B. Craven. Bone density and bone mineral content of adolescent soccer athletes and competitive swimmers. *Pediatr. Exerc. Sci.* 4:319–330, 1992.
85. McKay, H. A., D. A. Bailey, W. Wallace, A. A. Wilkinson. Site specificity in bone mineral accretion and bone mineral loss: Evidence from a generational study. 11th International Bone Densitometry Workshop, Oregon, 1995.

86. McKay, H., D. Bailey, A. Wilkinson, and C. Houston. Familial comparison of bone mineral density at the proximal femur and lumbar spine. *Bone Miner.* 24:95–107, 1994.
87. Meema, H. E. Cortical bone atrophy and osteoporosis as a manifestation of aging. *AJR Am. J. Roentgenol.* 89:1287–1295, 1963.
88. Miller, J. Z., C. W. Slemenda, F. J. Meaney, T. K. Reister, S. Hui, and C. C. Johnston. The relationship of bone mineral density and anthropometric variables in healthy male and female children. *Bone Miner.* 14:137–152, 1991.
89. Mora, S., W. G. Goodman, M. L. Loro, T. F. Roe, J. Sayre, and V. Gilsanz. Age-related changes in cortical and cancellous vertebral bone density in girls: assessment with quantitative CT. AJR *Am. J. Roentgenol.* 162:405–409, 1994.
90. Nichols, D. L., C. F. Sanborn, S. L. Bonnick, V. Ben-Ezra, B. Gendch, and N. DiMarco. The effects of gymnastics training on bone mineral density. *Med. Sci. Sports Exerc.* 26:1220–1238, 1994.
91. Nichols, D. L., C. F. Sanborn, S. L. Bonnick, B. Gench, and N. DiMarco. Relationship of regional body composition to bone mineral density in college females. *Med. Sci. Sports Exerc.* 27:178–182, 1995.
92. Nordin, B. E. C. Guidelines for bone densitometry. *Med. J. Aust.* 160:517–520, 1994.
93. Ohlsson, C., J. Isgaard, J. Tornell, A. Nilsson, O. Isaksson, and A. Lindahl. Endocrine regulation of longitudinal bone growth. *Acta. Paediatr. Suppl.* 391:119–125, 1993.
94. Ortolani, S., C. Trevisan, M. L. Bianchi, et al. Spinal and forearm bone mass in relation to ageing menopause in healthy Italian women. *Eur. J. Clin. Invest.* 21:33–39, 1991.
95. Ortolani, S., C. Trevisan, M. L. Bianchi, G. Gandolini, R. Cherubini, and E. E. Polli. Influences of body parameters on female peak bone mass and bone loss. *Osteoporos. Int.* 4:(Suppl. 1):S61–S66, 1993.
96. Parfitt, A. M. The two faces of growth: benefits and risks to bone integrity. *Osteoporos. Int.* 4:382–398, 1994.
97. Peacock, M. Calcium absorption efficiency and calcium requirements in children and adolescents. *Am. J. Clin. Nutr.* 54:S261–S265, 1991.
98. Ponder, S. W., D. P. McCormick, H. D. Fawcett, J. L. Palmer, and M. G. McKernan. Spinal bone mineral density in children aged 5 through 11.99 years. *Am. J. Dis. Child.* 144:1346–1348, 1990.
99. Preece, M. A. Prepubertal and pubertal endocrinologyy. F. Faulkner and J. Tanner (eds). *Human Growth: A Comprehensive Treatise,* Vol. 2: *Postnatal Growth: Neurobiology.* New York: Plenum Press, 1986, pp. 211–224.
100. Preece, M. A., and M. J. Baines. A new family of mathematical models describing the human growth curve. *Ann. Hum. Biol.* 5:1–24, 1978.
101. Preece, M. A., H. Pan, and S. G. Ratcliffe. Auxological aspects of male and female puberty. *Acta. Paediatr. Suppl.* 383:11–13, 1992.
102. Recker, R. R., K. M. Davies, S. M. Hinders, R. P. Heaney, M. R. Stegman, and D. B. Kimmel. Bone gain in young adult women. *J.A.M.A.* 268:2403–2408, 1992.
103. Rice, S., C. J. Blimkie, C. G. Webber, et al. Correlates and determinants of bone mineral content and density in healthy adolescent girls. *Can. J. Physiol. Pharmacol.* 72:923–930, 1993.
104. Rico, H., M. Revilla, L. F. Villa, E. R. Hernandez, M. Alvarez de Buergo, and V. Villa. Body composition in children and Tanner's stages: a study with dual-energy x-ray absorptiometry. *Metabolism* 42:967–970, 1993.
105. Ringe, J. D. Precision and clinical application of peripheral single photon absorptiometry. C. C. Johnston and J. Dequeker (eds). *Non-Invasive Bone Measurements: Methological Problems.* Oxford, England: IRL Press, 1982, pp. 47–54.
106. Risser, W., E. Lee, A. Leblanc, et al. Bone density in eumenorrheic female college athletes. *Med. Sci. Sports Exerc.* 22:570–574, 1990.
107. Robinson, T., C. Snow-Harter, D. Taafe, D.Gillis, J. Shaw, R. Marcus. Gymnasts exhibit higher bone mass than runners despite similar prevalence of amenorrhea and oligomenorrhea. *J. Bone Miner. Res.* 19(1):26–35, 1995.

108. Rodin, A., B. Murby, M. A. Smith, et al. Premenopausal bone loss in the lumbar spine and neck of femur: a study of 225 caucasian women. *Bone* 11:1–5, 1990.
109. Rubin, C. T., T. S. Gross, K. J. McLeod, and S. D. Bain. Morphologic stages in lamellar bone formation stimulated by a potent mechanical stimulus. *J. Bone Miner. Res.* 10:488–495, 1995.
110. Rubin, K., V. Schirduan, P. Gendreau, M. Sarfarazi, R. Mendola, and G. Dalsky. Predictors of axial and peripheral bone mineral density in healthy children and adolescents, with special attention to the role of puberty. *J. Pediatr.* 123:863–870, 1993.
111. Ruff, C. B., and W. C. Hayes. Subperiosteal expansion and cortical remodeling of the human femur and tibia with aging. *Science* 217:945–948, 1982.
112. Ruiz, J. C., C. Mandel, and M. Garabedian. Influence of spontaneous calcium intake and physical exercise on the vertebral and femoral bone mineral density of children and adolescents. *J. Bone Miner. Res.* 5:675–682, 1995.
113. Seeman, E. Reduced bone density in women with fractures: contribution of low peak bone density and rapid bone loss. *Osteoporos. Int. Suppl.* 1:19–25, 1994.
114. Sledge, C., and C. Rubin. Formation and resorption of bone. W. Kelley, E. Harris, S. Ruddy, and C. Sledge (eds). *Textbook of Rheumatology.* Philadelphia: W. B. Saunders, 1989, pp. 54–75.
115. Slemenda, C., J. Christian, C. Williams, J. Norton, and C. Johnston. Genetic determinants of bone mass in adult women: a reevaluation of the twin model and the potential importance of gene interaction on heritability estimates. *J. Bone Miner. Res.* 6:561–567, 1991.
116. Slemenda, C. W., and C. C. Johnston. High intensity activities in young women: site specific bone mass effects among female figure skaters. *Bone Miner.* 20:125–132, 1993.
117. Slemenda, C. W., J. Z. Miller, S. L. Hui, T. K. Reister, and C. C. Johnston. Role of physical activity in the development of skeletal mass in children. *J. Bone Miner. Res.* 6:1227–1233, 1991.
118. Slemenda, C. W., T. K. Reister, S. L. Hui, J. Z. Miller, J. C. Christian, and C. C. Johnston. Influences on skeletal mineralization in children and adolescents: evidence for varying effects of sexual maturation and physical activity. *J. Pediatr.* 125:201–207, 1994.
119. Smith, P., R. A. Bloom, and J. Berkowitz. Diachronic trends in humeral cortical thickness of Near Eastern populations. *J. Hum. Evol.* 13:603–611, 1984.
120. Snow-Harter, C. M. Bone health and prevention of osteoporosis in active and athletic women. *Athletic Woman* 13:389–404, 1994.
121. Snow-Harter, C., M. Bouxsein, B. Lewis, D. Carter, and R. Marcus. Effects of resistance and endurance exercise on bone mineral status of young women: a randomized exercise intervention trial. *J. Bone Miner. Res.* 7:761–769, 1992.
122. Snow-Harter, C. M., and R. Marcus. Exercise, bone mineral density and osteoporosis. *Exerc. Sport Sci. Rev.* 19:351–388, 1991.
123. Southard, R. N., J. D. Morris, J. Mahan, et al. Bone mass in healthy children: measurement with quantitative DXA. *Radiology* 179:735–738, 1991.
124. Sugimoto, T., M. Nishino, T. Tsunenari, et al. Radial bone mineral content of normal Japanese infants and prepubertal children: influence of age, sex and body size. *Bone Miner.* 24:189–200, 1994.
125. Talmage, R. U., and J. J. B. Anderson. Bone density loss in women: effects of childhood activity, exercise, calcium intake and estrogen therapy. *Calcif. Tissue Int.* 36:52, 1984.
126. Teegarden, D., W. R. Proulx, B. R. Martin, et al. Peak bone mass in young women. *J. Bone Miner. Res.* 10:711–715, 1995.
127. Theintz, G., B. Buchs, R. Rizzoli, et al. Longitudinal monitoring of bone mass accumulation in healthy adolescents: evidence for a marked reduction after 16 years of age at the levels of lumbar spine and femoral neck in female subjects. *J. Clin. Endocrinol. Metab.* 75:1060–1065, 1992.
128. Thomas, K. A., S. D. Cook, J. T. Bennett, T. S. Whitecloud, and J. C. Rice. Femoral neck

and lumbar spine bone mineral densities in a normal population 3–20 years of age. *J. Pediatr. Orthop.* 11:48–58, 1991.

129. Tothill, P. Methods of bone mineral assessment. *Phys. Med. Biol.* 34:543–572, 1989, 1992.

130. Turner, C. H., T. A. Woltman, D. A. Belongia. Structural changes in rat bone subjected to long-term, in vivo, mechanical loading. *Bone* 13:417–422, 1992.

131. Turner, J. G., N. L. Gilchrist, E. M. Ayling, A. J. Hassall, E. A. Hooke, and W. A. Sadler. Factors affecting bone mineral density in high school girls. *N.Z. Med. J.* 105:95–96, 1992.

132. Tylavsky, F., J. Anderson, R. Talmage, and T. Taft. Are calcium intakes and physical activity patterns during adolescence related to radial bone mass of college age females? *Osteoporos. Int.* 2:232–240, 1992.

133. Tylavsky, F. A., A. D. Bortz, R. L. Hancock, and J. J. Anderson. Familial resemblance of radial bone mass between premenopausal mothers and their college age daughters. *Calcif. Tissue Int.* 45:265–272, 1989.

134. United Nations. *Interpolated National Populations by Age and Sex: 1950–2025* (1992 Revision). New York: United Nations Population Division, United Nations, 1992.

135. Valimaki, M. J., M. Karkkainen, C. Lamberg-Allardt, et al. Exercise, smoking, and calcium intake during adolescence and early adulthood as determinants of peak bone mass. *Br. Med. J.* 309:230–235, 1994.

136. Virvidakis, K., I. Georgiou, A. Korkotsidis, K. Ntalles, and C. Proukakis. Bone mineral content of junior competitive weightlifters. *Int. J. Sports Med.* 11:244–246, 1990.

137. Wasnich, R. Bone mass measurement: prediction of risk. *Am. J. Med.* 95(5A):6S–10S, 1993.

138. Watson, R. Bone growth and physical activity in young males. R. Mazess (ed). *International Conference on Bone Mineral Measurements.* Washington, DHEW Publication, NIH 75–683, 1974, pp. 380–385.

139. Webber, C.E., C. L. Gordon, L. F. Chambers, J. Martin, C. J. Blimkie, and N. McCartney. Body composition and bone mass in female adolescents and elderly subjects entering exercise programs. K. Ellis and J. Estman (eds). *Human Body Composition.* New York: Plenum Press, 1993, pp. 259–262.

140. Welten, D. C., H. C. G. Kemper, G. B. Post, et al. Weight-bearing activity during youth is a more important factor for peak bone mass than calcium intake. *J. Bone Miner. Res.* 9:1089–1096, 1994.

141. White, C. M., A. C. Hergenroeder, and W. J. Klish. Bone mineral density in 15- to 21-year old eumenorrheic and amenorrheic subjects. *Am. J. Dis. Child.* 146:31–35, 1992.

142. Wolpoff, M. H. *Paleoanthropology.* New York: Knopf, 1980.

143. Yeager, K., R. Agostini, A. Nattiv, and B. Drinkwater. The female athlete triad: disordered eating, amenorrhea, osteoporosis. *Med. Sci.Sports Exerc.* 25:775–777, 1993.

144. Young, N., C. Formica, G. Szmukler, and E. Seeman. Bone density at weight-bearing and non-weight-bearing sites in ballet dancers: the effects of exercise, hypogonadism, and body weight. *J. Clin. Endocrinol. Metab.* 78:449–454, 1994.

145. Zanchetta, J. R., H. Plotkin, and M. L. Alvarez Filgueira. Bone mass in children: normative values for the 2–20 year-old population. *Bone* 16:393S–399S, 1995.

146. Zhang, J., P. J. Feldblum, and J. A. Fortney. Moderate physical activity and bone density among perimenopausal women. *Am. J. Public Health* 82:736–738, 1992.

9
Exercise Training and the Cross-Stressor Adaptation Hypothesis

MARK S. SOTHMANN, Ph.D., FACSM
JANET BUCKWORTH, Ph.D.
RANDAL P. CLAYTOR, Ph.D.
RON H. COX, Ph.D.
JILL E. WHITE-WELKLEY, Ph.D.
ROD K. DISHMAN, Ph.D., FACSM

Despite the difficulty in achieving consensus on "stress" as a scientific construct, the concept has shown remarkable tenacity and an intellectual resilience that has allowed it to persist for thousands of years and, in modern times, to conform to prevailing scientific and intellectual conditions. One example, of this is an emerging research thrust, suggesting that a stressor of sufficient intensity and/or duration will induce an adaptation of the stress response systems, which becomes apparent under other similarly taxing states. This is termed the "cross-stressor adaptation hypothesis," and it is being studied in the scientific disciplines of neurochemistry and neuroendocrinology, both in terms of the processes involved and its implications for health. Recently, exercise scientists have asked the very basic questions of whether exercise training may modify the physiological stress response to nonexercise stressors, under what conditions this may occur, and whether there are health outcomes. Although the questions are straightforward, as recent reviews suggest [10, 21, 27, 62, 78], the findings remain ambiguous. There is clearly a need for more focus on theoretical modeling, from which a few critical research questions may emanate.

The goal of this chapter is to articulate a paradigm that defines the cross-stressor adaptation hypothesis in specific operational terms, so that experimental studies of the future can more specifically address past limitations. The physiological stress response cannot be fully interpreted out of the context of behavior, environment, or phenomenology [49]. Nevertheless, principally, our focus herein is on how exercise-induced adaptation of an integrated physiological system may generalize to an organism's responsiveness to stressors other than exercise. To accomplish this objective, this chapter is comprised of four principal sections: 1) evolution of the physiological stress concept; 2) principal physiological stress mechanisms; 3) the cross-stressor adaptation hypothesis, as it applies to exercise training; and 4) new directions for research.

EVOLUTION OF THE PHYSIOLOGICAL STRESS CONCEPT

Although the term "stress" was first presented by Hans Selye [69], its development spans thousands of years. Previous reviews have articulated that evolution suggests that physiological disharmony is a natural, intrinsic process, necessary for survival [14]. Modern day theories of stress start with Claude Bernard who, in the 19th century, described the *milieu interieur* as an internal physiological equilibrium, necessary for maintaining health. In the early 1900s, Walter Cannon used the term "homeostasis" to refer to coordinated physiological processes that maintain the steady states of an organism. He further defined the "fight-or-flight" reaction as the first defense against threatening stimuli.

Selye credited these events in forming his definition of stress as a nonspecific response of the body to any demand [69]. He recognized that environmental challenges elicit physiological responses specific to a challenge. However, he contended that underlying this specificity, there are also nonspecific processes responsive to many different types of stressors and mediated by neuroendocrine mechanisms having whole system, integrative properties. Selye maintained that there are "diseases of adaptation" that have less specific causation than Pasteur's theory of disease (e.g., infection). Much of Selye's research with what he termed the "General Adaptation Syndrome" focused on nonspecificity of response, and it was instrumental in his view of a "sickness syndrome," which he held to be common physiological manifestations across very diverse disease states. In later years Selye articulated two additional dimensions to his stress concept. Hyper- and hypostress represent extremes of what would be considered optimal stress. Much medical attention has focused on hyperactivity of the stress response as a factor in diseases of the circulatory system, melancholic depression, panic anxiety, anorexia nervosa, and obsessive-compulsive disorders. Hypostress may be an element of obesity, atypical depression, posttraumatic stress disorder, and chronic fatigue syndrome [14]. The second is a dichotomy between negative (distress) and positive (eustress) factors precipitating the stress response and their relation to physiological outcome.

Although the notion of disequilibrium remains common to most contemporary treatments of the stress concept, considerable debate has evolved regarding the nature of the physiological compensatory response. The development of sophisticated techniques currently applied to the measurement of autonomic and endocrine effectors has revealed a closer match between challenge and response (i.e., greater specificity), thus encouraging some disillusionment with the notion of a generalized response [38]. At this point it is important to draw a distinction between Selye's view of a physiological response, which incorporated both specificity and nonspecificity, and "stress," which referred to just the nonspecific element. This is an important consideration for the cross-stressor adaptation of hypothesis in that its validity is dependent on there being nonspecific, generalized adaptations. In a recent biomedical review [14], stress was defined as threatened homeostasis, which can be specific or nonspecific to the stressor, with the latter occurring only when the magnitude of the threat to homeostasis exceeds a certain threshold. In this chapter we adopt that definition to develop a rationale for how physical training may modify the specific and nonspecific aspects of a physiological response to a nonexercise stressor.

PHYSIOLOGICAL STRESS SYSTEMS

Several physiological systems are involved in the stress response, and they can act synergistically. Prominent effector systems include the autonomic nervous system, sympathoadrenal system, hypothalamic-pituitary-adrenocortical axis (HPA), renin-angiotensin system, and systems involving vasopressin and endogenous opioids. This chapter will focus on the HPA and sympathoadrenal systems, because they have been the most consistently researched with exercise. Figure 9.1, from a review by Chrousos and Gold [14], illustrates the two systems.

Hypothalamic-Pituitary-Adrenocortical Axis

During a stress response signals from multiple pathways, including emotional stimuli via the limbic system, set into motion a coordinated series of physiological and behavioral responses, activated by the HPA axis. Summation of these signals, when stimulatory, results in the secretion of corticotropin-releasing hormone (CRH). CRH neurons are widespread throughout the brain, but within the hypothalamus they are most prominent in the parvocellular area of the paraventricular nucleus [63]. CRH axon terminals, located at the median eminence, release CRH into the hypothalamic hypophyseal portal vessels that lead to the anterior pituitary gland. CRH causes the precursor molecule proopiomelanocortin (POMC) to be released. Adrenocorticotropin hormone (ACTH), β-endorphin, and other neuropeptides are cleaved from the POMC molecule (see ref. 33 for review). Elevation of circulating ACTH stimulates the release of glucocorticoids at the adrenal cortex. The adrenal glands are paired organs situated at the top of each kidney and are comprised of two parts, namely, the cortex and the medulla. Species differences exist in the adrenal cortical response, with humans releasing cortisol and rats, corticosterone.

Precise changes and adjustments in HPA activity in response to external challenges are necessary for the survival of the organism. Negative feedback mechanisms exist at multiple levels to regulate the output of releasing factors and tropic hormones. Increased CRH or ACTH will inhibit CRH release in the hypothalamus. Heightened circulating cortisol can also inhibit

FIGURE 9.1

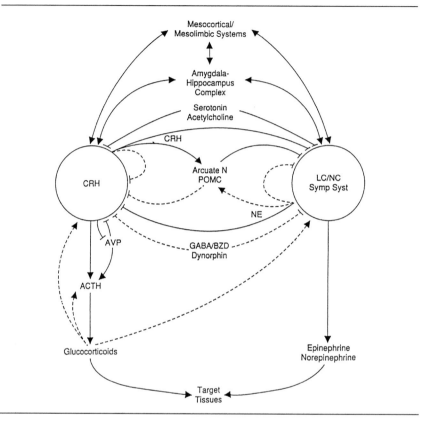

the release of ACTH and CRH. Also, there is a time element to the feedback. Fast feedback occurs at the anterior pituitary gland and hypothalamus and above [42], whereas a delayed feedback may take hours through corticosteroid action at glucocorticoid receptors in the hypothalamus, anterior pituitary gland, hippocampus, and throughout the brain. In these regions, glucocorticoid receptor (GR)-steroid complex binds to the DNA to act as an inhibitor of POMC transcription [42]. However, beyond the breadth of this review, it should be recognized, there are other physiological stress systems involved in this feedback process. For example, recently an interaction between CRH neurons and the immune system has been proposed. Glucocorticoids suppress the production of interleukin-1 whereas, conversely, interleukin-1 may function as one of the central regulators of CRH production and release, thereby indirectly activating the HPA axis [63].

Psychological stimuli, interpreted as alerting or threatening, potentiate the activation of the HPA via limbic (e.g., amygdala) input into the hypothalamus [83]. Moreover, elevated CRH may influence behavior, but the manifestations vary, depending on the environment and level of activation. In a familiar environment, CRH administered via intracerebroventricular injection produces marked behavioral activation, including increased locomotor activity, rearing, and grooming. In contrast, in more novel settings CRH administration is associated with decreased exploration in an open field, decreased feeding, and enhanced fear-induced freezing and fighting. At high doses CRH can suppress sexual behavior, feeding, and operant performance [46]. It is clear that if exercise training is to promote cross-stressor adaptation, the HPA axis is a critical mechanism by which this can occur.

Locus Ceruleus-Sympathetic-Adrenomedullary System

Efferent fibers project widely from the norepinephrine (NE)-containing neurons of the locus ceruleus, located adjacent to the fourth ventricle of the brain at the level of the pons [34]. Signals arising in other parts of the brain (e.g., hippocampus, amygdala, hypothalamus, and motor cortex) because of physical or psychological challenges serve as feed-forward activators of the locus ceruleus, which is a potent stimulus of central noradrenergic activation in particular and neuroendocrine release in general [43]. One prevalent hypothesis [5] is that locus ceruleus neurons are excited by sensory or spontaneous alertness. This enhanced activity then traverses the divergent efferent projections of the locus ceruleus, orienting the brain to physiological and behavioral states (e.g., arousal, vigilance) to respond preferentially to external events of phasically high priority. Suppressed locus ceruleus activity would allow more internally oriented, instinctual behavior (e.g., sleep, grooming, and eating).

Activation of the locus ceruleus stimulates release of NE from the sympathetic nervous system (SNS), and NE and epinephrine (E) from the adrenal medulla. Although not anatomically the same, the LC and SNS act in an analogous fashion during states of physiological arousal [1]. Tissue specificity in the SNS response is a well-documented phenomena. For example, NE turnover varies substantially across the heart, kidney, and liver of acutely exercised rats [52], and muscle sympathetic nerve activity (MSNA) may decrease in the arm while increasing in the leg during mental arithmetic [4].

Complex feedback mechanisms exist to regulate sympathetic activation during stress. As reviewed by Kjaer [43], the control can be exerted through metabolic or nonmetabolic signals (pressure, temperature, or volume) or afferent nerves as neural reflex mechanisms. Mechanical and chemosensitive receptors exist in a variety of tissue (e.g., skeletal, arterial, cardiac, and lung). The relative roles of central and peripheral factors in regulating SNS and hormonal response to acute exercise have been extensively studied. Moreover, as will be discussed in a subsequent section, this interaction forms the basis of one of the hypothetical mechanisms by which exercise training may influence cross-stressor adaptation.

Integration of the Physiological Stress Systems

Much of the stress-related research over the last decade has focused on the underlying mechanisms by which the HPA and locus-ceruleus-sympathetic-adrenomedullary systems interact to amplify whole system physiological arousal. Figure 9.1 demonstrates that the mechanisms for this dual activation are complex and multidimensional. Much more needs to be learned about the nature of the precipitants of dual-system activation, because dissociation of the systems' responses is a common observation [35]. The physiological results (e.g., redirection of nutrients to the central nervous system, increased blood pressure and heart rate, increased gluconeogenesis and lipolysis, and heightened respiration) differ in nature and/or magnitude, depending on the level of singular or dual activation. This is an important concept for understanding a threshold-mediated interaction of specific and nonspecific physiological responses inherent to the definition of the stress concept articulated by Chrousos and Gold [14]. As will be discussed later, acute exercise of sufficient intensity crosses that threshold, resulting in activation of both systems.

EXERCISE TRAINING AND CROSS-STRESSOR ADAPTATION

Cross-Stressor Adaptation Hypothesis

McCarty et al. [54] recently integrated the evolution of neuroendocrine research on cross-stressor adaptation with associative and nonassociative learning theory. Associative learning recognizes that there is a temporal component to the adaptation process. This occurs when an association is drawn between two stimuli (classical conditioning) or a stimulus and response (operant conditioning). For example, mastery of a task and avoidance are two behaviors that have been shown to have a profound impact on the neuroendocrine response to a stressor. Nonassociative learning implies an underlying neuroadaptation to repeatedly administered stimuli that cannot be attributed to classical or operant conditioning. The theoretical focus of this chapter, that exercise training promotes cross-stressor tolerance by adaptation of the physiological stress response systems, would be part of nonassociative learning theory.

Certain key concepts have emerged from research on nonassociative learning that are useful for understanding how adaptation of the neuroendocrine system enhances physiological coping with a stressor. "Habituation" refers to a decrease in the amplitude of a response with repeated exposure to an intermittent challenge. "Sensitization" describes the facilitation of a nonhabituated response to an intense or novel stimuli. Animals routinely exposed to a variety of stressors (e.g. footshock, restraint, and temperature) have been shown to habituate by manifesting a blunted neuroendocrine response. However, when the animal habituated to one stressor is presented with another novel stressor, there is an augmented response that often exceeds initial levels. This process of habituation and sensitization has been observed both centrally [2] and peripherally [45].

Kvetnansky [47] has proposed that habituation involves a tonic central nervous system inhibition that allows an animal to minimize the physiological response necessary to successfully meet a familiar (homotypic) challenge. However, this process of habituating also incorporates cellular adaptations, involving increased biosynthesis and storage of critical neurotransmitters. In the presence of a novel (heterotypic) or threatening challenge, CNS inhibition is overridden, allowing the animal's new neurochemical potential to be released, which results in a facilitated response, as compared to that of nonhabituated animals when they face a new stressor.

Using this paradigm, several investigators [15, 21, 78, 87] have argued that exercise training may be viewed as a homotypic stressor. This has led to research interest as to whether exercise training influences the physiological stress response to a nonexercise challenge during either an initial exposure (heterotypic) or after repeated exposure (homotypic).

Exercise Training and Stress System Adaptation

The first step in evaluating the theoretical potential of exercise training for promoting adaptation to either heterotypic or homotypic nonexercise stressors is in examining whether a physiological stress system adaptation is, in fact, induced by chronic exercise.

HYPOTHALAMIC-PITUITARY-ADRENOCORTICAL AXIS. Plasma levels of ACTH increase acutely during exercise in a manner dependent on duration and intensity at relative intensities exceeding 50% of aerobic capacity [80]. The responses of the HPA hormones typically habituate to exercise training. This is demonstrated by a decline in the magnitude of the response at a given absolute workload. Exercise-trained individuals, at the same absolute exercise intensity, have lower circulating HPA hormones than their sedentary counterparts but, when they are compared to sedentary individuals at the same relative intensities, responses are nearly the same or a bit higher in the trained. At maximal and supramaximal exercise, the trained have higher responses [43].

At rest, basal cortisol levels have been significantly higher in healthy male senior runners, compared to those in sedentary controls [40] after a CRH challenge. These findings suggest either an enhanced secretory capacity or sensitivity to CRH. Much more needs to be learned about the regulation and capacity of the HPA system after exercise training.

LOCUS CERULEUS-SYMPATHETIC-ADRENOMEDULLARY A SNS adaptation to exercise is suggested by animal studies demonstrating tissue-specific adaptations in NE turnover [52, 53] and increased NE concentration in selected sympathetic nerve endings [3]. Central noradrenergic activation with a stressor has been shown to be an analog to SNS activity [1]. Exercise training has been shown to increase brain NE concentrations (see refs. 12 and 33 for a review), although there is concern that these findings may be confounded by other stressors (e.g., forced vs. voluntary exercise). Peripheral NE "appearance rate" at rest, as measured by radioisotope dilution, may increase, decrease, or remain unchanged with exercise training, depending on the population studied [41, 64, 67, 68]. At maximal and supramaximal exercise, NE and E release has been shown to be augmented in exercise-trained subjects [43]. In humans, with E this has been attributed to heightened secretory capacity, because training status was not related to clearance. In animals, intense exercise training results in higher adrenal E content and higher weight [43]. With respect to regulation of the sympathetic nervous system, as early as 1978 Winder et al. [89] demonstrated a dissociation between the relative work rate and sympathoadrenal response to exercise with training. This is important, because it contradicts the suggestion that any observed change in circulating NE is attributable to the change in relative work and not a SNS adaptation per se [62].

AUTONOMIC NERVOUS SYSTEM. Training-induced bradycardia is observed at rest and during the same absolute exercise intensity. Whether this reflects a training-induced change in autonomic control has historically been an area of considerable debate. There is cross-sectional and longitudinal evidence for both a change in intrinsic heart rate and for higher vagal tone at rest and during sleep among more fit and exercise trained subjects [35, 37, 66, 74]. If the lower resting heart rate associated with fitness reflects greater parasympathetic tone, it has relevance to the cross-stressor adaptation hypothesis.

Adaptations involving the carotid baroreflex may be the origin for the putative enhancement of parasympathetic tone. However, an association between fitness or exercise training and changes in carotid baroreflex sensitivity has not been established [36]. It has been speculated [82] that aerobic training enhances the inhibitory effect of the cardiac afferent and does not change the baroreflex response per se. This has been supported by studies showing a vertical shift in the stimulus-response curve without changes in sensitivity [11, 39].

INTEGRATIVE MECHANISMS FOR EXERCISE TRAINING AND CROSS- STRESSOR ADAPTATION The previous sections suggest that the cardiovascular and neuroendocrine responses to acute exercise habituate with repeated exercise bouts (*i.e*, chronic exposure). Although beyond the scope of this review, it should be recognized that there are a myriad of other peripheral adaptations involving the cardiorespiratory, neuromuscular, and musculoskeletal [65, 66, 75] systems that, through integrative physiological functioning, are potentially involved in the stress response, depending on the nature and intensity of the stressor. Figure 9.2 presents one example of how exercise training may modify this integration at numerous levels of function in a manner that could influence the stress response to certain other stressors.

Emotion and associated cognitive processes (No. 1, in Fig. 9.2) have long been recognized as critical elements in the initiation of neuroendocrine and autonomic activation [57]. Moreover, changing such factors as stressor predictability and behavioral control can alter the nature and/or magnitude of the response [60]. Exercise training has been speculated to influence such cognitive processes as self-perception, attentional focus, appraisal of arousal, anger, etc., but the experimental evidence of it remains uncompelling because of limitations in research design and methods [13, 27].

Motor control (No. 2 in Fig. 9.2) represents the initiation of muscle activity and autonomic activity often referred to as "central command." Changes in motor unit recruitment patterns, synchronization, and cocontraction as a function of exercise training are well accepted. However, whether these motor alterations contribute to changes in physiological response when muscles not specifically trained are activated or "tensed," as may be the case with behavioral provocations, is more controversial. This is

FIGURE 9.2

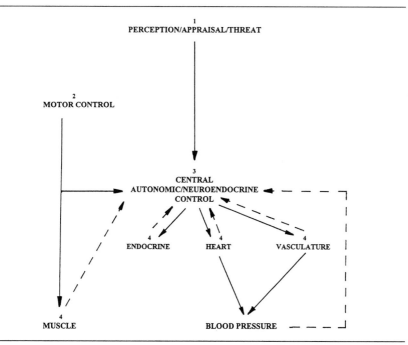

one important topic for which more basic research is required. Additionally, there is agreement that cardiovascular and muscle sympathetic nerve adaptations are manifested when an isometrically trained muscle is exercised. However, it is not clear whether cardiovascular or muscle sympathetic nerve adaptation to isometric exercise will be expressed when a nontrained muscle is exercised [50, 68].

The regulation of autonomic and neuroendocrine function (No. 3 in Fig. 9.2) at the level of the brain may also be influenced by exercise training. Adaptations in neurotransmitter concentration and/or activity have been observed with exercise training in critical brain regions integrating behaviors related to anxiety and depression (e.g., the pons/medulla, frontal cortex, and hippocampus), as well as with those involved in neuroendocrine and autonomic responses to behavioral challenges (e.g., hypothalamic and those of the locus ceruleus) [12; A. Dunn, personal communication, 1995]. Research is emerging that uses pharmacological blocking to determine the relative importance of central command and peripheral afferent feedback in regulating the cardiovascular and neuroendocrine response to exercise, as well as the changes that may occur with physical training (see ref. 43 for a detailed review). No comparable studies have been published that substantively evaluate linkage to cross-stressor tolerance.

There are a multitude of end-organ adaptations (No. 4 in Fig. 9.2) innervated by the autonomic nervous system that may influence physiological stress responses in two ways: 1) by means of functional changes within the organ (e.g., myocardial hypertrophy and receptor function) and 2) by alteration of feedback to central controlling sites (e.g., baroreceptor and muscle mechanical receptors). This is a complex integrative system of efferent (i.e., feed-forward) and afferent (i.e., feedback) neural communication that may be altered by exercise training at various junctures. Kjaer and Mitchell [43, 58] have reviewed the literature supporting the role of muscle in autonomic regulation during exercise and mediated by metabolic and mechanical receptor activity. However, it is not presently clear what role exercise training may have in influencing autonomic response to a nonexercise stressor via muscle afferent activity.

Of related interest is the important role of receptor function in modifying a cardiovascular response to a given level of central neuroendocrine/ autonomic activation. The literature regarding the effect of exercise training on receptor function is presently evolving and requires much more research. It should be noted, however, that the potential change in response is probably not unidimensional (i.e, blunted). In one study [81], the infusion of E was shown to result in a lower diastolic blood pressure but increased systolic pressure in the exercise-trained subject, as compared to results with the untrained. The chronotropic and inotropic responses to infused CA were not markedly changed as a function of training. A uniform change in receptor function cannot explain these results.

In summary, Figure 9.2 suggests that exercise training of sufficient intensity induces adaptations in each individual system (e.g., cardiorespiratory, muscular, and neural) but, more importantly, it promotes coordination between the systems to minimize the disruption to homeostasis in response to exercise, which has direct relevance to the issue of specificity and nonspecificity of response. An improved-response specificity is an important adaptation in that it minimizes the energy expenditure to successfully meet a challenge. However, there are also two important implications for the nonspecific element of the physiological response elicited by exercise. First, any specific adaptation of effector systems would be expected to be exhibited when those specific systems are challenged by other stressors. Secondly, when the exercise training is of sufficient intensity, a more generalized response pattern is activated, thus inducing generalized adaptations that would be manifested whenever the systems are provoked. Chrousos and Gold [14] argue that the nonspecific aspect of a stress response is achieved when a threshold is crossed. An example of a threshold is demonstrated when circulating neurotransmitters and hormones reach concentrations that initiate systemic physiological arousal. This concentration may be 50–100 pg/ml and 1800 pg/ml for E and NE, respectively [20,71], and these values are obtained with moderately strenuous physical exercise [89]. Thus, chronically eliciting this generalized response with exercise training could, theoretically, induce an adaptation in receptor function in tissues not directly involved in exercise-induced sympathetic arousal, thus promoting a generalized adaptation.

STUDIES ON EXERCISE AND CROSS-STRESSOR ADAPTATION

Previous reviews [10, 27, 78] have demonstrated the equivocal nature of the studies on exercise and cross-stressor adaptation, as well as their corresponding limitations. One of the principal problems has been the lack of developing experimental designs that emanate from a theoretical base. As such, the following review is limited to studies directly relevant to the cross-stressor adaptation hypothesis, as we have described it. This selective review will lead to what we consider to be critical research directions that need to be cultivated.

Hypothalamic-Pituitary-Adrenocortical Axis

In humans, enhanced cardiovascular fitness resulting from long-term exercise training has not yet been shown to modulate ACTH and cortisol to a cognitive/psychomotor challenge [8, 73, 76]. Thus, the limited human research has not supported either an attenuation or sensitization. In those studies the cognitive/psychomotor tasks could be considered a mild stressor, and the circulating hormone levels did not markedly increase. Significant activation of the HPA axis from amygdala input is marked when the psychological stimuli are threatening [83]. Thus, when exercise training modulates the HPA axis, it may be only under specific and, to date unknown, conditions.

In rodents, in which more extreme challenges can be induced, the results have been both positive and negative. Investigators have reported no alteration in corticosterone [22, 30, 61] or ACTH response [30, 61] to a heterotypic stressor after exercise training, whereas others have reported an attenuation (86; White-Welkley, personal communication 1995). In contrast, in estradiol-treated female rats, a sensitized (augmented) ACTH response after treadmill exercise has been demonstrated [87, 88].

Locus Ceruleus-Sympathetic-Adrenomedullary System

The majority of human studies on exercise and cross-stressor tolerance that have monitored NE and E response have been cross-sectional in nature and have focused on a healthy population. Those studies using novel, mild-intensity cognitive/psychomotor stressors have reported equivocal results [62, 73, 78]. In one study in which the subjects were familiarized with the stressor, a group of sedentary and markedly low-fit middle-aged males had an augmented NE response, as compared to their moderate and highly fit counterparts [76, 78]. Discrete aerobic fitness groups have not been shown to differ on plasma NE with orthostasis [44] or cold pressor [17]. Few longitudinal studies have been performed and, with one exception [9], researchers in conducting these investigations [19, 44, 72, 77] have failed to observe a significant change in venous CA response to a cognitive/psychomotor or orthostatic stressor after 3–4 mo of exercise training and a 10–20% improvement in VO_{2max}.

There is consistent evidence [43] that highly trained humans have an augmented E response to a variety of exercise (e.g., supramaximal) and nonexercise (e.g., hypoglycemia or hypercapnia) challenges. Three studies [16, 18, 76] with a behavioral challenge noted an augmented E response in highly trained subjects. However, exercise training for a few months has not been shown to increase E response [77].

In contrast to human training studies, swim training in the rat has been shown to reduce the development of hypertension and plasma NE response to a repeated footshock [22, 23]. The influence of exercise training on sensitization of the sympathoadrenal system is less clear. In a series of studies with a novel stressor, exercise trained rats did not manifest the expected augmented CA response and, in fact, had lower levels [23, 55, 56].

Cardiovascular System

In humans there is lower absolute heart rate (HR) at rest and during a provocation with training, but the relative change from baseline as a measure of "cardiovascular reactivity" remains controversial [10]. A metaanalysis of 34 studies pertaining to exercise and stress [24], which was dominated by studies in which a cognitive/psychomotor challenge was used and which focused principally on heart rate, indicated a 0.50 SD effect size for exercise-induced reductions in responsiveness. However, this finding should be interpreted with caution; the obvious limitation of a metaanalysis is that its inclusiveness incorporates research that by today's standards has serious methodological problems. A second concern is the task-specific nature of the HR response. For example, passive coping tasks elicit a decrease in HR and an increase in blood pressure. Under such conditions, HR would not be a true reflection of "cardiovascular reactivity." An additional concern is the lack of accounting for the theoretical perspective, supported by data [16, 18, 43, 76], that an augmented stress response is typical of increased fitness under certain conditions.

Training adaptations to other physical stressors have been examined. Although several studies have linked exercise training to impaired orthostatic tolerance, there remains controversy regarding this idea [36, 66]. Responses to cold tests as a function of fitness or training have been mixed [11, 32]. Changes in carotid-cardiac baroreflex with exercise training may be limited to a vertical shift in the stimulus-response curve at rest, but there is some evidence that fitness buffers a decrease in baroreflex sensitivity observed during a mental challenge in individuals with parental history of hypertension [11, 32].

Several investigators [15, 25, 70, 84] have argued that our understanding of cardiovascular adjustments is facilitated by the measurement of more than HR rate and blood pressure. Data from cross-sectional studies suggest that even though HR and blood pressure response to a challenge may be similar, cardiac output and stroke volume responses are attenuated in trained, as compared to untrained subjects [15]. Concomitantly, the reduction in peripheral vascular resistance during stress is lessened as a function of training [15, 70].

Novelty vs. familiarity with a behavioral stressor has also been shown to be a factor in the relationship between fitness and hemodynamic response. Although mean arterial pressure and cardiac output increased, the exercise-trained group exhibited significantly attenuated responses relative to their untrained counterparts with exposure to a familiar behavioral challenge [15, 70]. Additionally, the decrease in total peripheral resistance was minimally attenuated in the trained group across four sequential exposures to the same behavioral challenge. In contrast, HR reactivity was unaffected for either of the groups [15]. Such findings support the importance of measuring the underlying components of the blood pressure response to a behavioral provocation.

Animal studies of cardiovascular dynamics indicate enhanced blood pressure responsiveness to a novel stressor [22, 23, 48] with exercise training. Moreover, the effect of training on blood pressure reactivity is more pronounced in animals with a genetic background of hypertension [48]. Such findings in the animal model are consistent with a recent finding in humans of an augmented blood pressure response to a novel behavioral challenge with enhanced fitness [18].

Summary

There is evidence emerging from our laboratories and others to support the need to evaluate the cross-stressor adaptation hypothesis along a dimension of novelty and familiarity. In cross-sectional studies with humans, there is increasing evidence for an augmented E and blood pressure response in trained subjects with exposure to a novel stressor. How the blood pressure findings relate to potential changes in baroreceptor sensitivity with training [11, 32] requires further research. Conversely, repeated exposure to a stressor has resulted in an attenuated increase in NE and cardiac output in trained individuals, relative to untrained counterparts. No influence of fitness has been observed with the HPA axis in humans. To date, short-term, longitudinal exercise training studies have failed to significantly alter any stress response profile. However, cross-stressor studies with animals, which can use a more intense challenge, have provided clear evidence that the stress response is changed by exercise training, which is more consistent with the sympathoadrenal system than with the HPA axis. Plasma NE response in trained animals is reduced relative to untrained animals in a variety of stress paradigms. Second, the blood pressure response to novel stressors is augmented with training, particularly in those animals with a genetic background of hypertension. It is presently unclear as to what is mediating the lack of significant findings in human training studies, relative to the animal model, but intensity of training, the nature of training (forced vs. voluntary exercise), and intensity or predictability/controllability of the stressor are potential factors requiring further examination.

DIRECTIONS FOR FUTURE RESEARCH

Previous reviews [10, 27, 62] have articulated existing methodological problems contributing to the equivocal results on exercise and cross-stressor tolerance. In humans there have been few training studies of a true experimental nature with accurate measures of fitness, random assignment, appropriate control groups, assessment of reactivity to the same stressors before and after training, or documentation of postexercise training effects. Individual characteristics affecting reactivity are usually not considered [39]. Although these methodological issues are compelling and need to be resolved, in this part of the chapter we present what we consider to be significant research thrusts necessary to advance understanding of the postulated relationship between exercise training and cross-stressor adaptation.

Clinical Populations

Relatively short-term exercise intervention studies with humans have not demonstrated a marked change in the stress response to nonexercise stressors. However, those studies generally focused on healthy individuals, and experimental strategy has been to initiate an acute perturbation of the physiological stress response systems. There is clearly a need for more research on the potential of exercise training for promoting health in clinical populations in which a characteristic of the medical condition includes a more chronically compromised stress capability. Recent research [14] suggests that compromised stress system involvement in such medical conditions as depression, panic anxiety, hypertension, chronic fatigue syndrome, obesity, etc., may fall along a continuum of hyper- and hypoactivity. Critical issues to be addressed included determining whether exercise training induces a stress system adaptation in such clinical groups, whether that intervention is effective along the entire range of the stress continuum, and the implications for rehabilitation. Along this line, it is clear from the equivocal results of existing studies that more invasive and sophisticated techniques of measuring physiological adjustments must be used if we are to make progress.

Mechanisms

Three ongoing lines of investigation in exercise physiology have direct relevance to furthering our understanding of the mechanisms underlying the postulated role of exercise training in the cross-stressor adaptation hypothesis. Better understanding brain neurotransmitter synthesis and release with exercise training would help clarify whether chronic exercise may protect against dysregulation of the HPA and sympathoadrenal systems. For example, sedentary rats have been shown to have lower NE levels in the locus ceruleus, hippocampus, and central amygdala following footshock [29] and after immobilization, when compared with home cage control animals and chronic activity wheel animals [28]. These results are consistent with decreased responsiveness to both controllable and uncontrollable stressors or with increased NE storage for physically active animals, as compared to sedentary animals. Exercise studies are needed to examine specific aspects of synthesis and metabolism of brain neurotransmitters as they relate to peripheral stress system regulation.

Secondly, modification in the arterial baroreflex with exercise training has been implicated as a mechanism for cross-stressor adaptation of HR and blood pressure, but there has been limited work in this area [11], and the sites of adaptation (i.e., baroreceptor resetting, central integration, or end-organ response) have not been elucidated. Better defining baroreceptor function with exercise training (see ref. 36 for review) is critical to furthering our understanding of the control of HR and blood pressure. On a related issue, during an exercise challenge there is a coupled reciprocal response in which increases in HR and systolic blood pressure are matched to the metabolic needs to maintain tissue perfusion. However, with a mental stressor, there is evidence of an uncoupled response in which high levels of sympathetic nerve activity override the cardiac baroreflex response [7, 11, 31]. Blood pressure increases, but reflexive HR decreases are inhibited. Hypothesized mechanisms for this uncoupling include inhibition of the cardiac arm of the baroreflex by the hypothalamus or amygdala [7]. In uncoupled responses, the balance of the sympathetic and parasympathetic systems is a critical factor. Thus, determining the influence of fitness on the HR and blood pressure response to nonexercise stressors is enhanced with simultaneous assessment of parasympathetic and sympathetic function.

Finally, skeletal muscle makes up almost 40% of our body mass and is the source of copious metabolic and mechanical signals. Several lines of evidence support the notion that skeletal muscle and cardiovascular function are related (see ref. 6 for review). Because muscular activation or tension is a well-documented corollary of stress, there is no reason to assume that information from muscle is not being used in the orchestration of final autonomic nervous system outflow decisions. How the information from muscles might change with training and affect the physiological stress response is unknown. A reasonable supposition would be that there is less likelihood for the trained subject to respond in a manner that is not in proportion to the muscular requirement. The challenge for exercise scientists will be in devising the methodologies and techniques needed to address this issue.

Gender

Perhaps one of the most relevant limitations is the lack of research on females. A high incidence of autonomic disease and the possibility that neural control of circulation during a physical or behavioral challenge may be qualitatively and quantitatively different from those in males makes this an important consideration [59]. With respect to the HPA axis, there is a growing body of literature that indicates that the HPA and hypothalamic gonadal (HPG) axes interact to influence the neuroendocrine stress response [51]. For example, exercise-trained male rats showed an attenuated ACTH to immobilization (White-Welkley, personal communication 1995), whereas trained female rats primed with estrogen have exhibited a sensitized ACTH response [87, 88]. One line of human research in this area has focused on amenorrhea. Elevations in basal cortisol have been reported in amenorrheic female runners [84], but a blunted cortisol response after ACTH stimulation, despite mild hypercortisolism, suggests a possible limitation of adrenal secretory capacity [26]. More research is necessary to further elucidate the physiological stress response and regulation in females, the adaptation to exercise training, and the implications for cross-stressor tolerance. Moreover, the influence of the menstrual cycle on neuroen-docrine and hormonal response dictates rigorous experimental design.

CONCLUSION

The last 15 years has been a time of considerable research activity on the cross-stressor adaptation hypothesis, aided in large measure by the rapid development of sensitive analytical procedures. In many respects this research is the quintessential integrative research. Moreover, it highlights many of the classic questions in the exercise field (e.g., specificity vs. generality of training and central vs. peripheral adaptations), and it exposes the limits in our knowledge of exercise training adaptations.

REFERENCES

1. Abercrombie, E., and B. Jacobs. Single unit response of noradrenergic neurons in the locus coeruleus of freely moving cats. II. Adaptation to chronically presented stressful stimuli. *J Neurosci.* 7:2844–2848, 1987.
2. Abercrombie, E. D., L. K. Nisenbaum, and M. J. Zigmond. Impact of acute and chronic stress on the release and synthesis of norepinephrine in brain: microdialysis studies in behaving animals. R. Kvetnansky, R. McCarty, and J. Axelrod (eds). *Stress: Neuroendocrine and Molecular Approaches.* Philadelphia: Gordon & Breach, 1992, pp. 29–42.
3. Ahlo, H., J. Koistinaho, V. Kovanen, H. Suominen, and A. Hervonen. Effect of prolonged physical training on the histochemically demonstratable catecholamines in the sympathetic neurons, the adrenal gland and extra-adrenal catecholamine storing cells of the rat. *J. Auton. Nerv. Syst.* 10:181–191, 1984.
4. Anderson, E. A., B. G. Wallin, and A. L. Mark. Dissociation of sympathetic nerve activity in arm and leg muscle during mental stress. *Hypertension* 9 (Suppl. III): 114–119, 1987.
5. Aston-Jones, G. A., S. L. Foote, and F. B. Bloom. Anatomy and physiology of locus coeruleus neurons: functional implications. M. Ziegler and C. R. Lake (eds). *Norepinephrine.* Baltimore: Williams & Wilkins, 1984, pp. 92–116.
6. Basset, D. R. Skeletal muscle characteristics: relations to cardiovascular risk factors. *Med. Sci. Sports Exerc.* 26:957–966, 1994.
7. Berntson, G., J. T. Cacioppo, and K. Quigley. Autonomic determinism: the modes of autonomic control, the doctrine of autonomic space, and the laws of autonomic constraint. *Psychophysiology* 98:459–487, 1991.
8. Blaney, J., M. Sothmann, H. Raff, B. Hart, and T. Horn. Impact of exercise training on plasma adrenocorticotropin hormone response to a well learned vigilance task. *Psychoneuroendocrinology* 15:453–462, 1990.
9. Blumenthal, J. A., M. Fredrikson, C. Kuhn, R. Ulmer, M. Walsh-Riddle, and M. Applebaum. Aerobic exercise reduces levels of cardiovascular and sympathoadrenal responses to mental stress in subjects without prior evidence of myocardial ischemia. *Am. J. Cardiol.* 65:93–98, 1990.
10. Brown, D. R. Exercise, fitness, and mental health. C. Bouchard, R. J. Shephard, T. Stephens, J. R. Sutton, and B. D. McPherson (eds). *Exercise, Fitness, and Health: A Consensus of Current Knowledge.* Champaign, IL: Human Kinetics, 1990, pp. 607–626.
11. Buckworth, J., R. K. Dishman, and K. J. Cureton. Autonomic responses of women with parental hypertension: effects of physical activity and fitness. *Hypertension* 24:576–584, 1994.

12. Chaouloff, F. Physical exercise and brain monoamines: a review. *Acta Physiol. Scand.* 137:1–13, 1989.
13. Chodzko-Zajko, W., and K. A. Moore. Physical fitness and cognitive functioning in aging. *Exerc. Sport Sci. Rev.* 22:195–220, 1994.
14. Chrousos, C. P., and P. W. Gold. The concepts of stress and stress system disorders: overview of physical and behavioral homeostasis. *J.A.M.A.* 267:1244–1252, 1992.
15. Claytor, R. P. Stress reactivity: hemodynamic adjustments in trained and untrained humans. *Med. Sci. Sports Exerc.* 23:783–881, 1991.
16. Claytor, R. P., and R. H. Cox. Exercise training-induced enhancement in sympathoadrenal response to a behavioral challenge (Abstract). *Med. Sci. Sports Exerc.* 24 (Suppl.):S25, 1992.
17. Claytor, R. P., R. H. Cox, E. T. Howley, K. A. Lawler, and J. A. Lawler. Aerobic power and cardiovascular response to stress. *J. Appl. Physiol.* 65(3):1416–1423, 1988.
18. Claytor, R. P., R. Mallie, C. Canan, W. Mays and T. Kimball. Aerobically trained males exhibit greater cardiovascular and sympathoadrenal reactivity to a novel behavioral challenge (Abstract). *Med. Sci. Sports Exerc.* 26(Suppl.):S114, 1994.
19. Cleroux, J., F. Peronnet, and J. De Champlain. Sympathetic indices during psychological and physical stimuli before and after training. *Physiol. Behav.* 35:271–275, 1985.
20. Clutter, W. E., D. M. Bier, S. D. Shah, and P. E. Cryer. Epinephrine plasma clearance rates and physiologic thresholds for metabolic and hemodynamic actions in man. *J. Clin. Invest.* 66:94–101, 1980.
21. Cox, R. H. Exercise training and response to stress: insights from an animal model. *Med. Sci. Sports Exerc.* 23:853–859, 1991.
22. Cox, R. H., J. W. Hubbard, J. E. Lawler, B. J. Sanders, and V. P. Mitchell. Cardiovascular and sympathoadrenal responses to stress in swim trained rats. *J. Appl. Physiol.* 58:1207–1204, 1985a.
23. Cox, R. H., J. W. Hubbard, J. E. Lawler, B. J. Sanders, and V. P. Mitchell. Exercise training attenuates stress-induced hypertension in the rat. *Hypertension* 7:747–751, 1985b.
24. Crews, D. J., and D. M. Landers. A meta-analytic review of aerobic fitness and reactivity to psychological stressors. *Med. Sci. Sports Exerc.* 19(5):S114–S120, 1987.
25. de Geus, E. J., L. J. van Doornen, and J. F. Orlebeke. Regular exercise and aerobic fitness in relation to psychological makeup and physiological stress reactivity. *Psychosom. Med.* 55:341–363, 1993.
26. Desouza, M. J., A. A. Luciano, J. C. Arce, L. M. Demers, and A. B. Loucks. Clinical test explain blunted cortisol responsiveness but not mild cortisolism in amenorrheic runners. *J. Appl. Physiol.* 76:1320–1309, 1994.
27. Dishman, R. K. Biological psychology, exercise, and stress. *Quest.* 46:28–59, 1994.
28. Dishman, R. K., K. Renner, J. White, B. Bunnel, S. Youngstedt, and R. Armstrong. Effects of treadmill training on locus coeruleus monoamines following running and immobilization. (Abstract). *Med. Sci. Sports. Exerc.* 24(Suppl.):S525, 1992.
29. Dishman, R. K., K. J. Renner, S. D. Youngstedt, T. Reigle, K. Kedzie, B. Bunnell, and H. Yoo. Spontaneous physical activity moderates escape latency and brain monoamines after uncontrollable footshock. *Med. Sci. Sports. Exerc.* 25(Suppl.):590, 1993.
30. Dishman, R. K., J. M. Warren, S. D. Youngstedt, H. Yoo, B. N. Bunnell, E. H. Mougey, J. L. Meyerhoof, L. Jaso-Friedmann, and D. L. Evans. Activity-wheel running attenuates suppression of natural killer cell activity after footshock. *J. Appl. Physiol.* 78:1547–1554, 1995.
31. Ditto, B., and C. France. Carotid baroreflex sensitivity at rest and during psychological stress in offsprings of hypertensives and non-twin sibling pairs. *Psychosom. Med.* 52:610–620, 1990.
32. Dixon, E. M., M. V. Kamath, N. McCartney, and E. L. Fallen. Neural regulation of heart rate variability in endurance athletes and sedentary controls. *Cardiovasc. Res.* 26:713–719, 1992.
33. Dunn, A.L., and R. K. Dishman, Exercise and the neurobiology of depression. *Exerc. Sport Sci. Rev.* 19:41–98, 1991.

34. Foote, S. L., F. B. Bloom, and G. A. Aston-Jones. Nucleus locus ceruleus: new evidence of anatomical and physiological specificity. *Physiol. Rev.* 63:844–914, 1983.

35. Frankenhaeuser, M., V. Lundberg, and L. Forsmen. Dissociation between sympathetic-adrenal and pituitary-adrenal responses to an achievement situation characterized by high controllability: comparison between type A and type B females. *Biol. Psychol.* 10:79–91, 1980.

36. Geelen, G., and J. E. Greenleaf. Orthostasis: exercise and exercise training. *Exerc. Sport Sci. Rev.* 21:210–230, 1993.

37. Goldsmith, R. L., J. T. Bigger, R. C. Steinman, and J. L. Fleiss. Comparison of 24-hours parasympathetic activity in endurance-trained and untrained young men. *J. Am. Coll. Cardiol.* 20:552–558, 1992.

38. Goldstein, D. S. *Stress, Catecholamines, and Cardiovascular Disease.* New York: Oxford University Press, 1995, pp. 3–53.

39. Graham, R., A. Zeichner, L. J. Peacock, and R. K. Dishman. Bradycardia and cardiac vagal tone during autonomic challenge: cardiorespiratory fitness and hostility. *Psychophysiology* (in press), 1995.

40. Heuser, I. J., H. J. Wark, J. Keul, and F. Holsboer. Hypothalamic-pituitary-adrenal axis function in elderly endurance athletes. *J. Clin. Endocrinol. Metab.* 73:485–488, 1991.

41. Jennings, G., L. Nelson, P. Nestel, M. Esler, P. Korner, D. Burton, and J. Brazelmans. The effects of changes in physical activity on major cardiovascular risk factors, hemodynamics, sympathetic function, and glucose utilization in man: a controlled study of four levels of activity. *Circulation.* 73:30–40, 1986.

42. Jones M. T., and B. Gilliam. Factors involved in the regulation of adrenocorticotropic hormone/β-lipotropic hormone. *Physiol. Rev.* 68:743–818, 1988.

43. Kjaer, M. Regulation of hormonal and metabolic responses during exercise in humans. *Exerc. Sport Sci. Rev.* 20:161–184, 1992.

44. Kohrt, W. M., R. J. Spina, A. A. Ehsani, P. E. Cryer, and J. O. Holloszy. Effects of age, adiposity, and fitness level on plasma catecholamine responses to standing and exercise. *J. Appl. Physiol.* 75:1828–1835, 1993.

45. Konarska, M., R. E. Stewart, and R. McCarty. Habituation and sensitization of plasma catecholamine responses to chronic intermittent stress: effects of stressor intensity. *Physiol. Behav.* 47:647–652, 1990.

46. Koop, G. F. The behavioral neuroendocrinology of corticotropin-releasing factor, growth hormone-releasing factor, somatostatin, and gonadotropin releasing hormone. C. B. Nemeroff (ed). *Neuroendocrinology.* Boca Raton, FL: CRC Press, 1992, pp. 353–364.

47. Kvetnansky, R. Recent progress in catecholamines under stress. E. R. Usdin, R. Kvetnansky, and I. J. Kopin (eds). *Catecholamines and Stress: Recent Advances.* New York: Elsevier, 1980, pp. 1–7.

48. Lawler, J. E., S. K. Naylor, C. H. Wang, and R. H. Cox. Family history of hypertension, exercise training and reactivity to stress: a study in rats. in press, 1995.

49. Lazarus, R. S. *Emotion and Adaptation.* Oxford, England: Oxford Press, 1991, pp. 1–170.

50. Lewis, S., E. Nygaard, J. S. Sanchez, H. Egeblad, and B. Saltin. Static contraction of the quadriceps muscle in man: cardiovascular control and responses to one-legged strength training. *Acta Physiol. Scand.* 122:341–353, 1984.

51. Loucks, A. B., J. F. Mortola, L. Girton, and S. S. C. Yen. Alterations in the hypothalamic-pituitary-ovarian and the hypothalamic-pituitary adrenal axes in athletic women. *J. Clin. Endocrinol. Metab.* 68:402–411, 1989.

52. Mazzeo, R. S. Catecholamine responses to acute and chronic exercise. *Med. Sci. Sports Exerc.* 23:839–845, 1991.

53. Mazzeo, R. S., and P. A. Grantham. Norepinephrine turnover in various tissues at rest and during exercise: evidence for a training effect. *Metabolism* 38:479–483, 1989.

54. McCarty, R., M. Konarska, and R. E. Stewart. Adaptation to stress: a learned response? R. Kvetnansky, R. McCarty, and J. Axelrod (eds). *Stress: Neuroendocrine and Molecular Approaches.* Philadelphia: Gordon & Breach, 1992, pp. 521–535.

55. McCoy, D. E., J. E. Steele, R. H. Cox, and R. L. Wiley. Swim training alters sympathoadrenal and endocrine responses to hemorrhage in borderline hypertensive rats. *Am. J. Physiol.* 269:R124–R130, 1995.

56. McCoy, D. E., J. E. Steele, R. H. Cox, R. L. Wiley, and G. J. McGuire. Swim training alters renal and cardiovascular responses to stress in borderline hypertensive rats. *J. Appl. Physiol.* 75:1946–1954, 1994.

57. Mikhail, A. Stress: a psychophysiological conception. *J. Hum. Stress,* June:9–15, 1981.

58. Mitchell, J. H. Neural control of circulation during exerise. *Med. Sci. Sports Exerc.* 22:141–154, 1990.

59. Mitchell, J. H., and P. B. Raven. Cardiovascular adaptations to physical activity. C. Bouchard, R. J. Shephard, and T. Stephens (eds). *Physical Activity, Fitness, and Health: International Proceedings and Consensus Statement.* Champaign, IL: Human Kinetics, 1994, pp. 286–301.

60. Mormede, P., R. Dantzer, B. Michaud, K. Kelly, and M. Le Moal. Influence of stressor predictability and behavioral control on lymphocyte reactivity, antibody responses and neuroendocrine activation in rats. *Physiol. Behav.* 43:577–583, 1988.

61. Overton, M. J., K. C. Kregal, G. Gorman, D. Seals, C. M. Tipton, and L. A. Fisher. Effects of exercise training on responses to central injection of CRF and noise stress. *Physiol. Behav.* 49:3–98, 1991.

62. Peronnet, F., and A. Szabo. Sympathetic response to acute psychological stressors in humans: linkage to physical exercise and training. P. Seraganinan (ed). *Exercise Psychology: the Influence of Physical Exercise on Psychological Processes.* New York: John Wiley, 1993, pp. 172–217.

63. Petrusz, P., and I. Merchenthaler. The corticotropin-releasing factor system. C. B. Nemeroff (ed). *Neuroendocrinology.* Boca Raton, FL: CRC Press, 1992, pp. 129–183.

64. Poehlman, E. T., and E. Danforth. Endurance training increases metabolic rate and norepinephrine appearance rate in older individuals. *Am. J. Physiol.* 261:E233–E239, 1991.

65. Rogers, M. A., and W. J. Evans. Changes in skeletal muscle with aging: effects of exercise training. *Exerc. Sport Sci. Rev.* 21:65–102, 1993.

66. Rowell, L. B. *Human Cardiovascular Control.* New York: Oxford University Press, 1993.

67. Schwartz, R. S., L. F. Jaeger, R. C. Veith and S. Lakshminarayan. The effect of diet or exercise on plasma norepinephrine kinetics in moderately obese young men. *Int. J. Obes.* 14:1–11, 1989.

68. Seals, D. R., and R. G. Victor. Regulation of muscle sympathetic nerve activity during exercise in humans. *Exerc. Sport Sci. Rev.* 19:313–349, 1991.

69. Selye, H. The stress concept: past, present, and future. C. L. Cooper (ed). *Stress Research.* New York: Wiley, 1983, pp. 1–20.

70. Sherwood, A., K. C. Light, and J. A. Blumenthal. Effects of aerobic exercise training on hemodynamic responses during psychosocial stress in normotensive and borderline hypertensive type A men: a preliminary report. *Psychosom. Med.* 51:123–136, 1989.

71. Silverberg, A. B., S. D. Shah, M. W. Haymond, and P. E. Cryer. Norepinephrine: hormone and neurotransmitter in man. *Am. J. Physiol.* 234:E252–E256, 1978.

72. Sinyor, D., F. Peronnet, G. Brisson, and P. Seraganian. Failure to alter sympathoadrenal response to psychological stess following aerobic training. *Physiol. Behav.* 42:293–296, 1988.

73. Sinyor, D., S. Schwartz, F. Peronnet, G. Brisson, and P. Seraganian. Aerobic fitness level and reactivity to psychosocial stress: physiological, biochemical, and subjective measures. *Psychosom. Med.* 65: 205–217, 1983.

74. Smith, M. L., D. L. Hudson, H. M. Graitzer, and P. B. Raven. Exercise training bradycardia: the role of autonomic balance. *Med. Sci. Sports Exerc.* 21(1):40–44, 1989.

75. Snow-Harter, C. and R. Marcus. Exercise, bone mineral density, and osteoporosis. *Exerc. Sport Sci. Rev.* 19:351–388, 1991.

76. Sothmann, M.S., A. B. Gustafson, T. L. Garthwaite, T. S. Horn, and B. A. Hart. Cardiovas-

cular fitness and selected adrenal hormone responses to cognitive stress. *Endocr. Res.* 14:59–69, 1988.

77. Sothmann, M. S., B. A. Hart, and T. S. Horn. Sympathetic nervous system and behavioral responses to stress following exercise training. *Physiol. Behav.* 51:1097–1103, 1992.

78. Sothmann, M. S., T. S. Horn, and B. A. Hart. Plasma catecholamine response to acute psychological stress in humans: relation to aerobic fitness and exercise training. *Med. Sci. Sports Exerc.* 23:860–867, 1991.

79. Sothmann, M. S., T. S. Horn, B. A. Hart, and A. B. Gustafson. Comparison of discrete cardiovascular fitness groups on plasma catecholamine and selected behavioral responses to psychological stress. *Psychophysiology* 24:47–54, 1987.

80. Sutton, J. R., P. A. Farrell, and V. J. Harber. Hormonal adaptation to physical activity. C. Bouchard, R. J. Shephard, T. Stephens, J. R. Sutton, and B. McPherson (eds). *Exercise Fitness and Health: a Consensus Statement of Current Knowledge.* Champaign, IL: Human Kinetics, 1990, pp. 217–258.

81. Svedenhag, J., A. Martinsson, B. Ekblom, and P. Hjemdahl. Altered cardiovascular responsiveness to adrenaline in endurance trained subjects. *Acta Physiol. Scand.* 126:539–550, 1986.

82. Tipton, C. M. Exercise, training, and hypertension: an update. *Exerc. Sport Sci. Rev.* 19:446–505, 1991.

83. Van de Kar, L. D., R. A. Piechowski, P. A. Rittenhouse, and T. S. Gray. Amygdaloid lesions. Differential effect on conditioned stress and immobilization-induced increases in corticosterone and renin secretion. *Neuroendocrinology* 54:89–95, 1991.

84. van Doornen, L. J., and E. J. deGeus. Aerobic fitness and the cardiovascular response to stress. *Psychophysiology* 26:17–28, 1989.

85. Villaneau, A. L., C. Schlosser, B. Hopper, J. H. Liu, D. I. Hoffman, and R. W. Rebar. Increased cortisol production in women runners. *J. Clin. Endocrinol. Metab.* 63:133–136, 1986.

86. Watanabe, T., A. Morimoto, Y. Sakata, N. Tan, K. Morimoto, and N. Murakami. Running training attenuates the ACTH responses in rats to swimming and cage-switch stress. *J. Appl. Physiol.* 73:2452–2456, 1992.

87. White, J. E., R. K. Dishman, B. N. Bunnel, G. L. Warren, E. H. Mougey, and J. L. Meyerhoff. Chronic treadmill training moderates plasma ACTH responses to homotypic and heterotypic stress. *Med. Sci. Sports Exerc.* 25(Suppl.91):507, 1993.

88. White-Welkley, J. E., B. N. Bunnell, E. H. Mougey, J. L. Meyerhoff, and R. K. Dishman. Treadmill training and estradiol differentially modulate hypothalamic-pituitary-adrenal cortical responses to acute running and immobilization. *Physiol. Behav.* 57:533–540, 1995.

89. Winder, W. W., J. Hagberg, R. Hickson, A. Ehsani, and J. McLane. Time course for sympathoadrenal adaptation for endurance training in man. *J. Appl. Physiol.* 45:370–374, 1978.

10
Contractile Activity-Induced Mitochondrial Biogenesis in Skeletal Muscle

DAVID A. ESSIG, Ph.D.

Skeletal muscles adapt to regularly performed endurance exercise with an increase in the mass of the mitochondrial organelle. This observation, first reported in 1967 by Holloszy [39], has been central to our understanding the basis for improvement in muscle performance. A greater mass of mitochondria after training results in less disturbance of homeostasis during endurance exercise and occurs independent of changes in oxygen delivery [40]. However, the signals and the regulatory process that govern the assembly of more mitochondria during endurance training have remained largely unexplained.

In the last decade, enormous progress has been made in the molecular characterization of the genes encoding mitochondrial proteins. New proteins have been discovered that control transcription of mitochondrial genes, replication of mitochondrial DNA, and the intricate process of importing proteins into the mitochondria. Despite this progress, little of this information has been incorporated into understanding the molecular basis for training-induced mitochondrial biogenesis in muscle. The purpose of this review is to integrate recent molecular biological findings with the previous morphological and biochemical analysis of endurance training adaptations. A major goal will be to synthesize these data into a model that classifies the type of genes regulated at different stages of mitochondrial biogenesis. This review will consider, as much as possible, research that has used training, rather than chronic nerve stimulation, because the latter has been the major focus of recent reviews on mitochondrial assembly [32, 92].

INTRODUCTION TO MUSCLE MITOCHONDRION

The Basic Mitochondrial Structure

All mitochondria are composed of outer and inner phospholipid membranes, an intermembrane space, and an internal soluble matrix. Each compartment is associated with specialized functional capabilities. The outer membrane, for example, contains proteins involved in the import of incoming newly synthesized proteins. The inner membrane contains the protein complexes that function in oxidative phosphorylation and electron transport. In many mitochondria, including those in muscle, the inner membrane is folded into cristae to increase surface area. The soluble-matrix compartment contains the enzymes of the Krebs cycle, and β-oxidation is used in the generation of reducing equivalents for oxidative phosphorylation.

Mitochondria in various tissues have a somewhat differentiated phenotype [2, 67]. For example, liver mitochondria are equipped with the enzymes that allow high rates of fatty acid oxidation, as well as synthesis of ketone bodies, heme, glucose, and urea. In contrast, the muscle mitochondrial phenotype is more specialized toward synthesizing high rates of adenosine triphosphate (ATP). Compared to liver mitochondria, muscle mitochondria lack the enzymes for gluconeogenesis and urea cycle and have a greater surface area of cristae [67].

Muscle Mitochondria or Mitochondrion?

The classical view of the mitochondria in mammalian limb muscle is one of discrete spherically or elliptically shaped organelles [30]. However, based on more recent ultrastructural studies, the muscle mitochondrion may exist as a complete or partial reticulum [5, 6, 46]. Similar mitochondrial networks have also been recently described in cultured smooth muscle cells fixed for standard transmission electron microscopy but in the absence of plastic resin [66]. The original concept of a mitochondrial reticulum came from the morphological studies of Skulachev in the adult rat diaphragm muscle [6]. The slow oxidative fibers of the diaphragm, when serial sectioned in the transverse plane along the length of several sarcomeres, showed evidence of tubular mitochondrial profiles. These profiles were parallel to Z-lines and joined perpendicularly to columns of mitochondrial branches which ran parallel to the myofibrils [6]. Kirkwood et al. [47] have reported similar findings in several hindlimb muscles of the rat. On the other hand, Kayar et al. [46] showed evidence consistent with only a partial reticulum of mitochondria found in different cells from horse semitendinosus limb muscle. However, the extent of the reticulum increased in relation to the volume density of mitochondrial material in each cell. Thus, a more complete reticulum may have been found in the rodent muscle types, because the rate diaphragm and hindlimb muscles have a volume density of mitochondria higher than horse semitendinosus muscle [46].

RULES FOR MITOCHONDRIAL ASSEMBLY

Overview

The fundamental prerequisite for assembling more mitochondria is the presence of preexisting mitochondria [35]; a mitochondrion cannot be formed de novo. All or nearly all cells meet this requirement, because they ultimately derive their complement of mitochondria from the egg. It has been estimated that the unfertilized egg of xenopus laevis provides enough mitochondria to equip 100,000 cells with 1000 mitochondria [67]. The process of building an organelle such as the mitochondrion is exceedingly complex from a molecular standpoint. The majority of proteins are made outside of the mitochondrion in the cytosol and must be imported into a preexisting mitochondrion. Because the mitochondrion has its own genome, but has limited coding capacity, precise coordination must occur between the nuclear and mitochondrial genomes to assemble a mitochondrion containing the proper stoichiometry of proteins.

Mitochondrial DNA Transcription/Replication Is Linked

The most basic blueprint for the mitochondrion is derived from mitochondrial DNA (mit DNA). All mitochondria possess a closed circular double-stranded DNA molecule that codes for 13 mitochondrial proteins, all of which are subunits found in the respiratory complexes of the inner membrane. In addition, the mit DNA codes for a large and small ribosomal RNA and 22 transfer RNAs. This protein synthetic machinery is confined to mitochondria and is used to translate the mRNAs transcribed within the mitochondrias. The enzymes and other proteins needed for transcription, translation, and posttranslational processes are synthesized outside the mitochondrion and must be imported from the cytoplasm.

Transcription of most (12 of the 13) mit DNA protein coding genes proceeds from a single promoter, located in one of the two strands (H) of the mitochondrial DNA (Fig. 10.1). A single polycistronic mRNA is generated by the action of the mitochondrial RNA polymerase and the transcription factor, MtTFA [18]. This large mRNA is then cleaved into individual mRNAs by the action of RNA endonucleases. After each mRNA is polyadenylated and translated, the newly synthesized protein moves within the mitochondrion to be incorporated into multisubunit proteins of the inner membrane.

The mitochondrial DNA is present in multiple copies within the matrix compartment and can replicate at varying rates, depending on the species and tissue type [1]. From the standpoint of biogenesis, the most important feature of mit DNA replication is that it is dependent on previously initiated RNA transcription [14]. In a region of the mit DNA termed the D-loop (displacement), primers for replication of heavy-strand (H-strand) DNA are generated from previously initiated mit DNA transcription on the opposite or light strand (L strand) (Fig. 10.2). The mit DNA polymerase then proceeds to replicate the entire H strand. The decision to switch from RNA to DNA synthesis depends on the presence of limiting amounts of an RNA processing enzyme, MRP RNase [15, 18]. Once the H strand is duplicated, the L strand is then replicated by means of a similar priming mechanism.

The mit DNA only encodes 13 of the ~100 proteins required to assemble a mitochondria. However, all mitochondria, no matter the cell type, are

FIGURE 10.1

Major steps in transcription and translation within the mitochondrion. 1, The H-strand DNA codes for 12 proteins and is transcribed from a single transcriptional start site. The rate of transcription is regulated by the MtTFA transcription factor, which binds to the heavy-strand promoter (HSP). 2, The polycistronic RNA is cleaved into individual protein coding mRNAs by RNA endonucleases. 3, The individual mRNAs are translated, and the newly synthesized proteins are incorporated into multisubunit enzymes, such as cytochrome oxidase, located within the inner membrane. LSP, light-strand promoter; kb, kilobase; ds, double strand.

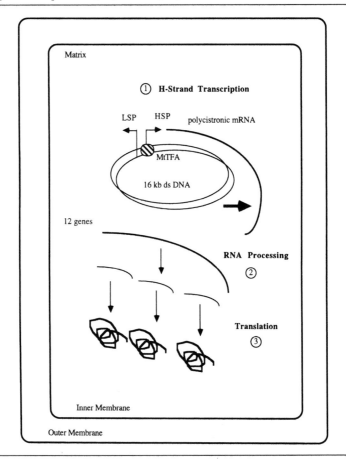

FIGURE 10.2

Mitochondrial DNA replication and the role of the mitochondrial RNA processing endonuclease (MRP RNAse). In the D (displacement) loop region of the mitochondrial DNA, RNA polymerase catalyzed transcription from the L-strand DNA occurs in the same region where heavy-strand (H-strand) DNA replication is initiated. RNA transcription proceeds, unless the content of MRP RNAse increases, in which case, the mit DNA switches to a replicative mode. The MRP RNAse cleaves the nascent RNA transcript, which then serves as an RNA primer for mit DNA polymerase. Open circle, RNA polymerase; filled circle, DNA polymerase.

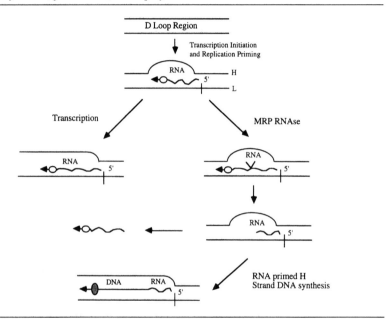

composed of this invariant set of proteins. On the other hand, it is the imposition of a larger set of nuclear gene products that ultimately determines the phenotype of the mitochondrion [2].

Nucleus-Encoded Mitochondrial Genes Have Coordinate Control Mechanisms

Genes encoding mitochondrial proteins found in the nucleus have a greater diversity of possible regulatory mechanisms than their mitochondrially encoded counterparts but, at the same time, appear to possess the capability for coordinated expression. The nuclear gene products include all enzymes of the Krebs cycle, β-oxidation, most of the respiratory complexes, ATP/ADP translocators, and the enzymes involved directly with assembly, such as heme biosynthesis, import of newly synthesized proteins, the mitochondrial DNA and RNA polymerases, and regulatory protein factors. The nucleus-encoded mitochondrial genes are all transcribed by RNA polymerase II (POL II), with exception of the RNA subunit of MRP RNAse (see below). A simplified POL II nuclear mitochondrial gene is illustrated in Figure 10.3. A variety of transcription factor DNA binding proteins bind the DNA in selected regions upstream of transcriptional initiation and interact with POL II to determine the overall rate of transcription. The binding of these factors is influenced by signaling pathways, which originate from the intra- or extracellular environment.

Several nuclear genes encoding mitochondrial proteins have been characterized, including cytochrome c [25, 26], cytochrome oxidase subunit IV [26], aminolevulinate synthase [13], mtTFA [82], cytochrome c_1 [78], ATP synthase β-subunit [17], and ADP/ATP translocator-one [50]. In general, these genes contain a spectrum of transcriptional control elements (transcription factor DNA binding sites) also found in other cellular genes. However, there are several transcription factors that are found predominantly in nuclear encoded mitochondrial genes. These factors are generally believed to function in the coordinated expression of nuclear mitochondrial genes. However, thus far, no single transcription factor has been found to bind and regulate all nuclear encoded genes. Rather, it would appear that many factors regulate overlapping subsets of genes.

The first such factors described were the nuclear respiratory factors 1 and 2 (NRF-1 and NRF-2), observed by Scarpulla and colleagues in rat cytochrome c gene [26]. Functional binding sites for NRF-1 are found in the 5'-flanking regions of at lease nine nuclear encoded mitochondrial genes, and they include cytochrome c; cytochrome oxidase subunited IV, Vb, and VIIa, uniquinone binding protein; ATP synthase β-subunit; MRP RNAase subunit RNA; 5'-aminolevulinate synthase (ALAS) and mtTFA [88]. Since the MRP RNAse RNA subunit and mtTFA play critical roles in mit DNA replication and transcription, respectively, the presence of NRF-1 regulation has been theorized to coordinate the mit DNA template availability (number of mit DNA copies) and the mit DNA transcription rate with that of various nuclear genes [88].

The NRF-1 mRNA has been cloned and sequenced [88]. Portions of the NRF-1 protein bear strong resemblance to developmental regulatory proteins in lower eukaryotes, suggesting that its functions may be more general. In addition to the nine mitochondrial genes identified, NRF-1 binding sites have also been identified in genes encoding proteins involved in signal transduction and control of protein synthesis. One common finding among all of the genes containing NRF-1 binding sites was that the protein functioned as the rate-limiting-step in a particular pathway. Thus, NRF-1-dependent mitochondrial genes appear to be linked to other genes that regulate cellular processes requiring long-term changes in energy provision.

NRF-2 has been found to bind and regulate the expression of two cytochrome oxidase subunit genes, IV and Vb, as well as the ATP synthase β-

FIGURE 10.3

Steps in the expression of a nucleus-encoded mitochondrial gene. 1, The mitochondrial gene is transcribed by RNA polymerase II (RNA Pol II). The activity of RNA polymerase is influenced by the binding of various DNA binding proteins (transcription factors) to the "promoter" or "enhancer" regions of the DNA, located upstream (to the left) of the start site of transcription (arrow). 2, The mRNA is translated in the cytoplasm on polysomes. 3, The amino terminus of the protein contains a short presequence that directs the protein to the outer mitochondrial membrane, in which the cyto HSP 70 chaperon proteins assist in unfolding of the protein. The protein moves through the outer and inner membranes in a process that is dependent on the presence of a membrane potential and ATP. 4, The protein, once across the inner membrane, has its presequence cleaved and binds with HSP 70, which "pulls" the protein into the matrix. 5, The refolding of the protein is facilitated via interactions with HSP60. 6, The protein has now assumed it native conformation.

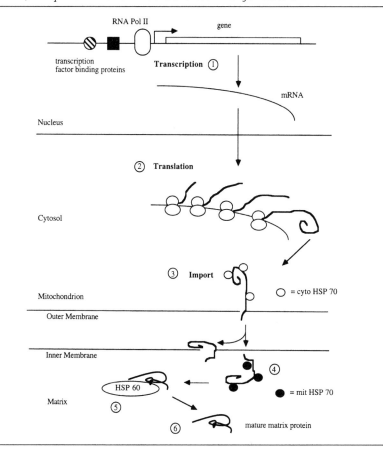

subunit gene [87]. NRF-2 is a multisubunit protein that contains a single DNA binding subunit identical to a previously described protein GA binding protein (GABP), which functions to activate viral promoters. The relative amount of binding and transcriptional activation may be determined by the formation of homo- or heterodimers with other NRF-2 subunits. Thus, in addition to facilitating the coordination of nuclear gene transcription products, the NRF-2 factors may also participate in determining the absolute levels of respiratory proteins (Virbasius) [87].

Two other less well characterized coordinating factors have also been reported that appear to have properties distinct from those of the NRFs. Tomura et al, [83] have described an enhancer element found in the nuclear genes for ATP synthase β-subunit, cytochrome c_1, and pyruvate dehydrogenase subunit E1α. The DNA element specifically bound protein in a gel retardation assay and was capable of conferring enhancement of transcription on an heterologous promoter in an orientation-independent manner. A second binding domain has been located in the promoter sequences of ADP/ATP translocator-1 and ATP synthase β-subunit genes [50]. Two transcription factor proteins termed OXBOX and REBOX, bind to the region in a tissue-specific manner [17]. The OXBOX binding factors were only found in extracts from myogenic cells whereas the REBOX binding factors were present in both muscle and nonmuscle cell extracts. The REBOX factor binding was sensitive to the redox status of the extracts, suggesting that these factors may be linked to the metabolic activity of the cell.

Nucleus-Encoded Mitochondrial Proteins Are Imported

After transcription of the nuclear genes, the mRNAs are translated on soluble polysomes in the cytoplasm and then imported into the mitochondria. All proteins destined for the mitochondria have a presequence (20–80 amino acids), located at the amino terminus, which directs the protein to the mitochondria and, ultimately, to a specific compartment within the mitochondrion. The import process has several general features, but they may differ, depending on the ultimate destination of the protein, i.e., outer membrane, intermembrane space, or inner membrane or matrix. In the case of matrix enzymes, it has recently been proposed that import involves two major steps [61] (see Fig. 10.3). First, the newly synthesized protein (also termed "immature protein" or preprotein") binds to a particular class of "chaperon" protein, known as HSP 70, which helps to maintain a transport-competent unfolded conformation. With the help of protein receptors (MOM 19 and 72), located in the outer membrane, and a general insertion protein (GIP), the presequences are inserted and translocated across the outer membrane. At the outside surface of the inner membrane, the presequence is further translocated in response to the membrane potential and, once in the matrix, the presequences are then cleaved with a peptidase. In the second stage, the unfolded protein binds with a mitochondrial HSP 70 isoform, which facilitates the transit of the remaining C-terminal portion of the protein into the matrix [28]. Once in the matrix, another chaperon protein, HSP 60, facilitates the folding of the protein into the native conformation. The overall process of import is energy dependent; ATP is required for releasing the proteins from the HSP 70 and 60 chaperons. The process is, nonetheless, rapid. It has been estimated that, in growing fungal cells, 50–150 proteins traverse the outer membrane of a mitochondrion per second [61].

Phospholipid Biosynthesis

The biosynthesis of the mitochondrial membranes is an essential step in mitochondrial biogenesis but has been less well studied in mammalian systems. The membranes of the mitochondria have a high protein to lipid content (3:1; see ref. 20), and within the lipid portion, three major types of phospholipids predominate. These include, in order of abundance, phosphotidylcholine (lecithin), phosphatidylethanolamine (cephalin) and diphosphatidylglycerol (cardiolipin) [45]. The latter is found nearly exclusively in the mitochondrial membranes [2]. The major precursor, phosphatidate (a derivative of diacylglycerol), is the same for phospholipids and triglycerides [34] and may account for the close proximity of triglyceride deposits and the mitochondrion commonly observed in the myocardium [64]. The phospholipids, in particular cardiolipin, are tightly associated with membrane proteins, such as cytochrome oxidase, and are necessary for optimal function [19]. Cells deficient in cardiolipin are characterized by reduced rates of oxygen consumption, increased glycolysis, and lowered levels of ATP [62].

The mitochondrion contains all the enzymes required for de novo synthesis of cardiolipin. The pathway involves five major enzymes, all of which have been well characterized in yeast but none of which have been completely purified to homogeneity from any mammalian source [36]. In the first step, glycerol-3-phosphate is acylated (long-chain fatty acid added) by an enzyme in the outer membrane to eventually form a phosphatide (PA). The PA is then converted via the action of PA:CTP cytidyltransferase into CDP diglyceride. CDP diglyceride is then converted by the combined action of PGP synthase and PGP phosphatase into phosphatidylglycerol (PG). In the final step, PG reacts with another molecule of CDP diglyceride via cardiolipin synthase to form cardiolipin (CL). The rate-limiting step in mammalian heart is the conversion of phosphatides into CDP glycerol [36]. The synthesis of CDP glycerol and CL have been shown to occur on the inner surface of the inner membrane, and suggesting that newly synthesized imported proteins destined for the inner membrane can associate with cardiolipin before insertion in the membrane [73].

STAGES OF MITOCHONDRIAL BIOGENESIS: INSIGHTS FROM ENDURANCE TRAINING STUDIES

Overview

In the nearly three decades that have passed since systematic study of the mitochondrial adaptations to endurance training, insights into the mechanisms involved are still elusive. However, a pattern of three sequential phases can be observed on examination of the time course of changes in protein expression during training. Identification of these stages may be insightful for future testing of mechanistic hypotheses. These stages can be described as follows and are illustrated in Figure 10.4:

1. Preexisting mitochondria direct the assembly of membrane projections to increase the connections between mitochondria.
2. Sequential phases
   a. *Early:* After 1–3 days of training, proteins involved in heme synthesis, phospholipid synthesis, and import are induced. These "assembly" genes are all encoded in nuclear DNA.
   b. *Middle:* After 5–7 days of training, proteins that participate in ATP yielding pathways increase in a slow, coordinated manner. These "metabolic enzyme genes" are encoded in both mit and nuclear DNA.
   c. *Late:* After 6 wk of training, mit DNA content is increased, presumably by an increased rate of replication.

Training Enhances Mitochondrial Connections

Because the muscle mitochondrion most likely exists as a single or partial reticulum, as opposed to existing as individual units [46], mitochondrial growth, as induced by training, most likely involves an elaboration of the reticulum. This is consistent with the tendency for the connectivity of the reticulum, either during development of the diaphragm [47] or across muscle types [46], to be highest when mitochondrial volume density is also high [46]. Evidence to support a reticular elaboration has been provided by Kirkwood, using high-voltage transmission electron microscopy (TEM). Rat hindlimb muscles from endurance-trained rats underwent a 60–90% increase in the density of their reticulum [48]. In the soleus and superficial portion of the vastus lateralis muscles, the increase in volume density occurred without a change in surface to volume ratio, suggesting that proliferation occurred by increasing the number of lateral projections or by lengthening already existing lateral projections. In the Type IIa fibers of the deep portion of the vastus lateralis, the increase in volume density occurred with a decrease in surface: volume ratio, indicating that the lateral projections increased in diameter, in addition to lengthening or increasing in number.

This morphological analysis suggests that preexisting mitochondrial ma-

FIGURE 10.4

The sequential phases of mitochondrial biogenesis during endurance training. 1, The nuclear genes that code for proteins involved in heme biosynthesis (ALAS), mit DNA transcription (MtTFA), mit RNA replication (MRP Rnase) and phospholipid biosynthesis are induced during the early phase (1–7 days of training). 2, Expression of mitDNA and nucleus encoded genes and nuclear DNA-encoded genes that code for metabolic enzyme proteins are increased slowly, in a coordinated manner, after 1 wk of training. Presumably, these proteins are targeted for the "biogenesis zone," in which membrane expansion is occurring to connect preexisting mitochondrion. 3, In what may be a final stage, mitDNA is replicated perhaps to accommodate the increased mitochondrial volume.

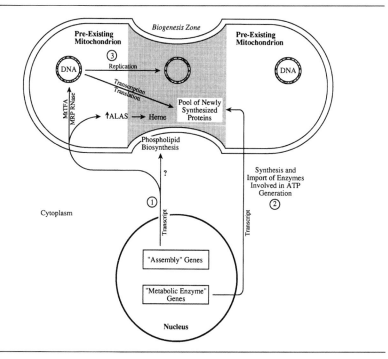

terial simply expands to achieve a greater structural unity as well as greater mass. The newly assembled mitochondrial material is likely to be similar in composition to the preexisting mitochondrion, given that protein: lipid ratios and the majority of mitochondrial enzyme-specific activities were essentially unchanged in mitochondria isolated from endurance-trained rats, as compared to control [20]. This model would predict that intramitochondrially synthesized proteins would simply diffuse into the growing branch sites (Fig. 10.4). Proteins synthesized outside of mitochondria would be directed to the nascent mitochondrial membranes or matrix space. However, direct evidence of biosynthetic activity in the vicinity of the lateral projections is not yet available. Future studies, using recent molecular cytological techniques developed for use in cell culture [37] or in situ hybridization procedures, could provide insights into the overall process of mitochondrial growth.

Evidence for the Sequential Assembly of the Mitochondrion

The increase in expression of proteins involved in mitochondrial ATP generation during the course of endurance training in rodents is a relatively slow adaptive process. Approximately 5–7 days of training or nerve stimulation are necessary before any statistically significant increase in the activities of several mitochondrial enzymes commonly used as markers of mitochondrial growth is observed (Table 10.1). The relatively slow increase is most likely a direct function of the relatively long half-life (5–7 days) for many mitochondrial proteins [4, 17, 81]. Proteins that have a longer half-life require a longer time to reach a new steady-state value for a given increase in synthesis rate. This slow increase is also likely a reflection of the sequential nature of mitochondrial assembly. Newly synthesized metabolic enzyme proteins must be presented with the proper "posttranslational environment." For example, apocytochrome proteins, such as cytochrome c, must bind heme in a reaction catalyzed by heme lyase to be retained in the mitochondrion after import [60]. Thus, sufficient heme must be synthesized before or during the initial week of training to ensure optimal uptake of this protein for subsequent mitochondrial growth. In terms of membrane formation, Takahashi and Hood [79] have shown that the mitochondrial phospholipid cardiolipin accumulated at a faster rate than the

TABLE 10.1.
Metabolic Enzyme Proteins First Increase after ~ 7 Days of Endurance Training or Nerve Stimulation

			DAYS											
Ref.	*Protein*	*Muscle*	*1*	*2*	*3*	*4*	*5*	*6*	*7*	*8*	*9*	*10*	*14*	*28–35*
84	CO	pln	1.0		1.2				1.4[a]					1.8[a]
42	cyt c	r-vtl	1.0	1.2				1.4[a]					1.6[a]	1.7[a]
81	cyt c	r-vtl					1.1					1.3[a]	1.3[a]	1.5[a]
44	CO[b]	ta			1.1				1.5[a]				2.5[a]	3.0[a]

CO, cytochrome oxidase; cyt c, cytochrome c; pln, plantaris; ta, tibialis anterior; r-vtl, red-vastus lateralis.
[a]Values from the endurance-trained or stimulated muscle were significantly higher than those of controls (P < .05).
[b]Data were obtained in studies with rats subjected either to endurance training or nerve stimulation. The numbers represent the fold increase in protein content or enzyme activity relative to control value.

increase in citrate synthase or cytochrome oxidase activities during the first 2 wk of chronic nerve stimulation to the tibialis anterior muscle. These data are consistent with a model in which newly synthesized enzyme proteins, such as cytochrome oxidase, must await the synthesis of phospholipid bilayer [2] or the arrival of specific phospholipids, such as cardiolipin [73] before insertion into the membrane. Proteins that likely direct the assembly process (membrane biogenesis, heme synthesis, and import) thus represent a unique class of nucleus-encoded genes that prepare for the impending coordinated increase in synthesis of proteins involved in ATP generation.

THE EARLY PHASE OF MITOCHONDRIAL BIOGENESIS

The expression of proteins that comprise pathways involved in the early phase have not been well studied during mitochondrial biogenesis in mammals. For example, there have been no studies published to date that have investigated the possible changes in expression of the enzyme proteins involved in phospholipid biosynthesis. However, at least three genes have been studied during training, 5'-aminolevulinate synthase, HSP 70, and the MRP RNAase RNA subunit, which likely comprise a class of "early-response" genes.

Expression of proteins involved in heme biosynthesis was first examined in 1979 by Holloszy and Winder [42]. These investigators showed that the activity of ALAS, a mitochondrial enzyme that catalyzes the first and rate-limiting enzyme in heme biosynthesis, was increased 2-fold in the red vastus lateralis muscle after a single day of repeated treadmill running sessions. This induction was transient, and the activity of ALAS had returned to control value by 48 hr postexercise. During this same time frame, cytochrome c content was unchanged, relative to that in controls. Similar results have been observed by Town and Essig [84] in the plantaris muscle. These data indicate that an increase in heme synthesis appears to precede the increase in the content of mitochondrial cytochromes and probably most, if not all other, enzymes that participate directly in energy provision. In yeast, heme serves not only as a prosthetic group for heme proteins but also as a transcriptional cofactor that permits the binding of the HAP-1 transcription to the cytochrome c gene and activates transcription [27]. Thus, it is possible that the increase in heme synthesis from the mitochondrion is a prerequisite signal for subsequent synthesis of apoproteins.

The chaperon proteins, such as cytoplasmic HSP 70, function in the unfolding of newly synthesized proteins destined for import into the mitochondria are also induced after 1–3 days of endurance exercise. In a recent study by Skidmore and associates [75], HSP 70 protein content was increased 2 to 5-fold in soleus and gastrocnemius immediately after an acute bout of treadmill running. Earlier studies [52, 70] also demonstrated a significant increase in the synthesis of a protein with a mass of ~70 kD after an acute bout of treadmill running exercise at normal room temperature. Although it is likely that an increased amount of HSP 70 may facilitate the import of mitochondrial proteins [89], this has not been directly demonstrated during conditions in which an increase in mitochondrial biogenesis is in progress. A greater content of HSP 70 may also be needed to protect newly synthesized proteins from damage or denaturation from proteotoxic agents generated during and after exercise, such as heat, lowered pH, reactive oxygen species (ROS), or some combination of these agents [52, 70, 75].

Increased synthesis of proteins that regulate the transcription and replication of mit DNA (MRP RNAse and MtTFA) is likely to play a key role in directing assembly of the mitochondrion [18]. Thus far, there have been no studies that have investigated the change in MtTFA expression in muscle. The mitochondrial RNA processing enzyme was increased during repetitive nerve stimulation as evidenced by the increased expression of the RNA subunit of the enzyme (MRP–RNA). The MRP RNAase RNA was increased to ~3 fold above control 24 hr after initiation of 10-Hz nerve stimulation and well before the increase in citrate synthase activity and mit DNA content [63]. This temporal relationship suggested that MRP RNase might be involved in preparing the mitochondrial DNA to switch from a transcriptional to a replicative mode [14, 63]. Whether a similar induction of the MRP RNA would occur with endurance training has yet to be demonstrated.

Middle Phase of Mitochondrial Biogenesis

The class of mitochondrial proteins most well studied by exercise physiologists is that which comprises the metabolic pathways that result in net ATP synthesis. These include enzymes in the Krebs cycle, starting with pyruvate dehydrogenase; β-oxidation, starting with carnitine palmitoyl transferase and ending with the multisubunit protein assemblies found in the electron transport chain. In general, the activities of these enzymes, when measured at V_{max} are increased to roughly the same extent (~2 fold) in mixed-fiber type skeletal muscle of the rat after a standard 10 to 20-wk endurance training regimen [10, 39, 40, 64; see Table 10.2]. This finding implies that the protein content of the enzymes was governed by a mechanism that allowed the expression of each gene (protein synthesis) to be increased in a proportional manner. The time course of the increase in the enzyme activities, with either endurance training or chronic nerve stimulation, demonstrates a reasonable degree of coordination (Table 10.3). This apparent coordination can be further appreciated when one considers that cytochrome oxidase activity alone requires synthesis and assembly of 13 different protein subunits.

TABLE 10.2
Most Metabolic Enzyme Proteins Increase to the Same Extent after 10–12 wk of Endurance Training

Ref.	Muscle	Mitochondrial Protein/Pathway	Fold Increase
20	Hindlimb	Pyruvate-malate oxidase	1.6
		Succinate oxidase	2.2
		Palmitoyl carnitine oxidase	2.4
		Succinate dehydrogenase	2.0
		NADH dehydrogenase	1.6
		Choline dehydrogenase	2.2
		Cytochrome c (+c1)	2.0
		Cytochrome a	2.0
65	gtn	Oligomycin ATPase	2.0
		Cytochrome c	2.2
		Adenylate kinase	1.0
		Creatine kinase	1.0
56	gtn/vtl	Palmitoyl CoA synthetase	2.3
		Carnitine palmitoyl transferase	1.9
		Palmitoyl CoA dehydrogenase	2.3
41	gtn/vtl	Citrate synthase	2.0
		Isocitrate dehydrogenase	1.9
		Succinate dehydrogenase	2.0
		Cytochrome c	2.0
		Malate dehydrogenase	1.5
		Glutamate dehydrogenase	1.3
		α-Ketoglutarate dehydrogenase	1.5

gtn, gastocnemius; vtl, vastus lateralis.

TABLE 10.3
Mitochondrial Metabolic Enzyme Proteins Increase in a Coordinate Manner

						Wk								
Ref.	Muscle	ET/Stim	Protein	1	2	3	4	5	6	7	8	9	10	11	12–17
8	sol/gtn	ET	SDH		1.1		1.4					2.0			2.4
			CO		1.3		1.5					1.7			2.0
			CRED		1.0		1.1					1.2			1.4
7	quad	ET	cyt a			1.1			1.3			1.3			1.4
			cyt c			1.1			1.2			1.2			1.3
44	ta	Stim	CO	1.5	2.5	2.7	3.0	2.8							
			CS	1.5	2.5	2.7	3.0	3.2							

Values are expressed as a fold difference (endurance-trained or stimulated value/control). All data are from studies conducted with the rat. sol, soleus; gtn, gastrocnemius; ta, tibialis anterior; quad, quadriceps; ET, endurance training; Stim, continuous nerve stimulation; SDH, succinate dehydrogenase; CO, cytochrome oxidase; CRED, cytochrome reductase; cytc, cytochrome c; cyt a, cytochrome a; CS, citrate synthase.

The genes that specify metabolic enzyme proteins are located both in the nuclear DNA and mitochondrial DNA. Thus, it is tempting to speculate that some of the aforementioned coordination factors, such as NRF-1, are involved in the coordinate expression of the metabolic enzyme genes during endurance training. It is known, for example, that the mRNAs for several of the subunits in both nuclear and mitochondrial DNA, are increased after long-term training (>4 wk) [54, 59], suggesting that, at least in principle, the transcription of these genes could be a site for coordination control.

The Late Phase of Mitochondrial Biogenesis

The major event associated with this phase is the apparent replication of mit DNA. Mit DNA in rat soleus muscle was at control value after 3 and 6 wk of endurance training but was significantly increased by 35%, after 12 wk [59]. This situation is analogous to the previously described 4 to 5-fold increase in mit DNA content observed with repetitive nerve stimulation in the rabbit tibialis anterior muscle, which occurred after 21 days [90, 94]. The increase in mit DNA content is presumably a mechanism that increases the coding capacity of mit DNA. This event may coincide with expansion of the mitochondrial volume, such that the rate of transcription of an individual mit DNA remains constant.

The three phases of mitochondrial biogenesis identified in the above discussion serve to underscore another level of regulation, namely, that of a temporal progression, which is in addition to the spatial or coordinate control mechanisms also discussed. To overcome the apparent limitations associated with simultaneous analysis of many genes, much can be gained in terms of these types of regulation by attempting first to understand in great detail the regulation of representative genes from each stage of mitochondrial biogenesis.

REGULATION OF SELECTED MITOCHONDRIAL GENES DURING ENDURANCE TRAINING

Early-Phase Genes

ALAS. The pathway for heme biosynthesis involves eight enzymes distributed in the mitochondrial matrix and cytosolic compartments. In most tissues, including muscle, the activity of ALAS, which catalyzes the first step in the pathway, determines the rate of heme synthesis [55, 74]. In the context of mitochondrial biogenesis, ALAS plays an important role in the provision of heme necessary for import and assembly of inner membrane cytochromes and cytochrome oxidase. The most dramatic illustration of this can be appreciated from investigations using yeast mutants that are deficient in ALAS activity. In these mutants, the native cytochrome structures are not formed, and selected subunits are lacking [71]. These data underline the possibly significant role of heme synthesis in the early phase of mitochondrial biogenesis.

In response to a variety of exercise stimuli, one of the most consistent findings is that ALAS activity is induced within 1–3 days after the onset of the training stimulus. Holloszy and Winder [42] showed that in previously untrained rats, ALAS activity was increased by 2-fold in the red portion of the vastus lateralis muscle 17 hr after a vigorous acute bout of exercise. No change in the level of cytochrome c content was noted in this time frame, and subsequent experiments showed that cytochrome c did not increase until after 6 consecutive days of treadmill running. Similar results were observed by using the chicken wing overload model [23]. ALAS activity was induced after 3 days of overload, but no significant increase in cytochrome oxidase was noted until after 7 days. In a recent training study, rats undergoing 28 days of treadmill running showed significant increases in plantaris muscle ALAS activity after 3, 7, and 28 days, but cytochrome oxidase activity did not increase until after 7 days of exercise [84].

With discontinuous exercise models such as the running rat, the induction of ALAS in the postexercise recovery period is rather short lived. ALAS activity was elevated at 17 hr postexercise but had returned to control value by 48 hr [42]. These results were extended in a recent study, using 3 hr of daily 10-Hz stimulation of rat tibialis anterior muscle [80]. Compared to control (contralateral) unstimulated values, there was a significant 70% increase in cytochrome oxidase activity, which was evident when measured either at 0, 18, or 48 hr poststimulation. In contrast, ALAS activity was the same as control immediately after stimulation but increased to 2-fold higher than contralateral control 18 hr poststimulation. This induction was reduced at 48 hr of recovery, but remained 1.6-fold greater than the contralateral, nonstimulated muscle. The simplest interpretation of these data is that cytochrome oxidase had undergone a gradual increase in activity over a 7-day period, whereas ALAS activity was likely reinduced in each recovery period between successive days of 3-hr stimulation.

Alterations in the level of ALAS activity appear to be determined by proportional changes in the concentration of the enzyme protein [55]. Because the half-life of ALAS is very short (90–120 min, as reviewed in ref. 55), a high rate of protein synthesis is required to sustain normal steady-state levels of the enzyme activity. ALAS is a mitochondrial matrix enzyme, and the newly translated polypeptide exists in precursor form with an aminoterminal prepeptide necessary for import into the mitochondria. As a result, many regulatory sites in the synthesis of the enzyme are possible, including transcription, mRNA stability, import of the preprotein precursor, and translation.

Several studies have determined the changes in ALAS mRNA expression that accompany induction by repetitive contractile activity [23, 80, 84]. The regulation of ALAS activity during chronic weight-bearing activity (over-load) in chicken skeletal muscle was investigated [23]. Maximal enzyme activity was increased 2.5- and 4.0-fold after 3 and 7 days of overload, respectively. The content of ALAS mRNA (in nanograms per milligram of total RNA) was not changed after 3 days but increased significantly after 7 days of overload. Normalizing the content of ALAS mRNA relative to the increase in total RNA indicated that ALAS mRNA increased by 1.6- and 2.0-fold at 3 and 7 days, respectively. On this basis, the increase in enzyme activity per gram of protein exceeding the increase in mRNA content per gram of protein by 60–70%. Thus, induction of ALAS activity was regulated largely by processes at the translational or posttranslational steps in the protein expression pathway. Similar patterns have been observed after endurance training or nerve stimulation [80, 84]. This type of regulation is separate from but can interact with the apparent transcriptional control of ongoing developmental and tissue-specific regulation of ALAS expression (reviewed in ref. 22). Further research will be necessary to clarify the exact site of this post-transcriptional regulation.

The induction of ALAS in liver cells has been explained by a negative feedback model (reviewed in ref. 55). The main evidence supporting this model is that exogenous heme or its precursors inhibit basal or induced ALAS activity. Furthermore, estimates of normal cellular levels of free heme suggest that ALAS activity is repressed. Induction is thought to occur by derepression when cellular heme levels are reduced by increased formation of heme-dependent proteins and/or increased degradation of heme by heme oxygenase.

The existence of this pathway has been confirmed in muscle by examining the changes in ALAS activity 12 hr after injection of heme precursor aminolevulinate (1.7 mg/g i.p.) into rats. The results showed a dramatic 90% decrease in plantaris muscle ALAS activity, in comparison to that of saline-injected animals [22]. These data provide preliminary evidence that a negative feedback pathway exists in skeletal muscle and extend previous work in rat heart [76].

If this general model is applicable to synthesis of mitochondrial cytochromes, one would predict that cytochrome oxidase or other heme proteins will be induced before ALAS. However, as described above, heme proteins in muscle are induced at the protein level several days after ALAS activity, which contrasts with findings in liver tissue in response to prophyrinogenic drugs in which cytochrome P_{450} proteins and mRNAs are coinduced with ALAS protein and mRNA [33]. In muscle, unlike liver, the free heme pool may not be decreased because of increased mitochondrial cytochrome formation. Instead, ALAS may be induced by a more direct mechanism to increase the synthesis of heme in preparation for the subsequent demands of cytochrome formation. This hypothesis must be regarded, however, as tentative, because it is also possible that levels of free heme could have been lowered by means of other mechanisms, such as an increase in myoglobin synthesis [85] or an increase in the rate of heme or hemeprotein turnover. Another possibility is that a large pool of apocytochromes may exist in the cytosol that rapidly binds the available free heme and, thereby, induces ALAS. A final, intriguing speculation is that heme oxygenase, which catalyzes the first and rate-limiting step in heme degradation, may be initially induced by exercise, such that ALAS is derepressed as a consequence of the lowered free heme pool. Interestingly, heme oxygenase has been shown to be highly inducible in several tissues and is also classified as a stress protein [68]. To test this hypothesis, Essig et al. [24] determined that the mRNA for one of the isoforms of heme oxygenase (HO-1) underwent a large induction (average, 5-fold), compared to that of controls, during and 6 hr after a single 3-hr bout of nerve stimulation in the tibialis anterior muscle of rats. These results suggested that a rapid increase in heme degradation may occur after muscle contractile activity which, in turn, may lead to derepression of ALAS activity.

HSP 70. The heat stress protein family of proteins with 70-kd molecular mass (HSP 70) is composed of three isoforms, each encoded by a separate gene [89]. Two isoforms, HSP 70 i and HSP 70 c, are found in the cytoplasm, and the third, HSP 70 m, is localized to the mitochondrial matrix. A major regulator of the HSP 70 i gene is the heat shock factor (HSF), which binds a conserved element (HSE) upstream of the gene in response to a variety of proteotoxic stresses, including heat, ROS, and hypoxia [57]. The mRNA for HSP 70 i has been shown to be strongly induced (5–10 fold) in both heart and skeletal muscle after a single bout of endurance running exercise [53, 70]. In the myocardium, the increase in mRNA was observable with as little as 40 min of running and was coincident with an increase in the binding activity of the HSF [53]. Although it has not been conclusively shown that increased HSF binding is necessary for the increase in HSP 70 i transcription, the data strongly suggest that metabolic signals generated during exercise can rapidly increase the transcription of a gene, which may be important in the early phase of biogenesis of the mitochondrion.

RNA SUBUNIT OF MITOCHONDRIAL RNA PROCESSING RNASE. The enzyme mitochondrial RNA processing RNAse (MRP RNAse) functions to cleave nascent transcripts generated from the L-strand promoter of the mitochondrial DNA for use as primers in DNA replication. Functional RNAse MRP, as purified from HeLa cell mitochondria, contains an endonuclease enzyme activity and a small RNA subunit. Both the endonuclease and RNA subunits are the products of nuclear genes [14]. The enzyme has been proposed as a control point for modulating the rate of mit DNA replication (see above; see also ref 16). Analysis of transcription and the 5'-flanking region of the human gene revealed that the MRP RNAse RNA is transcribed by RNA polymerase III [15]. Interestingly, the gene can bind transcription factors ordinarily found only in POL II genes, such as NRF-1. The MRP gene has been shown to be expressed in rabbit skeletal muscle in apparent proportion to oxidative capacity [63], with the highest levels found in the heart and the lowest levels in Type IIb skeletal muscle. The content of MRP RNA, as assessed by northern blotting is markedly increased by nerve stimulation between 1 and 14 days [63], but its expression has not been examined as of yet during endurance training. The potential regulatory sites for controlling the MRP RNA are somewhat unusual, because the gene does not code for a protein (the RNA is the functional molecule) and the RNA must be imported into the mitochondria [51]. Hence, future studies will need to address the transcription rate as it correlates to the actual mitochondrial content of the MRP RNA.

Middle-Phase Genes

CYTOCHROME C. Cytochrome c is a 104-amino acid hemeprotein found in the intermembrane space loosely attached to the outside of the inner membrane [69]. The protein functions in the catalytic transfer of electrons between respiratory complexes II and IV. One isoform of cytochrome c is in all somatic tissues, and a second is expressed only during spermatogenic differentiation [32]. The rat somatic cytochrome c gene directs the transcription of 1.4, 1.1, and 0.7 kb (kilobase) mRNAs, all of which code for the full-sized cytochrome c protein. The content of the three mRNAs roughly parallels differences in tissue-specific variations in cytochrome c protein in skeletal muscle fiber types and heart, suggesting pretranslational control of cytochrome c expression [49]. The content of cytochrome c progressively increases with training duration to a value approximately 1.5- to 3-fold higher than control in various muscle fiber types, depending on the intensity of running [21].

The initial increases in cytochrome c protein are observed after the 5th or 6th day of training in red quadriceps muscle (Table 10.1). In a series of studies by Booth and associates [10, 11, 49, 58], it has been determined that the initial increase in cytochrome c protein may be mediated by several sites in the gene expression pathway. In the first week of training, cytochrome c protein synthesis rate was unchanged, relative to that of controls after 1 and 4 days of training. On the 5th day of training, a 29% increase in cytochrome c protein synthesis rate was noted without a significant change in cytochrome c mRNA content. Hence, this initial increase in cytochrome c was inferred to occur at either a translational step (increased rate of translational initiation or elongation per unit of cytochrome c mRNA) or posttranslational steps, perhaps involving the enhanced import of stored apocytochrome c [10]. In the 2nd wk of training, when cytochrome c content is increased to approximately 1.5-fold higher in red vastus muscle [42], Morrison et al. [58] showed a similar increase in cytochrome c mRNA content in plantaris muscle, suggesting that with longer durations of training, a pretranslational mechanism may operate to increase cytochrome c protein synthesis rates. The mechanism of how the cytochrome c gene might be regulated to achieve the increase in mRNA expression has not been determined with endurance training. Ongoing investigations in the factors that control cytochrome c mRNA stability (F. Booth and Z. Yhan, personal communication 1995) and transcription [31, 87, 88] should provide insight into this question.

CYTOCHROME OXIDASE. The enzyme cytochrome oxidase (CO) is an inner membrane protein that oxidizes reduced cytochrome c during respiration. The cytochrome oxidase holoprotein is composed of hemes a and a3 and 13 nonidentical protein subunits synthesized both in the cytoplasm and mitochondria. Several of the nucleus-encoded subunit genes have been characterized [77, 86], in addition to the three subunits encoded in the mitochondrial DNA [9]. Most studies to date have focused on only a few subunits from nuclear genes (CO VIc and CO IV) and only one subunit from the mitochondrial genome (CO III). Repetitive nerve stimulation of the rat and rabbit tibialis anterior muscle demonstrated approximately 2-fold increases in CO VIc mRNA content after 21 days of stimulation [44, 93]. Hood and associates have also showed a similar increase in the mitochondrial DNA-encoded subunit CO III mRNA {44}, suggesting a coordinate increase in the expression of CO subunits from nuclear and mitochondrial genomes.

The increases in CO subunit mRNA content could not account for all of the increase in cytochrome oxidase activity. For example, in the study of Williams et al. [93], cytochrome oxidase activity increased 2-fold above the control value after 10 days of stimulation, but CO VIc mRNA content was not different from that of controls. Similarly, after 21 days of nerve stimulation, cytochrome oxidase activity increased 4-fold, but CO IV mRNA increased only 2-fold. Hence, in addition to a possible transcriptional control mechanism, there are indications from these nerve stimulation studies that translational or posttranslational regulatory events may also be involved.

A similar type of regulatory scheme seems to be evident, based on endurance training studies. Town and Essig [84] showed in the plantaris muscle of rats exposed to treadmill running that cytochrome oxidase activity increased significantly after 7 days and reached a value 80% higher than that of controls after 4 wk. However, the content of CO subunit mRNAs III and IV remained at control levels throughout the 28 days of training. In a subsequent study, in which the same mRNAs were measured in the plantaris but after 10 weeks of training, Marone et al. [54] found parallel 2-fold increases in the activity of cytochrome oxidase and CO subunits mRNAs. Thus, as observed in the nerve stimulation experiments cited above, increases in cytochrome oxidase could be mediated by training duration-dependent mechanisms. These results are also somewhat reminiscent of the pattern observed with cytochrome c (see above): thus, the muscle cell may choose to increase expression of the protein early in training by increasing the efficiency of mRNA use (translational or posttranslational steps such as protein import) and, later, by an increase in the capacity of mRNA translation through increases in mRNA concentration at the transcriptional step or by increasing mRNA stability.

CYTOCHROME B. Cytochrome b is an inner membrane hemeprotein that accepts electrons from cytochrome c_1 in the electron transport chain. The cytochrome b gene specifies the transcription of a $\sim$1.2-kb mRNA which encodes the only monomeric protein in the mitochondrial genome. The expression of cytochrome b protein has been shown to increase $\sim$2-fold with endurance training [20]. In a recent study Murakami et al. [59] showed that cytochrome b mRNA was increased $\sim$50% in the soleus muscle after 3, 6, and 12 wk of endurance training. Thus, at least a portion of the increase in cytochrome b protein content may be mediated by an increase in mitochondrial DNA transcription. Part of the increase in cytochrome b mRNA could also be attributed to a $\sim$30% increase in mitochondrial DNA content in what is a unique example of control of gene expression by gene dosage. This is analogous to the earlier finding by Williams [90] in nerve-stimulated rabbit skeletal muscle, in which mitochondrial DNA copy number correlated directly with changes in cytochrome b mRNA content.

POSSIBLE SIGNALING PATHWAYS FOR MITOCHONDRIAL BIOGENESIS

Introduction

The signals and pathways that lead to the changes in mitochondrial gene expression documented during endurance training can only be described in a preliminary or theoretical manner. From the previous section, the sites of control have been assigned for a number of genes, and now it is becoming possible to begin "working backward," toward the description of signaling pathways and possible signals. Before attempting a discussion of this topic, it will be useful to make some assumptions concerning the site of signal generation and the type of control mechanism at work here.

First, it is likely that intracellular metabolic signals provoked by the imposition of contractility activity are most important. The major evidence for this finding comes from a study [31] in which it was shown that animals devoid of either pituitary hormones, insulin, or thyroid hormones underwent similar percent increases in selected Krebs cycle and total mitochondrial protein. It is worth noting that the same hormones, in particular thyroxine, may have normal physiological function because, in the absence each of these hormones, the basal level of mitochondrial enzyme activity was less than that of controls [31]. In addition, thyroxine has been shown to increase the transcription of cytochrome c [72] and activity of ALAS [42]. Another line of evidence in support of intracellular factors is the well-known ability of continuously or intermittently applied 10-Hz electrical stimulation of motor neurons to dramatically increase mitochondrial biogenesis in the absence of any changes in circulating hormones [43]. It is not yet possible to rule out, however, the operation of autocrine or paracrine mechanisms, which may use the extracellular or intracellular hormone receptors and signaling pathways.

A second assumption is that mitochondrial biogenesis is part of a larger homeostatic negative feedback loop in which the daily energetic demands of a particular motor unit are precisely matched to mitochondrial capacity to generate ATP [43]. The daily metabolic disturbance forms a signal for mitochondrial biogenesis, leading to an adaptive increase in mitochondrial gene expression, which is followed by an increase in the density of the mitochondrial reticulum, thereby reducing the metabolic disturbance and slowing the rate of mitochondrial biogenesis. Direct support for this concept is limited but comes mainly from the well-known pattern of changes in mitochondrial protein expression that follow saturation kinetics in response to a constant training stimulus [21, 81]. The concept of a homeostatic loop, in which intracellular signaling may predominate, is illustrated in Figure 10.5. Using this diagram as a framework, the forthcoming discussion will attempt to provide evidence for potential signals, signal pathways and possible links to specific genes.

Potential Signals: Insights from Studies in ATP Homeostasis

The signal or signals for mitochondrial biogenesis [44, 91] probably reflect a disparity in the inability to generate ATP relative to its demand by the cellular ATPases. Hochachka and associates quantified ATP turnover in relation to ATP synthesis during relatively high-intensity aerobic exercise [38]. The percent change in energy imbalance, defined as [ATP]/total ATP turnover, was remarkably small, on the order of 0% for both Type I and Type II muscles. The major determinant of the changes in ATP turnover during exercise was flux through the myosin ATPase [29], suggesting that when a motor unit is recruited, oxidative metabolism must be able to react precisely to the metabolic demands of the particular isoform of myosin ATPase (either fast or slow).

The percent imbalance is less precise (2–5%) in fast-twitch muscles, especially at near maximal rates of shortening during exercise demanding greater than 50% of ATP synthesis by means of anaerobic glycolysis [3]. However, it is this type of high-intensity sprint interval training that recruits IIB motor units and causes the largest relative increases (3 to 4-fold) in mitochondrial biogenesis reported in the literature [21]. It could be speculated that this is attributable to the relatively poor degree of energy coupling that occurs when this motor unit type is recruited in a repetitive manner. Thus, it is hypothesized that: 1) small but chronic changes in ATP energy homeostasis may represent the primary intracellular disturbance

FIGURE 10.5

ATP homeostasis and negative feedback control of mitochondrial biogenesis: a theo-
retical model. 1, An unidentified intracellular error signal is generated from an im-
balance in the supply of ATP relative to the demand for ATP by myosin ATPase. 2,
This signal may use signaling pathways that directly or indirectly (autocrine?) affect
the rate of nuclear gene expression. The role of endocrine signaling pathways may not
be as important for this adaptive process. 3, The intracellular signals initiate and
control the sequential phases of mitochondrial biogenesis, resulting in an increase in
mitochondrial mass. 4, As the mitochondrial mass and resultant increase in ATP
synthesizing capacity increases, the error signal decreases, and biogenesis slows to
basal levels.

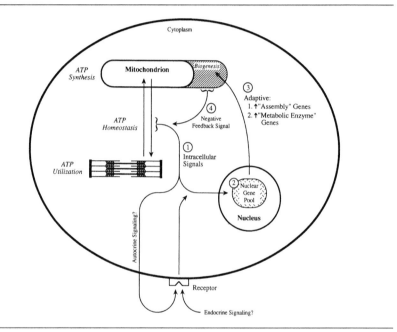

leading to changes in mitochondrial biogenesis; 2) for a given motor unit
that is recruited, the extent of coupling will be affected by parameters on
both the demand (ATPase activity, exercise duration/frequency) and supply (preexisting mitochondrial density); and 3) with training, the increased
capacity for ATP generation as a result of mitochondrial biogenesis will lead
to a better coupling of ATP turnover to ATP synthesis.

If it is the extent of coupling that determines the need to increase the capacity for mitochondrial ATP synthesis, how might that be translated into
a signal? Unfortunately, there is not a clear-cut answer to this question, and
the search for a solution will continue to be a topic of future investigation.

However, it would seem prudent to consider signals that can account for the tight control of ATP supply and demand, not only during acute contractile activity but also during long-term maintenance of ATP homeostasis, when the muscle may encounter daily disturbances, such as exercise training.

Potential Signals and Pathways: Insight from Selected Genes

Signaling pathways must link changes in ATP homeostasis with proteins that regulate expression of mitochondrial genes. As our understanding of mechanisms of gene regulation progresses at all levels (transcription, translational, and posttranslational steps), so does the potential to link these events with already-known signaling pathways. The list below details progress made thus far at finding possible signal transduction pathways using this approach. These mitochondrial genes are known to be increased by training or nerve stimulation and they have a transcription factor that binds to the gene that has been linked to a signaling pathway.

CYTOCHROME C GENE. In certain cell types cytochrome c [31] but not cytochrome oxidase subunit IV transcription can be induced by raising cyclic adenosine monophosphate (cAMP) levels. This induction was mediated by increasing protein kinase A activity, resulting in the phosphorylation of the cyclic AMP response element binding protein (CREB). Because exercise may cause an increase in cAMP (reviewed in ref. 12), this may represent one pathway by which the previously demonstrated increases in cytochrome c mRNA expression observed with endurance training.

ATP SYNTHASE β AND ADP/ATP TRANSLOCATOR-1. Several putative DNA binding activities are associated with the REBOX and OXBOX regions of these genes [17]. The REBOX binding activities were responsive to the presence of reducing agents, such as nicotinomide adenine dinucleotide (NADH). This suggests that for these two genes, direct sensing (no second messenger required) of metabolism may be possible via changes in the NADH/NAD ratio.

NRF-1-DEPENDENT GENES. While a great deal is known about this factor (contained within ref. 88), there has yet to be a signaling pathway established. However, it has been suggested that NRF-1-dependent increase in transcription may be induced by growth- or differentiation-transducing signals that affect not only mitochondrial genes but also other cellular genes involved in protein synthesis.

SUMMARY AND FUTURE DIRECTIONS

The biogenesis of mitochondria in muscle is an important adaptation underlying improvements in exercise performance after training. The overall process involves the quantitative expansion of the preexisting mitochondrial reticular structure into a more dense network of branch-like connections. With training, this assembly process can be divided into three sequential phases. In the first, nuclear genes coding for proteins that have no direct role in ATP generation are expressed. These protein products function in pathways of heme synthesis, phospholipid synthesis, or in protein import to provide the necessary environment for newly synthesized metabolic pathway enzymes. In the second phase, a slow coordinated rise in the synthesis of mitochondrial proteins from both nuclear and mitochondrial genomes occurs to supply the nascent mitochondrial structure with proper stoichiometric quantities of enzymes for optimal ATP generation. Finally, the replication of mit DNA occurs, perhaps to fill the growing mitochondrion with additional template to maintain a constant rate of mit DNA transcription. Several genes characteristic of the early and middle phases of mitochondrial biogenesis have been studied, and putative regulatory sites are beginning to unfold. There is some evidence suggesting the need for training duration-dependent types of gene regulation. Translational and posttranslational control mechanisms may predominate early, whereas pretranslational types of regulation may function later in training.

A lack of basic knowledge is still preventing us from attaining further progress in the field. Exercise scientists need to direct attention to identifying the protein factors that mediate the temporal (sequential phases) and spatial (coordinate) types of regulation noted above. Although it is possible that some of these factors may be those already identified for some genes (e.g., NRF-1, NRF-2), many of these transcription factors have been isolated in cellular contexts that might give rise to developmental, rather than metabolic, signals. Thus, strategies need to be developed to examine gene regulation during metabolic disturbances in adult tissues. This type of effort could be especially fruitful by focusing on the regulation of the *early-phase* genes, which are likely to accept the initial signals generated from a disturbance in ATP homeostasis.

ACKNOWLEDGMENTS

The author thanks Yevette Johnson for help in the literature research and Darrell Borger for his drawing expertise.

REFERENCES

1. Annex, B. H., and R. S. Williams. Mitochondrial DNA structure and expression in specialized subtypes of mammalian striated muscle. *Mol. Cell Biol.* 10:5671–5678, 1990.
2. Aprille, J. R. Perinatal development of mitochondria in rat liver. G. Fiskum (eds). Mitochondrial Physiology and Pathology. New York: Van Nostrand Reinhold 1986, pp. 66–99.
3. Arthur, P. G., T. G. West, R. W. Brill, P. M. Schulte, and P. W. Hochachka. Recovery metabolism of skipjack tuna white skeletal muscle: rapid and parallel changes in lactate and phosphocreatine after exercise. *Can. J. Zool.* 70:1230–1239, 1992.

4. Aschenbrenner, V, R. Druyan, R. Albin, and M. Rabinowitz. Haem a, cytochrome c and total protein turnover in mitochondria from rat heart and liver. *Biochem. J.* 119:157–160, 1970.

5. Bakeeva I. K., Y. S. Chentsov, and V. P. Skulachev. Ontogenesis of mitochondrial reticulum in rat diaphragm muscle. *Eur. J. Cell Biol.* 25:175–181, 1981.

6. Bakeeva, I. K., Y. S. Chentsov, and V. P. Skulachev. Mitochondrial framework (reticulum mitochondriale) in rate diaphragm muscle. *Biochim. Biophys. Acta* 501:349–369, 1978.

7. Barnard, R. J., and J. B. Peter. Effect of exercise on skeletal muscle. III. Cytochrome changes. *J. Appl. Physiol.* 32:904–908, 1971.

8. Benzi, G., P. Panceri, M. De Bernardi, R. Villa, E. Arcelli, L. d'Angelo, and F. Berte. Mitochondrial enzymatic adaptation of skeletal muscle to endurance training. *J. Appl. Physiol.* 38:565–569, 1975.

9. Bibb, M. J., R. A. Van Etten, C. T. Wright, M. W. Walberg, and D. A. Clayton. Sequence and gene organization of mouse mitochondrial DNA. *Cell* 26:167–180, 1981.

10. Booth, F. W. Cytochrome c protein synthesis rate in rat skeletal muscle. *J. Appl. Physiol.* 71:1225–1230, 1991.

11. Booth, F. W., and J. O. Holloszy. Cytochrome c turnover in rat skeletal muscles. *J. Biol. Chem.* 252:416–419, 1977.

12. Booth, F. W., and D. B. Thomason. Molecular and cellular adaptations of muscle in response to exercise: perspectives of various models. *Physiol. Rev.* 71:541–574, 1991.

13. Braidotti, G., I. A. Borthwick, and B. K. May. Identification of regulatory sequences in the gene for 5- aminolevulinate synthase from rat. *J. Biol. Chem.* 268:1109–1117, 1993.

14. Chang, D. D., and D. A. Clayton. A mammalian mitochondrial RNA processing enzyme contains nucleus encoded RNA. *Science* 235:1178–1184, 1987.

15. Chang, D. D. and D. A. Clayton. Mouse RNAse MRP RNA is encoded by a nuclear gene and contains a decamer sequence complementary to a conserved region of mitochondrial substrate. *Cell* 56:131–139, 1989.

16. Chang, D. D., W. W. Hauswirth, and D. A. Clayton. Replication priming and transcription initiate from precisely the same site in mouse mitochondrial DNA. *EMBO J.* 4:1559–1567, 1985.

17. Chung, A. B., G. Stepien, Y. Harguchi, K. Li, and D. Wallace. Transcriptional control of nuclear genes for the mitochondrial ADP/ATP translocator and the ATP synthase β subunit. Multiple factors interact with the OXBOX/REBOX promoter sequences. *J. Biol. Chem.* 267:21154–21161, 1992.

18. Clayton, D. A. Transcription and replication of animal mitochondrial DNAs. *Int. Rev. Cytol.* 141:217–232, 1992.

19. Daum, G. Lipids of mitochondria. *Biochim. Biophys. Acta* 822:1–42, 1985.

20. Davies, K. J. A., L. Packer, and G. A. Brooks. Biochemical adaptation of mitochondria, muscle, and whole-animal respiration to endurance training. *Arch. Biochem. Biophys.* 209:539–554, 1981.

21. Dudley, G. A., W. M. Abraham, and R. L. Terjung. Influence of exercise intensity and duration on biochemical adaptations in skeletal muscle. *J. Appl. Physiol.* 53:844–850, 1982.

22. Essig, D. A. Exercise induction of 5'-aminolevulinate synthase: a mitochondrial enzyme in the heme biosynthetic pathway. Y. Sato, J. Poortmans, I. Hashimoto, Y. Oshida (eds). *Integration of Medical and Sports Sciences.* Basel, Switzerland: Karger, 1992, pp. 299–308.

23. Essig, D. A., J. M. Kennedy, and L. A. McNabney. Regulation of 5'-aminolevulinate synthase activity in overloaded skeletal muscle. *Am. J. Physiol.* 259:C310–C314, 1990.

24. Essig, D. A., D. A. Jackson, and D. Borger. A heme oxygenase mRNA is induced in skeletal muscle following 3 hours of nerve stimulation. *Med. Sci. Sports Exerc.* 26:S94, 1994.

25. Evans, M. J., and R. Scarpulla. Both upstream and intron sequence elements are required for elevated expression of the rat somatic cytochrome c gene in COS cells. *Mol. Cell. Biol.* 8:35–41, 1988.

26. Evans, M. J., and R. Scarpulla. Interaction of nuclear factors with multiple sites in the so-

matic cytochrome c promoter. Characterization of upstream NRF-1, ATF, and intron Sp1 recognition sequences. *J. Biol. Chem.* 264:14361–14368, 1989.

27. Forsburg, S. L., and L. Guarente. Communication between mitochondria and nucleus in regulation of cytochrome genes in the yeast *Saccharomyces cervisiae*. *Annual Rev. Cell Biol.* 5:153–180, 1989.

28. Glick, B. S. Can HSP 70 proteins act as force generating motors? *Cell* 80:11–14, 1995.

29. Gollnick, P. D., and C. D. Ianuzzo. Hormonal deficiencies and the metabolic adaptations of rats to training. *Am. J. Physiol.* 223:278–282, 1972.

30. Gollnick, P. D., and D. W. King. Effect of exercise and training on mitochondria of rat skeletal muscle. *Am. J. Physiol.* 216:1502–1509, 1969.

31. Gopalakrishnan, L., and R. Scarpulla. Differential regulation of respiratory chain subunits by a CREB-dependent signal transduction pathway. *J. Biol. Chem.* 269:105–113, 1994.

32. Hake, L. E., A. A. Alcivar, and N. B. Hecht. Changes in mRNA length accompany translational regulation of the somatic and testis specific cytochrome c genes during spermatogenesis in the mouse. *Development* 110:249–257, 1990.

33. Hamilton, J. W., B. W. J. Bement, P. R. Sinclair, J. F. Sinlair, and K. E. Wetterhann. Expression of 5'- aminolevulinate synthase and cytochrome P-450 mRNAs in chicken embryo hepatocytes in vivo and in culture: Effects of porphyrinogenic drugs and haem. *Biochem. J.* 255:267–275, 1988.

34. Harper, H. *Review of Physiological Chemistry*. Los Altos, CA: Lange, 1975, p. 290.

35. Hartl, F.-U., N. Pfanner, D. W. Nicholson, and W. Neupert. Mitochondrial protein import. *Biochim. Biophys. Acta* 988:1–45, 1989.

36. Hatch, G. M. Cardiolipin biosynthesis in the isolated heart. *Biochem. J.* 297:201–208, 1994.

37. Hayashi, J-I, M. Takemitsu, Y. Gota, and I. Nonaka. Human mitochondria and mitochondrial genome function as a single dynamic cellular unit. *J. Cell Biol.* 125:43–50, 1994.

38. Hochachka, P. W., M. Bianconcini, W. S. Parkhouse, and G. P. Dobson. Role of actomyosin ATPase in metabolic regulation during intense exercise. *Proc. Natl. Acad. Sci. (U. S. A.)* 88:5764–5768, 1991.

39. Holloszy, J. O. Biochemical adaptations in muscle. *J. Biol. Chem.* 242:2278–2282, 1967.

40. Holloszy, J. O., and E. F. Coyle. Adaptations of skeletal muscle to endurance exercise and their metabolic consequences. *J. Appl. Physiol.* 56:831–838, 1984.

41. Holloszy, J. O., L. B. Oscai, I. J. Don, and P. A. Mole. Mitochondrial citric acid cycle and related enzymes: adaptive response to exercise. *Biochem. Biophys. Res. Commun.* 40:1368–1373, 1970.

42. Holloszy, J. O., and W. W. Winder. Induction of δ-aminolevulinic acid synthetase in muscle by exercise or thyroxine. *Am J. Physiol.* 236:R180–R183, 1979.

43. Hood, D. A., A. Balaban, M. K. Connor, E. E. Craig, M. L. Nishio, M. Rezvani, and M. Takahashi. Mitochondrial biogenesis in striated muscle. *Can. J. Appl. Physiol.* 12–48, 1994.

44. Hood, D. A., R. Zak, and D. Pette. Chronic stimulation of rat skeletal muscle induces coordinate increases of mitochondrial and nuclear mRNAs of cytochrome c oxidase subunits. *Eur J. Biochem.* 179:275–280, 1989.

45. Jakovcic, S., J. Haddock, G. S. Getz, M. Rabinowitz, and H. Swift. Mitochondrial development in liver of foetal and newborn rats. *Biochem. J.* 121:341–347, 1971.

46. Kayar, S. R., H. Hoppeler, L. Mermod, and E. R. Weibel. Mitochondrial size and shape in equine skeletal muscle: a three dimensional reconstruction study. *Anat. Rec.* 222:333–339, 1988.

47. Kirkwood, S. P., E. A. Munn, and G. A. Brooks. Mitochondrial reticulum in limb skeletal muscle. *Am. J. Physiol.* 251:C395–C402, 1986.

48. Kirkwood, S. P., L. Packer, and G. A. Brooks. Effects of endurance training on a mitochondrial reticulum in limb skeletal muscle. *Arch. Biochem. Biophys.* 255:80–88, 1987.

49. Lai, M. M., and F. W. Booth. Cytochrome c mRNA and α-actin mRNA in muscles of rats fed β-GPA. *J. Appl. Physiol.* 69:843–848, 1990.

50. Li, K., J. A. Hodge, and D. C. Wallace. OXBOX, a positive transcriptional element of the heart-skeletal muscle ADP/ATP translocator gene. *J. Biol. Chem.* 265:20585–20588, 1990.
51. Li, K., C. S. Smagula, W. J. Parsons, J. A. Richardson, M. Gonzalez, H. K. Hagler, and R. S. Williams. Subcellular partitioning of MRP RNA assessed by ultrastructural and biochemical analysis. *J. Cell Biol.* 124:871–882, 1994.
52. Locke, M., E. Noble, and B. Atkinson. Exercising mammals synthesize stress proteins. *Am. J. Physiol.* 258:C723–C729, 1990.
53. Locke, M., E. G. Noble, R. M. Tanguay, M. R. Feild, S. E. Ianuzzo, and C. D. Ianuzzo. Activation of heat shock transcription factor in rat heart following heat shock and exercise. *Am. J. Physiol.*, in press, 1995.
54. Marone, J. R., M. T. Falduto, D. A. Essig, and R. C. Hickson. Effects of glucocorticoids and endurance training on cytochrome oxidase expression in skeletal muscle *J. Appl . Physiol.* 77:1685–1690, 1994.
55. May, B. K., I. A. Borthwick, G. Srivastava, B. A. Piroloa, and W. H. Elliott. Control of 5'-aminolevulinate synthase in animals. *Curr. Top. Cell Regul.* 28:233–262, 1987.
56. Mole, P. A., L. B. Oscai, and J. O. Holloszy. Adaptation of muscle to exercise. Increase in levels of palmityl CoA synthetase, carnitine palmityltransferase, and palmityl CoA dehydrogenase, and in the capacity to oxidize fatty acids. *J. Clin. Invest.* 50:2323–2330, 1971.
57. Morimoto, R. I. Cells in stress: transcriptional activation of heat shock genes. *Science.* 259:1409–1410, 1993.
58. Morrison, P. R., R. B. Biggs, and F. W. Booth. Daily running for 2 wk and mRNAs for cytochrome c and α-actin in rat skeletal muscle. *Am. J. Physiol.* 257:C936–C939, 1989.
59. Murakami, Y., Y. Shimomura, N. Fujitsuka, N. Nakai, S. Sugiyama, T. Ozawa, M. Sokabe, S. Horai, K. Tokuyama, and M. Suzuki. Enzymatic and genetic adaptation of soleus muscle to physical training in rats. *Am. J. Physiol.* 267:E388–E395, 1994.
60. Nicholson, D. W., and W. Neupert. Import of cytochrome c into mitochondria: Reduction of heme mediated by NADH and flavin nucleotides is obligatory for its covalent linkage to apocytochrome c. *Proc. Natl. Acad. Sci. U. S. A.* 86:4340–4344, 1989.
61. Neupert, W., F.-U. Hartl, E. A. Craig, and N. Pfanner. How do polypeptides cross the mitochondrial membranes? *Cell* 63:447–450, 1990.
62. Ohtsuka, T., M. Nishijima, K. Suzuki, and Y. Akamatsu. Mitochondrial dysfunction of a cultured Chinese hamster ovary cell mutant deficient in cardiolipin. *J. Biol. Chem.* 268:22914–22919, 1993.
63. Ordway, G. A., K. Li, G. A. Hand, and R. S. Williams. RNA subunit of mitochondrial-processing enzyme is induced by contractile activity in striated muscle. *Am. J. Physiol.* C1511–C1516, 1993.
64. Oscai, L. B., D. A. Essig, and W. K. Palmer. Lipase regulation of muscle triglyceride hydrolysis. *J. Appl. Phsyiol.* 69:1571–1577, 1990.
65. Oscai, L. B., and J. O. Holloszy. Biochemical adaptations in muscle. *J. Biol. Chem.* 246:6968–6972, 1971.
66. Penman, S. Rethinking cell structure. *Proc. Natl. Acad. Sci. U. S. A.* 92:5251–5257, 1995.
67. Pollack, J. K., and R. Sutton. The differentiation of animal mitochondria during development. *Trends in Biochemical Sciences.* 5:23–27, 1980.
68. Raju, V. S., and M. D. Maines. Coordinated expression and mechanism of induction of HSP 32 (heme oxygenase-1) mRNA by hyperthermia in rat organs. *Biochim. Biophys. Acta* 1217:273–280, 1994.
69. Salemme, F. R. Structure and function of cytochrome c *Annu. Rev. Biochem.* 46:299–329, 1977.
70. Salo, D. C., C. Donovan, and K. J. A. Davies. HSP 70 and other possible heat shock or oxidative stress proteins are induced in skeletal muscle, heart and liver during exercise. *Free Radic. Biol. Med.* 11:239–246, 1991.

71. Saltzgaber-Muller, J., and G. Schatz. Heme is necessary for the accumulation and assembly of cytochrome c oxidase subunits in *Saccharomyces cervisiae. J. Biol. Chem.* 253:305–310, 1978.

72. Scarpulla, R. C., M. C. Kilar, and K. M. Scarpulla. Coordinate induction of multiple cytochrome c mRNAs in response to thyroid hormone. *J. Biol. Chem.* 261:4660–4662, 1986.

73. Schlame, M., and D. Haldar. Cardiolipin is synthesized on the matrix side of the inner membrane in rat liver membrane. *J. Biol. Chem.* 268:74–79, 1993.

74. Sedman, R., G. Ingall, G. Rios, and T. R. Tephly. Heme biosynthesis in the heart. Biochem. Pharmacol. 32:761–766, 1982.

75. Skidmore, R., J. A. Gutierrez, V. Guerriero, and K. C. Kregel. HSP 70 induction during exercise and heat stress in rats. Role of internal temperature. *Am. J. Physiol.* 268:R92–R97, 1995.

76. Srivastava, G., I. A. Borthwick, D. J. Maguire, V. J. Elfernick, M. J. Bawden, J. F. B. Mercer, and B. K. May. Regulation of 5'-aminolevulinate synthase mRNA in different rat tissues. *J. Biol. Chem.* 263:5202–5209, 1988.

77. Suske, G., C. Enders, A. Schlerf, and B. Kadenbach. Organization and nucleotide sequence of two chromosomal genes for rat cytochrome c oxidase subunit Vic: a structural and a processed gene. *DNA:* 7:163–171, 1988.

78. Suzuki, H., Y. Hosokawa, M. Nishikimi, and T. Ozawa. Structural organization of the human mitochondrial cytochrome c1 gene. *J. Biol. Chem.* 264:1368–1374, 1989.

79. Takahashi, M., and D. A. Hood. Chronic stimulation- induced changes in mitochondria and performance in rat skeletal muscle. *J. Appl. Physiol.* 74:934–941, 1993.

80. Takahashi, M., D. T. M. McCurdy, D. A. Essig, and D. A. Hood. δ-aminolevulinate synthase expression in muscle after contractions and recovery. *Biochem. J.* 291:219–223, 1993.

81. Terjung, R. The turnover of cytochrome c in different skeletal muscle fiber types of the rat. *Biochem. J.* 178:569–674, 1979.

82. Tominaga, K. S. Akiyama, Y. Kagawa, and S. Ohta. Upstream region of a genomic gene for human mitochondrial transcription factor 1. *Biochim. Biophys. Acta* 1131:217–219, 1992.

83. Tomura, H., H. Endo, Y. Kagawa, and S. Ohta. Novel regulatory element in the nuclear gene of the human mitochondrial ATP synthase β subunit. *J. Biol. Chem.* 265:6525–6527, 1990.

84. Town, G. P., and D. A. Essig. Cytochrome oxidase in muscle of endurance trained rats: subunit mRNA contents and heme synthesis. *J. Appl. Physiol.* 74:192–196, 1993.

85. Underwood, L. E., and R. S. Williams. Pretranslational regulation of myoglobin gene expression. *Am. J. Physiol.* 252:C450–C453, 1987.

86. Virbasius, J. V., and R. Scarpulla. The rat cytochrome c oxidase subunit IV gene family: tissue specific and hormonal differences in subunit IV and cytochrome c mRNA expression. *Nucleic Acids Res.* 18:6581–6586, 1990.

87. Virbasius, J. V., C. A. Virbasius, and R. Scarpulla. Identity of GABP with NRF-2, a multisubunit activator of cytochrome oxidase expression, reveals a cellular role for an ETS domain activator of viral promoters. *Genes Dev.* 7:380–392, 1993.

88. Virbasius, C. A., J. V. Virbasius, and R. Scarpulla. NRF-1, an activator involved in nuclear-mitochondrial interactions, utilizes a new DNA-binding domain conserved in a family of developmental regulators. *Genes Dev.* 7:2431–2445, 1993.

89. Welch, W. J. Mammalian stress response: cell physiology structure/function of stress proteins and implications for medicine and disease. *Physiol. Rev.* 72:1063–1077, 1992.

90. Williams, R. S. Mitochondrial gene expression in mammalian striated muscle. Evidence that variation in gene dosage is the major regulatory event. *J. Biol. Chem.* 261:12390–12394, 1986.

91. Williams, R. S. Frontiers of exercise research: a search for the molecular basis of the exercise training effect in skeletal muscle. R. S. Williams and A. Wallace (eds). *Biological Effects of Physical Activity.* Champaign, IL: Human Kinetics, 1989, pp. 139–148.

92. Williams, R. S. Genetic mechanisms that determine oxidative capacity of striated muscles. Circulation 82:319–331, 1990.
93. Williams, R. S., M. Garcia-Moll, J. Mellor, S. S. Salmons, and W. Harlan. Adaptation of skeletal muscle to increased contactile activity. Expression of nuclear genes encoding mitochondrial proteins. *J. Biol. Chem.* 262:2764–2767, 1987.
94. Williams, R. S., S. Salmons, E. A. Newsholme, R. E. Kaufman, and J. Mellor. Regulation of nuclear and mitochondrial gene expression by contractile activity in skeletal muscle. *J. Biol. Chem.* 261:376–380, 1986.

11
Thyroid Hormone: Modulation of Muscle Structure, Function, and Adaptive Responses to Mechanical Loading

VINCENT J. CAIOZZO, Ph.D.
FADIA HADDAD, Ph.D.

One of the major roles of skeletal muscle is to produce mechanical work and power during activities like cycling, rowing, running, and swimming. Such activities require skeletal muscle to perform repetitive cyclic contractions that consist of shortening and lengthening phases. During the shortening phase, the muscle produces positive mechanical work, whereas during the lengthening phase, mechanical work is done on the muscle (i.e., negative mechanical work).

At the level of the contractile machinery (see Fig. 11.1), the net mechanical work produced by skeletal muscle is determined by a complex interaction of at least six major factors. The factors controlling the ability of skeletal muscle to produce positive mechanical work include: 1) the rate of activation; 2) the force-velocity relationship; 3) the rate of relaxation; and 4) the length-tension relationship. In contrast, the factors that influence the amount of negative work include: 5) the amount of tension present during the lengthening phase and 6) the passive compliance of the muscle being lengthened.

Any perturbation that alters some or all of these factors will influence the mechanical work and power production of skeletal muscle. Over the past 25 years, it has become apparent that some skeletal muscles are highly malleable. Specifically, it has been shown that the thyroid hormone can exert a powerful influence over a number of key phenotypic properties of skeletal muscle. Given the importance of the thyroid hormone, this review will focus on the following issues: 1) the molecular basis of thyroid hormone cellular action; 2) thyroid hormone modulation of key skeletal muscle protein isoforms; and 3) the translation of altered protein phenotype into altered muscle function. Ultimately, skeletal muscle function is dependent on the protein composition of the sarcomere. Hence, mechanisms controlling the rate of synthesis and degradation of these key proteins can have a profound influence over the function of skeletal muscle. As shown in Figure 11.1, the myosin molecule and the sarcoplasmic reticulum (SR) play central roles in determining the production of mechanical work and power. Consistent with these roles, a substantial body of literature exists regarding the effects of the thyroid hormone on these systems. In contrast,

FIGURE 11.1.

Conceptual schematic illustrating the various factors that determine the ability of skeletal muscle to produce mechanical work and power.

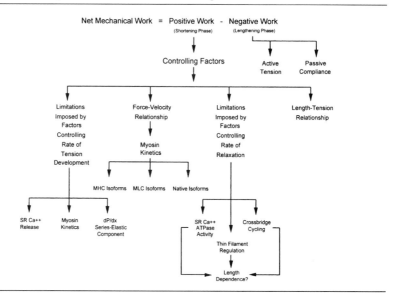

very little is known about the effects of the thyroid hormone on other sarcomeric proteins, such as tropomyosin and troponin. As a consequence, this review will be primarily directed at describing the effects of the thyroid hormone on the expression of myosin isoforms and key proteins of the SR.

GENETIC AND CELLULAR ACTION OF THYROID HORMONE

The thyroid hormone exerts its biological effects largely by influencing gene expression. The major form of the thyroid hormone secreted into the bloodstream is thyroxine (T4), which is peripherally transformed into tri-iodothyronine (T3), the most biologically active form of the hormone. In some tissues, such as the pituitary gland and the cerebral cortex, the major source of T3 is derived from the intracellular deiodination of T4. In other tissues, such as skeletal muscle, however, the major source of T3 is derived from plasma. T3 is transported into the nucleus of target cells, where it interacts with high-affinity binding proteins, known as thyroid hormone receptors (TRs). This interaction triggers cell-specific T3 effects (Fig. 11.2).

The Nuclear TRs and the 10^{-10} to 10^{-11} erbA Genes

TRs are nuclear proteins that bind T3 with high-affinity (Kd=$10^{-10} - 10^{-11}$ M) and specificity, and they are tightly associated with the chromatin. TRs

FIGURE 11.2.

T3 cellular action results from T3 interaction with its high-affinity nuclear receptor (TR) which is strongly bound to a cis regulatory element called thyroid response element (TRE) located upstream of thyroid-responsive genes. The interaction between T3 and TR-TRE alters the transcriptional activity of specific genes that are translated into proteins; these proteins manifest the T3 effects. Also shown is that these proteins can, in turn, affect protein expression at any of the highlighted levels in the cascade of protein synthesis. BP, plasma T3 binding proteins; CTBP, cytosolic T3 binding protein.

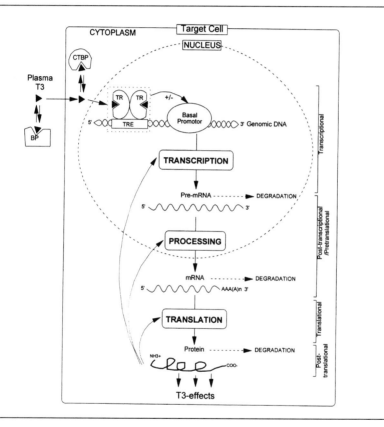

are expressed in most mammalian tissues, and they form a heterogeneous population, with molecular sizes ranging from 48 to 70 kDa (see ref. 105 for review). The biological action of the thyroid hormone has been well correlated with its interaction with nuclear TRs. Also tissue thyroid hormone responsiveness is dependent upon nuclear T3 binding capacity.

After cloning the cDNAs encoding TRs in 1986 [121, 149], considerable progress has been made in understanding the molecular action of T3 and TRs in living cells. It has been demonstrated that the thyroid receptors are the products of the c-erbA protooncogene family, which also encodes for a superfamily of nuclear receptors that include the steroid hormones, vitamin D, and retinoic acid receptors. Analysis of the amino acid sequence of this superfamily has shown that these receptors possess conserved structural regions and that each receptor can be divided into four functional domains (see Fig. 11.3): 1) the N-terminal domain (A/B), which has the most variability in both length and amino acid sequence and plays a role in transactivation; 2) the DNA binding domain (C), which is the most highly conserved region of this superfamily and plays a role in nuclear localization; 3) the hinge region (D), which is also variable in length and amino acid se-

FIGURE 11.3.
Panel A depicts the diverse forms of rat TRs and related proteins: These isoforms are dissected into their functional domains. The number in the rectangle refers to % homology of the particular domain in reference to TR-β1. Domains with completely unique sequences are depicted with a different shading pattern. The numbers above the rectangles represent the number of the amino acid (see test for further details). Panel B depicts the structure of the rev-erb A-α cDNA in comparison to that of erbA-α2 cDNA. Notice the existence of 269 in common sequence but in reverse direction. Arrow = initiation codon; UGA, translation termination codon.

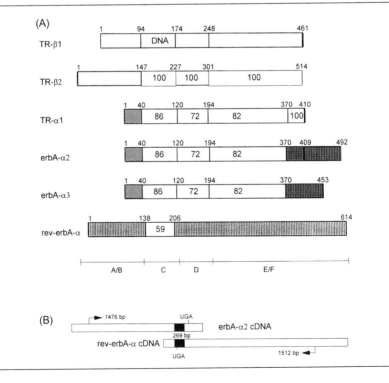

quence and plays a role in homodimerization and heterodimerization of the receptors; and 4) the C-terminal domain (E/F), which is specialized for ligand binding and plays a role in protein-protein interaction and transactivation. This C-terminal domain is highly conserved across different species and isoforms of each receptor [75, 126].

Two distinct erbA genes, α and β, encoding for the TRs have been characterized (see Table 1) and are reported to be located on different chromosomes. The α gene encodes multiple mRNA species that are generated by alternative splicing giving expression to at least three species, erbA-α1, erbA-α2, and erbA-α3 [60, 77, 78, 89, 90, 96, 142]. The amino acid sequence of the rat erbA-α1, -α2, and -α3 proteins is identical for the first 370 residues (Fig. 11.3). The last 40 amino acids for α1 are replaced by 122 amino acids in α2. The α3 protein is identical to α2, but it lacks the first 39 amino acids of the 122 amino acid extension at the C terminus. The erbA-α1 isoform is a high-affinity TR (TR-α1), whereas the erbA-α2 and α3 isoforms do not bind T3 but can associate, like the TR-α1, with high-affinity DNA binding sites designated as thyroid-responsive elements (TREs), located upstream from the start site of T3-responsive genes. In addition, transcription from the opposite strand of the α gene yields a related protein, rev-erbA-α (Fig. 11.3), which is of unknown function and also binds to TRE but does not bind T3 [76]. The erbA-β gene encodes at least two different mRNA species that give expression to two distinct proteins erbA-β1 (TR-β1) and erbA-β2 (TR-β2). The TR-β2 isoform is identical to the TR-β1 isoform, except that the N-terminal region is 53 residues longer (Fig. 11.3). Both of the β forms are high-affinity TRs. Although TR-β1 is expressed in most tissues found in the rat, the TR-β2 is expressed only in the pituitary gland rats [75, 142]. Recently, a novel nuclear receptor, rev-erb-β, was cloned from mouse liver cDNA [41]. This rev-erb-β, also referred to as RVR [115], is highly homologous to rev-erbA-α, which makes it a new member of the TR family. Rev-erb-β binds to DNA elements, but it lacks transactivation activity and is thought to act as a negative transcriptional regulator.

TABLE 11.1.
Listing of the Known erbA Gene Protein Products and Their Characteristics

	T3 Binding	TRE Binding	Effect on T3-responsive Gene Transcription
TR-α1	Yes	Yes	Positive
erbA-α2	No	Yes	Negative
erbA-α3	No	Yes	Negative
rev-erbA-α	No	Yes	Negative
TR-β1	Yes	Yes	Positive
TR-β2	Yes	Yes	Positive
rev-erb-β	No	Yes	Negative

Several studies have demonstrated that TR-α1, erbA-α2, and TR-β1 are widely distributed among tissues and that the level of mRNA expression for erbA products is highly variable and is differentially regulated in a tissue-specific manner. For example, TR-α1 mRNA is downregulated by T3 in multiple tissues, such as the heart, skeletal muscle, kidney, and pituitary gland, but not in the brain [52]. ErbA-α2 mRNA is particularly abundant in brain tissue and is downregulated by T3 in a manner similar to that of TR-α1 mRNA [52]. TR-β1 mRNA expression is upregulated in skeletal muscle in response to T3 (V. J. Caiozzo and F. Haddad, unpublished data). Both rev-erbA-α and rev-erb-β mRNA are widely expressed in tissues, and they are particularly abundant in skeletal muscle [41, 76, 115]. Recently, Hoffman et al. [53] reported that TR mRNA isoform expression is also muscle type-specific and is regulated differentially during development and in response to both thyroid hormone treatment and denervation. Importantly, investigators reported that no correlation was found between the amount of TR-α1 and TR-β1 mRNA expression and the nuclear T3 binding capacity in a tissue [132], which suggests the existence of both translational and post-translational regulation of TR protein expression. Based on these findings, it is important to study both TR protein expression and mRNA expression to obtain meaningful interpretation of TR gene regulation.

These findings suggest that the multiple physiological effects of thyroid hormone are mediated by a family of highly specialized receptors. The significance of these diverse forms of expression for the TR is not yet completely understood; however, their differential expression and regulation in different tissue clearly point to their important role in the regulatory mechanisms involved in the complex eukaryotic system.

T3 Modulation of Gene Expression

Protein expression in living cells generally involves the following steps: 1) transcription into a primary RNA transcript; 2) processing of this primary transcript into mature mRNA, and 3) translation of that mRNA into proteins. The control of gene expression can occur at any of the following levels during the cascade of protein synthesis: 1) the transcriptional level; 2) the posttranscriptional/pretranslational level; 3) the translational level; and 4) the posttranslational level. Transcriptional regulation can occur by increasing or decreasing the gene transcription rate into RNA. Posttranscriptional/pretranslational regulation involves changes in either RNA processing rate (capping, excision of introns, and polyadenylation) or mRNA stability. Translational regulation affects the rate of protein synthesis at constant mRNA concentration. Finally, protein concentration is affected not only by its synthesis rate but also by its degradation rate, i.e., by what is referred to as posttranslational regulation (Fig. 11.2). The thyroid hormone could affect gene expression in skeletal muscle at any of the above steps [2, 11, 12, 23, 27, 49, 58, 62, 85, 105, 135, 144]. Transcriptional regulation by thyroid hormone is probably the best understood of these processes, given the identification of TREs in the regulatory region of promoters found in most thyroid-responsive genes [75, 126]. However, the thyroid hormone is also known to affect muscle protein expression at the posttranscriptional/ pretranslational, translational, and posttranslational levels. The exact mechanism of this posttranscriptional regulation is not yet clear. However, it could be via induction of expression of specific proteins involved in these processes.

TRANSCRIPTIONAL REGULATION. The most powerful evidence that TRs are directly involved in the regulation of gene transcription comes from the identification of specific response elements in target genes that bind the TR with high affinity. Mutation or deletion of these sequences abolishes both TR binding and T3 responsiveness.

Direct vs. Indirect Transcriptional Regulation. The thyroid hormone can alter the transcription rate of a gene by direct interaction with a TR-TRE located in the vicinity of the promoter of the target gene. Specifically, TREs have been found in the promoter regulatory regions of several genes expressed in skeletal muscle, including those genes for Type I myosin heavy-chain (MHC), α-actin, and the SR Ca^{2+} ATPase pump [36, 48, 97]. Thus, it is likely that T3 causes a direct transcriptional regulation of the expression of these genes. In some cases, the thyroid hormone affects the transcription of a gene lacking a TRE, which is referred to as indirect regulation by T3. This indirect regulation of gene transcription is possible when T3 modulates the expression of a nuclear factor that, in turn, acts as a direct transcriptional factor for a particular target gene (Fig. 11.4). For example, a TRE has been identified on both the MyoD and the myogenin genes [31, 98]. These two proteins are muscle-specific transcriptional factors that act as transcriptional activators/silencers of several muscle genes, including the MHC genes, and are directly under the control of thyroid hormones. Thus, MHC gene expression might be indirectly regulated by T3 via MyoD/myogenin-mediated action.

T3 can modulate gene expression by having either a positive or a negative effect on RNA transcription. Under certain conditions, T3 differentially regulates the expression of a particular gene in a tissue-specific fashion, i.e., it increases its expression in one tissue and decreases it in another. For example, T3 increases the expression of the MHC Type IIA gene in slow muscles like the soleus (SOL) and the vastus intermedius (VI), whereas it decreases the expression of this same gene in fast muscles, such as the plantaris (PLAN) and the medial gastrocnemius (MG; see ref. 61). This characteristic of bi-directional regulation is the result of a complex interplay of several *cis* regulatory elements and *trans* acting factors on the gene in question.

TRE Characteristics. The TRs are hormone-dependent transcriptional factors. In order to modulate transcription of target genes, these TRs must

FIGURE 11.4.
Direct and indirect T3 transcriptional regulation. T3 modulates Gene I protein expression via a direct interaction with a TRE located upstream of the promotor (P). Protein I is a transcription factor for gene II, thus modulating Protein II transcription. Protein II is indirectly regulated by T3 via Protein I. IRE, Protein I response element.

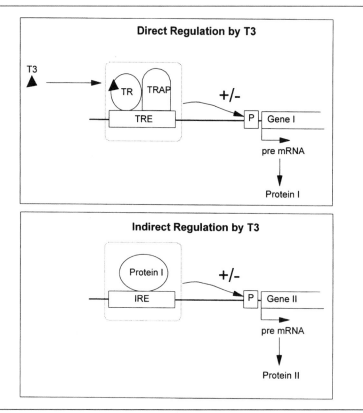

bind to specific DNA sequences, TRE, which are located on target genes (Fig. 11.2 and 11.4). TREs belong to the class of *cis* acting genetic elements known as enhancers or repressors, which can impart T3 responsiveness to heterologous genes. As more TREs are identified, it has become clear that the rules that govern their design are much more complex than was initially believed. Several investigators have shown that these elements are repeats of a half-site consensus motif, $(A/G)GG(A/T)CA$ [28]. The binding properties and transcriptional activity of TRs for a particular TRE appear to be determined by the orientation of the half-sites and the number of nucleotides separating them. The TRs interact at these sites as monomers, homodimers, and/or heterodimers, in association with nuclear proteins such as thyroid receptor auxiliary proteins (TRAPs) [95], and retinoid-X receptors (RXRs; see refs. 125 and 159). This complexity has created a diversity in the TR regulation of gene transcription. For example, it has been shown that the different isoforms of RXR can dictate whether T3-regulated and TR-α-mediated transcription is either positive or negative [59]. Furthermore, T3 concentration can decrease the homodimer, but not the heterodimer, binding properties to some of the TREs [5, 155, 156]. The existence of different TR and RXR isoforms also adds to the complexity and diversity of this regulation process.

POSTTRANSCRIPTIONAL/PRETRANSLATIONAL REGULATION. Very few studies have dealt with striated muscle RNA stability under altered thyroid status. However, indirect evidence supports the idea that T3 can act on gene expression by changing its RNA stability. For example, studies have shown that T3 regulates, in a tissue-specific fashion, the malic enzyme gene by: 1) increasing its transcription rate in the heart and liver; and/or 2) stabilizing its primary transcript only in the liver [32]. A similar dual regulatory mechanism involving T3 has been reported for the spot 14 gene [66], the 3-hydroxy-3-methylglutaryl-coenzyme A reductase gene [128], and the RXR-α and RXR-γ genes [85].

TRANSLATIONAL AND POSTTRANSLATIONAL CONTROL. T3 is also thought to affect gene expression by exerting an influence on the rates of both protein synthesis and degradation. Protein levels could either increase or decrease as a result of a change in translation efficiency or protein stability. For example, studies of protein turnover in skeletal muscles show that thyroid hormone causes increases in both global protein synthesis and degradation rates [2, 11, 12, 24, 68, 135, 158]. These respective increases could be disproportionated in time, thereby resulting in a negative net protein balance, i.e., a net loss of protein. These studies also show that slow muscles are more sensitive to thyroid hormone changes than fast muscles.

EFFECTS OF THYROID STATE ON MYOSIN IN SKELETAL MUSCLE

The Myosin Molecule

Myosin is the principal component that makes up the contractile system, accounting for approximately 25% of the total protein found in skeletal muscle fibers. Myosin was initially discovered in 1864 by Kuhne [148], who showed that high salt concentrations extracted a substance from skeletal muscle that Kuhne called "myosin." The central role of myosin in the contractile process was elucidated many years later by Engelhardt and Ljubimowa [148] and Szent-Gyorgyi [148]. Today, it is known that the myosin molecule is a complex hexameric molecule that is composed of two heavy chains and two pairs of light chains [86]. Each MHC has a molecular weight of ~230 kDa and is composed of two distinct domains, the rod region and globular head. The rod regions of the two heavy chains originate at the C-terminus and fold together to form a coiled-coil alpha helix. This region of the MHC constitutes approximately 50% of the amino acid sequence and plays a key structural role in the assembly of myosin into thick filaments. The S-1 globular head of the MHC contains three distinct proteolytic domains (i.e., 25, 50, and 20 kd), containing approximately 850 amino acids [86]. Residues 1–212 constitute the 25-kd domain that is known to contain the ATP binding site. The 50-kd segment (213–645) contains the docking domain specific for actin. This domain is thought to exist close to the 50 kDa–20-kDa joint region. Finally, the 20-kD segment (amino acid residues 646–849) not only is partially responsible for binding to actin but also contains the binding sites for the light chains. Recently, Rayment et al. [109] published the three-dimensional structure of the S-1 subunit and reported that the regulatory light chain binds in the region of residues 808–840, whereas the essential light chain interacts with residues 783–806 [109].

Historically, two classes of light chains have been distinguished in skeletal muscle. These have been categorized as the *essential* and *regulatory* light chains [84]. Initial experiments demonstrated that when the so-called essential light chains were removed from myosin, there was a complete loss of ATPase activity [131], hence, the designation "essential." The regulatory light chains derive their name from the fact that they could be used to replace Ca^{2+}-binding regulatory light chains found in molluscan muscle [131]. Additionally, the regulatory light chains are also known to act as substrates for myosin light chain kinase and, consequently, have also been called "P-light chains" [131]. More recently, light chains have been identified according to their molecular weight. On this basis, the two essential light chains have been identified as light chain-1 (LC1) and light chain-3 (LC3). These two light chains have respective molecular weights of approximately 21.5 and 16 kD. The regulatory light chain with a molecular weight of approximately 18 kD has been designated as light chain-2 (LC2; see ref. 146).

MHC, MLC, AND NATIVE ISOFORMS. Slow and fast muscles are known to differ substantially with respect to contractile properties, such as the force-velocity relationship and maximal shortening velocity (V_{max}). Both of these parameters are thought to reflect cross-bridge cycling rates and adenosine triphosphate (ATP) hydrolysis. Consequently, it seems reasonable to suspect that there might be different isoforms of myosin in slow and fast skeletal muscle. In fact, a number of isoforms have been identified. Using gel electrophoretic and immunological techniques, at least 8 isoforms of the MHC have been identified to date in skeletal muscle, and it has been suggested that there may be as many as 22 different MHC isoforms. The eight different MHC isoforms have been designated as embryonic, neonatal, extraocular, adult slow Type I, adult fast Type IIA, adult fast Type IIX, adult fast Type IIB, and the so-called "super-fast" MHC [108, 124].

In mammalian skeletal muscle, three different essential light chain isoforms have been identified. These have been identified as slow light chain-1 (SLC1), fast light chain-1 (FLC1), and fast light chain-3 (FLC3). As derived from their classification, SLC1 is associated with muscle fibers containing the slow Type I MHC isoform, whereas FLC1 and FLC3 are found in fibers containing the fast MHC isoforms (see Table 11.2). Currently, two regulatory light-chain isoforms have been identified in mammalian skeletal muscle. These have been categorized as slow light chain-2 (SLC2) and fast light chain-2 (FLC2).

As described above, native myosin isoforms exist as hexameric molecules, and at least five different native myosin isoforms have been identified previously in adult rodent skeletal muscle [146]. These native isomyosins have been separated on polyacrylamide gel by electrophoresis under non-denaturing conditions and have been designated as slow myosin (SM), intermediate myosin (IM), fast myosin-3 (FM3), fast myosin-2 (FM2), and fast myosin-1 (FM1), in order of their increased electrophoretic mobility.

The heavy- and light-chain isoform composition of these different native isoforms is shown in Table 11.2. The scheme presented in table 2 is based on the work of Tsika et al. [146]. It should be noted that at the time this scheme was published, the fast Type IIX MHC isoform had not been identified. Based on data obtained from the white region of the MG muscle, [21], the fast Type IIX MHC protein isoform is probably a component of the FM3 and, possibly, FM2 native isoforms. Although most muscles are thought to contain at least one of the native isoforms described above in Table 11.1, it is theoretically possible that a number of hybrid native isoforms might exist under altered physiological conditions [108]. Consistent with this suggestion, recent studies have reported the existence of so-called hybrid fibers that contain polymorphic expressions of the MHC isoforms [108].

FUNCTIONAL SIGNIFICANCE OF MYOSIN HEAVY CHAIN ISOFORMS. There is an intricate interaction between the operational state of a cross-bridge (i.e., attached or detached) and the biochemical events involved in converting the chemical energy of ATP into mechanical work and heat (i.e., ATP hydrolysis). Consequently, it seems logical to assume that the V_{max} of skeletal

TABLE 11.2.
MHC and MLC Composition of Various Native Myosin Isoforms

Native Isoform	MHC Isoform	Essential MLC Isoform	Regulatory MLC Isoform
SM	Slow MHC I homodimer	SLC 1 homodimer	SLC2 homodimer
IM	Fast MHC IIA homodimer	SLC1/FLC1 heterodimer	FLC2 homodimer
FM3	Fast MHC IIB homodimer	FLC1 homodimer	FLC2 homodimer
FM2	Fast MHC IIB homodimer	FLC1/FLC3 heterodimer	FLC2 homodimer
FM1	Fast MHC IIB homodimer	FLC3 homodimer	FLC2 homodimer

muscle must be related to the myosin ATPase activity of muscle. The relationship between V_{max} and myosin ATPase activity was firmly established by the classical study by Barany [4].

Given the ATPase properties of the MHC, Reiser and colleagues [111–114] performed a more stringent test of the relationship between V_{max} and MHC isoform composition by examining this relationship at the single-fiber level. Reiser et al. [113, 114] initially demonstrated that the maximal unloaded shortening velocity (V_o) of single fibers from the SOL muscle was correlated with the fraction of fast MHC found in these fibers. Subsequently, Reiser and colleagues [111–114] performed a series of studies that examined this relationship in animals undergoing developmental and hypokinetic manipulations. In each case, the V_o-MHC relationship was confirmed. Consistent with the findings of Reiser and colleagues, Caiozzo et al. [22] reported a high correlation between the V_o and the fast Type IIA MHC isoform composition of the SOL muscle.

More recently, Bottinelli and colleagues [6, 7] examined V_o across distinct populations of single fibers containing slow Type I, fast Type IIA, fast Type IIX, or fast Type IIB MHC isoforms. The findings of these investigators demonstrated that single fibers expressing the slow Type I MHC isoform had mean V_o values of 1.05 FL $\cdot$ s^{-1}. In contrast, fibers expressing either the fast Type IIA, IIX, or IIB MHC isoforms had mean V_o values of 2.33, 3.07, and 3.69 FL $\cdot$ s^{-1}, respectively. It is important to note that there was a high degree of overlap between the V_o values of the fast single fibers.

FUNCTIONAL SIGNIFICANCE OF MYOSIN LIGHT CHAINS. Several studies have tested the concept that the essential light-chain isoform composition of skeletal muscle also influences maximal shortening velocity [6, 34, 65, 74, 137]. The findings from these studies have been equivocal in nature. Sweeney et al. [137] examined the V_o of fast Type IIB fibers from rabbit psoas and tibialis anterior (TA) muscles. These muscles are thought to have similar MHC isoform compositions (i.e., fast Type IIB MHC) but different myosin light chain (MLC) isoform compositions. It was found that fast Type IIB fibers containing only fast LC3 had higher V_o values than those containing the fast LC1/LC3 heterodimer [137]. Consistent with the concept that MLC isoforms do play a role in determining maximal shortening velocity, Bottinelli et al. [6] found that the relative fast MLC3 isoform content was directly correlated with V_o in fast Type IIA, IIX, and IIB fibers. Interestingly, the correlation between V_o and the fast LC3 was also dependent on the predominant MHC isoform. Fibers containing the fast Type IIB MHC isoform had a greater dependence on the relative fast LC3 content than fibers containing either the fast Type IIA or IIX MHC isoforms. In contrast to the findings of Sweeney et al. [137] and Bottinelli et al. [6], Larsson and Moss [74] did not observe a correlation between V_o and essential light-chain isoform composition in single muscle fibers taken from biopsies of the human vastus lateralis muscle. Whether this represents a species-specific difference is currently not clear.

Effects of Thyroid State on MHC Gene Expression

HYPOTHYROIDISM. Hypothyroidism (a reduction in circulating T3) induces alterations in MHC phenotypes consisting of an increased expression of the slow Type I MHC isoform, coupled with a decreased expression of the fast Type IIB MHC [19, 20, 61, 101]. Bidirectional shifts have been observed in Types IIA/IIX MHC expression in response to hypothyroidism, depending on muscle type (see refs. 61 and 108 and *unpublished data*). For example, in rodent slow muscles, such as the SOL and VI, hypothyroidism causes a decrease in the expression of IIA/IIX MHCs. In fact, hypothyroidism causes all of the IIA/IIX fibers of the SOL muscle (approximately 10–15% of the total fiber pool) to express only the Type I MHC isoform. This apparently homogeneous fiber composition in the hypothyroid SOL is also observed in overloaded SOL muscles [57]. In the VI, not all the IIA and IIX fibers shift to Type I fibers (V. J. Caiozzo and F. Haddad, unpublished data). In fast muscles, such as the PLAN and the MG, hypothyroidism induces a small increase in Type I MHC expression, coupled with a small decrease in IIB MHC expression. As for the IIA and IIX MHC response to hypothyroidism in these fast muscles, it appears that it differs depending on regions of the muscle. For example, in the red inner core regions of muscles like the PLAN, hypothyroidism causes an increase in Types I and IIA MHCs and a decrease in Types IIX and IIB MHCs. In contrast, in the white superficial regions of fast muscles like the PLAN, hypothyroidism causes an increase in IIX expression and a decrase in IIB MHC expression (V. J. Caiozzo and F. Haddad, unpublished data). These observations are consistent with the findings of Petrof et al. [107], showing that hypothyroidism in rats resulted in an increase in Type I and IIA MHC expression, coupled with a decrease in IIX and IIB MHC expression in the pharyngeal dilator muscle, a fast-twitch muscle (90% Type II). It is important to note that results reported earlier [18–20, 22, 30, 40] were controversial because most studies used electrophoretic techniques that did not separate the fast IIA and IIX MHC isoforms from one another. These findings suggest that there are a limited number of fibers within both the slow SOL and the red regions of the fast muscles (likely transformable Type IIA and/or IIX fibers) that revert to the expression of Type I MHC in the absence of sufficient levels of circulating T3, whereas a small proportion of the IIB fibers in the superficial region of fast muscle revert to the expression of IIX MHC.

The above findings concerning hypothyroidism effects on the PLAN muscle are particularly interesting, because this muscle responds to compensatory overload with a greater capacity for upregulating Type I MHC, as compared to that of experimental conditions involving hypothyroidism [57, 139]. Thus, the transformable IIA and IIX pool in the PLAN and other fast muscles may be differentially responsive to increased loading, as compared to that of hypothyroidism. This stimulus-dependent responsiveness might occur because this IIX-IIa pool is derived, in part, from two different types of transformable fibers: 1) transformed Type I fibers, which are believed to be sensitive to both thyroid and loading state; and 2) untransformed IIA and IIX fibers (and, possibly, some IIB fibers in the inner core of the muscle) that are particularly responsive to elevations in mechanical loading independent of thyroid state.

HYPERTHYROIDISM. Hindlimb skeletal muscle response to hyperthyroidism is opposite to that occurring in response to hypothyroidism. This response is remarkably similar in pattern to that induced by chronic states of unloading. The key observations are as follows: 1) there is upregulation of IIA/IIX MHC expression in approximately 30–35% of the fibers of the SOL muscle, whereas the remaining Type I fibers appear to be unresponsive [22, 124]; 2) a prolonged state of hyperthyroidism (20 wk) does not result in Type IIB MHC expression in the SOL muscle [19, 22]; and 3) in the PLAN, VI, and red MG muscles, there is a decrease in both the Type I and IIA/IIX MHC isoforms, as well as a concomitant increase in the expression of the Type IIB MHC isoform, but these transformations are relatively small (a 12–15% change). Interestingly, these findings further suggest that because IIA and IIX fibers are abundantly expressed in these faster muscles, there must be a large number of IIA and IIX fibers that are unresponsive to hyperthyroidism. Presently, it is unresolved as to whether unloading exerts a greater influence than hyperthyroidism in upregulating the expression of the faster MHCs in these relatively fast muscles. Also, it is not known whether the same population of fibers is responsive to both unloading and hyperthyroidism, or whether these different stimuli affect different populations of fibers.

MOLECULAR BASIS OF THYROID HORMONE ACTION ON THE MHC GENES. *Direct Thyroid Control of MHC Gene Expression.* Studies to date concerned with T3 regulation of muscle gene expression have largely focused on the MHC isoforms expressed in cardiac muscle [16, 17, 36, 60, 72, 103, 104, 116, 133, 134, 138]. Cardiac muscle expresses two MHC genes, one encoded for an α (fast) MHC and the other for a β (slow) MHC, respectively. Interestingly, the slow β-MHC gene in cardiac muscle is identical to the slow Type I MHC gene expressed in skeletal muscle. These α- and β-MHCs form native isomyosins V1 (αα), V2 (αβ), and V3 (ββ) that are responsible for the intrinsic functional properties of the cardiac cell. The contractile properties of the cardiac V1 and V3 isoforms are analogous with the fast and slow contractile properties found in skeletal muscle. Available evidence suggests the existence of thyroid response element(s) (TRE) in the regulatory region of both the α- and β-MHC genes that binds T3-TR complexes. The regulatory region of the β-MHC gene is depicted below [36, 143].

Studies have shown that the interactions of T3-TR-TRE exert positive and negative transcriptional control on the α- and the β-MHC genes, respectively. These findings suggest that the level of TRs maintained in the cell, as well as the level of TRAP proteins, may play an important role in the regulation of Type I MHC expression in different types of muscle, both under control conditions and in response to hormonal, metabolic, and mechanical intervention. In highlighting the role of TRs and TRAPs in MHC gene regulation, the study by Swoap et al. [138] showed that chronic energy deprivation, which upregulates cardiac β-MHC gene transcription while concomitantly decreasing cardiac α-MHC gene transcription (determined by nuclear run-on assays), is associated with a 2-fold decrease in the expression of TRs and TRAPs. These reported changes in cardiac β-MHC expression occurred without significant changes in circulating T3 levels [138]. Thus, the T3 axis, independent of circulating thyroid hormone level, can alter MHC expression in those MHC genes containing a TRE.

Indirect Control of Thyroid Hormone on MHC Genes. Studies of the effects of thyroid states on MHC expression in skeletal muscles demonstrate the responsiveness of the fast MHCs to T3 [57, 58, 61, 139]. The exact mechanism of this responsiveness is not clear, because the regulatory regions for IIA and IIX genes have not been isolated yet. Recently, the promoter region of the mouse Type IIB MHC gene was isolated [140]. Sequence analyses of the isolated region demonstrated the lack of a TRE, however this observation does not exclude the existence of a TRE upstream to the region analyzed. The figure below is a schematic representation of the promoter region of the mouse IIB MHC gene [140].

Myo-D, a myogenic protein, can exert positive transcriptional control on the IIB MHC promoter (via interaction with the MEF-1 site) when transfected into quail myotubes [140]. Furthermore, it has been shown that the promoter of the myo-D gene contains a TRE that enhances transcriptional activity when bound by T3-TR [98]. Because detectable levels of Myo-D have been measured in adult fast IIX and IIB fibers [55], it is possible that some of the modulatory influences of T3 on fast muscle fibers may be mediated via T3-induced expression of MyoD or possibly other nuclear factors that, in turn, act on either positive or negative regions of MHC gene promoters. Interestingly, it is apparent that the development of IIB MHC expression is significantly blunted when rodents are made hypothyroid during the neonatal period of muscle development [15].

Effects of Thyroid State on MLC Expression in Skeletal Muscle

HYPOTHYROIDISM. In response to hypothyroidism, both fast and slow skeletal muscle exhibit a general pattern of upregulating the slow essential and regulatory MLC isoforms. Specifically, Ianuzzo et al. [58] reported that hypothyroidism increased the relative SLC1 and SLC2 content of the PLAN muscle. Consistent with this observation, Fitzsimons et al. [40] and Caiozzo et al. [20] found that hypothyroidism increased the relative content of these two MLC isoforms in the red region of the MG and the PLAN muscles, respectively. Fitzsimons et al. [40], however, did not observe any influence of hypothyroidism on the MLC isoform distribution in the white region of the MG muscle. The slow SOL muscle is known to contain approximately 15% fast Type IIA fibers, and these fibers express the FLC1 and FLC2 isoforms. Hypothyroidism has been shown to repress the expression of these MLC isoforms [20, 40].

HYPERTHYROIDISM. In contrast to the fast-to-slow MLC transitions observed under conditions of hypothyroidism, hyperthyroidism has been shown to upregulate the expression of fast MLC isoforms in both fast and slow skeletal muscle. Fitzsimons et al. [40] and Caiozzo et al. [19] reported that hyperthyroidism downregulated the expression of the slow MLCs and upregulated the expression of the fast MLCs in the red region of the MG and the PLAN muscles, respectively. In contrast, however, it should be noted that Larsson et al. [73] recently reported that hyperthyroidism downregulated the relative FLC3 content in the extensor digitorum longus (EDL) and this appeared to be more pronounced in old animals. With respect to the slow skeletal muscle, it has been uniformly reported that hyperthyroidism increases the expression of FLC1 and FLC2 [19, 40, 58, 73].

EFFECTS OF THYROID STATE UPON THE SARCOPLASMIC RETICULUM

The SR plays a central role in the cyclic nature of activation-relaxation during skeletal muscle activity [88]. The three key properties of the SR that are essential for the cyclical activity of skeletal muscle are: 1) Ca^{2+} release; 2) Ca^{2+} uptake; and 3) Ca^{2+} storage. Release of Ca^{2+} from the SR is known to be dependent on the density of Ca^{2+} release channels, also known as ryanodine receptors [102]. Currently, two isoforms of the ryanodine receptor have been identified and categorized as cardiac and skeletal muscle isoforms [102]. With respect to the second SR process, Ca^{2+} uptake, it has been known for some time that this process is dictated by the amount and type of the 110-kd sarcoplasmic/endoplasmic reticulum Ca^{2+}-ATPase pump (SERCA) [8, 9, 14, 44, 83]. This protein represents approximately 60–70% of the protein content of the SR membrane. Currently, three SERCA genes have been identified and classified as SERCA1, SERCA2, and SERCA3 [44]. The SERCA1 gene is known to produce two protein isoforms (SERCA1a and SERCA1b) via alternative splicing [44]. The SERCA1a and SERCA1b protein isoforms have been found in adult fast skeletal muscle and neonatal skeletal muscle, respectively. The SERCA2 gene also is known to undergo alternative splicing, producing the SERCA2a and SERCA2b protein isoforms that are found, respectively, in slow/cardiac and smooth muscle [1, 153]. The SERCA3 protein isoform is found in a variety of nonmuscle tissue. The SR Ca^{2+}-ATPase activity of cardiac and slow skeletal muscle has been shown to be sensitive to a small transmembrane protein in the SR known as phospholamban. The nonphosphorylated form of phospholamban is thought to inhibit the SR Ca^{2+}-ATPase activity by altering its Km. In contrast, the phosphorylated form of phospholamban significantly increases the Ca^{2+}-ATPase activity of the SR [3, 110]. Finally, within the lumen of the SR, calsequestrin [154] has been shown to act as an important Ca^{2+} buffer, lowering the free Ca^{2+} concentration within the lumen and reducing the gradient against which the Ca^{2+}-ATPase pump must work. Two isoforms of calsequestrin have been discovered and identified as cardiac/slow and fast isoforms [51, 54].

Effects of Thyroid State on Ca^{2+} Uptake and SR Ca^{2+}-ATPase Activity

The Ca^{2+}-ATPase pump is thought to expend 1 molecule of ATP for every 2 Ca^{2+} taken up by the SR [54, 88]. The energy cost of the SR Ca^{2+}-ATPase pump has been reported to represent $\sim 25\%$ of the metabolic expenditure during contractile activity [150].

HYPOTHYROIDISM. The effect of thyroid state upon the SR Ca^{2+}-ATPase pump has been examined by several investigators [3, 38, 71, 82, 100, 129, 136, 147, 157]. The study by Farnburg [38] was one of the first to examine the influence of thyroid state on the Ca^{2+} uptake rate and Ca^{2+}-ATPase activity of the SR. Farnburg [38] reported that 4 wk of hypothyroidism (induced by propylthiouracil) reduced the Ca^{2+} uptake rate of fragmented SR (FSR) preparations by approximately 30%. In contrast, however, Farnburg did not observe any changes in the Ca^{2+}-ATPase activity of the FSR. It should be noted, however, that the FSRs that were prepared by Farnburg were obtained from the entire hindlimb musculature. Given the potential role of fiber type-specific responses to thyroid state, it is not surprising that the Ca^{2+}-ATPase activity of the FSR preparations were unaltered.

HYPERTHYROIDISM. Subsequently, Fitts and colleagues [39] examined the effect of hyperthyroidism on the Ca^{2+}-ATPase activity and Ca^{2+} uptake rate of the SR in slow and fast skeletal muscle. Initially, Fitts et al. [39] examined the effects of hyperthyroidism on the SR properties in the SOL muscle. Per gram of muscle, they found a 2-fold increase in the SR protein yield, a 3-fold increase in the Ca^{2+} ATPase activity, and a 2- to 3-fold increase in total Ca^{2+} uptake. Subsequently, this group of investigators reported that hyperthyroidism increased the Ca^{2+} uptake rate in the slow SOL muscle (+90%) but had no effect in the fast deep and superficial regions of the vastus lateralis. Consistent with these findings, it was noted that hyperthyroidism increased the yield of FSR by approximately 2.3-fold in the SOL muscle [37, 69].

At the single-fiber level, Muller et al. [94] have observed immunohistochemically that in the SOL muscle, hyperthyroidism decreased the percentage of fibers containing the slow SERCA2a protein isoform from a control value of ~80 to ~65%. This finding is consistent with those of Schiaffino et al. [123] and Caiozzo et al. [22], who reported that only a subpopulation of slow fibers in the SOL muscle was capable of upregulating the fast MHC protein isoform content under hyperthyroid conditions.

Effects of Thyroid State on SERCA mRNA Levels

HYPOTHYROIDISM. Table 11.3 represents a summary of the effects of hypothyroidism on SERCA mRNA isoform expression in different types of skeletal muscles. These data show that hypothyroidism affects SERCA mRNA expression in both slow and fast muscles (Table 11.3). In the slow SOL muscle, both fast SERCA1 and slow SERCA2 mRNA were reduced, although the reduction in the fast isoform was more prominent [122, 130]. In the fast EDL, there is general agreement that the fast SERCA1 mRNA expression is decreased under hypothyroid conditions [122, 130].

In contrast, the slow SERCA2 mRNA expression in the EDL was reported to be either undetected [130] or increased by 75% [122]. The reason for this discrepancy is not clear. It could be attributable to differences in the rat strain used (Wistar vs. Sprague-Dawley) or to a difference in hybridization methodology. When detected, this slow isoform constitutes only a very small percentage of the total SERCA mRNA expressed in EDL (5–10%; see ref. 122). Note that in the rabbit, slow SOL muscle, fast SERCA1 mRNA could not be detected in either the control or hypothyroid state [3]. This observation suggests the existence of both species-specific and tissue-specific expression of the SERCA genes.

HYPERTHYROIDISM. Table 11.4 provides a summary of the effects of hyperthyroidism on SERCA mRNA isoform expression in different types of skeletal muscles. These data show that, in the slow SOL muscle, the fast SERCA1 mRNA isoform expression was increased in response to hyperthyroidism, whereas no change could be detected in the fast SERCA1 expression in fast EDL. These results correlate well with the Ca^{2+} ATPase activity

TABLE 11.3.
Hypothyroidism Effects on SERCA1 and SERCA2 mRNA Levels in Slow (SOL) and Fast (EDL) Muscles

	Slow (SOL)	*Fast (EDL)*
Fast SERCA1 mRNA	↓78% [130] ↓77% [122] ND [3][a]	↓[130] ↓40% [122]
Slow SERCA2 mRNA	↓75% [130] ↓50% [122] ↓25% [3]	ND [130] ↑75% [122]

[a]ND, not detected; ↑, increases by; ↓, decreases by. Refs. are in brackets.

TABLE 11.4.
Hyperthyroidism Effects on SERCA1 and SERCA2 mRNA Levels in Slow (SOL) and Fast (EDL) Muscles

	Slow (SOL)	Fast (EDL)
Fast SERCA1 mRNA	↑10× [130][a] ↑152% [122] ↑ [3]	↔ [122, 130]
Slow SERCA2 mRNA	↔ [130] ↓29% [122] ↑40–90% [3]	ND [130] ↓40% [122]

[a]ND, not detected; ↔, no change; ↑, increases; ↓, decreases. Refs. are in brackets.

of these muscles [130]. The reported effects of hyperthyroidism on the slow SERCA2 mRNA isoform expression are equivocal. For example, in the slow SOL muscle, hyperthyroidism has been shown to cause either no change, a decrease, or an increase in the SERCA2 mRNA expression (Table 11.4). The reason for these differences is not clear. It could be attributable to differences in either the species examined or the technical conditions used. Furthermore, in the fast EDL muscle, slow SERCA2 isoform was reported to be either undetected or decreased in the hyperthyroid fast EDL (Table 11.4).

These collective findings suggest that SERCA mRNA isoform expression is regulated by thyroid hormone in skeletal muscle in a muscle-type specific manner (fast vs. slow). As reported above for the regulation of the myosin heavy chain, the same isoform could be either upregulated or downregulated by thyroid hormone, according to muscle type. This specificity in regulation is likely the result of a complex interplay among multiple tissue-specific nuclear factors interacting in a coordinated fashion with TREs on T3 responsive genes. More information is necessary about this tissue-specific regulation, because it is one of the most important and common mechanisms involved in skeletal muscle adaptation.

Modulation of SERCA Gene Transcription by Thyroid Hormone

In one of the initial studies that examined transcriptional modulation of SERCA genes by the thyroid hormone, Rohrer et al. [117] demonstrated that the slow SERCA2 gene was sensitive to as little as 1–10 pM T3, and that induction can be observed in as little as 8 hr after the onset of T3 exposure. Rohrer et al. [117] concluded further that these in vitro findings were very similar to the sensitivity and time-course observed under in vivo conditions.

In addition to the effects of T3 on expression of the slow SERCA2 gene, Rohrer et al. [118] also examined the separate influence of retinoic acid (RA). Although RA was capable of upregulating the expression of the SERCA2 gene, it had a much lower EC_{50} than that of T3 (2 nM vs. 30 pM, respectively).

Rohrer et al. [118] identified a region 60 nucleotides long that was -322 to -262 from the transcription start site. This sequence was found to have a high degree of homology with a known TRE found in the growth hormone gene. A subsequent study by Hartong et al. [48] examined the promoter region of the SERCA2 gene in more detail and yielded the following key results. First, three separate TREs were identified and designated as TRE1 (-481 to -458), TRE2 (-310 to -289), and TRE3 (-219 to -194). These TREs were found to differ from one another in spacing, orientation, and nucleotide sequence of the half-sites. Secondly, each TRE was found to exhibit specific binding properties with regard to TR isoforms. For example, TR-α1 isoforms bind to TRE1 as monomers, whereas TR-β isoforms bind as homodimer. TRE2 and TRE3 were both found to bind TR-α as a homodimer. Finally, with respect to TR-RXR complexes, RXRs were found to enhance the binding of TR-α and TR-β to TRE1 in the form of RXR-TR heterodimers, whereas there was a preferential homodimeric complex binding on TRE2 and TRE3 in the presence of RXR [48]. Despite differences in their binding properties, it was found that all three TREs conferred similar T3 responsiveness on promoters of reporter genes [48]. This finding on the presence of multiple TREs on the SERCA2 gene with different specificity for TR isoforms and homodimers/heterodimer binding might have important physiological significance. It allows for a complex interplay between the TRs and other transcriptional factors in order to achieve optimal regulation of the SERCA2 gene expression under diverse pathophysiological conditions.

EFFECTS OF THYROID STATE ON MECHANICAL PROPERTIES OF SKELETAL MUSCLE

The Force-Velocity Relationship

When skeletal muscle contracts against heavy loads, it shortens slowly. Conversely, when skeletal muscle contracts against light loads, it shortens rapidly. This property of skeletal muscle is known as the force-velocity relationship and can be described by the Hill equation:

$$(P + a)(V + b) = b(P_o + a)$$

where P_o is maximal isometric tension, P is isotonic tension, V is shortening velocity, and a and b are constants with the dimensions of force and velocity, respectively. The ratio of $a{:}P_o$ describes the extent of the curvature in the force-velocity relationship (e.g., the lower this ratio, the more curved the force-velocity relationship). The force-velocity relationship represents one of the most important contractile properties of skeletal muscle because it: 1) describes the spectrum of possible force-velocity interactions; 2) determines the mechanical work and power output of skeletal muscle; 3) determines the enthalpy change (Δheat + Δwork) during contraction; 4) determines the rate of ATP hydrolysis; 5) dictates the efficiency of contraction; and 6) reflects the basic molecular events responsible for generating tension.

From a mechanistics perspective, Huxley [56] proposed that cross-bridges operated within two realms: 1) x/h>0; and 2) x/h<0. Within the first realm, cross-bridges act to generate a positive force. However, as the velocity of contraction increases, it is postulated that a progressive number of cross-bridges are swept into the negative force x/h < 0 region. Here, cross-bridges are to retard those attached in the positive force region. At V_{max}, it is believed that the forces generated by the cross-bridges attached in the positive region just balance those in the negative region, resulting in zero force.

Based on this explanation, muscles with faster ATPase activities should have a higher V_{max}, because at any given shortening velocity, fewer cross-bridges would have been swept into the negative force region. Consistent with this speculation, the study of Barany [4] was the first to demonstrate across a wide diversity of muscles that there is a high correlation between V_{max} and ATPase activity. Subsequently, it was found that multiple isoforms of myosin existed. Over the last 10 years, investigators have shown [6, 7, 22, 111–114], at both the whole-muscle and single-fiber level, that there is a good correlation between myosin isoform content and maximal shortening velocity.

THE EFFECTS OF ALTERED THYROID STATES ON THE FORCE-VELOCITY RELATIONSHIP OF SKELETAL MUSCLE.

Maximal Shortening Velocity. The study by Gold et al. [43] was the first to demonstrate, in skeletal muscle, that thyroid state influences the isotonic contractile properties of slow skeletal muscle. Using an afterload condition that represented approximately 3% of P_o Gold et al. [43] found that under hyperthyroid conditions, the shortening velocity of the SOL muscle was approximately 20% greater than normal. Under hypothyroid conditions, Gold et al. [43] found that the shortening velocity of the SOL muscle was only 60% of normal. Subsequently, Caiozzo et al. [19] and Montgomery [92] found, respectively, that hyperthyroidism produced 27 and 50% increases in V_{max}. Also, consistent with the initial findings of Gold et al. [43], both Caiozzo et al. [20] and Montgomery [92] reported that hypothyroidism reduced V_{max} by approximately 20%. In contrast to the findings of Gold et al. [43], Montgomery [92], and Fitts et al. [39] reported that hyperthyroidism did not increase V_{max} in the SOL muscle. This finding is somewhat surprising because Fitts et al. [39] found changes in the isometric twitch properties and a large increase in the fast Type IIC fiber population.

It should be emphasized that the impact of thyroid state on the maximal shortening velocity is dependent upon the method used to measure maximal shortening velocity. Measurements of maximal shortening velocity have classically been determined by extrapolation of force-velocity data. Because the low force region of the force-velocity relationship deviates from a hyperbola, measurements of V_{max} underestimate the true maximal shortening velocity of skeletal muscle. Edman [35] developed the slack test, which provides a measurement of the unloaded maximal shortening velocity of skeletal muscle (V_o). It has been shown that V_o [19, 20, 22] is typically greater than V_{max}, but this difference is dependent upon the myosin isoform composition of skeletal muscle.

Consistent with this perspective, it has been shown in the SOL muscle that hyperthyroidism increased V_{max} by 27%, while V_o was increased by 54%, respectively [19, 22]. In contrast, hypothyroidism decreased V_{max} and V_o by 20% and 32% respectively in the same muscle [19, 22].

The effects of altered thyroid state on V_{max} and V_o have also been studied in the PLAN muscle. Hyperthyroidism did not affect either of these two measurements. In contrast, hypothyroidism reduced V_{max} and V_o in the PLAN by approximately 6 and 19%, respectively. Consistent with the alterations in maximal shortening velocity, a decrease in the fast native isoforms and a concomitant increase in the SM1 native isoform were also found [19, 20].

Maximal Isometric Tension. The amount of isometric force that can be produced by a muscle is thought to be dependent on the amount of contractile protein in parallel. Hypothyroidism has been shown to retard the rate of muscle growth. Hence, muscle mass from hypothyroid animals is usually less than that from control animals. Therefore, maximal isometric tension of a muscle is reduced in a hypothyroid state; however, when maximal isometric tension is normalized to cross-sectional area (i.e., specific tension), the effects of thyroid state were not significant.

The Force-Frequency Relationship

The force that a muscle fiber produces is not only dependent on the amount of contractile protein in parallel but also on the relationship between force and frequency of stimulation. The shape and position of the force-frequency relationship is determined, in part, by the rate of relaxation. In muscles composed predominantly of slow Type I fibers, relaxation occurs at a slow rate. In muscles composed primarily of fast muscle fibers, the kinetics of relaxation are much faster. As a result, the force-frequency relationship of slow muscle fibers is shifted to the left of that found in fast muscle fibers.

As mentioned above, hyperthyroidism has been shown, in the SOL muscle, to produce a conversion of some slow Type I fibers to fast Type IIA/IIX fibers. Consistent with this conversion of slow to fast fibers, the force-frequency relationship of the SOL muscle is shifted to the right [19].

In contrast, hypothyroidism has been shown to completely repress the expression of fast fibers in the SOL muscle. Although the SOL muscle only contains approximately 15% fast muscle fibers, this conversion of the fast fibers to slow fibers has been shown to produce significant alterations in the force-frequency relationship. This finding suggests that the small relative population of fast fibers in the SOL muscle plays an important role in determining the mechanical properties of this muscle.

Fast muscles like the PLAN have been shown to be much less sensitive to thyroid state. Hence, the force-frequency relationship of fast muscles appears to be relatively insensitive to thyroid state [19, 20, 22].

Relaxation Kinetics

The relaxation properties of skeletal muscle have classically been described with the use of isometric twitch data. The time required for tension to decay 50% from the peak of the isometric twitch is known as one-half relaxation time (1/2RT). From a mechanistic perspective, it has been suggested that relaxation as described by 1/2RT is dependent on the rate Ca^{2+} sequestration, and not Ca^{2+} dissociation from troponin-C or cross-bridge detachment.

As with V_{max}, the thyroid hormone has been found to exert an influence over the relaxation properties that appears to be muscle specific. Fitts et al. [39], Caiozzo et al. [19], Montgomery [92], and Larsson and Moss [73] each reported that hyperthyroidism decreased the 1/2RT of the SOL muscle by approximately 30–50%. In contrast, hyperthyroidism has been found to produce smaller changes in 1/2RT of fast muscles like the PLAN [19] and extensor digitorum longus [73]. With respect to hypothyroidism, Caiozzo et al. [20] and Montgomery [92] found that the 1/2RT of the SOL muscle was increased by approximately 100%. The effects of hypothyroidism on fast skeletal muscle are not as uniform. For example, Caiozzo et al. [20] and Dulhunty [33] reported that hypothyroidism did not affect the relaxation rate of the PLAN and EDL muscles, respectively. In contrast, Leijendekker and van Hardeveld [81] reported that hypothyroidism increased 1/2RT of the rodent gastrocnemius muscle by approximately 70%.

From a mechanistic perspective, Dulhunty [33] correlated the density of Ca^{2+} ATPase pumps with relaxation rates under euthyroid and hyperthyroid conditions. A high correlation between the Ca^{2+} ATPase content of the SOL muscle and its rate of relaxation after tetanus was reported [33]. However, Dulhunty [33] was not able to demonstrate a similar relationship with respect to the tension decay in fast-twitch muscle (EDL).

The rate of relaxation is known to be dependent on muscle length. Interestingly, the length dependence of relaxation can be modified by altering the thyroid state. As shown in Figure 11.5 the mean 1/2RT of control SOL muscles was ~40 ms at a muscle length that corresponded to -3 mm L_o. At a muscle length that was 3 mm beyond L_o, the mean 1/2RT increased to a value of 70 ms. In contrast to the relaxation rate of the control muscles, the hypothyroid data presented in Figure 11.5 indicates that over this same range of muscle length, 1/2RT increased by 100 ms. Currently, it is unclear

FIGURE 11.5.

The relationship between one-half relaxation time and muscle length is depicted here. So that researchers could gain some insight regarding the importance of fiber type, a group of animals underwent thyroidectomy and injections of propylthiouracil. Hypothyroidism causes the SOL to become a truly slow muscle with no fast fibers. In contrast, the control SOL muscles contain approximately 15% fast muscle fibers. Note that, for both the hypothyroid and control groups, 1/2RT is dependent on muscle length. The dependence of 1/2RT on muscle length, however, was much greater for the hypothyroid SOL muscle.

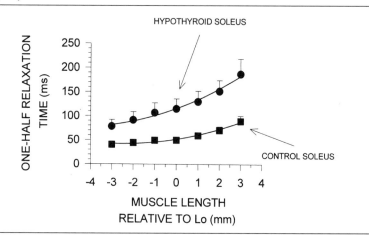

as to whether this increased length dependence of relaxation in the SOL muscle is attributable to fast fibers transforming into slower fibers, or whether all muscle fibers have an increased length dependence of relaxation.

Postetanic Twitch Potentiation

Potentiation of isometric twitch tension can be produced after various levels of tetany. Currently, it is believed that the extent of twitch potentiation is governed by the level of P-light chain phosphorylation. P-light chain phosphorylation is regulated by a Ca^{2+}-calmodulin system that modulates the level of myosin light-chain kinase (MLCK) activity. Slow muscles such as the SOL are known to have low levels of MLCK, whereas fast muscles contain large amounts of this enzyme. The causal relationship between twitch potentiation and MLCK activity is supported by the observation that slow muscles such as the SOL have low levels of MLCK and twitch potentiation, whereas fast muscles like the gastrocnemius contain high levels of MLCK and exhibit high degrees of twitch potentiation [93, 106].

Given the potential relationship between P-light chain phosphorylation and twitch potentiation, Leijendekker and van Hardeveld [81] found that hypothyroidism reduced the degree of P-light chain phosphorylation. They found that the isometric twitch potentiation of the hypothyroid gastrocnemius (GAST) muscle was less than that of the euthyroid muscles. Consistent with these mechanical findings, they reported that hypothyroidism reduced the degree of P-light chain phosphorylation.

The Work Loop Technique: an Integrative Contractile Measurement

The work loop technique (see Fig. 11.6), as studied by Josephson and Stokes [63, 64], represents a powerful approach for investigating the capacity of skeletal muscle to produce mechanical work and power. This technique allows the investigator to impose various waveforms of length change on a muscle, attempting to simulate the shortening-lengthening cycles that occur under normal in vivo conditions. Each of the factors described in Figure 11.1 potentially can affect measurements of mechanical work and, using the work loop method, it is possible to identify the theoretical mechanical work (based on force-velocity data) and realized mechanical work (i.e., that work actually measured). The difference between theoretical and actual mechanical work represents limitations imposed by either activation or relaxation.

Under conditions of hypothyroidism, the ability of slow muscles such as the SOL to produce mechanical work is reduced for several reasons (see Fig. 11.7). First, the force-velocity relationship is altered in such a way that at any level of force, the shortening velocity will be less. Hence, the theoretical capacity of muscle is reduced. Secondly, activation occurs at a slower rate. As a consequence, the amount of mechanical work unrealized because of factors controlling the rate of activation is increased. Thirdly, relaxation occurs at a slower rate. Hence, a greater duration of the shortening phase must be devoted to relaxation, minimizing the realization of mechanical work.

INTERACTION OF THYROID STATE AND LOADING CONDITIONS ON MHC PHENOTYPE

The phenotypic expression of myosin appears to be under the control of neural, hormonal, and mechanical factors [13, 29, 30, 40, 46, 61, 120]. Recently, the interaction of the thyroid hormone with altered mechanical loading states has been studied [21, 30, 57, 70]. Mechanical unloading, as induced by hindlimb suspension or microgravity, has been shown to increase the relative fast myosin isoform content and population of fast fibers. In contrast, increased mechanical loading induced by synergistic ablation or high-resistance training has been shown to upregulate the slower myosin isoforms and fiber types [21, 139]. As mentioned by Ianuzzo et al. [57], some investigators have suggested that activity predominates over hor-

FIGURE 11.6.

Illustration of work loop technique. Top panel illustrates sinusoidal length change that is imposed on the muscle. Muscle length is expressed relative to L_o (= 0 mm). In this example, the amplitude of sinusoidal length change is 4 mm and has a frequency of 1 Hz. The muscle is stimulated at the peak of the sine wave, and force is produced (middle panel). The duration of stimulation was set so that the muscle was completely relaxed by the onset of the subsequent lengthening phase. The force observed during the lengthening phase is attributable to the passive compliance of the muscle. The force-length relationship, obtained from the top and middle panels, is plotted in the bottom panel and represents a work loop. The area under the force-length curve during the shortening phase (from + 2 mm to − 2 mm) represents total positive mechanical work. The area under the force-length curve during the lengthening phase (from − 2 mm to + 2 mm) represents negative mechanical work. The difference between total positive and negative work is net mechanical work and is represented by the area within the work loop.

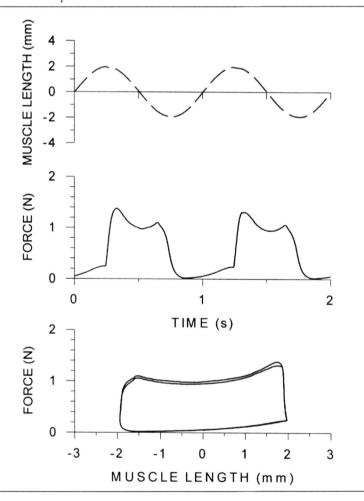

FIGURE 11.7.
Theoretical (solid line) and actual (dashed line) work loops produced by control (left panel) and hypothyroid (right panel) soleus muscles. The theoretical work loops were determined from force-velocity data, whereas the actual work loops were measured while having the muscles perform sinusoidal length changes with a strain of approximately 14% L_0 and a frequency of 1 Hz. Note that the capacity of the hypothyroid soleus to produce mechanical work is reduced because: 1) it has less theoretical capacity, as determined by alterations in the force-velocity relationship; and 2) the muscle has slower relaxation kinetics and must begin relaxation earlier than the control muscle. As a result of this earlier initiation of relaxation, a greater amount of mechanical work is unrealized in the hypothyroid soleus muscle.

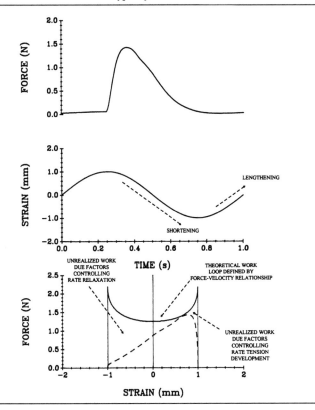

monal influences. The findings described below are diametric to this supposition.

Hyperthyroidism vs. Functional Overload

When studied independently, hyperthyroidism and overload produce opposite effects on MHC adaptations. When the two interventions were placed in competition against one another, the hyperthyroid state was able to completely block the overload-induced increase in Type I expression in both SOL and PLAN muscles [57, 139]. Thus, elevations in thyroid hormone can block the mechanical stimulus that normally results in up-regulation of Type I MHC expression in those responsive fibers. However, hyperthyroidism does not appear to be capable of fully blunting the down-regulation of IIB MHC expression that is associated with functional overload of the PLAN [139]. The relative changes at mRNA level paralleled those observed at the protein level, suggesting that the influence of thyroid state, under these experimental conditions, occurs at a pretranslational/transcriptional level. This same response was observed in the superficial GAST muscle, when hyperthyroidism was competed with heavy-resistance training, i.e., hyperthyroidism was partially effective in blunting the down-regulation of Type IIB MHC [18].

The chronic low frequency stimulation (CLFS) model that has been used by Pette and Staron [108] represents another method by which the mechanical activity of a muscle can be modulated. The CLFS model has been shown to be a powerful modulator of myosin isoform expression. Kirschbaum et al. [70] reported that CLFS reduced the relative fast Type IIB MHC protein isoform of rodent TA muscle from a control value of 67 to 15% of the total MHC protein isoform pool. When CLFS was combined with hyperthyroidism, it was found that this reduction in fast Type IIB MHC protein isoform was blunted.

Hypothyroidism vs. Hindlimb Unloading

These two interventions also independently produce opposite effects on MHC adaptations [29, 30, 141]. Consequently, when animals were subjected simultaneously to hypothyroidism and hindlimb suspension, the hypothyroid state completely prevented the unloading-induced transformations in the various MHC phenotypes that occurred in the euthyroid SOL, VI, and PLAN muscles [30]. Furthermore, relative changes at the mRNA level paralleled those occurring at the protein level, further suggesting that the influence of thyroid state, under these experimental conditions, is occurring at a pretranslational/transcriptional level [30].

Collectively, the responses summarized in this section raise the question as to whether adaptations involving Type I MHC phenotype in response to mechanical activity are mediated via thyroid control of the Type I gene. For example, hindlimb unloading might produce an increase in the Type IIX (and IIA) content of slow SOL muscle by increasing the sensitivity of a portion of the slow fibers in this muscle to circulating T3. Similarly, functional overload might upregulate transformed Type I/IIA fibers by causing these muscle fibers to become less sensitive to circulating T3 levels, i.e., they revert to expressing primarily Type I MHC in the presence of mechanical stress.

FUTURE RESEARCH

Studies of Gene Regulation In Vivo

Elucidation of the intracellular signals and the regulatory factors controlling muscle adaptation as a result of altered mechanical activity or of hormonal change has been a major focus in research for the past several decades, and it will continue to be a challenge for future researchers. Advances in molecular biology metholodogy can be applied to study the role of certain genes in muscle physiology and adaptation. Much of the information on the molecular basis of T3 action and the role of TRs and other transcription factors in the regulation of gene transcription comes from in vitro studies. This in vitro research involves the introduction into cell cultures of the 5' regulatory sequences linked to reporter genes with or without expression vectors for a specific receptor. However, cell culture systems do not represent precisely what goes on in a physiological setting in the whole animal. In fact, fundamental differences exist on how genes are regulated in vivo vs in vitro [16, 17]. One approach to studying either transcriptional regulation of a gene or the function of a particular gene in intact animals is the use of both transgenic animals and direct gene transfer methods.

TRANSGENIC ANIMALS. Transgenic mouse technology has been widely used for the study of gene function and regulation in many areas of biomedicine (see refs. 87 and 145 for review). Transgenic mice can be produced by microinjection of DNA constructs in the male pronucleus, i.e., the larger of the two pronuclei, of fertilized eggs that are then retransferred into the oviducts of pseudopregnant females and allowed to develop to term. A proportion of the offspring have the foreign DNA sequences permanently integrated into their genome and thus become transgenic. Using transgenic mice became a more powerful technique with the development of gene targeting via the embryonic stem cell system [87]. While initial trangenic mice development involved random integration of the foreign DNA into the host genome, in gene targeting technology, homologous recombination between input and host DNA is exploited to introduce a specific alteration to a particular host gene. Embryonic stem (ES) cells are derived from the inner cell mass of early mouse embryos (blastocyst). These ES cells can be grown in culture and can be reimplanted into the mouse embryo, where they can contribute to the development of a chimeric animal (part from the host embryo and part from ES cells). When a specific gene alteration is introduced to the ES cells in culture, the resulting targeted gene can be one part of the chimeric animals' germline and, thus, can be transmitted to future generations. Usually, contribution of the ES gametes to an animal and transmission into future generations are monitored, using a coat-colored genetic marker [87]. Using these methods, one can produce mice with any desired genetic alteration.

The regulation of gene expression in vivo can be studied by producing transgenic mice, whereby the transgene is composed of the regulatory sequences of a gene of interest driving the expression of a reporter gene. To delineate DNA sequences necessary for tissue-specific expression and regulation of a certain gene, transgenic mice can be produced that contain several deletions or mutations of the 5' flanking sequence linked to a prokaryotic reporter gene (chloramphenicol transferase). Using this approach, the regulation of β-myosin heavy-chain gene expression in the heart and skeletal muscle and its regulation by thyroid hormone were studied [116]. It was demonstrated that the region located in the 600 bp upstream of the β-MHC gene is sufficient for skeletal muscle-specific expression [116]. In contrast, for cardiac-specific expression of the β-MHC gene, a region located in the 5600 bp upstream was required [116]. This study also points out that thyroid hormone regulation requires elements that are not identical, in cardiac vs skeletal muscles. Similar approaches were used in studying thyroid regulation of the α-MHC gene [133, 134] and the tissue-specific expression of the cardiac myosin LC2 gene [79, 80].

Furthermore, using transgenic animals allows one to obtain the overexpression of genes, which can be targeted to the muscle using muscle-specific promoters, which provides more insight into the functional significance of a particular protein. For example, muscles overexpressing the glucose transporter protein GLUT 1 exhibited an increase in their basal glucose transport, but insulin did not stimulate glucose uptake any further [45]. Also, overexpression of Glut 4 significantly improved the diabetic state in dbdb mice [42, 47]. Muscle creatine kinase-B isoform overexpression did not significantly alter the metabolic state of the muscle [10], whereas overexpression of the dystrophin gene in muscle eliminated the dystrophic symptoms without adverse effects in mice [25]. This approach was also used to study the role of activated protein kinase C in the regulation of β-MHC gene expression in cardiac muscle and the induction of cardiac hypertrophy [67]. The above studies demonstrate that the overexpression of genes in skeletal muscles is possible and can be used not only to gain further insight into the functional aspect of a protein but also can be applied in clinical aspect, such as for gene therapy.

A more radical way of studying the function of a particular gene is by studying the consequences of its loss of function. Specific genes can be "knocked out" or turned off by homologous recombination and gene targeting [87, 127, 145]. A series of gene knockout experiments has contributed to the understanding of the role of basic helix loop helix (bHLH) transcription factors in the control of muscle development. MyoD, a member of the bHLH family, was initially thought to be a key protein in differentiation of myoblasts into myotubes, which is based on the fact that MyoD is expressed in muscle and can activate the transcription of several muscle-specific genes [119]. On the basis of MyoD properties, one would think that a MyoD knock out mouse would not develop mature muscle. However, it turned out that MyoD knockout developed normal muscle [119]. Targeting myf-5, another member of the bHLH family, also did not stop the development of muscle, but mice died at birth because of defective respiratory muscles [119]. However, targeting myogenin, a third member of the bHLH family, resulted in development of mice with very little muscle [50, 99, 119], pointing out the important role of myogenin in muscle differentiation. In the context of these studies, it would be interesting to create specific MHC isoform knockout or a specific TR isoform knockout to see what the effect would be on muscle fiber development and muscle phenotype.

The ability to readily assess the role of a particular gene in transgenic mice in vivo represents a major advance, bridging molecular biology and whole-animal physiology. However, for practical purpose, this approach is limited to small mammals, i.e., the mouse; therefore, it cannot be used in all situations, especially in studying rat muscle adaptation and, more importantly, human gene regulation.

DIRECT GENE TRANSFER. The demonstration of gene transfer in intact animals by simple injection of plasmid DNA into skeletal muscle is a tremendous development that provides convenient alternative ways to study gene regulation that combine the advantages of in vitro transfection assays and of the transgenic animal model. Straited muscles have the unique ability to uptake and express foreign DNA injected into their mass; this property is thought to be attributable to the existence of the T-tubule system [151]. One of the advantages in using direct gene transfer in muscles is that the uptaken DNA can be maintained episomally almost indefinitely, and expression can be studied at various times. This property has to do with the fact that after differentiation, muscles are in a postmitotic stage.

One drawback of this method, however, is the variability of expression. This variability can be overcome by coinjection of a constitutively expressed gene, in addition to the gene of interest. Activity for the gene of interest can be normalized relative to that of the constitutive gene.

Heterologous gene constructs consist of a promoter regulatory sequence of the gene of interest linked to a reporter gene that is usually not expressed in eukaryotic cells (such as chloramphenicol transferase, luciferase, or β-galactosidase). These constructs can be injected into a rat cardiac or skeletal muscle. Under altered functional or hormonal states, the transcriptional activity of the promoter can be tracked in either a whole muscle or at the single-fiber level, using immunohistochemistry.

This method is simpler, faster, and more economic than producing transgenic mice. Of greater importance is that this approach has proved promising in providing insight on how genes are regulated in vivo. For example, this approach was used to study the regulation of the α-MHC gene promoter in cardiac muscle under altered thyroid state and under pressure overload [17, 72, 91, 103, 104]. Ojamaa and Klein [103, 104] have shown that the α-MHC sequence (−613 to +421) is not sufficient to confer thyroid hormone regulation identical to what is observed normally in vivo. However, this sequence was able to confer tissue-specific expression, as no activity of the reporter gene was found when the gene construct was injected into skeletal muscle [72]. Other studies showed that mutation of the M-CAT and A-rich binding sites inhibits expression of the α-MHC enhancer/promoter in vivo, and pressure overload is associated with increased binding activity on these two binding sites [91]. One of the advantages of using this method over transgenic animals is that it can be applied to muscles of any species, including rats and, more importantly, to that of humans. Because of its potential use, it is important to find conditions that improve DNA transfer efficiency into skeletal muscle. This issue seems to be a concern of several laboratories [26, 152].

Refractory Fibers

One of the most intriguing aspects of studying muscle fiber adaptations to hormonal or mechanical stimuli is the existence of a subset of unresponsive fibers that have been classified as refractory Type I fibers [22]. These nonadaptive fibers were observed in the SOL in response to either hyperthyroidism, denervation, or high-frequency stimulation [22, 123]. Using immunohistochemical techniques, it was demonstrated that rat SOL muscle contains two populations of Type I fibers, which are similar in their phenotype but are different in their responsiveness to thyroid hormone and mechanical stimuli. The exact mechanism behind the existence of this refractory Type I subpopulation of fibers is not clear and remains to be explored in future studies. Do these refractory fibers lack specific nuclear factors necessary for fast MHC expression? Do they lack TRs or TRAPs? In order to better characterize these nonadaptive subpopulations of fibers, in situ hybridization and immunohistochemical methods provide powerful tools in this characterization. With respect to the origin of these subpopulation of fibers, it has been speculated that nonadaptive fibers and responsive fibers are different in their developmental history with respect to MHC expression, i.e., they originate from different myoblasts [22, 123]. Whether this differential response is attributable to developmental programs, difference in TR, or other mechanisms remains to be explored.

CONCLUSIONS

Our knowledge of muscle plasticity and adaptation in response to thyroid hormone and altered mechanical activity has expanded dramatically over the past decade. Altered gene expression for specific isoforms is a pivotal process in muscle adaptation. Recent studies have provided a wealth of information concerning muscle plasticity and regulation of muscle gene expression by thyroid hormone and mechanical activity. However, most of these studies focused their attention on the MHC and SR genes. It has been shown that both thyroid hormone and mechanical activity can induce rapid quantitative and qualitative alterations in muscle protein expression. This remodeling may have a significant impact on muscle functional properties. As for the molecular signaling involved in these adaptations, it is well established by now that thyroid hormone exerts its effects by altering the transcription of specific genes via direct interaction with nuclear receptors. Further research is needed in order to elucidate the precise mechanisms by which mechanical stimuli are converted into biochemical signals that lead to altered protein expression.

With the rapid progress and advances in molecular biology techniques, it is likely that in the future there will be a better understanding of the molecular basis of the complex process of muscle adaptation in response to both hormonal and mechanical stimuli.

ACKNOWLEDGMENTS

The authors are greatly indebted to Kenneth M. Baldwin for his guidance, support, and encouragement. This work was funded in part by NIH AR30346 (K.M.B.).

REFERENCES

1. Anger, M., J. L. Samuel, F. Marotte, F. Wuytack, L. Rappaport, and A. M. Lompre. In situ mRNA distribution of sarco(endo)plasmic reticulum Ca(2+)-ATPase isoforms during ontogeny in the rat. *J. Mol. Cell. Cardiol.* 26(4):539–550, 1994.
2. Angeras, U., and P. O. Hasselgren. Protein turnover in different types of skeletal muscle during experimental hyperthyroidism in rats. *Acta Endocrinol.* 109(1):90–95, 1985.
3. Arai, M., K. Otsu, D. H. Maclennan, N. R. Alpert, and M. Periasamy. Effect of thyroid hormone on the expression of mRNA encoding sarcoplasmic reticulum proteins. *Circ. Res.* 69:266–276, 1991.
4. Barany, M. ATPase activity of myosin correlated with speed of muscle shortening. *J. Gen. Physiol.* 50S:197–216, 1967.
5. Bendik, I., and M. Pfahl. Similar ligand-induced conformational changes of thyroid hormone receptors regulate homo- and heterodimeric functions. *J. Biol. Chem.* 270(7):3107–3114, 1994.
6. Bottinelli, R., R. Betto, S. Schiaffino, and C. Reggiani. Unloaded shortening velocity and myosin heavy chain and alkali light chain isoform composition in rat skeletal muscle fibres. *J. Physiol.* 478:341–349, 1994.
7. Bottinelli, R., S. Schiaffino, and C. Reggiani. Force-velocity relations and myosin heavy chain isoform compositions of skinned fibres from rat skeletal muscle. *J. Physiol.* 437:655–672, 1991.
8. Brandl, C. J., S. deLeon, D. R. Martin, and D. H. Maclennan. Adult forms of the Ca(2+)-ATPase of sarcoplasmic reticulum. *J. Biol. Chem.* 262(8):3768–3774, 1987.
9. Brandl, C. J., N. M. Green, B. Korczak, and D. H. Maclennan. Two Ca(2+)-ATPase genes:

homologies and mechanistic implications of deduced amino acid sequences. *Cell* 44:597–607, 1986.

10. Brosnan, M. J., S. P. Raman, L. Chen, and A. P. Koretsky. Altering creatine kinase isoenzymes in transgenic mouse muscle by overexpression of the B subunit. *Am. J. Physiol.* 264(Part 1):C151–160, 1993.

11. Brown, J. G., and D. J. Millward. Dose response of protein turnover in rat skeletal muscle to triiodothyronine treatment. *Biochim. Biophys. Acta.* 757:182–190, 1983.

12. Brown, J. G., P. C. Bates, M. A. Holliday, and D. J. Millward. Thyroid hormones and muscle protein turnover. *Biochem. J.* 194:771–782, 1981.

13. Buller, A. J., J. C. Eccles, and R. M. Eccles. Interactions between motoneurons and muscles in respect to the characteristic speeds of their responses. *J. Physiol.* 150:417–439, 1960.

14. Burk, S. E., J. Lytton, D. H. Maclennan, and G. E. Shull. cDNA cloning, functional expression, and mRNA tissue distribution of a third organellar $Ca(2+)$-pump. *J. Biol. Chem.* 264(31):18561–18568, 1989.

15. Butler-Browne, G. S., D. Herlicoviez, and R. G. Whalen. Effects of hypothyroidism on myosin isozyme transitions in developing rat muscle. *F.E.B.S. Lett.* 166:71–75, 1984.

16. Buttrick, P. M., M. L. Kaplan, R. N. Kitsis, and L. A. Leinwand. Distinct behavior of cardiac myosin heavy chain gene constructs in vivo. Discordance with in vitro results. *Circ. Res.* 72(6):1211–1217, 1993.

17. Buttrick, P. M., A. Kass, R. N. Kitsis, M. L. Kaplan, and L. A. Leinwand. Behavior of genes directly injected into the rat heart in vivo. *Circ. Res.* 70(1):193–198, 1992.

18. Caiozzo, V. J., M. J. Baker, C. Carmody, and K. M. Baldwin. The competitive interaction of high resistance training and thyroid hormone on myosin heavy chain isoform expression. *Med. Sci. Sports Exerc.* 27(5):S124, 1995.

19. Caiozzo, V. J., R. E. Herrick, and K. M. Baldwin. The influence of hyperthyroidism on the maximal shortening velocity and myosin isoform distribution in slow and fast skeletal muscles. *Am. J. Physiol.* 261:C285–295, 1991.

20. Caiozzo, V. J., R. E. Herrick, and K. M. Baldwin. Response of slow and fast muscle to hypothyroidism: maximal shortening velocity and myosin isoforms. *Am. J. Physiol.* 263(*Cell Physiol.* 32):C86–C94, 1992

21. Caiozzo, V. J., E. Ma, S. A. McCue, E. Smith, R. E. Herrick, and K. M. Baldwin. A new animal model for modulating myosin isoform expression by altered mechanical activity. *J. Appl. Physiol.* 73(4):1432–1440, 1992.

22. Caiozzo, V. J., S. Swoap, M. Tao, D. Menzel, and K. M. Baldwin. Single fiber analyses of type IIA myosin heavy chain distribution in hyper- and hypothyroid soleus. *Am. J. Physiol.* 265:C842–C850, 1993.

23. Carter, W. J., W. S. van der Weijden Benjamin, and F. H. Faas. Effect of thyroid hormone on protein turnover in cultured cardiac myocytes. *J. Mol. Cell. Cardiol.* (9):897–905, 1985.

24. Cote, C., and D. Boulet. The translation system of rat heart muscle mitochondria is stimulated following treatment with L-triiodothyronine. *Biochem. Biophys. Res. Commun.* 128(3):1425–1433, 1985.

25. Cox, G. A., N. M. Cole, K. Matsumura, S. F. Phelps, S. D. Hauschka, K. P. Campbell, J. A. Faulkner, and J. S. Chamberlain. Overexpression of dystrophin in transgenic mdx mice eliminates dystrophic symptoms without toxicity. *Nature* 364(6439):725–729, 1993.

26. Davis, H. L., R. G. Whalen, and B. A. Demeneix. Direct gene transfer into skeletal muscle in vivo: factors affecting efficiency of transfer and stability of expression. *Hum. Gene Ther.* (2):151–159, 1993.

27. Demartino, G. N., and A. L. Goldberg. Thyroid hormones control lysosomal enzyme activities in liver and skeletal muscle. *Proc. Natl. Acad. Sci. U.S.A.* 75(3):1369–1373, 1978.

28. Desvergne, B. How do thyroid hormone receptors bind to structurally diverse response elements? *Mol. Cell. Endocrinol.* 100(1–2):125–131, 1994.

29. Diffee, G. M., V. J. Caiozzo, R. E. Herrick, and K. M. Baldwin. Contractile and biochemi-

cal properties of rat soleus and plantaris following hindlimb suspension. *Am. J. Physiol.* 260:C528–C534, 1991.

30. Diffee, G. M., F. Haddad, R. E. Herrick, and K. M. Baldwin. Control of myosin heavy chain expression: interaction of hypothyroidism and hindlimb suspension. *Am. J. Physiol.* 261:C1099–C1106, 1991.

31. Downes, M., R. Griggs, A. Atkins, E. N. Olson, and G. E. Muscat. Identification of a thyroid hormone response element in the mouse myogenin gene: characterization of the thyroid hormone and retinoid X receptor heterodimeric binding site. *Cell Growth Differ.* 4(11): 901–909, 1993.

32. Dozin, B., M. A. Magnuson, and V. M. Nikodem. Thyroid hormone regulation of malic enzyme synthesis. Dual tissue-specific control. *J. Biol. Chem.* 261(22):10290–10302, 1986.

33. Dulhunty, A. F. The rate of tetanic relaxation is correlated with the density of calcium ATPase in the terminal cisternae of thyrotoxic skeletal muscle. *Pflügers Arch.* 415(4): 433–439, 1990.

34. Eddinger, T. J., and R. L. Moss. Mechanical properties of skinned single fibres of identified types from rat diaphragm. *Am. J. Physiol.* 253:C210–C218, 1987.

35. Edman, K. A. The velocity of unloaded shortening and its relation to sarcomere length and isometric force in vertebrate muscle fibres. *J. Physiol.* 291:143–159, 1979.

36. Edwards, J. G., J. J. Bahl, I. L. Flink, Y. S. Cheng, and E. Morkin. Thyroid hormone influences beta myosin heavy chain (beta MHC) expression. *Biochem. Biophys. Res. Commun.* 199(3):1482–1488, 1994.

37. Everts, M. E. Effects of thyroid hormone on $Ca(2+)$ efflux and $Ca(2+)$ transport capacity in rat skeletal muscle. *Cell Calcium* 11:343–352, 1990.

38. Farnburg, B. L. Calcium transport by skeletal muscle sarcoplasmic reticulum in the hypothyroid rat. *J. Clin. Invest.* 47:2499–2506, 1968.

39. Fitts, R. H., W. W. Winder, M. H. Brooke, K. K. Kaiser, and J. O. Holloszy. Contractile, biochemical, and histochemical properties of thyrotoxic rat soleus muscle. *Am. J. Physiol.* 238(1):C14–C20, 1980.

40. Fitzsimons, D. P., R. E. Herrick, and K. M. Baldwin. Isomyosin distribution in rodent skeletal muscles: effects of altered thyroid state. *J. Appl. Physiol.* 69:321–327, 1990.

41. Forman, B. M., J. Chen, B. Blumberg, S. A. Kliewer, R. Henshaw, E. S. Ong, and R. M. Evans. Cross-talk among ROR alpha 1 and the Rev-erb family of orphan nuclear receptors. *Mol. Endocrinol.* 9:1253–1261, 1994.

42. Gibbs, E. M., J. L. Stock, S. C. McCoid, H. A. Stukenbrok, J. E. Pessin, R. W. Stevenson, A. J. Milici, and J. D. McNeish. Glycemic improvement in diabetic db/db mice by overexpression of the human insulin-regulatable glucose transporter (GLUT4). *J. Clin. Invest.* 4:1512–1518, 1995.

43. Gold, H. K., J. F. Spann, and E. Braunwald. Effect of alterations in the thyroid state on the intrinsic contractile properties of isolated rat skeletal muscle. *J. Clin. Invest.* 49:849–854, 1970.

44. Grover, A. K., and I. Khan. Calcium pump isoforms: diversity, selectivity and plasticity. *Cell Calcium* 13(1):9–17, 1992.

45. Gulve, E. A., J. M. Ren, B. A. Marshall, J. Gao, P. A. Hansen, J. O. Holloszy, and M. Mueckler. Glucose transport activity in skeletal muscles from transgenic mice overexpressing GLUT1. Increased basal transport is associated with a defective response to diverse stimuli that activate GLUT4. *J. Biol. Chem.* 269(28):18366–18370, 1994.

46. Haddad, F., R. E. Herrick, G. R. Adams, and K. M. Baldwin. Myosin heavy chain expression in rodent skeletal muscle: effects of exposure to zero gravity. *J. Appl. Physiol.* 75(6):2471–2477, 1993.

47. Hansen, P. A., E. A. Gulve, B. A. Marshall, J. Gao, J. E. Pessin, J. O. Holloszy, and M. Mueckler. Skeletal muscle glucose transport and metabolism are enhanced in transgenic mice overexpressing the Glut4 glucose transporter. *J. Biol. Chem.* 270(4):1679–1684, 1995.

48. Hartong, R., N. Wang, R. Kurokawa, M. A. Lazar, C. K. Glass, J. W. Apriletti, and W. H. Dill-

mann. Delineation of three different thyroid hormone-response elements in promoter of rat sarcoplasmic reticulum Ca(2+) ATPase gene. *J. Biol. Chem.* 269(17):13021–13029, 1994.

49. Hasselgren, P. O., I. W. Chen, J. H. James, M. Sperling, B. W. Warner, and J. A. Fischer. Studies on the possible role of thyroid hormone in altered muscle protein turnover during sepsis. *Ann. Surg.* 206(1):18–24, 1987.

50. Hasty, P., A. Bradley, J. H. Morris, D. G. Edmondson, J. M. Venuti, E. N. Olson, and W. H. Klein. Muscle deficiency and neonatal death in mice with a targeted mutation in the myogenin gene. *Nature* 364:501–506, 1993.

51. Hersberg, A. Z., L. Fliegel, and D. H. Maclennan. Structure of the rabbit fast-twitch skeletal muscle calsequestrin gene. *J. Biol. Chem.* 263(10):4807–4812, 1988.

52. Hodin, R. A., M. A. Lazar, and W. W. Chin. Differential and tissue-specific regulation of the multiple rat c-erbA messenger RNA species by thyroid hormone. *J. Clin. Invest.* 85(1):101–105, 1990.

53. Hoffman, R., M. Lazar, N. Rubinstein, and A. Kelly. Differential expression of α1, α2 and β1 thyroid hormone genes in developing rat skeletal muscle. *J. Cell. Biochem.* 18D:517, 1994.

54. Holguin, J. A. Cooperative effects of Ca2+ and Sr2+ on sarcoplasmic reticulum adenosine triphosphatase. *Arch. Biochem. Biophys.* 251(1):9–16, 1986.

55. Hughes, S. M., J. M. Taylor, S. J. Tapscott, C. M. Gurley, W. J. Carter, and C. J. Peterson. Selective accumulation of myoD and myogenin mRNAs in fast and slow adult skeletal muscle is controlled by innervation and hormones. *Development* 118:1137–1147, 1993.

56. Huxley, A. F. Muscle structure and theories of contraction. *Prog. Biophys. Biophysical Chem.* 7:255–317, 1957.

57. Ianuzzo, C. D., N. Hamilton, and B. Li. Competitive control of myosin expression: hypertrophy vs. hyperthyroidism. *J. Appl. Physiol.* 70(5):2328–2330, 1991.

58. Ianuzzo, C. D., P. Patel, V. Chen, and P. O'Brien. A possible thyroidal trophic influence on fast and slow skeletal muscle. *Plasticity of Muscle.* Berlin, 1980.

59. Ikeda, M., M. Rhee, and W. W. Chin. Thyroid hormone receptor monomer, homodimer, and heterodimer (with retinoid-X receptor) contact different nucleotide sequences in thyroid hormone response elements. *Endocrinology* 135(4):1628–1638, 1994.

60. Izumo, S., and V. Mahdavi. Thyroid hormone receptor alpha isoforms generated by alternative splicing differentially activate myosin HC gene transcription. *Nature* 334(6182):539–542, 1988.

61. Izumo, S., B. Nadal-Ginard, and V. Mahdavi. All members of the MHC multigene family respond to thyroid hormone in a highly tissue-specific manner. *Science* 231:597–600, 1993.

62. Jepson, M. M., P. C. Bates, and D. J. Millward. The role of insulin and thyroid hormones in the regulation of muscle growth and protein turnover in response to dietary protein in the rat. *Br. J. Nutr.* 59:397–415, 1988.

63. Josephson, R. K. Mechanical power output from striated muscle during cyclic contraction. *J. Exp. Biol.* 114:493–512, 1985.

64. Josephson, R. K., and D. R. Stokes. Strain, muscle length and work output in a crab muscle. *J. Exp. Biol.* 145:45–61, 1989.

65. Julian, F. J., R. L. Moss, and P. J. Reiser. Mechanical properties and myosin light chain composition of skinned muscle fibers from adult and new-born rabbits. *J. Physiol.* 311:201–218, 1981.

66. Jump, D. B. Rapid induction of rat liver S14 gened transcription by thyroid hormone. *J. Biol. Chem.* 264(8):4698–4703, 1989.

67. Kariya K., L. R. Karns, and P. C. Simpson. An enhancer core element mediates stimulation of the rat beta-myosin heavy chain promoter by an alpha 1-adrenergic agonist and activated beta-protein kinase C in hypertrophy of cardiac myocytes. *J. Biol. Chem.* 269(5):3775–3782, 1994.

68. Kayali, A. G., N. M. Goodman, J. Lin, and V. R. Young. Insulin- and thyroid hormone-in-

dependent adaptation of myofibrillar proteolysis to glucocorticoids. *Am. J. Physiol.* 259 (22):E699–E705, 1990.

69. Kim, D. H., F. A. Witzman, and R. H. Fitts. Effect of thyrotoxicosis on sarcoplasmic reticulum in rat skeletal muscle. *Am. J. Physiol.* 243(12):C151–C155, 1982.

70. Kirschbaum, B. J., H. Kucher, A. Termin, A. M. Kelly, and D. Pette. Antagonistic effects of chronic low frequency stimulation and thyroid hormone on myosin expression in rat fast twitch muscle. *J. Biol. Chem.* 23:13974–13980, 1990.

71. Kiss, E., G. Jakab, E. G. Kranias, and I. Edes. Thyroid hormone-induced alterations in phospholamban protein expression. *Circ. Res.* 75(2):245–251, 1994.

72. Kitsis, R. N., P. M. Buttrick, E. M. McNally, M. L. Kaplan, and L. A. Leinwand. Hormonal modulation of a gene injected into rat heart in vivo. *Proc. Natl Acad. Sci. U.S.A.* 88(10): 4138–4142, 1991.

73. Larsson, L., X. Li, A. Teresi, and G. Salviati. Effects of thyroid hormone on fast- and slow-twitch skeletal muscles in young and old rats. *J. Physiol. (Lond.)* 481(1):149–161, 1994.

74. Larsson, L., and R. L. Moss. Maximum velocity of shortening in relation to myosin isoform composition in single fibres from human skeletal muscle. *J. Physiol. (Lond.)* 472:595–614, 1993.

75. Lazar, M. A., and W. W. Chin. Nuclear thyroid hormone receptors. *J. Clin. Invest.* 86:1777–1782, 1990.

76. Lazar, M. A., R. A. Hodin, G. Cardona, and W. W. Chin. Gene expression from the c-erbA alpha/Rev-ErbA alpha genomic locus. Potential regulation of alternative splicing by opposite strand transcription. *J. Biol. Chem.* 265(22):12859–12863, 1990.

77. Lazar, M. A., R. A. Hodin, D. S. Darling, and W. W. Chin. Identification of a rat c-erbA alpha-related protein which binds deoxyribonucleic acid but does not bind thyroid hormone. *Mol. Endocrinol.* 2(10):893–901, 1988.

78. Lazar, M. A., R. A. Hodin, D. S. Darling, and W. W. Chin. A novel member of the thyroid/steroid hormone receptor family is encoded by the opposite strand of the rat c-erbA alpha transcriptional unit. *Mol. Cell Biol.* 9(3):1128–1136, 1989.

79. Lee, K. J., R. Hickey, H. Zhu, and K. R. Chien. Positive regulatory elements (HF-1a and HF-1b) and a novel negative regulatory element (HF-3) mediate ventricular muscle-specific expression of myosin light-chain 2-luciferase fusion genes in transgenic mice. *Mol. Cell. Biol.* 14(2):1220–1229, 1994.

80. Lee, K. J., R. S. Ross, H. A. Rockman, A. N. Harris, T. X. O'Brien, M. van Bilsen, H. E. Shubeita, R. Kandolf, G. Brem, and J. Price. Myosin light chain-2 luciferase transgenic mice reveal distinct regulatory programs for cardiac and skeletal muscle-specific expression of a single contractile protein gene. *J. Biol. Chem.* 267(22):15875–15885, 1992.

81. Leijendekker, W. J., and C. van Hardeveld. Structural and functional aspects of the actomyosin complex from fast-twitch muscle of euthyroid and hypothyroid rats. *Pflügers Arch.* 410:48–54, 1987.

82. Limas, C. J. Calcium transport ATPase of cardiac sarcoplasmic reticulum in experimental hyperthyroidism. *Am. J. Physiol.* 235(6):H745–H751, 1978.

83. Lytton, J., M. Westlin, S. E. Burk, G. E. Shull, and D. H. Maclennan. Functional comparisons between isoforms of the sarcoplasmic or endoplasmic reticulum family of calcium pumps. *J. Biol. Chem.* 267(20):14483–14489, 1992.

84. Manning, D. R., and T. J. Stull. Myosin light chain phosphorylation and phosphorylase A activity in rat extensor digitorum longus muscle. *Biochem. and Biophys. Res. Commun.* 90(1):164–170, 1979.

85. Mano, H., R. Mori, T. Ozawa, K. Takeyama, Y. Yoshizawa, R. Kojima, Y. Arao, S. Masushige, and S. Kato. Positive and negative regulation of retinoid X receptor gene expression by thyroid hormone in the rat. Transcriptional and post-transcriptional controls by thyroid hormone. *J. Biol. Chem.* 269(3):1591–1594, 1994.

86. McLachlan, A. D. Structural implications of the myosin amino acid sequence. *Ann. Rev. Biophys. Bioeng.* 13:167–189, 1984.

87. Melton, D. W. Gene targeting in the mouse. *Bioessays* 16(9):633–638, 1994.
88. Mermier, P., and W. Hasselbach. Comparison between strontium and calcium uptake by the fragmented sarcoplasmic reticulum. *Eur. J. Biochem.* 69(1):79–86, 1976.
89. Mitsuhashi, T., and V. M. Nikodem. Regulation of expression of the alternative mRNAs of the rat alpha-thyroid hormone receptor gene. *J. Biol. Chem.* 264(15):8900–8904, 1989.
90. Mitsuhashi, T. G., E. Tennyson, and V. M. Nikodem. Alternative splicing generates messages encoding rat c-erbA proteins that do not bind thyroid hormone. *Proc. Natl. Acad. Sci. U.S.A.* 85(16):5804–5808, 1988.
91. Molkentin, J. D., and B. E. Markham. An M-CAT binding factor and an RSRF-related A-rich binding factor positively regulate expression of the alpha-cardiac myosin heavy-chain gene in vivo. *Mol. Cell. Biol.* (8):5056–5065, 1994.
92. Montgomery, A. The time course of thyroid-hormone-induced changes in the isotonic and isometric properties of rat soleus muscle. *Pflügers Arch.* 421:350–356, 1992.
93. Moore, R. L., and J. T. Stull. Myosin light chain phosphorylation in fast and slow skeletal muscles in situ. *Am. J. Physiol.* 247(16):C462–C471, 1984.
94. Muller, A., G. C. van der Linden, M. J. Zuidwijk, W. S. Simonides, W. J. van der Laarse, and C. van Hardeveld. Differential effects of thyroid hormone on the expression of sarcoplasmic reticulum. Ca^{++}-ATPase isoforms in rat skeletal muscle fibers. *Biochem. Biophys. Res. Commun.* 203(2):1035–1042, 1994.
95. Murray, M. B., and H. C. Towle. Identification of nuclear factors that enhance binding of the thyroid hormone receptor to a thyroid hormone response element. *Mol. Endocrinol.* 3(9):1434–1442, 1989.
96. Murray, M. B., N. D. Zilz, N. L. McCreary, M. J. MacDonald, and H. C. Towle. Isolation and characterization of rat cDNA clones for two distinct thyroid hormone receptors. *J. Biol. Chem.* 263(25):12770–12777, 1988.
97. Muscat, G. E., R. Griggs, M. Downes, and J. Emery. Characterization of the thyroid hormone response element in the skeletal alpha-actin gene: negative regulation of T3 receptor binding by the retinoid X receptor. *Cell Growth Differ.* 4(4):269–279, 1993.
98. Muscat, G. E., L. Mynett-Johnson, D. Dowhan, M. Downes, and R. Griggs. Activation of myoD gene transcription by 3,5,3'-triiodo-L-thyronine: a direct role for the thyroid hormone and retinoid X receptors. *Nucleic Acids Res.* 22(4):583–591, 1994.
99. Nabeshima, Y., K. Hanaoka, M. Hayasaka, E. Esumi, S. Li, I. Nonaka, and Y. Nabeshima. Myogenin gene disruption results in perinatal lethality because of severe muscle defect. *Nature* 364(6437):532–535, 1993.
100. Nagai, R., A. Z. Herzberg, C. J. Brandl, J. Fujii, M. Tada, D. H. Maclennan, N. R. Alpert, and M. Periasamy. Regulation of myocardial Ca^{++}-ATPase and phospholamban mRNA expression in response to pressure overload and thyroid hormone. *Proc. Natl Acad. Sci. U.S.A.* 86:2966–2970, 1989.
101. Nwoye, L., and W. F. Mommaerts. The effects of thyroid status on some properties of rat fast-twitch muscle. *J. Muscle Res. Cell Motil.* 2:307–320, 1981.
102. Ogawa Y. Role of ryanodine receptors. *Crit. Rev. Biochem. Mol. Biol.* 29(4):229–274, 1994.
103. Ojamaa, K., and I. Klein. Thyroid hormone regulation of alpha-myosin heavy chain promoter activity assessed by in vivo DNA transfer in rat heart. *Biochem. Biophys. Res. Commun.* 179(3):1269–1275, 1991.
104. Ojamaa, K., and I. Klein. In vivo regulation of recombinant cardiac myosin heavy chain gene expression by thyroid hormone. *Endocrinology* 132(3):1002–1006, 1993.
105. Oppenheimer, J. H., and H. H. Samuels. *Molecular Basis of Thyroid Hormone Action.* New York: Academic Press, 1983.
106. Persechini, A., J. T. Stull, and R. Cooke. The effect of myosin phosphorylation on the contractile properties of skinned rabbit skeletal muscle fibers. *J. Biol. Chem.* 260(13):7951–7954, 1985.
107. Petrof, B. J., A. M. Kelly, N. A. Rubinstein, and A. I. Pack. Effect of hypothyroidism on

myosin heavy chain expression in rat pharyngeal dilator muscles. *J. Appl. Physiol.* 73(1):179–187, 1992.

108. Pette, D., and R. S. Staron. Cellular and molecular diversities of mammalian skeletal muscle fibers. *Rev. Physiol. Biochem. Pharmacol.* 116:1–76, 1990.

109. Rayment, I., W. R. Rypniewski, K. Schmidt-Base, R. Smith, D. R. Tomchick, M. M. Benning, D. A. Winkelmann, G. Wesenberg, and H. M. Holden. Three-dimensional structure of myosin subfragment-1: a molecular motor. *Science* 261(5117):50–58, 1993.

110. Reddy, L. G., L. R. Jones, S. E. Cala, J. J. O'Brian, S. A. Tatulian, and D. L. Stokes. Functional reconstitution of recombinant phospholamban with rabbit skeletal $Ca(2+)$-ATPase. *J. Biol. Chem.* 270(16):9390–9397, 1995.

111. Reiser, P. J., C. E. Kasper, M. L. Greaser, and R. L. Moss. Functional significance of myosin transitions in single fibers of developing soleus muscle. *Am. J. Physiol.* 254(23):C605–C613, 1988.

112. Reiser, P. J., C. E. Kasper, and R. L. Moss. Myosin subunits and contractile properties of single fibers from hypokinetic rat muscles. *J. Appl. Physiol.* 63(6):2293–2300, 1987.

113. Reiser, P. J., R. L. Moss, G. G. Giulian, and M. L. Greaser. Shortening velocity in single fibers from adult rabbit soleus muscles is correlated with myosin heavy chain composition. *J. Biol. Chem.* 260:9077–9080, 1985.

114. Reiser, P. J., R. L. Moss, G. G. Giulian, and M. L. Greaser. Shortening velocity and myosin heavy chains of developing rabbit muscle fibers. *J. Biol. Chem.* 260:14403–14405, 1985.

115. Retnakaran, R., J. Flock, and G. V. Giguere. Identification of RVR, a novel orphan nuclear receptor that acts as a negative transcriptional regulator. *Mol. Endocrinol.* (9):1234–1244, 1994.

116. Rindt, H., J. Gulick, S. Knotts, J. Neumann, and J. Robbins. In vivo analysis of the murine beta-myosin heavy chain gene promoter. *J. Biol. Chem.* 268(7):5332–5338, 1993.

117. Rohrer, D., and W. H. Dillmann. Thyroid hormone markedly increases the mRNA coding for sarcoplasmic reticulum Ca^{++}-ATPase in the rat heart. *J. Biol. Chem.* 263(15):6941–6944, 1988.

118. Rohrer, D. K., R. Hartong, and W. H. Dillmann. Influence of thyroid hormone and retinoic acid on slow sarcoplasmic reticulum Ca^{++}-ATPase and myosin heavy chain alpha gene expression in cardiac myocytes. *J. Biol. Chem.* 266(13):8638–8646, 1991.

119. Rudnicki, M. A., and R. Jaenisch. The MyoD family of transcription factors and skeletal myogenesis. *Bioessays* 17(3):203–209, 1995.

120. Salmons, S., and F. Sreter. Significance of impulse activity in the transformation of skeletal muscle type. *Nature* 263:30–34, 1976.

121. Sap, J., A. Munoz, K. Damm, Y. Goldberg, J. Ghysdael, A. Leutz, H. Beug, and B. Vennstrom. The c-erb-A protein is a high-affinity receptor for thyroid hormone. *Nature* 324(6098):635–640, 1986.

122. Sayen, M. R., D. K. Rohrer, and W. H. Dillmann. Thyroid hormone response of slow and fast sarcoplasmic reticulum Ca^{++} ATPase mRNA in striated muscle. *Mol. Cell Endocrinol.* 87:87–93, 1992.

123. Schiaffino, S., L. Gorza, S. Ausoni, R. Bottinelli, C. Regiani, L. Larsson, L. Edstrom, K. Gunderson, and T. Lomo. Muscle fiber types expressing different myosin heavy chain isoforms: their functional properties and adaptive capacity. *The Dynamic State of Muscle Fibers.* New York: Walter de Gruyter, 1990.

124. Schiaffino, S., L. Gorza, S. Sartore, L. Saggin, S. Ausoni, M. Vianello, K. Gundersen, and T. Lomo. Three myosin heavy chain isoforms in type 2 skeletal muscle fibers. *J. Muscle Res. Cell Motil.* 10:197–205, 1989.

125. Schrader, M., and C. Carlberg. Thyroid hormone and retinoic acid receptors form heterodimers with retinoid X receptors on direct repeats, palindromes, and inverted palindromes. *DNA Cell Biol.* 13(4):333–341, 1994.

126. Schwartz, H. L., K. A. Strait, and J. H. Oppenheimer. Molecular mechanisms of thyroid hormone action. A physiologic perspective. *Clin. Lab. Med.* 3:543–561, 1993.

127. Shastry, B. S. More to learn from gene knockouts. *Mol. Cell. Biochem.* 136(2):171–182, 1994.

128. Simonet, W. S., and G. C. Ness. Transcriptional and posttranscriptional regulation of rat hepatic 3-hydroxy-3-methylglutaryl-coenzyme A reductase by thyroid hormones. *J. Biol. Chem.* 263(25):12448–12453, 1988.

129. Simonides, W. S., and C. van Hardveld. The effect of hypothyroidism on sarcoplasmic reticulum in fast-twitch muscle of the rat. *Biochim. Biophys. Acta* 844:129–141, 1985.

130. Simonides, W. S., G. C. van der Linden, and C. van Hardeveld. Thyroid hormone differentially affects mRNA levels of Ca-ATPase isozymes of sarcoplasmic reticulum in fast and slow skeletal muscle. *F.E.B.S. Lett.* 274:73–76, 1990.

131. Squire, J. M. *Muscle: Design, Diversity, and Disease.* Benjamin Cummings, 1986.

132. Strait, K. A., H. L. Schwartz, A. Perez-Castillo, and J. H. Oppenheimer. Relationship of c-erbA mRNA content to tissue triiodothyronine nuclear binding capacity and function in developing and adult rats. *J. Biol. Chem.* 265(18):10514–10521, 1990.

133. Subramaniam, A., J. Gulick, J. Neumann, S. Knotts, and J. Robbins. Transgenic analysis of the thyroid-responsive elements in the alpha-cardiac myosin heavy chain gene promoter. *J. Biol. Chem.* 268(6):4331–4336, 1993.

134. Subramaniam, A., W. K. Jones, J. Gulick, S. Wert, J. Neumann, and J. Robbins. Tissue-specific regulation of the alpha-myosin heavy chain gene promoter in transgenic mice. *J. Biol. Chem.* 266(36):24613–24620, 1991.

135. Sugden, P. H., and S. J. Fuller. Regulation of protein turnover in skeletal and cardiac muscle. *Biochem. J.* 273:21–37, 1991.

136. Suko, J. The calcium pump of cardiac sarcoplasmic reticulum. Functional alterations at different levels of thyroid state in rabbits. *J. Physiol. (Lond.)* 228:563–582, 1973.

137. Sweeney, H. L., M. J. Kushmerick, K. Mabuchi, F. A. Streter, and J. Gergely. Myosin alkali light chain and heavy chain variations correlate with altered shortening velocity of isolated skeletal muscle fibers. *J. Biol. Chem.* 263:9034–9039, 1988.

138. Swoap, S. J., F. Haddad, P. Bodell, and K. M. Baldwin. Effect of chronic energy deprivation on cardiac thyroid hormone receptor and myosin isoform expression. *Am. J. Physiol.* 266:E254–260, 1994.

139. Swoap, S. J., F. Haddad, V. J. Caiozzo, R. E. Herrick, S. A. McCue, and K. M. Baldwin. Interaction of thyroid hormone and functional overload on skeletal muscle isomyosin expression. *J. Appl. Physiol.* 77(2):621–629, 1994.

140. Takeda, S., D. L. North, M. M. Lakich, S. G. Russell, and R. G. Whalen. A possible regulatory role for conserved promoter motifs in an adult-specific muscle myosin gene from mouse. *J. Biol. Chem.* 267(24):16957–16967, 1992.

141. Thomason, D. B., R. E. Herrick, D. Surdyka, and K. M. Baldwin. Time course of soleus myosin expression during hindlimb suspension and recovery. *J. Appl. Physiol.* 62:2180–2186, 1987.

142. Thompson, C. C., Weinberger, R. Lebo, and R. M. Evans. Identification of a novel thyroid hormone receptor expressed in the mammalian central nervous system. *Science* 237(4822):1610–1614, 1987.

143. Thompson, W. R., B. Nadal-Ginard, and V. Mahdavi. A Myod1-independent muscle-specific enhancer controls the expression of the beta-myosin heavy chain gene in skeletal muscle and cardiac muscles. *J. Biol. Chem.* 266:22678–22688, 1991.

144. Towle, H. C., and C. N. Mariash. Regulation of hepatic gene expression by lipogenic diet and thyroid hormone. *Fed. Proc.* 45(9):2406–2411, 1986.

145. Tsika, R. W. Transgenic animal models. *Exerc. Sport Sci. Rev.* 22:361–388, 1994.

146. Tsika, R. W., R. E. Herrick, and K. M. Baldwin. Subunit composition of rodent isomyosins and their distribution in hindlimb skeletal muscles. *J. Appl. Physiol.* 63(5):2101–2110, 1987.

147. van der Linden, G. C., W. S. Simonides, and C. van Hardeveld. Thyroid hormone regu-

lates Ca^{++}-ATPase mRNA levels of sarcoplasmic reticulum during neonatal development of fast skeletal muscle. *Mol. Cell. Endocrinol.* 90:125–131, 1992.

148. Warrick, H. M., and J. A. Spudich. Myosin structure and function in cell motility. *Annu. Rev. Cell Biol.* 3:379–421, 1987.

149. Weinberger, C., C. C. Thompson, E. S. Ong, R. Lebo, D. J. Gruol, and R. M. Evans. The c-erb-A gene encodes a thyroid hormone receptor. *Nature* 324(6098):641–646, 1986.

150. Woledge, R. C., N. A. Curtin, and E. Homsher. *Energetic Aspects of Muscle Contraction.* New York: Academic Press, 1985.

151. Wolff, J. A., R. W. Malone, P. Williams, W. Chong, G. Acsadi, A. Jani, and P. L. Felgner. Direct gene transfer into mouse muscle in vivo. *Science* 247(4949 Part 1):1465–1468, 1990.

152. Wolff, J. A., P. Williams, G. Acsadi, S. Jiao, A. Jani, and W. Chong. Conditions affecting direct gene transfer into rodent muscle in vivo. *Biotechniques* 11(4):474–485, 1991.

153. Wuytack, F., H. Raeymaekers, J. A. De Smedt, and L. Eggermont. Ca(2+)-transport ATPases and their regulation in muscle and brain. *Ann. N. Y. Acad. Sci.* 671:82–91, 1992.

154. Yano, K., and A. Zarain-Herzberg. Sarcoplasmic reticulum calsequestrins: structural and functional properties. *Mol. Cell. Biochem.* 135(1):61–70, 1994.

155. Yen, P. M., J. H. Brubaker, J. W. Apriletti, J. D. Baxter, and W. W. Chin. Roles of 3,5′,3′-triiodothyronine and deoxyribonucleic acid binding on thyroid hormone receptor complex formation. *Endocrinology* 134(3):1075–1081, 1994.

156. Yen, P. M., D. S. Darling, R. L. Carter, M. Forgione, P. K. Umeda, and W. W. Chin. T3 decreases binding to DNA by T3 receptor homodimers but not receptor-auxiliary protein heterodimers. *J. Biol. Chem.* 267:3565–3568, 1992.

157. Zarain-Herzberg, A., J. Marques, D. Sukovich, and M. Periasamy. Thyroid hormone receptor modulates the expression of the rabbit cardiac sarco (endo) plasmic reticulum Ca(2+)-ATPase gene. *J. Biol. Chem.* 269(2):1460–1467, 1994.

158. Zeman, R. J., P. L. Bernstein, R. Ludemann, and J. D. Etlinger. Regulation of Ca^{++}-dependent protein turnover in skeletal muscle by thyroxine. *Biochem. J.* 240:269–272, 1986.

159. Zhang, X. K., B. Hoffmann, P. B. Tran, G. Graupner, and M. Pfahl. Retinoid X receptor is an auxiliary protein for thyroid hormone and retinoic acid receptors. *Nature* 355(6359):441–446, 1992.

12
Strength and Power Training: Physiological Mechanisms of Adaptation

WILLIAM J. KRAEMER, Ph.D.
STEVEN J. FLECK, Ph.D.
WILLIAM J. EVANS, Ph.D.

The stimulus of resistance exercise activates multiple physiological mechanisms related to the ability of the skeletal muscle(s) to meet the external force demands of a task [79, 85]. The specific type of heavy resistance exercise protocol performed helps to define the type of physiological mechanisms stimulated [35, 96, 101]. Ultimately, repeated exposure to a specific type of exercise stimuli results in the initiation of adaptations in the physiological mechanisms that are activated with training [8, 26].

Much of what we understand about the differential nature of various resistance exercise protocols has been gained through the examination of the acute physiological responses to various protocols. A resistance exercise protocol can be described by five acute program variables: 1) choice of the exercise; 2) order of the exercise; 3) resistance or intensity used; 4) number of sets; and 5) the rest period length between sets and exercises [33, 97]. Differences in the acute physiological and psychological responses to resistance exercise can be linked to differences in these acute program variables [95, 98, 100, 103, 152]. Historically, the use of a specific type of resistance exercise protocol to affect a specific type of physiological adaptation has been one of the basic training principles in program development [34, 91, 93, 96].

Because the resistance exercise protocols can be differentially configured (i.e., acute program variables) to present a variety of exercise demands, training adaptations have been thought to be specific to the type of exercise protocols used in a training program. This specificity is related to the specific pattern of neuromuscular activation required to perform a resistance exercise [52, 53]. In turn, this neuromuscular stimulation activates a variety of other systems (e.g., endocrine), which act to support the adaptive changes of the neuromuscular system [86, 87, 89]. The sequence of adaptational events is initiated with the first exercise session and follows a time course of adaptation that is specific to the individual and the type of exercise protocol used in the training program [120].

The primary purposes of this chapter will be to review adaptations of the neuromuscular system to heavy resistance training and examine the adaptational time course for these changes.

PROGRESSIVE OVERLOAD AND NEUROMUSCULAR ADAPTATIONS

Progressive Overload: an Old Concept

Bodily adaptations observed because of resistance training are dependent on the increased demands placed on the neuromuscular system. For more than a century, the concept of increasing the demands placed on the body to enhance strength performance has been a basic principle of resistance training [129]. Although advances over the last 30 yr in redefining the implementation of this concept (i.e., periodization) have occurred, it has become fundamental that, in order to obtain muscular strength and size gains, the training stimulus must be consistently increased [53].

Magnetic resonance images (MRI) allow for the visualization of whole muscle groups [38–40, 156]. Activated muscle can be observed via the exercise-induced contrast shifts in spin-spin relaxation time (T_2)-weighted images, which are reflective of concentric muscle use [1, 2, 32, 128, 137]. This contrast shift has been shown to be directly related to force development from muscle contractions evoked by both voluntary and surface electromyostimulation [2, 128]. A representative transaxial (T_2)-weighted MRI before and after heavy resistance exercise is shown in Figure 12.1.

Ploutz et al. [128] used MRI technology and a specific program that was designed to increase strength with little or no change in muscle size over a 9-week training period. Training was performed 2 days/wk. Each session consisted of high-intensity single-knee extension exercise using the left quadriceps for 3–6 sets of 12 repetition maximum loads. Exercise-induced contrast shifts were evoked by using 5 sets of 10 knee extensions for each intensity load of 50, 75, and 100% of the maximum pretraining load that could be lifted for 5 sets of 10 repetitions. The results demonstrated that one repetition maximum (RM) strength increased by 14% over the training period in the trained left thigh musculature and by 7% in the right untrained thigh musculature. The left quadriceps femoris muscle increased by 5% in cross-sectional area whereas the right one demonstrated no changes. This indicated that neural factors mediated much of the improvement in 1 RM strength. Interestingly, the amount of muscle that is needed to be activated in the posttraining test was less than that required to perform the same exercise protocol before training. This reduction in the amount of muscle needed to lift a given resistance in the posttraining state demonstrated that unless the resistance used is progressively increased over a training period, less muscle will be activated as muscular strength increases with training.

These data also give insights as to why a classic modification of the concept of progressive overload, specifically, periodized training [113] (i.e., variation in resistances and exercise volume used in training) may, in fact, be effective in providing recovery for certain muscle fibers. With increasing muscle strength over a training program, the use of heavy, moderate, and

FIGURE 12.1.
Preexercise and postexercise MRIs of the things are presented. The lighter white areas represent muscle that has been activated. Courtesy of Dr. Gary Dudley, University of Georgia, and Dr. Lori Ploutz, Ohio University.

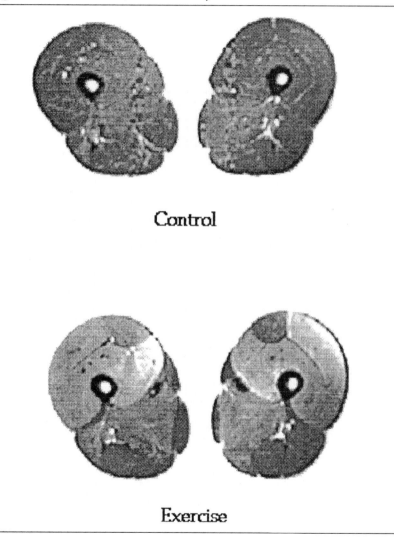

Control

Exercise

light resistances in training will allow for specific muscle fibers not to be taxed by the lifting requirement on light- and moderate-training days. Yet, the increased stress per cross-sectional unit area of activated muscle could potentially elicit a physiological stimulus for strength gains and tissue growth [128]. The heavy-training days would maximally activate the available musculature, but by alternating the intensities over time, overtraining or a lack of recovery could be minimized [45, 46]. Such periodized training manipulations have been found to be important, especially as the level of training becomes more demanding [52, 55, 57, 58, 101, 102].

The Neuromuscular System

Theoretical paradigms for the various interactions of neuromuscular system with strength and power training have been proposed by several investigators [27, 53, 131]. Figure 12.2 presents a flow chart that overviews the basic proposed interactions and relationships among components of the neuromuscular system. The stimulus for muscle activation comes from the generation of a high-level central control command signal. This signal is then sent to a lower level controller (spinal cord or brainstem) and transformed into a specific pattern of motor unit activation. The motor units activated meet the demands of force production by activating their associated muscle fibers [115, 131, 132]. Various feedback loops exist that can help modify force production as well as provide communication to other physiological systems (e.g., endocrine) [55, 57–59]. The high-level and low-level commands can be modified by feedback from both the peripheral sensory and the high-level central-command controller. Various adaptations in systems-level communications among the various neuromuscular systems can be observed

FIGURE 12.2.
Theoretical relationships among the various components of the neuromuscular system. EMG, electromyogram.

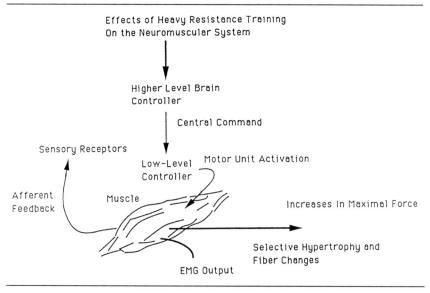

Effects of Heavy Resistance Training
On the Neuromuscular System

Higher Level Brain
Controller

Central Command

Sensory Receptors

Low-Level   Motor Unit Activation
Controller

Afferent   Muscle
Feedback   Increases In Maximal Force

Selective Hypertrophy and
Fiber Changes
EMG Output

with resistance training [53, 80, 83]. Differences in training programs can influence the type of adaptational changes (e.g., very heavy resistance can elicit increases in strength with little changes in muscle size [128]).

Motor Unit Activation

The functional unit of the neuromuscular system is the "motor unit" [125]. It consists of the motoneurone and the muscle fibers it innervates. Motor units range in size from one that contains only a few to those that contain several hundred muscle fibers. Muscle fibers from two different motor units can be anatomically situated next to each other, which means that it is possible for one to be actively generating force and the other only moving passively because of no direct neural stimulation. When the maximal possible force is desired from a muscle, all of the available motor units must be activated. How muscle force is affected by different types of motor unit firing rates or frequencies is also an adaptive mechanism affected by heavy resistance training [53, 125, 131, 132].

   The activation of motor units is also influenced by a concept called the "size principle," which is based on the observed relationship between motor unit twitch force and recruitment threshold [21]. Specifically, motor units are recruited according to their recruitment thresholds and firing rates, which results in a continuum of voluntary force in the agonist muscle [65]. Thus, with most muscles containing a range of motor units (with both Type I and Type II fibers), force production can span from very low levels of force production to maximal force production [126]. Maximal force production requires not only the recruitment of all motor units, including the "high-threshold" motor units, but also, these motor units must be recruited at a high enough firing rate to produce maximal force [131]. It has been theorized that untrained individuals may not be able to voluntarily recruit the highest threshold motor units or maximally activate their muscles. Furthermore, electrical stimulation has been shown to be more effective in eliciting gains in untrained or injury rehabilitation scenarios, suggesting further inability to successfully activate all of the available tissue [22, 135]. Thus, part of the training adaptation is to develop the ability to recruit all motor units when needed to perform a task.

   Few exceptions to the size principle are believed to exist. However, some advanced lifters or athletes may not require the order of recruitment stipulated by the size principle. It may be possible to inhibit lower threshold (i.e., slow) motor units and still activate the higher threshold motor units, in an attempt to enhance rate of force development and power production of the musculature. This idea has been derived from observations made during very rapid stereotyped movements and during voluntary eccentric muscle action in humans [23, 115, 121]. Dudley et al. [23] also demonstrated that the activation of knee extensors by the central nervous system (CNS) during maximal efforts depends on the speed and type of muscle action. The CNS is also capable of limiting force by engaging inhibitory mechanisms that may be protective in nature. Thus, training may also result in changes of the order of fiber recruitment or reduced inhibition, which may help in the performance of certain types of muscle actions.

Morphological Plasticity in the Neuromuscular System with Exercise

Little is understood concerning responses to exercise training of the different morphological structures in the nervous system. Future work will require examination of this aspect to help explain the more global events observed with nervous system function. The neuromuscular junction is an important and representative structure of the nervous system, which mediates the process of nervous system excitation and consequent contraction of skeletal muscle [20]. Although it has been the subject of study since the turn of the century, limited data exist as to the effects of exercise. Understanding the potential for adaptations in the neuromuscular junction (NMJ) represents an important aspect in the study of exercise training, as it is the interface between the nervous system and skeletal muscle. Only limited data are available as to the molecular mechanisms involved with neural adaptations to general exercise training in young animals [4, 20]. The majority of morphological data have examined the impact of exercise training as it relates to a prophylactic effect on NMJ alterations associated with aging, which have shown different results, when compared to responses of young animals. For example, contrary to the results observed in senescent mice, an 8-wk program of endurance exercise resulted in an increased presynaptic nerve terminal area in young adult mice [4]. Morphological changes in the nervous system of humans with heavy resistance training remain unknown!

Insights into the plasticity of NMJ morphological changes with different intensities of exercise were demonstrated by Deschenes et al. [20], who examined the effects of high- vs. low-intensity treadmill exercise training on NMJ adaptations in the soleus muscle of rats. A detailed image of the NMJ was obtained with a laser scanning microscopy system. Fluorescent histochemical staining allowed an accurate approximation of the density of acetylcholine (ACH) vesicles and receptor clusters. In addition, nerve terminal branching was evaluated. Both high- and low-intensity exercise running produced increased area of the NMJ. Although NMJ hypertrophic responses were observed in both groups, the high-intensity group was associated with more dispersed, irregularly shaped synapses, whereas the low-intensity training resulted in more compact, symmetrical synapses. The high-intensity training group also exhibited a greater total length of branching, when compared to low-intensity and control groups. Thus, it might be hypothesized that heavy resistance exercise training would produce morphological changes in the NMJ and that these changes may be of much greater magnitude than adaptations attributable to endurance training because of the differences in required quanta of neurotransmitter involved with the recruitment of high-threshold motor units.

Time Course of Neural Changes with Resistance Training

As we have seen in the development of the progressive overload concept in resistance training, it is possible for neural factors to mediate a large portion of the strength increases attributable to resistance training without large increases in cross-sectional muscle area [119, 128]. This appears to be most obvious in the early phases (2–8 wk) of training, where strength gains are much greater than that which can be explained by muscle hypertrophy. In addition, the ability to activate all of the available motor units may also be enhanced in the early phases of training, when trainees are "learning" how to exert force in various resistance exercises. The specific type of program used may be one of the most important factors in initial strength gains attributable to neural factors, because those programs that are of very high intensity (>90% of 1 RM) but are low in total exercise volume (low number of sets × reps) may not be an adequate stimulus for muscle tissue growth [131]. Therefore, strength gains may be more dependent on neural factors in these types of programs. When a program does promote muscle tissue growth, it may diminish the contribution of the initial neural adaptations to strength and power gains. However, typically muscle fiber hypertrophy has been shown to require more than 16 workouts to produce significant increases [143]. Thus, while it may be possible that various types of training may be able to enhance the hypertrophy of muscle more quickly in the early phases (1–8 wk) of training, thereby enhancing the hypertrophic contribution to the strength and power gains, this has been observed only in a few studies [12,13, 48, 154]. The large majority of studies have demonstrated that, in the early phases of a heavy resistance training program, increased voluntary activation of muscle is the largest contributor to strength increases observed (for reviews, see refs. 52, 53, 117, 119, 131).

The neural component may also play a major role in mediating strength gains in advanced lifters. In a study by Häkkinen et al. [58], minimal changes in muscle fiber size was observed in competitive Olympic weightlifters, but strength and power increased over 2 yr of training. EMG data demonstrated that voluntary activation of muscle was enhanced over the training period. Thus, even in advanced resistance-trained athletes, the mechanisms of strength and power improvement may be related to neural factors. It must be kept in mind that the subjects in this investigation were competitive weightlifters who compete in body mass classification groups, and gains in muscle mass may not necessarily enhance their competitive advantage. Furthermore, the types of programs used by Olympic weightlifters are primarily related to strength and power development [49, 102]. Other types of programs (e.g.; emphasizing hypertrophy or specific sport movements) for body builders and sport athletes may have some similar characteristics related to power development but be designed differently with regard to exercise, sets and intensities used to meet muscle mass and/or specific sport performance needs [47, 67–69, 84, 124]. Thus, training goals and specific protocols used to meet them play a key role in the adaptational response to resistance training.

Sale et al. [131] have described this dynamic interplay of neural and hypertrophic factors (see Fig. 12.3). A dramatic increase in the adaptation of neural factors is observed over the time course (e.g., 6–10 wk) used for most resistance training studies in the literature. As the duration of training increases (>10 wk), muscle hypertrophy eventually takes place and contributes more than neural adaptations to the strength and power gains observed. However, eventually, muscle hypertrophy also reaches a maximum and levels off. It is interesting to note that increases in cross-sectional area of muscle fibers range from about 20 to 45% in most training studies with some greater than 50% [144]. Few studies have demonstrated increases in muscle fiber size greater than 50% and this may be due to the pre-training size of the fiber, the program used and/or the duration of training. With the development of whole muscle image systems (MRI, CT scans), the mus-

FIGURE 12.3.

Theoretical interplay of contributions of neural factors and hypertrophic factors over time with resistance training.

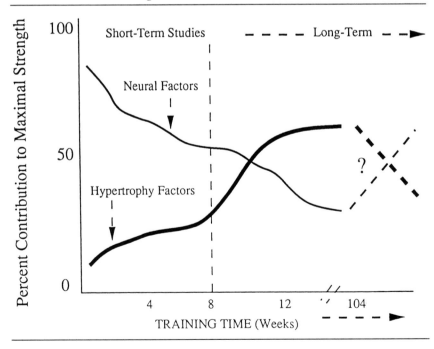

cle fiber changes in one specific area may not necessarily reflect the magnitude of changes in the whole muscle, which must be stimulated, many times, with several different angles of movement, to activate all of the available tissue over its cross-sectional area [128]. However, strength and power gains derived from the "progressively and properly" loaded and activated musculature appear to be bounded by a genetic upper limit of neuromuscular adaptation [52, 53].

CHANGES IN SKELETAL MUSCLE FIBERS WITH RESISTANCE TRAINING

Time Course of Changes

The time course of changes in muscle fibers with heavy resistance training must be viewed from the vantage point of both a "quality" and "quantity" of the contractile proteins (i.e., actin and myosin). With the initiation of a heavy-resistance training program, changes in the types of muscle proteins (e.g., myosin heavy chains) start to take place within a couple of workouts. As training continues, the quantity of contractile proteins starts to increase as muscle fibers develop increased cross-sectional areas. Muscle fiber hypertrophy appears to require a longer period of training time (>16 workouts) to sufficiently increase the contractile protein content in muscle cells [143].

It has become evident that a great deal of plasticity exists with regard to changes in muscle after exercise. This is attributable in part to the complex, yet readily adaptable, group of myosin contractile and regulatory proteins that is encoded by a highly conserved multigene family [142]. A lot of the work that has been done with resistance exercise has focused on the myosin molecule and examination of fiber types, based on the use of the histochemical myosin adenosine triphosphatase (mATPase)-staining activities at different pHs. This semiqualitative technique has been the method of choice in numerous investigations and has subsequently revealed a continuum of muscle fiber types [139, 141, 144, 145]. The continuum of muscle fiber types (human) is shown in Figure 12.4 going from the most oxidative, Type I, to the least oxidative, Type IIB [140]. The basis for the proposed continuum of seven human skeletal muscle fiber types is determined by different preincubation at various pH values [140].

As overviewed by Staron and Johnson [142], three different major types of polypeptide chains make up the myosin molecule, including heavy chains (approximately 200 kd) and two different types of light chains (alkali or essential and P, also referred to as regulatory, phosphorylatable, or 5,5'-dithiobis-2 nitrobenzoic acid (DTNB) light chains, each about 20 kd). The single myosin molecule is a hexamer that contains two identical myosins in heavy chains (HC), two identical P light chains (LC2), and either two identical (LC1/LC1 or LC3/LC3) or nonidentical (LC1/LC3) al-

FIGURE 12.4.
Muscle fiber type continuum is presented. As provided by Dr. Robert S. Staron, Ohio State University.

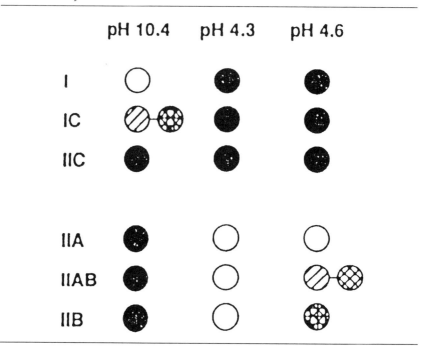

kali light chains. Figure 12.5 shows an example of the electrophoretic analysis of myosin heavy-chain content. The complexity of the system allows for the different expression of isomyosin forms that have different heavy- and light-chain compositions. The differential myosin expression has been of interest, because it is related to muscle function and adaptation to physiological demands [127].

A link between the mATPase fiber type distribution and myosin heavy-chain content in skeletal muscle has been undertaken by a number of investigators examining relationships for entire biopsy samples or single fibers [3, 139, 140, 143, 144]. Recently, Fry et al. [44] examined muscle fiber biopsy samples every 2 wk of an 8-wk, high-intensity resistance training program. Six muscle fiber types (I, IC, IIAC, IIA, IIAB, and IIB) were determined, using mATPase staining techniques and electrophoretic techniques were used to separate and quantify the percentage of myosin heavy chain (MHC) content in these same samples. MHC percentage (MHC I, MHC IIa, MHC IIb) and percentage of fiber type area (I, IIA, IIB) were shown to have high correlations with only 13–36% of the variance unaccounted for under various conditions of training in men and women. This unaccounted variance was suggested to be attributable to three possible sources of error, in-

FIGURE 12.5.
Example of the electrophoretic analysis of myosin heavy-chain content related to mAT-Pase stained fibers. Numbered, histochemically defined fibers (after preincubation at pH4.6 (A) and specific myosin heavy-chain analysis (B) Bar = 100 μm. Courtesy of Dr. Robert S. Staron, Ohio State University.

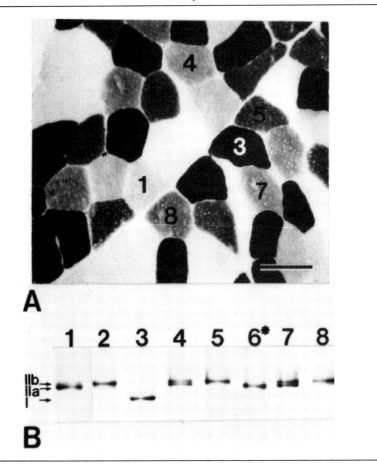

cluding compression of six fiber types into three in order to match the MHCs, lack of measurement of all cross-sectional areas of muscle fiber types, and exact determination of MHC IIa and IIb because of their close molecular weight. Nevertheless, changes in muscle mATPase muscle fiber types do give an indication of associated changes in the MHC content as well.

It has become apparent that, with resistance training, changes in the muscle fiber type continuum and associated MHC occur early in the training program. Figure 12.6 shows the transformation or movement of muscle

FIGURE 12.6.

Transformation or movement of muscle fiber subtypes with training and detraining.

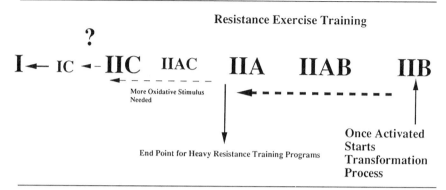

fiber subtypes with training and detraining. It is interesting to note that although transformation within the muscle fiber subtypes appears quite typical, any transformation from Type I to Type II muscle fiber types appears less probable. Whether transformation of Type I to Type II fibers or Type II to Type I is possible at all remains debatable [127, 142]. Figure 12.7 depicts the histochemical profile of such changes with concomitant changes in the MHC. In a study by Staron et al. [143], a high-intensity resistance training protocol was used by men and women two times/wk for 8 wk. This protocol focused on the thigh musculature of several exercises, with heavy multiple sets of 6–8 RM on one day and 10–12 RM on the other day (squat, leg press, and knee extensions). Two-minute rest periods were used to allow for adequate rest between sets and exercises but also induce hormonal increases with the exercise protocol [95, 103]. Maximal dynamic strength increased over the 8-wk training period without any significant changes in muscle fiber size or fat-free mass in men or women. This supports the concept of neural adaptations being the predominant mechanism in the early phase of training. It is interesting to note that a significant decrease in the Type IIB percentage was observed in women after just 2 wk of training (i.e., four workouts) and in the men after 4 wk of training (i.e., eight workouts). Over the 8-wk training program (16 workouts), the Type IIB muscle fiber types decreased to about 7% of the total muscle fibers in both men and women. The alteration in the muscle fiber types was supported by MHC analyses, with the replacement in this early phase of training of MHC IIB with MHC IIA chains. This was the first study to establish the time course of specific muscular adaptations in the early phase of a resistance training program for men or women. It is not known to what extent this remodeling of the muscle fibers may have contributed to muscle strength; however, gradual increases in the number and size of myofibrils and, perhaps, the fast

FIGURE 12.7.

Histochemical profile of muscle fiber subtype changes and myosin heavy-chains changes with resistance training. Male control subject (a–c) at the beginning of a training program and the end (d–f) of 8-wk training program. Male strength trained at beginning (g–i) and the end (j–l) of high-intensity strength training program. Arrows, scattered atrophic fibers, I, Type I; IC, Type Ic; C, Type IIac; A, Type IIa; AB, Type IIab; B, Type IIb. Bottom, Myosin heavy-chain analysis form biopsies obtained from female training and control subject. Note gradual loss of MHC IIb over time for training woman. Courtesy of Dr. Robert S. Staron, Ohio State University.

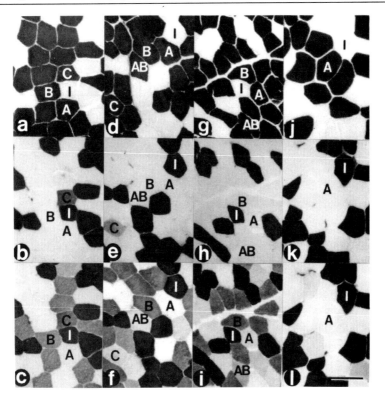

fiber type conversions of Type IIB to IIA might contribute to force production. In addition, this study demonstrated that changes in hormonal factors (testosterone and cortisol interactions) are correlated with such changes in the muscle fibers (e.g., percentage shift in Type IIA) and may help to mediate such adaptations. The data from this study demonstrates that although nervous system alterations may be the most dramatic effects mediating strength and power changes early in a training program, many other changes are taking place in the remodeling of the muscle fibers in the early phase of training that may have an influence when hypertrophy reaches a critical threshold. Thus, the "quality" of the protein type being generated because of the influence of resistance training is an important aspect of muscular development.

Longer periods of heavy resistance training have also examined changes in muscle fiber type and cross-sectional size with training. Staron et al. [144] examined changes in skeletal muscle in women who had trained for 20 wk, detrained for 30–32 wk, and then retrained for 6 wk. They observed dramatic increases in the cross-sectional muscle fiber size of all of the major fiber types. They also observed a decrease in the percentage of Type IIB muscle fibers with the 20 wk of training, using a program 2 days/wk, as reported above. The percentage of Type IIB fibers went down to 0.9%. This study also demonstrated that detraining did not result in muscle fiber returning to pretraining values of muscle fiber cross-sectional areas, but a conversion in the percentage Type IIA to Type IIB fibers toward pretraining values did occur. In addition, it was demonstrated that retraining resulted in a quicker change in muscle size and conversion to Type IIA fibers than when occurred when subjects started in an untrained condition. Such findings prompted the authors to suggest that, because the Type IIA fibers were as a group more oxidative than the Type IIB fibers in human muscles, a shift to the IIA fibers with training represents an increase in the oxidative capacity of strength-trained muscle. This has been supported by data from Frontera et al. [42], demonstrating that a significant increase in capillaries per fiber and citrate synthase activity in the vastus lateralis muscle of strength-trained older men. This adaptation may depend on the training status of the individual and the type of strength training program used. It might be postulated that the Type IIB fibers are a nonrecruited pool of fibers which, when recruited for high-threshold types of activities (i.e., heavy-resistance exercise), improve in oxidative ability, and changes in the histochemical profile are initiated and continue until few, if any, Type IIB fibers remain.

Several studies have also examined long-term heavy-resistance training programs in only men. In a group of studies using the same population of subjects, Dudley et al. [25] examined the impact of the type of muscle action on strength and muscle morphology. Hather et al. [63] examined the histochemical responses of the training program, and Adams et al. [3] examined the heavy-chain responses. Healthy men (36 yr old) acted as controls or performed heavy-resistance training (Groups: con [concentric training only] 4–5 sets of 6–12 reps, con/con [double concentric repetitions] 8–10 sets for 6–12 reps, and con/ecc [concentric and eccentric repetitions], 4–5 sets 6–12 reps) for 19 weeks, with some groups using con actions and another group using con/ecc actions. Three RM strength gains were made by all groups, but strength was significantly related to the total resistance used per day (partial r = 0.75). Biopsy samples from the vastus lateralis were obtained both before and after the training period. Increases in fiber area occurred in the con/con and con/ecc groups but not in the control and con only groups. Capillaries per fiber and capillaries per unit area were observed with training along with a concomitant increase in Type IIA muscle fibers [25, 63]. The proportion of Type I muscle fibers remained unchanged in all groups with training. Minor changes in strength were observed in the control group. The changes in the fiber subtypes was again paralleled by alterations in the MHC proteins, with a reduction in the MHC IIB content from 19% pretraining to 7% posttraining; MHC IIA content increased from 48 to 60%. The group means for percentage of Type IIB fibers decreased from approximately 18 to 1%, whereas the Type II A muscle fiber percentage increased from 46 to 60%. No changes were observed in the MHC I composition or fiber-type percentage [3]. Thus, transition of muscle fiber types that are associated with MHC content make dramatic changes with resistance training.

Kraemer et al. [105] examined changes in muscle fiber morphology over the course of a 3-mo training program in physically fit male subjects. Training took place 4 days/wk for 3 mo. Both high-intensity strength and endurance training programs were varied throughout the week to provide a "periodized" training program to enhance recovery from a high-volume exercise program to prevent overtraining (i.e., a decrease in performance). Thus, the weight-training program had 2 "heavy days" (i.e., 5 RM) and 2 "moderate days" (10 RM)/wk, and the endurance training program consisted of 2 "interval training" days and 2 "long duration" run days per week. Five groups of subjects were used to evaluate the muscle fiber changes in the vastus lateralis muscle, with training as follows: the S group performed a total body strength training program; the C group performed the same total body strength training program but also performed a high-intensity endurance training program; the UB group performed only the upper body strength training program and the high-intensity endurance training program; the E group performed only the high-intensity endurance training; and a control group performed no training. The data from the muscle fiber profile is shown in Table 12.1. The same response in the shift of muscle fiber types from Type IIB to Type IIA was again observed. It is doubtful that the Type IIB fibers, detected after training, were truly IIB, because of the lack of any measurement of the Type IIAB subtype. Ploutz et al. [128]

TABLE 12.1.
Muscle Fiber Characteristics Pre- and Posttraining

Group	C[a] (Pre-)	(n = 9) Post	S (Pre-)	(n = 9) (Post)	E (Pre-)	(n = 8) Post	UC (Pre-)	(n = 9) Post	Control (n = 5) (Pre-)	Control (n = 5) Post
% Type I	55.6 (±11.1)[b]	57.7 (±11.1)	55.21 (±11.7)	55.44 (±11.5)	54.1 (±5.9)	54.6 (±5.3)	50.6 (±8.0)	51.1 (±7.9)	52.0 (±11.5)	52.8 (±10.8)
IIC	1.9 (±2.2)	1.8 (±2.7)	2.4 (±1.6)	2.0 (±1.3)	0.9 (±0.6)	2.5[c] (±2.0)	1.3 (±1.0)	3.0[c] (±2.2)	1.6 (±0.9)	1.3 (±1.3)
IIA	28.4 (±15.4)	39.4[c] (±11.1)	23.3 (±11.5)	40.5[c] (±10.6)	25.75 (±4.8)	34.1[c] (±3.9)	25.5 (±4.2)	34.2[c] (±6.9)	25.6 (±1.6)	26.6 (±4.6)
IIB	14.11 (±7.2)	1.6[c] (±0.8)	19.1 (±7.9)	1.9[c] (±0.8)	19.2 (±3.6)	8.8[c] (±4.4)	22.6 (±4.9)	11.6[c] (±5.3)	20.8 (±7.6)	19.2 (±6.4)
Area I (μm²)	5008 (±874)	4756 (±692)	4883 (±1286)	5460[c] (±1214)	5437 (±970)	4853[c] (±966)	5680 (±535)	5376 (±702)	4946 (±1309)	5177 (±1344)
IIC	4157 (±983)	4658 (±771)	3981.2 (±1535)	5301[c] (±1956)	2741 (±482)	2402[c] (±352)	3050 (±930)	2918 (±1086)	3733 (±1285)	4062 (±1094)
IIA	5862 (±997)	7039[c] (±1151)	6084 (±1339)	7527[c] (±1981)	6782 (±1267)	6287 (±385)	6393 (±1109)	6357 (±1140)	6310 (±593)	6407 (±423)
IIB	5190 (±712)	4886 (±1171)	5795 (±1495)	6078 (±2604)	6325 (±1860)	4953 (±1405)	6052 (±1890)	5855 (±867)	5917 (±896)	6120 (±1089)

From ref. 105.
[a] Groups: C, combined; S, strength; E, endurance; UC, upper-body combined.
[b] Mean (±SD).
[c] $P < .05$ from corresponding pretraining value.

has shown that if the presence of IIAB fibers has not been determined, the remaining Type IIB fibers after high-intensity resistance training may not be true IIB fibers, as they each have been shown to have higher concentrations of aerobic enzymes. From this study it is obvious that the number of Type IIB muscle fibers is lower after high-intensity strength training, when compared to that of high-intensity endurance training, including interval training. This may be attributable to the greater recruitment of high-threshold motor units with heavy resistance training.

From an oxidative perspective it is interesting to note the small changes in the Type IIC population of muscle fibers. The use of just upper body strength training appears to also negate the decreases in Type I muscle fiber size in the legs with endurance training. This may be attributable to the isometric muscle actions of the legs that is needed to support the upper body for exercise. Changes in the muscle fiber areas (methods included measuring all available muscle fiber areas) demonstrate that changes occurred differentially across the continuum of exercise training modalities and that combination was dictated by the type or combination of training stimuli to which the muscle was exposed. It is interesting to note that the muscle fiber adaptations observed in the C group were different from those of either the S or the E groups, indicating that when two high-intensity training programs are used, with one focusing on high-intensity endurance training and the other on high-intensity strength training, the adaptive response of the combined group at the level of the muscle fiber is not the same as that of the single-mode training groups. In this study, power was compromised in the C group, and the rate of strength development appeared to demonstrate a trend toward a compromised state in the C group as well. Consistent with the results of several other studies, maximum oxygen consumption was not diminished by the performance of both a high-intensity strength and endurance training program [72, 114]. Thus, the mechanisms of adaptation to resistance exercise will depend on the global exercise stimuli presented to the activated musculature, and such changes may start to impact on performance in about 3 mo. It is also interesting that the changes in the fast fiber-type conversions have typically not been linked to the rate at which changes in the muscle fiber cross-sectional area take place, which appears to be the case over both the short- and long-term study durations.

Hypertrophy of Muscle Proteins

Muscle fibers must be activated to stimulate hypertrophy of intact muscle. Heavy resistance training has been shown to activate high-threshold motor units and, based on the size principle, typically stimulates all available motor units to meet the demands of heavy lifting. Thus, low-threshold to high-threshold motor units, containing both Type I and Type II muscle fibers, are recruited and are, therefore, presented with a potent stimulus for adaptation. Thus, resistance training typically results in increases in both the

Type I and Type II muscle fiber areas, as previously discussed. This fiber hypertrophy is translated to increases in the cross-sectional size of the intact muscle, which can be observed over several months [8, 9]. An upper limit of muscle cell growth has not been determined, but it has been suggested that an "optimal size" or ceiling of adaptation may exist for individual muscle fibers after a prolonged period of strength training. Alterations in the neural patterns of activation within the muscle to recruit all the available fibers may also be of importance for the intact muscle to achieve maximal hypertrophy [64]. The possibility of using hyperplasia as a potential adaptive strategy still exists [7], but the extent and frequency of the adaptive response remain topics of debate. It may be that hyperplasia exists but that the magnitude of its contribution, even in exceptional situations, may not be great (<5%). In addition, hyperplasia may not occur equally in all individuals [111].

The increase in muscle fiber hypertrophy is thought to occur by means of a remodeling of protein within the cell and an increase in the size and number of myofibrils [111]. Furthermore, increases in the number of the actin and myosin filaments, along with sarcomere addition, contribute to the increase in muscle fiber size and, ultimately, the intact muscle. It has been suggested that the packing density of actin increases, but not that of myosin, as the contractile proteins are added to the outside of the myofibril without altering the cross-bridge configurations [7, 111]. Also, the impact of con/ecc actions may play a role in optimization of training responses [15, 25].

The mechanisms and biochemical alterations that mediate the net changes observed with heavy-resistance exercise training remain an intense topic of study. The signals (e.g., hormonal) provided by the heavy-resistance exercise appear to stimulate the uptake of amino acids, yet their incorporation into the contractile unit is not guaranteed. Enhanced synthesis of contractile proteins appears to be primarily involved with those athletes who are not already highly adapted to the resistance exercise stimulus (e.g., as is the case competitive lifters). It is possible that contractile proteins accumulate in the muscle fiber, either by means of an increased synthesis or a decreased rate of breakdown or some combination of both. This also may be fiber specific with Type I reducing degradation and Type II increasing synthesis [50]. It is clear that muscle fibers are disrupted and certain fibers damaged with intense resistance exercise [95]. The extent of this damage is less in trained individuals than it is in untrained individuals. The repair process of remodeling the muscle fiber may well involve a host of regulatory mechanisms (e.g., hormonal and metabolic), interacting with the training status of the individual, as well as the availability of protein.

Although the protein needs of individuals who engage in heavy-resistance exercise may be great only during the period of time during which the majority of muscle hypertrophy is taking place in the muscle, that level of protein need may not be maintained but rather lowered in more advanced trained individuals, in whom a reduction in the rate of protein degradation in some fibers may suffice to support the maintenance of hypertrophic gains [29, 50]. This process would follow the adaptational events of muscle fiber hypertrophy and, when fully stimulated with an adequate muscle protocol, will be greatest in the first 6 months to a year of training in healthy adults. One factor that may determine the amount of needed protein is the type of heavy-resistance training program used (e.g., single-exercise, low-volume protocol vs. multiple-exercise high-volume protocol). The greater the total amount of stimulated muscle fibers in a program, the greater the potential protein requirement for the adaptive period of time for the program. Total-body protocols may have a longer requirement for greater amounts of protein because of a larger amount of muscle mass being remodeled. It is interesting that a multitude of sizes of muscle fibers exist even in highly trained individuals suggesting all fibers (within a type) have not met a maximal size limit due to neuromuscular recruitment.

STRENGTH TRAINING IN THE ELDERLY

Loss of muscle mass with age in humans has been demonstrated both indirectly and directly [58, 59, 75, 92]. The excretion of urinary creatinine, reflecting muscle creatine content and total muscle mass, decreases by nearly 50% between the ages of 20 and 90 [155]. Computed tomography of individual muscles shows that, after age 30, there is a decrease in cross-sectional areas of the thigh, along with decreased muscle density associated with increased intramuscular fat. These changes are most pronounced in women [74]. Muscle atrophy may result from a gradual and selective loss of muscle fibers. The number of muscle fibers in the midsection of the vastus lateralis of autopsy specimens is lower by about 110,000 in elderly men (ages 70–73) than it is in young men (ages 19–37), a 23% difference [110]. The decline is more marked in Type II muscle fibers, which fall from an average of 60% in sedentary young men to below 30% after the age of 80 [107], and it is significantly related to age-related decreases in strength ($r = .54$, $P < .001$). This age-associated reduction in muscle mass has been termed sarcopenia [29].

A reduction in muscle strength is a major component of normal aging. Data from the Framingham [76] study indicate that 40% of the female population at ages 55–64, almost 45% of women at ages 65–74, and 65% of women at ages 75–84 were unable to lift 4.5 kg. In addition, a similarly high percentage of women in this population reported that they were unable to perform some aspects of normal household work. Larsson et al. [109] studied 114 men between the ages of 11 and 70 yr and found that isometric and dynamic strength of the quadriceps increased up to age of 30 yr and decreased after age of 50. They saw reductions in strength between ages 50 and 70 that ranged from 24 to 36%. They concluded that much of the reduction in strength was attributable to a selective atrophy of Type II muscle fibers, which were 36% smaller in diameter, when compared to those of 40-yr-old subjects. It appears that muscle strength losses are most dramatic after age of 70. Knee extensor strength of a group of healthy 80-yr-old men and women studied in the Copenhagen City Heart Study [17] was found to be 30% lower than that in a previous population study [5] of 70-yr-old men and women. Thus, cross-sectional, as well as longitudinal data indicate that muscle strength declines by approximately 15% per decade in the sixth and seventh decades and by about 30% thereafter [17, 61, 108, 119]. Frontera et al. [41] examined more than 200 men and women between the ages of 45 and 78 yr old. Isokinetic and isometric strength of the upper and lower body were significantly different between men and women and decreased with advancing age. However, when corrected to total-body muscle mass (from urinary creatinine excretion), no significant age or gender associated differences in strength were seen.

As a result of these age-associated changes in muscle mass and strength, a great deal of attention has been focused on strategies for prevention and/or reversal. For this reason, resistance training has been demonstrated to be an effective means of increasing strength and improving functional status in the elderly. Aniansson and co-workers [5] demonstrated that a low-intensity resistance training regimen produce limited results, leading to the conclusion of some authors that the elderly have a lower capacity to respond to strengthening exercises than do younger people. Moritani and DeVries [118] examined a higher intensity training program in older men (yr) and concluded that the capacity for the elderly to increase strength is preserved; however, they also concluded that skeletal muscle has a reduced capacity for hypertrophy. Although they were unable to detect any evidence of muscle hypertrophy, their methods were indirect only. They used limb circumference and skinfold determinations to estimate muscle size. Frontera and co-workers used a high-intensity resistance training regimen (3 sets of 8 reps at 80% of 1 RM, 3 days/wk, for 12 wk) in a group of previously sedentary older men (ages 60–72 yrs) [43] and demonstrated substantial strength gains (up to a 200% increase in 1 RM of the knee extensors) and evidence of muscle hypertrophy from CAT and muscle biopsy analysis. The biopsy results demonstrated increases in both Type I and II fibers.

This increase in muscle size was also associated with an increase in 3-methylhistidine excretion, indicating that muscle hypertrophy is also associated with an increase in muscle protein degradation. This capacity for high-intensity resistance training to increase muscle fiber size has also been demonstrated in older women. Charrette and co-workers [14] examined muscle biopsies taken before and after 12 wk of high-intensity resistance training and demonstrated an increase in Type II fiber area with no significant change in Type I area. Fiatarone et al. [30] examined a group of very old (87–96 yr) men and women. They used a training stimulus that was similar to that of Frontera et al. [43]; however, their subjects trained only the knee extensors for only 8 wk. This study was the first to demonstrate that the capacity for muscle strength improvement is preserved, even in the oldest elderly person. This study also examined CT scans taken before and after training and demonstrated a significant increase in muscle size. However, as can be seen from Figure 12.8, the variability of this hypertrophic response is remarkable. More recently, this group of investigators [31] examined a larger group of very old, frail men and women and demonstrated

FIGURE 12.8.
Muscle mass changes (estimated from CT scans), resulting from 8 wk of high-intensity resistance training of eight very old nursing home subjects. Each bar represents changes experience by an individual. This graph of individual changes demonstrates the remarkable variability of response seen in the very old. Drawn from ref. 30.

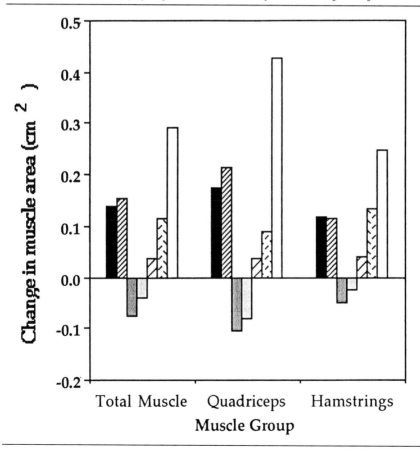

that high-intensity resistance training (80% of 1 RM for 10 wk) is safe for this population and produced significant increases in strength but no significant increase in muscle size. It is important to note that the increase in strength was associated with an increase in gait speed, stair-climbing power, balance, and overall spontaneous activity.

Recent research efforts have focused on the effects of resistance training on muscle protein metabolism. Campbell and co-workers [11] examined nitrogen balance before and after 12 wk of high-intensity resistance training (3 sets of 8 reps, 80% of 1 RM, upper and lower body exercises) in a group of older men and women. They found that resistance training increases nitrogen retention and, thus, lower dietary protein needs. In addition, a primed constant infusion of 1-[^{13}C]leucine revealed that training resulted in a significant increase in the rate of whole-body protein synthesis. Yarasheski and co-workers [158] determined the rate of quadriceps muscle protein synthesis, using the in vivo rate of incorporation of intravenously infused [^{13}C]leucine into mixed-muscle protein in both younger (24 yr) and older (63–66 yr) men and women before and at the end of 2 wk of resistance exercise training (2–4 sets, of 4–10 repetitions at 60–90% of 1 RM, 5 days/wk). They found that although the older subjects have a lower rate of muscle protein synthesis before training, the resistance exercise resulted in a significant increase in muscle protein synthetic rate in both groups of subjects. It is interesting to note that, although growth hormone (GH) administration has been suggested as an anabolic agent [130], when GH administration is combined with resistance training, it does not cause any greater increase in muscle mass than training alone [157].

Although many resistance training studies have examined short-term adaptations in the elderly, a few have examined strength and body composition changes after 52 wk or longer. Morganti et al. [116] examined 39 healthy postmenopausal women (59 ± 0.9 yr) who were randomized to either a control group or a progressive resistance training group (3 sets of 8 reps, 80% of 1 RM, upper and lower body exercises) that trained twice weekly for 12 mo. Strength continued to improve, with no evidence of a plateau during the 12 mo of the study. With the lateral pull-down, knee extension, and double-leg press, the greatest changes in strength were seen in the first 3 mo of the study. However, smaller, but statistically significant, changes were seen in the second 6 mo of the study (Fig. 12.9). These data support previous studies demonstrating large increases during the initial weeks of resistance exercise training. Using the same population of women, Nelson et al. [123] also demonstrated that high-intensity resistance training had significant effects on bone health, with increases reported in femoral and lumbar spine density after 1 yr of training. In addition to its effects on bone, resistance training was demonstrated to improve balance, total levels of physical activity, and muscle mass. Thus, resistance training has an effect on most of the major risk factors for an osteoporotic bone fracture.

FIGURE 12.9.
Mean percentage strength gains seen in a group of postmenopausal women during 1 yr of high-intensity resistance training (3 sets of 8 rep, 2 × wk, 80% of 1 RM, 52 wk)

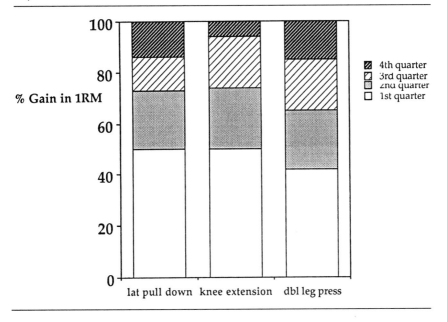

It is clear that the capacity to adapt to increased levels of physical activity is preserved even in the oldest elderly person. Regularly performed exercise has been demonstrated to result in a remarkable number of positive changes in elderly men and women. Because scrappiness and weakness may be an almost universal characteristic of advancing age, strategies for preserving or increasing muscle mass in the elderly should be implemented. With increasing muscle strength, increased levels of spontaneous activity have been seen in both healthy, free-living older subjects and very old and frail men and women. Resistance training, in addition to its positive effects on insulin action, bone density, energy metabolism, and functional status, may also be an important way of increasing levels of physical activity in the elderly. Resistance training may be one of the most effective and least costly means of intervention used to preserve independence that is available to a wide segment of the population.

ADDITIONAL SUPPORT SYSTEMS FOR MUSCLE ADAPTATION

Enzymes involved with oxidative metabolism obtained from weight-trained pooled muscle fiber types have not demonstrated increased activity [90,

147]. Nevertheless, increases in oxidative enzymes have been shown to be higher in Type IIA fibers than in Type IIB fibers [128]. Bodybuilders use programs of greater volume, with short rest periods between sets and exercises, and moderate-intensity training loads have been shown to have higher citrate synthase activity in fast-twitch fibers than those used by other types of lifters, who use heavier loads and longer rest periods between sets [147]. Thus, the type of program may influence the magnitude of aerobic enzyme changes in the muscle.

Little change in the nonglycolytic enzymes (e.g., creatine kinase or myokinase) have been observed with resistance exercise training [147]. Myosin ATPase has also shown only minor changes in pooled muscle fibers [147]. The fact that various isoforms of myosin ATPase exist and are altered with strength training may implicate the type of isoform as being more important than the absolute concentration change, especially when it is not accounted for by individual fiber analyses. Anaerobic-glycolytic enzymes (e.g., phosphofructokinase or lactate dehydrogenase) have been shown to be unaffected by heavy-resistance exercise training [71, 82, 149, 150, 154]. It again appears that the type of lifting protocol impacts the concentrations of such enzymes, because bodybuilders, swimmers, and physically active students all showed similar levels of PFK activity [150].

Muscle Substrate Stores

Glycogen content of skeletal muscle has been shown to increase with resistance training or to show no change [150]. Resistance training does not increase adenosine triphosphatase (ATP) or creatine phosphate concentrations in muscle [150]. Such findings for ATP and creatine phosphate may be attributable to the lack of significant amounts of muscle fiber hypertrophy, yet normal levels have been observed in athletes with dramatic hypertrophy [150]. The recent practice of using creatine supplementation and its effects on strength and power production, even in trained individuals, appears to support the concept that training alone induces only small changes but that muscle is still capable of enhanced energy stores with supplementation [51].

The enhancement of lipid stores in muscles with resistance training remains equivocal, as increases have been observed in the triceps muscle of the arm but not in the quadriceps muscles after training. The type of program, dietary profile, and potential differential responses of the upper vs. lower body could all help to explain differences between studies.

Myoglobin content in the muscle after a strength training program may be decreased [147]. Thus, it has been postulated that long-term strength training may depress myoglobin content and, therefore, the ability of muscle fibers to extract oxygen. Thus, a few changes occur in the metabolic substrate support systems, but few alterations beyond basic activities occur when strength training is specifically directed toward strength and power adaptations only. Again, the initial state of training, as well as the specific type of program that is used, can influence the variables mentioned above.

Capillary Supply and Mitochondrial Density

Oxidative metabolism is supported by capillary supply to the exercising muscle and the availability of cellular mitochondria to carry out oxidative metabolic cycles. Improved capillary structures have been observed to be enhanced with resistance training in untrained subjects [43, 63, 145, 150]. Hather et al. [63] demonstrated that, with all types of training (i.e., combinations of con/ecc muscle actions), capillaries per unit area and per fiber were significantly increased in response to heavy-resistance training, even with expansion of fiber areas. When comparing various types of lifters reflective of very specific types of training programs and performance outcomes, Olympic weightlifters and power lifters have showed lower and body builders higher capillary density when compared to untrained men. This may be in part attributable to the larger fibers exhibited by weight lifters and power lifters, contributing to an area dilution. Furthermore, how much blood flow is needed may be a function of the type of protocol used in training.

It has been shown that bodybuilders use moderate-intensity (e.g., 10RM), high-volume (many sets), and short-rest (1 min or less between sets and exercises) protocols, which result in lactate concentrations beyond 20 mmol $\cdot$ L^{-1} [98]. The higher capillary density may increase the ability to remove lactate from the muscle to the blood, thereby allowing better performance under such high lactate conditions [104]. Kraemer et al. [104] demonstrated that body builders had a greater capacity to use heavier loads under the same lactate conditions, as compared to that of power lifters, which suggests that greater clearance and buffering took place to allow for the superior strength performance in the lifting protocol. Because blood lactate levels observed with heavy-resistance protocols used by power lifters and weightlifters are rarely above 4 mmol $\cdot$ L^{-1}, the physiological stimulus to increase capillary increases may not be as great. As stated before, improved capillary density may be a function associated with the activation of a particular motor unit and, thus, may be dependent on the protocol and conditions under which the exercise is being performed (e.g., acid-base status).

The time course of such changes in capillary density appears to be unclear, as studies have shown that 6–12 wks may not stimulate capillary growth beyond normal untrained levels [147, 148, 150]. With extreme changes in muscle hypertrophy, capillary neoformation is typically smaller, muting the changes observed. As we have shown, studies have observed changes in capillary density with resistance training. Several factors may help explain the various results, including the possibility that such changes may depend on the method of analysis used, activated vs. nonactivated fibers may vary, and/or the initial training status may influence the potential for changes in those fibers. Thus, a base level of capillarization may exist for activated muscle fibers and, with further training, may be increased to address the functional demands of the fibers by means of the resistance training program.

Mitochondrial density has been shown to decrease with strength training because of the dilution effects of muscle fiber hypertrophy [112]. The observation of decreased mitochondrial density with strength and power training is consistent with the demands for oxidative metabolism placed upon the musculature. Furthermore, oxidative enzymes, although probably necessary in a minimal threshold concentration in activated fibers, are not necessary in higher amounts to enhance or mediate exercise performance.

Hormonal Factors

Endocrine factors play an important support function for adaptational mechanisms in skeletal muscle, ultimately leading to enhanced force production [86, 88, 89, 99, 106]. The primary mechanisms through which hormones mediate changes are related to their metabolic or trophic effects on the target cells of the body (i.e., nerve and muscle cells). It is well established that anabolic hormones (e.g., testosterone, insulin, insulin-like-growth Factor 1 and growth hormone) play various roles in enhancing tissue status. In addition, gender differences (i.e., testosterone responses) in these hormonal concentrations and responses to exercise do exist [98, 100]. The key sequence of events is related to the effective stimulation of an endocrine, paracrine, and/or autocrine endogenous response by the exercise protocol. These signals must then be received by the receptor mechanisms at or in the target tissues. The alteration of metabolism (typically, protein) and the molecular mechanisms associated with a cell transport phenomenon must then be translated into synthesis, reduced degradation, or augmentation of the cells' functional structure or secretory products, leading to enhanced muscle mass and/or improved force production.

The complexity of the neuroendocrine system has just started to be realized as a myriad of interactions occur among hormones and hormonal factors. Furthermore, endocrine function is highly integrated with nutritional status, nutritional intake, and other external factors (e.g., stress, sleep, and disease), which affect the remodeling and repair processes in the body. Much of the work in the area of hormonal changes with resistance exercise has focused on the alteration of hormonal concentrations in circulation [88, 89]. Differential alterations in hormones have been observed to be a function of the type of exercise protocol followed and its associated physiological demands.

How autocrine and paracrine changes are affected by heavy-resistance training remains unknown, and methodological considerations make it difficult to determine with greater sensitivity needed to assess such small local changes in cells or various intercellular spaces. Furthermore, our view of

FIGURE 12.10.

Responses of androgen receptors to training (maximum binding capacity). It is theorized that maximal binding of the androgen receptors in Type I muscles decreases to maintain optimal cell size and that Type II androgen receptors increase binding. Drawn from ref. 19.

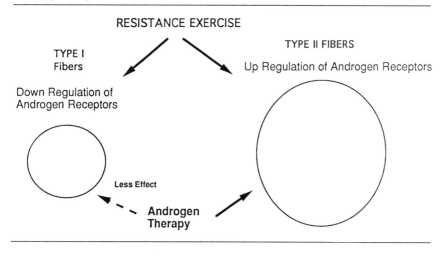

the endocrine system in response to resistance exercise has been somewhat limited to those molecular forms, which can be detected with an antibody mediated assay (immunoreactive molecular forms), thus eliminating from view the various molecular forms that are not immunoreactive (e.g., various forms of growth hormone). Finally, our understanding of the receptors on the target tissue for various hormones is just starting to develop [66]. We now understand that the receptors can be differentially regulated in different fiber types in response to exercise of different types [10, 19]. These responses at the target level determine whether a hormonal message is realized at the level of the individual cells. Figure 12.10 overviews responses of androgen receptors to resistance exercise.

SUMMARY

Adaptations in resistance training are focused on the development and maintenance of the neuromuscular unit needed for force production [97, 136]. The effects of training, when using this system, affect many other physiological systems of the body (e.g., the connective tissue, cardiovascular, and endocrine systems) [16, 18, 37, 77, 83]. Training programs are highly specific to the types of adaptation that occur. Activation of specific patterns of motor units in training dictate what tissue and how other physiological systems will be affected by the exercise training. The time course of the development of the neuromuscular system appears to be dominated in the early phase by neural factors with associated changes in the types of contractile proteins. In the later adaptation phase, muscle protein increases, and the contractile unit begins to contribute the most to the changes in performance capabilities. A host of other factors can affect the adaptations, such as functional capabilities of the individual, age, nutritional status, and behavioral factors (e.g., sleep and health habits). Optimal adaptation appears to be related to the use of specific resistance training programs to meet individual training objectives.

REFERENCES

1. Adams, G. R., M. R. Duvoisin, and G. A. Dudley. Magnetic resonance imaging and electromyography as indexes of muscle function. *J. Appl. Physiol.* 73:1578–1583, 1992.
2. Adams, G. R., R. T. Harris, D. Woodard, and G. A. Dudley. Mapping of electrical muscle stimulation using MRI. *J. Appl. Physiol.* 74(2):532–537, 1993.
3. Adams, G. R., B. M. Hather, K. M. Baldwin, and G. A. Dudley. Skeletal muscle myosin heavy chain composition and resistance training. *J. Appl. Physiol.* 74(2):911–915, 1993.
4. Andonian, M. J., and M. A. Fahim. Effects of endurance exercise on the morphology of mouse neuromuscular junctions during aging. *J. Neurocytol.* 16:589–599, 1987.
5. Aniansson, A., G. Grimby, Hedberg, M., and M. Krotkiewski. Muscle morphology, enzyme activity and muscle strength in elderly men and women. *Clin. Physiol.* 1:73–86, 1981.
6. Aniansson, A., and E. Gustafsson. Physical training in elderly men with special reference to quadriceps muscle strength and morphology. *Clin. Physiol.* 1:87–98, 1981.
7. Antonio, J., and W. J. Gonyea. Muscle fiber splitting in stretch-enlarged avian muscle. *Med. Sci. Sports Exerc.* 26(8):973–977, 1994.
8. Billeter, R., and H. Hoppeler. Muscular basis of strength. Komi, P. (ed). *Strength and Power in Sports. The Encyclopaedia of Sports Medicine.* Oxford, England: Blackwell, 1992, pp. 39–63.
9. Booth, F. W., and D. B. Thomason. Molecular and cellular adaptation of muscle in response to exercise: perspective of various models. *Physiol. Rev.* 71:541–585, 1991.
10. Bricourt, V. A., P. S. Germain, B. D. Serrurier, and C. Y. Guezennec. Changes in testosterone muscle receptors: effects of an androgen treatment on physically trained rats. *Cell Mol. Biol.* 40:291–294, 1994.
11. Campbell, W. W., M. C. Crim, V. R. Young, L. J. Joseph, and W. J. Evans. Effects of resistance training and dietary protein intake on protein metabolism in older adults. *Am. J. Physiol.* 268:E1143–E1153, 1995.
12. Cannon, R., and E. Cafarelli. Neuromuscular adaptations to training. *J. Appl. Physiol.* 63:2396–2402, 1987.
13. Carolan, B., and E. Cafarelli. Adaptations in coactivation after isometric resistance training. *J. Appl. Physiol.* 73:911–917, 1992.
14. Charette, S. L., L. McEvoy, G. Pyka, C. Snow-Harter, D. Guido, R. A. Wiswell, and R. Marcus. Muscle hypertrophy response to resistance training in older women. *J. Appl. Physiol.* 70:1912–1916, 1991.
15. Colliander, E. B., and P. A. Tesch. Effects of eccentric and concentric muscle actions in resistance training. *Acta Physiol. Scand.* 140:31–39, 1990.
16. Conroy, B. P., W. J. Kraemer, C. M. Maresh, G. P. Dalsky, S. J. Fleck, M. H. Stone, P. Miller, and A. C. Fry. Bone mineral density in elite junior weightlifters. *Med. Sci. Sports Exerc.* 25(10):1103–1109, 1993.
17. Danneskoild-Samsoe, B., V. Kofod, J. Munter, G. Grimby, P. Schnohr, and G. Jensen. Mus-

cle strength and functional capacity in 77–81 year old men and women. *Eur. J. Appl. Physiol.* 52:123–135, 1984.

18. Deschenes, M., W. J. Kraemer, C. M. Maresh, and J. F. Crivello. Exercise-induced hormonal changes and their effects upon skeletal muscle tissue. *Sports Med.* 12(2):80–93, 1991.

19. Deschenes, M. R., C. M. Maresh, L. E. Armstrong, J. M. Covault, W. J. Kraemer, and J. F. Crivello. Endurance and resistance exercise induce muscle fiber type specific responses in androgen binding capacity. *J. Steroid Biochem. Mol. Biol.* 50(3/4):175–179, 1994.

20. Deschenes, M. R., C. M. Maresh, J. F. Crivello, L. E. Armstrong, W. J. Kraemer, and J. Covault. The effects of exercise training of different intensities on neuromuscular junction morphology. *J. Neurocytol.* 22:603–615, 1993.

21. Desmedt, J. E. The size principle of motoneuron recruitment in ballistic or ramp-voluntary contractions in man. J. E. Desmedt (ed). *Progress in Clinical Neurophysiology*, Vol. 9: *Motor Unit Types, Recruitment and Plasticity in Health and Disease*. Basel, Switzerland: Karger, 1981, pp. 250–304.

22. Dudley, G. A., and R. T. Harris. Use of electrical stimulation in strength and power training. Komi, P. (ed). *Strength and Power in Sports. The Encyclopaedia of Sports Medicine*. Oxford, England: Blackwell, 1992, pp. 329–337.

23. Dudley, G. A., R. T. Harris, M. R. Duvoisin, B. M. Hather, and P. Buchanan. Effect of voluntary vs. artificial activation on the relationship of muscle torque to speed. *J. Appl. Physiol.* 69(6):2215–2221, 1990.

24. Dudley, G. A., R. S. Staron, T. F. Murray, F. C. Hagerman, and A. Luginbuhl. Muscle fiber composition and blood ammonia levels after intense exercise in humans. *J. Appl. Physiol.* 54:582–586, 1983.

25. Dudley, G. A., P. A. Tesch, B. J. Miller, and P. Buchanan. Importance of eccentric actions in performance adaptations to resistance training. *Aviat. Space Environ. Med.* 62:543–550, 1991.

26. Edman, K. A. P. Contractile performance of skeletal muscle fibers. Komi, P. (ed). *Strength and Power in Sports. The Encyclopaedia of Sports Medicine*. Oxford, England: Blackwell, 1992, pp. 96–114.

27. Enoka, R. Muscle strength and its development: new perspectives. *Sports Med.* 6:146–168, 1988.

28. Essen, R., E. Jansson, J. Henriksson, A. W. Taylor, and B. Saltin. Metabolic characteristics of fibre types in human skeletal muscle. *Acta Physiol. Scand.* 95:153–165, 1975.

29. Evans, W. J., and W. W. Campbell. Sarcopenia and age-related changes in body composition and functional capacity. *J. Nutr.* 123:465–468, 1993.

30. Fiatarone, M. A., E. C. Marks, N. D. Ryan, C. N. Meredith, L. A. Lipstiz, and W. J. Evans. High-intensity strength training in nonagenarians. Effects on skeletal muscle. *J.A.M.A.* 263:3029–3034, 1990.

31. Fiatarone, M. A., E. F. O'Neill, N. D. Ryan, K. M. Clements, G. R. Solares, M. E. Nelson, S. B. Roberts, J. J. Kehayias, L. A. Lipsitz, and W. J. Evans. Exercise training and nutritional supplementation for physical frailty in very elderly people. *N. Engl. J. Med.* 330(25):1769–1775, 1994.

32. Fisher, M. J., R. A. Meyer, G. R. Adams, J. M. Foley, and E. J. Potchen. Direct relationship between proton T_2 and exercise intensity in skeletal muscle MR images. *Invest. Radiol.* 25:480–485, 1990.

33. Fleck, S. J., and W. J. Kraemer. *Designing Resistance Training Programs*. Champaign, IL: Human Kinetics, 1987.

34. Fleck, S. J., and W. J. Kraemer. Resistance training: basic principles. *Phys. Sportsmed.* 16(3):160–171, 1988.

35. Fleck, S. J., and W. J. Kraemer. Resistance training: physiological adaptations. *Phys. Sportsmed.* 16(4):108–124, 1988.

36. Fleck, S. J., and W. J. Kraemer. Resistance training: physiological adaptations. *Phys. Sportsmed.* 16(5):63–76, 1988.

37. Fleck, S. J., P. M. Pattany, M. H. Stone, J. T. Kearney, W. J. Kraemer, J. Thrush, and K. Wong. Magnetic resonance imaging determination of left ventricular mass in elite Junior Olympic weightlifters. *Med. Sci. Sports Exerc.* 25(4):522–527, 1993.

38. Fleckenstein, J. L., L . A. Bertocci, R. L. Nunnally, R. W. Parkey, and R. M. Peschock. Exercise-enhanced MR imaging of variations in forearm muscle anatomy and use: importance in MR spectroscopy. *Am. J. Roentgenol. Radium Ther. Nucl. Med.* 153:693–698, 1991.

39. Fleckenstein, J. L., R. G. Haller, S. F. Lewis, B. T. Archer, B. R. Barker, J. Payne, R. W. Parkey, and R. M. Peschock. Absence of exercise-induced MRI enhancement of skeletal muscle in McArdle's disease. *J. Appl. Physiol.* 71:961–969, 1991.

40. Fleckenstein, J. L., D. Watumull, L. A. Bertocci, R. W. Parkey, and R. M. Pershock. Finger-specific flexor recruitment in humans: depiction by exercise-enhanced MRI. *J. Appl. Physiol.* 72:1974–1977, 1992.

41. Frontera, W. R., V. A. Hughes, and W. J. Evans. A cross-sectional study of upper and lower extremity muscle strength in 45–78 year old men and women. *J. Appl. Physiol.* 71:644–650, 1991.

42. Frontera, W. R., C. N. Meredith, K. P. O'Reilly, and W. J. Evans. Strength training and determinants of VO_2max in older men. *J. Appl. Physiol.* 68:329–333, 1990.

43. Frontera, W. R., C. N. Meredith, K. P. O'Reilly, H. G. Knuttgen, and W. J. Evans. Strength conditioning in older men: skeletal muscle hypertrophy and improved function. *J. Appl. Physiol.* 64:1038–1044, 1988.

44. Fry, A. C., C. A. Allemeier, and R. S. Staron. Correlation between percentage fiber type area and myosin heavy chain content in human skeletal muscle. *Eur. J. Appl. Physiol.* 68:246–251, 1994.

45. Fry, A. C., W. J. Kraemer, M. H. Stone, B. J. Warren, S. J. Fleck, J. T. Kearney, and S. E. Gordon. Acute endocrine responses to over-reaching before and after 1 year of weightlifting training. *Can. J. Appl. Physiol.* 19(4):400–410, 1994.

46. Fry, A. C., W. J. Kraemer, F. van Borselen, J. M. Lynch, J. L. Marsit, N. T. Triplett, and L. P. Koziris. Catecholamine responses to short-term, high intensity resistance exercise overtraining. *J. Appl. Physiol.* 77(2):941–946, 1994.

47. Fry, A. C., W. J. Kraemer, C. A. Weseman, B. P. Conroy, S. E. Gordon, J. R. Hoffman, and C. M. Maresh. The effects of an off-season strength and conditioning program on starters and non starters in women's intercollegiate volleyball. *J. Appl. Sport Sci. Res.* 5(4):174–181, 1991.

48. Garfinkel, S., and E. Cafarelli. Relative changes in maximal force, EMG, and muscle cross-sectional area after isometric training. *Med. Sci. Sports Exerc.* 24:1220–1227, 1992.

49. Garhammer, J., and B. Takano. Training for weightlifting. P. Komi (ed). *Strength and Power in Sports. The Encyclopaedia of Sports Medicine.* Oxford, England: Blackwell, 1992, pp. 357–369.

50. Goldspink, C. Cellular and molecular aspects of adaptation in skeletal muscle. P. Komi (ed). *Strength and Power in Sports. The Encyclopaedia of Sports Medicine.* Oxford, England: Blackwell, 1992, pp. 211–229.

51. Greenhaff, P. L., A. Casey, A. H. Short, R. Harris, K. Söderlund, and E. Hultman. Influence of oral creatine supplementation on muscle torque during repeated bouts of maximal voluntary exercise in man. *Clin. Sci.* 84:565–571, 1993.

52. Häkkinen, K. Neuromuscular and hormonal adaptations during strength and power training. A review. *J. Sports Med.* 29:9–26, 1989.

53. Häkkinen, K. Neuromuscular adaptation during strength training, again, detraining and immobilization. *Crit. Rev. Phys. Rehabil. Med.* 6(3):161–198, 1994.

54. Häkkinen, K., M. Alén, and P. V. Komi. Changes in isometric force- and relaxation-time, electromyographic and muscle fibre characteristics of human skeletal muscle during strength training and detraining. *Acta Physiol. Scand.* 125:573–585, 1985.

55. Häkkinen, K., and P. Komi. Training-induced changes in neuromuscular performance under voluntary and reflex conditions. *Eur. J. Appl. Physiol.* 55:147, 1986.

56. Häakkinen, K., P. V. Komi, and P. A. Tesch. Effect of combined concentric and eccentric strength training and detraining on force-time, muscle fiber and metabolic characteristics of leg extensor muscles. *Scand. J. Sports. Sci.* 3:50–58, 1981.
57. Häkkinen, K., and A. Pakarinen. Acute hormonal responses to two different fatiguing heavy-resistance protocols in male athletes. *J. Appl. Physiol.* 74(2):882–887, 1993.
58. Häkkinen, K., and A. Pakarinen. Muscle strength and serum testosterone, cortisol and SHBG concentrations in middle-aged and elderly men and women. *Acta. Physiol. Scand.* 148:199–207, 1993.
59. Häkkinen, K., and A. Pakarinen. Serum hormones and strength development during strength training in middle-aged and elderly males and females. *Acta Physiol. Scand.* 150:1–9, 1994.
60. Häkkinen, K., A. Pakarinen, M. Alén, H. Kauhanen, and P. V. Komi. Neuromuscular and hormonal adaptations in athletes to strength training in two years. *J. Appl. Physiol.* 65:2406–2412, 1988.
61. Harries, U. J., and E. J. Bassey. Torque-velocity relationships for the knee extensors in women in their 3rd and 7th decades. *Eur. J. Appl. Physiol.* 60:187–190, 1990.
62. Hather, B. M., C. E. Mason, and G. A. Dudley. Histochemical demonstration of skeletal muscle fiber types and capillaries on the same transverse section. *Clin. Physiol.* 11:127–134, 1991.
63. Hather, B. M., P. A. Tesch, P. Buchanan, and G. A. Dudley. Influence of eccentric actions on skeletal muscle adaptations to resistance training. *Acta Physiol. Scand.* 143:177–185, 1991.
64. Hay, J. G. Mechanical basis of strength expression. P. Komi (ed). *Strength and Power in Sports. The Encyclopaedia of Sports Medicine.* Oxford, England: Blackwell, 1992, pp. 197–210.
65. Henneman, E., G. Somjen, and D. O. Carpenter. Functional significance of cell size in apinal motoneurones. *J. Neurophysiol.* 28:560–580, 1985.
66. Hickson, R. C., and J. R. Marone. Exercise and inhibition of glucocorticoid-induced muscle atrophy. *Exer. Sport Sci. Rev.* 21:135–168, 1993.
67. Hoffman, J. R., A. C. Fry, R. Howard, C. M. Maresh, and W. J. Kraemer. Strength, speed, and endurance changes during the course of a Division I basketball season. *J. Appl. Sport Sci. Res.* 5(3):144–149, 1991.
68. Hoffman, J. R., W. J. Kraemer, A. C. Fry, M. Deschenes, and M. Kemp. The effects of self-selection for frequency of training in a winter conditioning program for football. *J. Appl. Sport Sci. Res.* 4(3):76–82, 1990.
69. Hoffman, J. R., C. M. Maresh, L. E. Armstrong, and W. J. Kraemer. The effects of off-season and in-season resistance training programs on collegiate male basketball team. *J. Hum. Muscle Perform.* 1(2):48–55, 1991.
70. Hoppeler, H. Exercise-induced ultrastructural changes in skeletal muscle. *Int. J. Sports Med.* 7:187–204, 1986.
71. Houston, M. E., E. A. Froese, S. P. Valeriote, H. J. Green, and D. A. Ramey. Muscle performance, morphology and metabolic capacity during strength training and detraining: a one leg model. *Eur. J. Appl. Physiol.* 51:25–35, 1983.
72. Hunter, G., R. Demment, and D. Miller. Development of strength and maximum oxygen uptake during simultaneous training for strength and endurance. *J. Sports Med. Phys. Fitness.* 27:269–275, 1987.
73. Ikai, M., and T. Fukunaga. A study of training effect on strength per unit cross sectional area of muscle by means of ultrasonic measurement. *Int. Z. Angew. Physiol. Einschl. Arbeitsphysol.* 28:173–180, 1970.
74. Imamura, K., H. Ashida, T. Ishikawa, and M. Fujii. Human major psoas muscle and scrospinalis muscle in relation to age: a study by computed tomography. *J. Gerontol.* 38:678–681, 1983.
75. Israel, S. Age-related changes in strength and special groups. P. Komi (ed). *Strength and Power in Sports. The Encyclopaedia of Sports Medicine.* Oxford, England: Blackwell, 1992, pp. 319–328.

76. Jette, A. M., and L. G. Branch. The Framingham disability study: II. Physical disability among the aging. *Am. J. Public Health* 71:1211–1216, 1981.
77. Jones, D. A., and O. M. Rutherford. Human muscle strength training: the effects of three different training regimes and the nature of the resultant changes. *J. Physiol. Lond.* 391:1–11, 1987.
78. Jones, D. A., O. M. Rutherford, and D. F. Parker. Physiological changes in skeletal muscle as a result of strength training. *Q. J. Exp. Physiol.* 74:233–256, 1989.
79. Knuttgen, H. G., and W. J. Kraemer. Terminology and measurement in exercise performance. *J. Appl. Sport Sci. Res.* 1:1–10, 1987.
80. Komi, P. V. Training of muscle strength and power: interaction of neuromotoric, hypertrophic, and mechanical factors. *Int. J. Sports Med.* 7:10–15, 1986.
81. Komi, P. V. How important is neural drive for strength and power development in human skeletal muscle? *Biochem. Exerc.* 16:515–529, 1986.
82. Komi, P. V., J. Karlsson, P. Tesch, H. Suominen, and E. Heikkinen. Effects of heavy resistance and explosive-type strength training methods and mechanical, functional and metabolic aspects of performance. P. V. Komi (ed). *Exercise and Sports Biology. International Series on Sports Sciences*, Vol. 12. Champaign, IL: Human Kinetics, 1982, pp. 99–102.
83. Komi, P., J. Viitasalo, R. Rauamaa, and V. Vihko. Effect of isometric strength training on mechanical, electrical, and metabolic aspects of muscle function. *Eur. J. Appl. Physiol.* 40:45–55, 1978.
84. Kraemer, W. J. Strength development for collision sports. A. Weltman and C. G. Spain, (eds). *Proceedings of the White House Symposium on Physical Fitness and Sports Medicine.* Washington, D.C.: President's Council on Fitness and Sports, 1983, pp. 60–62.
85. Kraemer, W. J. Measurement of strength. A. Weltman and C. G. Spain (eds). *Proceedings of the White House Symposium on Physical Fitness and Sports Medicine.* Washington, D.C.: President's Council on Fitness and Sports, 1983, pp. 35–36.
86. Kraemer, W. J. Endocrine responses to resistance exercise. *Med. Sci. Sports Exerc.* 20(Suppl.):S152–S157, 1988.
87. Kraemer, W. J. Physiological and cellular effects of exercise training. W. B. Leadbetter, J. A. Buckwalter, and S. L. Gordon (eds). *Sports-Induced Inflammation.* Park Ridge, IL: American Academy of Orthopaedic Surgeons, 1990, pp. 659–676.
88. Kraemer, W. J. Hormonal mechanisms related to the expression of muscular strength and power. P. V. Komi (ed). *The Encyclopaedia of Sports Medicine: Strength and Power.* Oxford, England: Blackwell, 1992, pp. 64–76.
89. Kraemer, W. J. Endocrine responses and adaptations to strength training. P. Komi (ed). *The Encyclopaedia of Sports Medicine: Strength and Power.* Oxford, England: Blackwell, 1992, pp. 291–304.
90. Kraemer, W. J. General adaptations to resistance and endurance training programs. T. R. Baechle (ed). *Essentials of Strength and Conditioning.* Champaign, IL: Human Kinetics, 1994, pp. 127–150.
91. Kraemer, W. J. Neuroendocrine responses to resistance exercise. T. R. Baechle (ed). *Essentials of Strength and Conditioning.* Champaign, IL: Human Kinetics, 1994, pp. 86–107.
92. Kraemer, W. J. The physiological basis for strength training in mid-life. S. L. Gordon (ed). *Sports and Exercise in Midlife.* Park Ridge, IL: American Academy of Orthopaedic Surgeons, 1994, pp. 413–433.
93. Kraemer, W. J., and T. R. Baechle. Development of a strength training program. F. L. Allman, and A. J. Ryan, (eds). *Sports Medicine*, 2nd ed. Orlando, FL: Academic Press, 1989, pp. 113–127.
94. Kraemer, W. J., M. R. Deschenes, and S. J. Fleck. Physiological adaptations to resistance exercise: implications for athletic conditioning. *Sports Med.* 6:246–256, 1988.
95. Kraemer, W. J., J. E. Dziados, L. J. Marchitelli, S. E. Gordon, E. A. Harman, R. Mello, S. J. Fleck, P. N. Frykman, and N. T. Triplett. Effects of different heavy-resistance exercise protocols on plasma β-endorphin concentrations. *J. Appl. Physiol.* 74(1):450–459, 1993.

96. Kraemer, W. J., and S. J. Fleck. Resistance training: exercise prescription. *Phys. Sportsmed.* 16(6):69–81, 1988.

97. Kraemer, W. J., S. J. Fleck, and M. Deschenses. A review: factors in exercise prescription of resistance training. *Nat. Strength Cond. Assoc. J.* 10:36–41, 1988.

98. Kraemer, W. J., S. J. Fleck, J. E. Dziados, E. A. Harman, L. J. Marchitelli, S. E. Gordon, R. Mello, P. N. Frykman, L. P. Koziris, and N. T. Triplett. Changes in hormonal concentrations following different heavy resistance exercise protocols in women. *J. Appl. Physiol.* 75(2):594–604, 1993.

99. Kraemer, W. J., A. C. Fry, B. J. Warren, M. H. Stone, S. J. Fleck, J. T. Kearney, B. P. Conroy, C. M. Maresh, C. A. Weseman, N. T. Triplett, and S. E. Gordon. Acute hormonal responses in elite junior weightlifters. *Int. J. Sports Med.* 13(2):103–109, 1992.

100. Kraemer, W. J., S. E. Gordon, S. J. Fleck, L. J. Marchitelli, R. Mello, J. E. Dziados, K. Friedl, E. Harman, C. Maresh, and A. C. Fry. Endogenous anabolic hormonal and growth factor responses to heavy resistance exercise in males and females. *Int. J. Sports Med.* 12(2):228–235, 1991.

101. Kraemer, W. J., and L. P. Koziris. Muscle strength training: techniques and considerations. *Phys. Ther. Pract.* 2(1):54–68, 1992.

102. Kraemer, W. J., and L. P. Koziris. Olympic weightlifting and power lifting. D. R. Lamb, H. G. Knuttgen, and R. Murray (eds). *Physiology and Nutrition for Competitive Sport.* Carmel, IN: Cooper Publishing, 1994, pp. 1–54.

103. Kraemer, W. J., L. Marchitelli, D. McCurry, R. Mello, J. E. Dziados, E. Harman, P. Frykman, S. E. Gordon, and S. J. Fleck. Hormonal and growth factor responses to heavy resistance exercise. *J. Appl. Physiol.* 69(4):1442–1450, 1990.

104. Kraemer, W. J., B. J. Noble, B. W. Culver, and M. J. Clark. Physiologic responses to heavy-resistance exercise with very short rest periods. *Int. J. Sports Med.* 8:247–252, 1987.

105. Kraemer, W. J., J. Patton, S. E. Gordon, E. A. Harman, M. R. Deschenes, K. Reynolds, R. U. Newton, N. T. Triplett, and J. E. Dziados. Compatibility of high intensity strength and endurance training on hormonal and skeletal muscle adaptations. *J. Appl. Physiol.* 78(3):976–989, 1995.

106. Kraemer, W. J., J. F. Patton, H. G. Knuttgen, C. J. Hannan, T. Kittler, S. Gordon, J. E. Dziados, A. C. Fry, P. N. Frykman, and E. A. Harman. The effects of high intensity cycle exercise on sypatho-adrenal medullary response patterns. *J. Appl. Physiol.* 70:8–14, 1991.

107. Larsson, L. Morphological and functional characteristics of the aging skeletal muscle in man. *Acta Physiol. Scand. Suppl.* 457:1–36, 1978.

108. Larsson, L. Histochemical characteristics of human skeletal muscle during aging. *Acta Physiol. Scand.* 117:469–471, 1983.

109. Larsson, L. G., G. Grimby, and J. Karlsson. Muscle strength and speed of movement in relation to age and muscle morphology. *J. Appl. Physiol.* 46:451–456, 1979.

110. Lexell, J., K. Henriksson-Larsen, B. Wimblod, and M. Sjostrom. Distribution of different fiber types in human skeletal muscles: effects of aging studied in whole muscle cross sections. *Muscle Nerve* 6:588–595, 1983.

111. MacDougal, J. D. Hypertrophy or hyperplasia. P. Komi (ed). *Strength and Power in Sports. The Encyclopaedia of Sports Medicine.* Oxford, England: Blackwell, 1992, pp. 230–238.

112. MacDougall, J. D., D. G. Sale, J. R. Moroz, G. C. B. Elder, J. R. Sutton, and H. Howard. Mitochondrial volume density in human skeletal muscle following heavy resistance training. *Med. Sci. Sports* 11:164–166, 1979.

113. Mateyev, L. *Periodisierang des sportlichen Training* (in German). Berlin: Berles & Wernitz, 1972.

114. McCarthy, J. P., J. C. Agre, B. K. Graf, M. A. Pozniak, and A. C. Vailas. Compatibility of adaptive responses with combining strength and endurance training. *Med. Sci. Sports Exerc.* 27(3):429–436, 1995.

115. Mellah, S., L. Rispal-Padel, and G. Riviere. Changes in excitability of motor units during preparation for movement. *Exp. Brain Res.* 82:178–186, 1990.

116. Morganti, C. M., M. E. Nelson, M. A. Fiatarone, G. E. Dallal, C. D. Economos, B. M. Crawford, and W. J. Evans. Strength improvements with 1 yr of progressive resistance training in older women. *Med. Sci. Sports Exerc.* 27:906–912, 1995.

117. Moritani, T., and H. A. deVries. Neural factors versus hypertrophy in the time course of muscle strength gain. *Am. J. Phys. Med.* 58:115–130, 1979.

118. Moritani, T., and H. A. deVries. Potential for gross muscle hypertrophy in older men. *J. Gerontol.* 35:672–682, 1980.

119. Moritani, T. Time course of adaptations during strength and power training. P. Komi (ed). *Strength and Power in Sports. The Encyclopaedia of Sports Medicine.* Oxford, England: Blackwell, 1992, pp. 266–278.

120. Murray, M. P., E. H. Duthie, S. T. Gambert, S. B. Sepic, and L. A. Mollinger. Age-related differences in knee muscle strength in normal women. *J. Gerontol.* 40:275–280, 1985.

121. Nardone, A., C. Romano, M. Schieppati. Selective recruitments of high-threshold human motor units during voluntary isotonic-lengthening of active muscles. *J. Physiol.* 409:451–471, 1989.

122. Narici, N., G. Roi, L. Landoni, A. Minetti, and P. Cerretelli. Changes in force, cross-sectional area and neural activation during strength training and detraining of the human quadriceps. *Eur. J. Appl. Physiol.* 59:310–319, 1989.

123. Nelson, M. E., M. A. Fiatarone, C. M. Morganti, I. Trice, R. A. Greenberg, and W. J. Evans. Effects of high-intensity strength training on multiple risk factors for osteoporotic fractures. *J.A.M.A.* 272:1909–1914, 1994.

124. Newton, R. U. and W. J. Kraemer. Developing explosive muscular power: implications for a mixed methods training strategy. *J. Strength Cond.* 16(5):20, 1994.

125. Noth, J. Motor units. P. Komi (ed). *Strength and Power in Sports. The Encyclopaedia of Sports Medicine.* Oxford, England: Blackwell, 1992, pp. 21–28.

126. Patton, J. F., W. J. Kraemer, H. G. Knuttgen, and E. A. Harman. Factors in maximal power production and in exercise endurance relative to maximal power. *Eur. J. Appl. Physiol.* 60:222–227, 1990.

127. Pette, D. and R. S. Staron. Cellular and molecular diversities of mammalian skeletal muscle fibers. *Rev. Physiol. Biochem. Pharmacol.* 116:2–75, 1990.

128. Ploutz, L. L., P. A. Tesch, R. L. Biro, and G. A. Dudley. Effect of resistance training on muscle use during exercise. *J. Appl. Physiol.* 76(4):1675–1681, 1994.

129. Roux, W. Gesammelte Abhandlugen über Entwicklungsmechanik der Organismen. Leipzig, Austria: Band I Funktionelle Anpassung, 1895.

130. Rudman, D., A. G. Feller, H. S. Nagraj, G. A. Gergans, P. Y. Lalitha, A. F. Goldberg, R. A. Schlenker, L. Cohn, I. W. Rudman, and D. E. Mattson. Effects of human growth hormone in men over 60 years old. *N. Engl. J. Med.* 323(1):1–6, 1990.

131. Sale, D. G. Neural adaptation to strength training. P. Komi (ed). *Strength and Power in Sports. The Encyclopaedia of Sports Medicine.* Oxford, England: Blackwell, 1992, pp. 249–265.

132. Sale, D. G., J. D. MacDougall, A. R. M. Upton, and A. J. McComas. Effect of strength training upon motorneuron excitability in man. *Med. Sci. Sports Exerc.* 15:57–62, 1983.

133. Schantz, P. Capillary supply in hypertrophied human skeletal muscle. *Acta Physiol. Scand.* 114:635–637, 1982.

134. Schantz, P. Capillary supply in heavy-resistance trained nonpostural human skeletal muscle. *Acta Physiol. Scand.* 117:153–155, 1983.

135. Schmidtbleicher, D. Training for power events. P. Komi (ed). *Strength and Power in Sports. The Encyclopaedia of Sports Medicine.* Oxford, England: Blackwell, 1992, pp. 381–396.

136. Sharp, M. A., E. A. Harman, B. E. Boutilier, M. W. Bovee, and W. J. Kraemer. Progressive resistance training program for improving manual materials handling performance. *Work* 3(3):63–69, 1993.

137. Shellock, F. G., T. Fukunaga, J. H. Mink, and V. R. Edgerton. Acute effects of exercise on MR imaging of skeletal muscle: concentric vs eccentric actions. *Am. J. Roentgenol. Radium Ther. Nucl. Med.* 156:765–768, 1990.

138. Smith, D. O., and J. L. Rosenheimer. Decreased sprouting and degeneration of nerve terminals of active muscles in aged rats. *J. Neurophysiol.* 48:100–109, 1982.

139. Staron, R. S. Correlation between myofibrillar ATPase activity and myosin heavy chain composition in single human muscle fibers. *Histochemistry* 96:21–24, 1991.

140. Staron, R. S., and R. S. Hikida. Histochemical, biochemical, and ultrastructural analyses of single human muscle fibers with special reference to the C fiber population. *J. Histochem. Cytochem.* 40:563–568, 1992.

141. Staron, R. S., R. S. Hikida, F. C. Hagerman, G. A. Dudley, and T. F. Murray. Human skeletal muscle fiber type adaptability to various workloads. *J. Histochem. Cytochem.* 32:146–152, 1984.

142. Staron, R. S., and P. Johnson. Myosin polymorphism and differential expression in adult human skeletal muscle. *Comp. Biochem. Physiol.* 106B(3):463–475, 1993.

143. Staron, R. S., D. L. Karapondo, W. J. Kraemer, A. C. Fry, S. E. Gordon, J. E. Falkel, F. C. Hagerman, and R. S. Hikida. Skeletal muscle adaptations during the early phase of heavy-resistance training in men and women. *J. Appl. Physiol.* 76(3):1247–1255, 1994.

144. Staron, R. S., M. J. Leonardi, D. L. Karapondo, E. S. Malicky, J. E. Falkel, F. C. Hagerman, and R. S. Hikida. Strength and skeletal muscle adaptations in heavy-resistance trained women after detraining and retraining. *J. Appl. Physiol.* 70:631–640, 1991.

145. Staron, R. S., E. S. Malicky, M. J. Leonardi, J. E. Fakel, F. C. Hagerman, and G. A. Dudley. Muscle hypertrophy and fast fiber type conversions in heavy resistance-trained women. *Eur. J. Appl. Physiol.* 60:71–79, 1989.

146. Tesch, P. A. Acute and long-term metabolic changes consequent to heavy-resistance exercise. *Med. Sports Sci.* 26:67–89, 1987.

147. Tesch, P. A. Short- and long-term histochemical and biochemical adaptations in muscle. P. Komi (ed). *Strength and Power in Sports. The Encyclopaedia of Sports Medicine.* Oxford, England: Blackwell, 1992, pp. 239–248.

148. Tesch, P. A., H. Hjort, and U. I. Balldin. Effects of strength training on G tolerance. *Aviat. Space Environ. Med.* 54:691–695, 1983.

149. Tesch, P. A., P. V. Komi, and K. Häkkinen. Enzymatic adaptations consequent to long-term strength training. *Int. J. Sports Med.* 8(Suppl.):66–69, 1987.

150. Tesch, P. A., A. Thorsson, and E. B. Colliander. Effects of eccentric and concentric resistance training on skeletal muscle substrates, enzyme activities and capillary supply. *Acta Physiol. Scand.* 140:575–580, 1990.

151. Tesch, P. A., A. Thorsson, and P. Kaiser. Muscle capillary supply and fiber type characteristics in weight and power lifters. *J. Appl. Physiol.* 56:35–38, 1984.

152. Tharion, W. J., T. M. Rausch, E. A. Harman, and W. J. Kraemer. Effects of different resistance exercise protocols on mood states. *J. Appl. Sci. Res.* 5(2):60–65, 1991.

153. Thomas, C. C., B. H. Ross, and B. Calanicie. Human motor unit recruitment during isometric contractions and repeated dynamic movements. *J. Neurophysiol.* 57:311–324, 1987.

154. Thorstensson, A., J. Karlsson, J. Viitasalo, P. Luhtanen, and P. Komi. Effect of strength in training on EMG of human skeletal muscle. *Acta Physiol.* 98:232–236, 1976.

155. Tzankoff, S. P., and A. H. Norris. Longitudinal changes in basal metabolic rate in man. *J. Appl. Physiol.* 33:536–539, 1978.

156. Weidman, E. R., H. C. Charles, R. Negro-Vilar, J. J. Sullivan, and J. R. MacFall. Muscle activity localization with ^{31}P spectroscopy and calculated T_2-weighted ^1H images. *Invest. Radiol.* 26:309–316, 1991.

157. Yaresheski, K. E., J. A. Campbell, K. Smith, M. J. Rennie, J. O. Holloszy, and D. M. Bier. Effect of growth hormone and resistance exercise on muscle growth in young men. *Am. J. Physiol.* 262:E261–E267, 1992.

158. Yarasheski, K. E., J. J. Zachwieja, and D. M. Bier: Acute effects of resistance exercise on muscle protein synthesis rate in young and elderly men and women. *Am. J. Physiol.* 265 (*Endocrinol. Metab.* 28):E210–E214, 1993.

13
Response of the Neuromuscular Unit to Spaceflight: What Has Been Learned from the Rat Model

ROLAND R. ROY, Ph.D.,
KENNETH M. BALDWIN, Ph.D.
V. REGGIE EDGERTON, Ph.D.

In the past few years, the opportunity for investigating the effects of microgravity on the mammalian organism has increased significantly. Results from a number of short-term spaceflights (4–22 days) have provided valuable insights into the adaptive potential of several mammalian systems, particularly in humans, monkeys, and rats. This chapter focuses on the functional, metabolic, and morphological adaptations occurring in the neuromuscular unit, i.e., skeletal muscles and the associated efferent and afferent neural elements associated with actual spaceflight in the rat model, and will highlight the functional implications of these adaptations. There are data in Table 13.1 that summarize flights on which some element of the rat neuromuscular unit has been studied. The readers also are directed to a number of published related reviews [15–17, 34, 35, 43, 58, 63, 68]. Spaceflight will be considered as a model of decreased activity and use, because the skeletal muscles are presumably chronically unloaded under conditions of weightlessness. However, no quantitative data have been published on either the activation electromyogram (EMG) patterns) or the loading (muscle forces) characteristics of rat muscles during spaceflight. Because there are significant differences in the usage patterns across muscles at $1g$, data on the activation and loading patterns of individual muscles, and probably other physiological perturbations induced at $0g$, will be necessary to determine the events in spaceflight that trigger muscle adaptations. Some initial observations of rats flown on a 14-day mission (STS-58), beginning 6 hr after landing, suggest an extreme dorsiflexion during posture maintenance and gait [19]. This "flexor dominance" (also seen in humans after spaceflight; see ref. 14 for a review) could have an impact on adaptations that may occur during the time interval between landing and tissue removal. In addition, these data will become more essential for the interpretation of muscle adaptations as the duration of spaceflight increases and the techniques for studying muscle adaptations become more sophisticated or refined.

When assessing the adaptations of skeletal muscle to spaceflight, factors such as the age, sex, and strain of the rats; the conditions under which

TABLE 13.1.
Summary of Flights on Which Some Element of the Rat Neuromuscular Unit Was Studied

Flight Identification	Duration (Days)	Tissue Removal (Hr after Landing)	Species (Wt at Launch)	Muscle or Neural Tissues Studied [ref]	Muscle Wet Wt. (% of Synchronous Control)
Cosmos 605	22	24 / 48	Wistar male	Spinal ganglia, ventral horn cells [22, 53] Sol, Gastroc, EDL, QF, BB, diaphragm [28]	Sol (−32), EDL (−12) all others (nc)
Cosmos 690	20.5	24 / 48	Wistar male	Sol, Plt [52, 53] Sol, EDL [48] Sol [21] MG, QF [20] Sol, Gastroc, EDL, BB [29]	Sol (−25), Gastroc (−19), EDL (nc), BB (nc)
Cosmos 936	18.5	4–9	Wistar male (SPF)[a] (~200 g)	Sol [7] Gastroc [11] Sol, Plt [52] Sol, Gastroc [62]	Sol (−40), EDL (−29); brachialis: (−22); TBmed: (−24)
Cosmos 1129	18.5	6–10	Wistar male (SPF) (300–360 g)	Sol, EDL, brachialis, TBmed [57, 67]	Sol (−17), Plt (−17), LG (−24)
Cosmos 1514	5	6–8	Wistar female pregnant (SPF) (~300–350 g)	Sol, Plt, LG [26] Sol, MG, EDL, brachialis, TBmed [56]	Sol (−17); MG (−11); EDL (−4); brachialis (−20); TBmed: (−7)
Cosmos 1667	7	4–8	Wistar male (SPF) (330–350 g)	Sol, EDL [13] Sol, Plt, LG [26] Sol, Gastroc, QF, BB [27] Sol, Gastroc, diaphragm [54] Sol, MG, EDL, brachialis, TBmed [56] Sol, Gastroc, diaphragm [3]	Sol (−23), EDL (−11) Sol (−29), Plt (−14), LG (−9) Sol (−23), Gastroc (−11), QF (nc); BB (−12) Sol (−29); MG (−11), EDL (−8); brachialis: (−17); TBmed: (−4)

Mission			Animal	Structures studied [ref]	Results
Cosmos 1887	12.5	48–53	Wistar male (SPF) (~300 g)	Spinal ganglia, ventral horn cells [36, 37, 50]	nc in any muscle
				Sol [8]	
				Sol; Gastroc; QF; BB [28]	
				Sol, Gastroc, diaphragm [55]	
				Sol, TA [38]	Sol (−15); MG (−16)
				Sol, MG [42]	
				VI, VL [5]	VI (−23); VL: (+8)
				Sol, AL, Plt, EDL [61]	
				TB [69]	
				Sol, Gastroc, diaphragm [3]	
Cosmos 2044	14	6–11	Wistar male (SPF) (~320 g)	Lumbar motoneurons, spinal ganglia [36, 37, 50]	
				Ventral horn cells [33]	
				AL [12]	AL (nc); EDL (−7)
				Sol, LG, EDL [66]	VM (nc)
				AL, Plt, EDL [59]	Sol (−25)
				VM [45]	MG (−13), TA (−4)
				Sol [49]	
				MG, TA [31]	
				Sol, TA [10]	
				VI, LG, TB [69]	
SLS-1 (Columbia)	9	3–6	Gastroc crush-injured	Gastroc [64]	
		6	Taconic albino male (SPF) (~330 G)	VI, VL, TA [6]	VI (−23); VL (−15), TA (−7)
				VI, VL, TA [24]	VI (−22); VL (−5), TA (−1)
SLS-2 (STS-58)	14	~5	Taconic Albino male (SPF) (130–155 g)	Sol, EDL [18]	
				Ventral horn cells (Ishihara et al., unpublished observations)	
				Sol [1]	Sol [−29]

TABLE 13.1.—*continued*

Flight Identification	Duration (Days)	Tissue Removal (Hr after Landing)	Species (Wt at Launch)	Muscle or Neural Tissues Studied [ref]	Muscle Wet Wt. (% of Synchronous Control)
SL-3	7	11–17	Taconic albino male (SPF)	Sol, AL, MG, Plt, EDL,TA [39]	(small rats)
				Sol, AL, MG, Plt, EDL [41]	(small rats)
				Sol, AL, Gastroc, Plt, EDL, TA [23]	(small rats)
				Sol,EDL [44]	(large rats)
				Sol, EDL [60]	(large rats)
				Sol, Gastroc, EDL [65]	(large rats)
			(360–410 g)	Sol, Gastroc, Plt EDL, TA [71]	Large rats: Sol (−24), AL (nc); Gastroc (−14), Plt (−11), EDL (−10), TA (−9)
			(190–250 g)		Small rats: Sol (−36); AL (−26); Gastroc (−21), Plt: (−22) EDL (−16), TA (−11)
STS-41 (PSE-1) (Discovery)	4	4–6	Taconic albino male (SPF) (125–135 g)	BB [4] Plt [70] Sol [32]	Sol (−37)
STS-48 (Discovery)	5.4	2–3'15"	Taconic albino female (SPF) (50–65 g)	Sol, Gastroc, Plt, TA, EDL [72]	Sol (−38); Gastroc: (−16); Plt (−24); TA: (nc); EDL: (−5)
STS-54	6	3–9	Taconic albino male (SPF) (~250 g)	Sol, EDL [25] Sol [9]	Sol (−38); EDL: (−4) Sol (−27)

[a]SPF, specific pathogen-free; nc, no change (no values reported). Muscle weights are absolute values, except for those flights in which the body weights of the flight and control rats were significantly different after flight (STS-41, STS-48), and the muscle weights are expressed relative to body weight.

control rats are maintained; the mode of landing; and the amount of time that the rats are at $1g$ before the muscles are tested and/or harvested must be considered. Most of the data used for comparison with flight rats are derived from synchronous control rats, i.e., rats of the same age, sex and strain, obtained at the same time as the flight rats and kept under housing conditions as "similar" as possible to those of the flight rats. Many of these variables are summarized for individual flights in Table 13.1. In addition, because of unavoidable constraints placed on individual spacecrafts and on sharing of tissues among investigators, the number of rats studied is usually lower than that which would give maximum power for statistical analyses. Thus in many instances, the sample sizes are limited, and some of the results are discussed in terms of trends, rather than significant differences.

BODY WEIGHT, MUSCLE WEIGHT, AND FIBER SIZE ADAPTATIONS

In general, the body weights of control and flight rats have not been significantly different at the time of muscle removal following these relatively short duration flights, at least in rats that are flown after their rapid growing stage of development. Thus in most cases, comparisons of the absolute muscle weights between control and flight rats are appropriate (Table 13.1). Whether longer flights will affect the muscle weight: body weight ratios remains to be determined.

A decrease in muscle mass and/or a reduction in growth generally occurs with spaceflight (Table 13.1). The relative response of individual muscles or muscle groups within any study appears to be related, in part, to one or more factors. The hindlimb muscles having primarily an extensor function (e.g., soleus (Sol), medial gastrocnemius (MG), plantars (Plt), and vastus intermedius (VI) are affected more than muscles having a primary flexor function (e.g., tibialis anterior (TA) and extensor digitorum longus (EDL). Within primary extensor groups, the degree of atrophy appears to be related to the fiber type composition of the individual muscles comprising the functional group, i.e., muscles having the highest proportion of slow fibers show the largest amount of atrophy. For example, in the calf the Sol (~90% slow fibers) atrophies more than the lateral (MG) gastrocnemius or Plt (MG), (LG), (all having less than 15% slow fibers) [2]. Similarly, in the thigh, the VI (~60% slow fibers) atrophies more than the vastus lateralis (VL) or vastus medialis (VM) (all having less than 10% slow fibers) [2]. In general, hindlimb muscles comprised predominantly of slow fibers show a large degree of atrophy, e.g., Sol, VI, and adductor longes (AL). The limited data on muscles in the forelimb show a different pattern (Table 13.1). The elbow flexors (brachialis and biceps brachii (BB)) appear to show greater atrophy than the elbow extensors (the triceps brachii (TB)), despite the fact that the most commonly studied extensor (the medial head of the TB, (or TB med) has a relatively high percentage of slow fibers. This apparent difference in the atrophic response of hindlimb and forelimb muscles may be related to the changes in the motor functions under spaceflight conditions. In any case, this issue needs further study.

Rat muscles have been studied during spaceflights as short as 4 days and as long as 22 days. The amount of muscle atrophy (whole muscle wet weight) observed has been quite variable,with little relationship to the duration of the flight. For example, Sol muscle atrophy has ranged from ~15 to 40%, with one of the largest atrophic responses reported after a 4-day flight [32]. However, this variability can be attributed, at least in part, to the presence of interstitial edema, a factor that appears to be related to the muscle type (slow muscles are affected more than fast muscles), to flight conditions, and to the amount of time lapsing between landing and the removal of the muscles (see ref. 14 for a discussion). Significant edema has been shown to occur rapidly in muscles exposed to weightlessness. For example, Henriksen et al. [25] reported a 52% increase in the interstitial fluid volume (defined by the insulin space, expressed in microliters per 100 mg of muscle) in the Sol of rats flown for ~5 days (STS-48), compared to that of ground-based controls. In contrast, no change in interstitial fluid volume was observed in the EDL of the same rats.

Fiber size changes also have shown some variability across studies: however, some of this variability can be attributed to differences in techniques for determining fiber size and, perhaps, to the extent of fiber disruption related to the amount of time reloading is allowed before muscle removal. The single fiber size data from the Sol clearly show that there is rapid period of atrophy (within the first 4–14 days), followed by a plateau (Table 13.2). In addition, the data show that both slow and fast fibers atrophy, with the slow fibers showing a response similar to or larger than that of the fast fibers. The fiber type specific atrophic response in predominantly fast muscles has been quite variable. One generalization that appears to be consistent for both slow and fast muscles is that the largest fibers atrophy the most.

Recently, Allen et al. [1] determined the number of myonuclei in mechanically isolated single-fiber segments from the Sol of 14-day flight (SLS-2) rats, using confocal microscopy. Compared to that of controls, the number of myonuclei per mm fiber length was decreased by 17 and 20% in Type I and hybrid (expressing both Type I and II MHCs) fibers. No change was observed in fibers expressing only Type II MHCs. Mean fiber size decreased by 44 and 33% in Type I and hybrid fibers and was unchanged in Type II fibers after flight. Because the decreases in fiber size were larger than the reductions in nuclear number, nuclear domains (cytoplasmic volume/myonucleus) were decreased by 29 and 16% in Type I and hybrid fibers, respectively. The mechanism(s) associated with the reduction in myonuclear number is (are) unknown. These results suggest that adaptation of skeletal muscle fibers to changes in function involves not only a modulation of the

TABLE 13.2.
Cross-Sectional Area Adaptations of Slow and Fast Fibers of the Sol to Spaceflight

Flight	STS-41	STS-54	Cosmos 1667	SL-3[a]	SL-3[b]	SL-3[b]	Cosmos 1887	Cosmos 1887	Cosmos 2044	Cosmos 690	Cosmos 605
Duration (days)	4[c]	6	7	7	7	7	12.5	12.5	14	20.5	22
Fiber type											
Slow	70	76	86	64	~60	68	53	54	70	77	73
Fast	82	97	82	64	~70	78	76	61	84	64	79
Reference	(32)	(9)	(29)	(41)	(44)	(60)	(42)	(30)	(49)	(27)	(28)

[a]Small rats from SL-3.
[b]Large rats from SL-3.
[c]Values are expressed as percent of ground-based synchronous control. Values for Musacchia et al. [44] are estimated from their Figure 1.

pattern and/or amount of gene expression among existing myonuclei but also an alteration in the total number of myonuclei available for gene expression modulation.

PROTEIN, AMINO ACID, DNA, AND RNA ADAPTATIONS

Spaceflight has been shown to have a significant effect on skeletal muscle composition. Noncollagenous protein content decreased in predominantly slow (Sol, AL) and fast (MG, Plt, TA, and EDL) muscles after 7 days of flight (SL-3), whereas the concentration decreased only in slow muscles [39]. In general, the losses were greater in slow than in fast muscles, thus paralleling the relative changes in muscle mass. The changes in collagen content and concentration were much less consistent. For the slow muscles, the Sol showed a decrease in content, whereas the AL showed a decrease in concentration. For the fast muscles, the Plt had lower values for both measures, and the EDL had a lower content after spaceflight. These data indicate that collagenous and/or noncollagenous protein loss can account for some of the weight loss associated with weightlessness. The protein changes appear to be muscle specific in that in some muscles, the primary loss of mass resulted from a change in the noncollagenous protein pool (AL, MG, and TA), whereas in other muscles (Sol, EDL, and Plt), a reduction in the collagenous protein pool was an additional contributing factor. Because the group of rats was relatively young (190–250 g at launch), Tischler et al. [71] calculated the growth rate of individual muscles in these same rats. Compared to a growth rate of 21–26% for all muscles studied in control rats, that of the Sol showed atrophy (-11%); the Plt ($+14\%$), gastrocnemius (Gastroc) ($+11\%$), and EDL ($+14\%$) showed reduced growth, and the TA showed normal growth ($+21\%$) during the 7-day flight. These data emphasize the need to interpret muscle mass changes in unloaded conditions relative to body weight changes, particularly in young growing animals.

In muscles from older rats (360–410 g at launch) flown on the same mission (SLS-3), total protein concentrations were unaffected in the Sol, Gastroc, and EDL, whereas total protein content was reduced (46%) in the Sol [65]. Myofibrillar and sarcoplasmic protein content were decreased in the Sol and the Gastroc but not in the EDL. The only significant change in concentration was a 15% increase in the sarcoplasmic protein pool of the Sol. There was a tendency for an increase in total DNA concentration in all muscles, with the Sol showing the only significant effect. Total RNA content was reduced in the Sol and Gastroc but not in the EDL. Total DNA content and RNA concentration were unaffected by 7 days of flight in any muscle studied. Similar results were obtained for the VM after 14 days of flight, i.e., no changes in protein, RNA, or DNA contents or concentrations were observed in this predominantly fast extensor [45]. Myofibrillar protein content and concentration in the VI were decreased by 34 and 46%, respectively, after 12.5 days of flight [5]. In contrast, these parameters were unaffected in the VL. After a 9-day flight, total muscle and myofibrillar protein content were unchanged in the VI or in a high oxidative or a low oxidative region of the VL [24]. However, there was a tendency for the myofibrillar yield to be somewhat depressed (an 8% decrease). Sarcoplasmic and myofibrillar (called actomyosin) protein content also decreased by ~46% in the Sol [21] but did not change in the quadriceps femoris (QF) [20] after 20.5 days of flight (Cosmos 690). Thus, adaptations in the total amount and concentration of muscle protein can occur with spaceflight, with the more marked effects in slow muscles.

The Sol content of several amino acids (asparagine/aspartate, glutamine/glutamate, glycine, histidine, and lysine) was reduced (range, 17–63%), whereas that of others was unchanged (alanine, arginine, serine, threonine, and taurine) after 7 days of flight (SL-3) in adult rats [65]. The only change in the Gastroc and EDL was a decrease in glutamine/glutamate. In the relatively young rats flown on the same flight, Tischler et al. [71] reported an increase in glutamine/glutamate and a decrease in aspartate levels in the Sol and Plt. These latter amino acids represent the only direct comparisons that can be made between these two studies. In these young rats, a decrease in fumarate and malate was observed in the Sol, whereas tyrosine was elevated in the Sol and unchanged in the Plt. These data suggest an age-specific effect of spaceflight on amino acid metabolism. All of these results demonstrate that total protein metabolism in skeletal muscle is adversely affected by spaceflight, especially in predominantly slow muscles. These findings are consistent with known effects of altered protein turnover, involving ground-based models of simulated microgravity [68].

FIBER TYPE AND CONTRACTILE PROTEIN ADAPTATIONS

Standard qualitative histochemical and quantitative histochemical and immunohistochemical techniques have been used to study the fiber type composition of a variety of muscles in control and spaceflight rats. In general, the data show a trend for an increase in the percentage of fast and/or hybrid fibers after flights as short as 4–6 days, particularly in predominantly slow muscles such as the Sol. For example, the percentage of "pure" slow fibers (either expressing only the slow MHC isoform or staining darkly and lightly for myofibrillar ATPase at an alkaline and acid preincubation, respectively) in the Sol decreased from 68 to 64% after 6 (STS-54) [9], from 85 to 79% after 7 (Cosmos 1667) [13], from 78 to 60% after 12.5 (Cosmos 1887) [42], from 80 to 66% (Cosmos 2044) [49] and from 75 to 61% (SLS-

2) [1] after 14 days of flight. Similar changes have been reported for other predominantly slow muscles: e.g., the percentage of slow fibers in the AL decreased from 80 to 54% after 7 (SL-3) [41], from 83 to 63% after 12.5 (Cosmos 1887) [61], and from 90 to 65% after 14 (Cosmos 2044) [59] days of flight. Combined with the trend for a greater atrophy in slow, as compared to fast fibers, these fiber type adaptations result in a larger percent of the cross-sectional area of these slow muscles, having fast fiber characteristics after, as compared to before, spaceflight. Predominantly fast muscles, such as the EDL (7 days, Cosmos 1667 [13]; 12.5 days, Cosmos 1887 [61]; MG (12.5 days, Cosmos 1887 [42]), and Plt (12.5 days, Cosmos 1887 [61]) show a much less dramatic effect after spaceflight.

Recent results using immunohistochemical procedures have shown a decrease in the percentage of fibers expressing only Type I MHC isoform, increases in the percentage of fibers expressing Types IIa and IIx isoforms, and a de novo expression of Type IIb and neonatal isoforms in the Sol muscle after spaceflight [1, 9]. A similar trend toward an increased proportion of fast and/or hybrid fibers and a shift toward faster MHC isoforms has been observed in other predominantly slow muscles, such as the AL [41] and VI [5]. Adaptations in MHC composition have also been observed in predominantly fast muscles, such as the VL [5], in that there appears to be a shift toward a higher percentage of fibers expressing faster MHC isoforms, particularly in the regions of the muscles containing the highest proportion of slow fibers. Similar trends in the MHC composition separated by gel electrophoresis have been observed. The Type I, IIa, and IIx MHC composition of the Sol of control and 6-day flight rats was 73:26:0% and 69:21:10%, respectively [9]. Haddad et al. [24] reported a slight shift from Type I to Type IIa-IIx MHC and a de novo expression of Type IIb MHC in the VI of rats flown for 9 days (SLS-1). In addition, the high oxidative red portion of the VL showed a significant shift from Type IIa-IIx to IIb MHC. No changes were observed in the low oxidative portion (no Type I MHC detected) of the VL or the TA. These studies suggest that there is a downregulation of slow myosin and an upregulation of of fast myosin associated with spaceflight, at least in some fibers of these slow muscles, and that there is a shift towards the faster isoforms in some regions of the fast muscles.

Recently, evidence has been accumulating that some of the adaptation in the myosin molecule occurs at a pretranslational level. For example, Haddad et al. [24] reported significant decreases in Type I (68% of control) and IIa (22% of control) MHC mRNA and a concomitant increase in Type IIb MHC mRNA (204% of control) in the VI after 9 days of flight. Furthermore, the high oxidative portion of the VL showed a significant decrease in Type IIa (38% of control) and an increase in Type IIb (220% of control) after flight. No changes were observed in the low oxidative portion of the VL or the TA. Although the changes in the message were consistent with the adaptations in the MHC composition, some discrepancies were evident. For example, the reduction in Type IIa mRNA was in the opposite direction of the increase in the Type IIa protein content. Also, the reduction in Type I MHC protein (~40%) exceeded the reduction in the corresponding mRNA signal (~2%). These apparent dissociations between the mRNA and protein levels indicate that posttranslational events must be contributing to the net protein accumulation in a rapidly adapting muscle.

Other contractile-related proteins have been studied at pre- and posttranslational levels in muscles from spaceflight rats. Caiozzo et al. [9] reported an increase in the relative content of fast light chain-1 and chain-2 in the Sol after a 6-day flight, and Riley et al. [59] reported an increase in the relative content of all fast light chains and a decrease in all slow light chains in the AL after 14 days of flight. Whether these relative changes were attributable to actual increases in fast light chains or solely to the differential atrophy of slow, as compared to fast fibers, is unknown. Esser et al. [18] studied the accumulation of mRNAs for myosin light chains, troponin, and tropomyosin isoforms in the Sol and EDL muscles after 9 days of spaceflight. Although the data could not be statistically analyzed because of the necessity to pool the samples, the data showed some interesting trends. Most fast mRNA levels were increased after flight in both the Sol (170–1100%) and the EDL (23–232%). In contrast, the slow mRNA levels were unaffected in the EDL and showed a variable response in the Sol, with some levels increasing up to 58% and some decreasing up to 86%. Thomason et al. [69] found 25 and 36% decreases in α-actin mRNA in the VI and LG, respectively, after 14 days of flight. In contrast, no change in skeletal α-actin mRNA occurred in the TB in these same rats. Steady-state levels of α-actin mRNA were also reduced in the BB after a 4-day flight [4]. These data indicate some level of pretranslational control for this muscle contractile protein during weightlessness, at least in some muscles that normally have a weight-supporting function at $1g$. Together, these results indicate that the transition to a faster phenotype associated with spaceflight may be regulated, at least in part, by transcript accumulation of several contractile-related proteins.

Myofibrillar ATPase activities appear to be elevated in predominantly slow muscles and unchanged in predominantly fast muscles after spaceflight. For example, Baldwin et al. [5] reported a 21% increase in myofibrillar ATPase activity in the VI and no change in the VL after 12.5 days of flight. Similarly, Martin et al. [41] showed a significant increase in the myofibrillar ATPase activity in the soleus but not the EDL after a 7-day flight. At the single-fiber level, ATPase activity appears to be minimally affected in either the slow or fast fibers of the Sol, MG, or TA after 14 days of flight [31, 49]. Thus, it appears that the increase in myofibrillar ATPase observed in muscle hemogenates can be attributed largely to the increase in the percentage of fast and/or hybrid fibers associated with spaceflight.

CONTRACTILE PROPERTIES

Whole Muscle Studies

Few studies have determined the in situ contractile properties of skeletal muscle after spaceflight. In the most thorough study published to date, Caiozzo et al. [9] found a significant decrease in tension capabilities and a significant increase in speed properties of the Sol muscle tested within 3–9 hr after a 6-day spaceflight. Although the maximum tetanic tension of the muscle decreased by 28%, the tension per unit cross-sectional area (specific tension) was unaffected. The isometric twitch properties, frequency-tension response, and maximum rate of shortening all shifted toward those normally observed in a "faster" muscle. In addition, the Sol became more fatigable after spaceflight. These data indicate that adaptations in the mechanical properties of the Sol occur rapidly under weightlessness conditions: similar data are needed from longer flights. Some data on the in situ mechanical properties of the Sol and EDL are available from early Cosmos flights and have been reviewed by Oganov and Potapov [48].

Single-Fiber Studies

Holy and co-workers [26, 66] have studied the effects of 5 (Cosmos 1514), 7 (Cosmos 1667), and 14 (Cosmos 2044) days of flight on the contractile properties of mechanically skinned (glycerinated) single fibers from a variety of muscles. The fibers were tested in vitro under maximum calcium activation conditions. After 7 days of flight, Sol fibers (not identified by type) were significantly atrophied (14%) and showed a 28% decrease in maximum tetanic tension [26]. However, specific tension was not significantly affected. Measures reflecting the speed of response, i.e., calcium threshold for activation and time to achieve maximum tetanic tension, indicated that the Sol fibers were faster after than before flight. In a subsequent 14-day study, individual fibers were typed based on their differences in Ca^{2+} and Sr^{2+} activation [66]. A population of fast fibers was observed in the Sol of flight but not in that of control rats. Compared to slow fibers in control rats, the mean diameter of slow and fast fibers in the Sol of flight rats was reduced by 45 and 33%, respectively. Maximum tetanic tension was reported to have decreased by 75 and 60%, respectively, but specific tension was not affected significantly. The slow fibers in the Sol of flight rats had speed-related properties similar to those of slow fibers in control rats. In contrast, the fast fibers of the Sol showed a significant adaptation in almost all properties studied and, in many instances, the values were similar to those observed in fast fibers of fast muscles (i.e., compared to those of the LG and EDL). Mean fiber sizes in fast muscles (Plt, LG, and EDL) were affected minimally (<10% atrophy) [26, 66], with the only significant difference found for the LG fibers after 5 days of flight [26]. Maximum tetanic tension was reduced in the LG after 5 (22%) [26] and 14 (35%) [66] days of flight.

Specific tensions were quite variable, with only the LG fibers showing a significant decrease (40%) after 14 days of flight [66]. The fibers in the predominantly fast extensor muscles, the LG and Plt, had slower activation properties after flight, i.e., the muscle fibers became "slower" after, as compared to before, flight. The fibers in the EDL, a fast flexor muscle, showed no effects of spaceflight. These data appear to be consistent with the single-fiber results from flights of longer duration [47]. One interesting observation from these longer flights was a reduction in the maximum tetanic tension capability of fibers from the brachialis (a relatively fast muscle) but not in the medial head of the TB (a relatively slow muscle) [57].

All of these data indicate that some fibers in the Sol muscle acquire faster mechanical properties after spaceflight. In addition, it appears that some fibers can atrophy significantly, while maintaining their intrinsic tension-producing capabilities. These data on single fibers from the Sol are consistent with the adaptations in the fiber type composition, the protein contents and concentrations, and the morphological properties of the Sol after spaceflight discussed in other sections of this review. The apparent "slowing" of a population of fibers in fast muscles after flight is surprising. To understand fully the functional capacity of muscles after weightlessness, both whole muscle and single-fiber mechanical data are needed. Both levels of analyses are needed for longer duration flights on fast and slow muscles from the hindlimb and forelimb.

METABOLIC PROPERTIES

Vascularity

The effects of weightlessness on the vascularity of muscles have been estimated, using light and electron microcopic investigations of muscle capillarity. Desplanches et al. [13] reported no change in capillary density (capillaries per square millimeter) or capillaries per fiber in the Sol after a 7-day flight (Cosmos 1667). Musacchia et al. [45] found a 21% increase and no change in the capillary density in a deep and a superficial region of the VM, respectively, after 14 days of flight (Cosmos 2044). In addition, there was no change in the number of capillaries per fiber in either portion of the muscle. After 7 days of flight, Musacchia et al. [44] reported an increase of 53 and 21% in capillary density in the Sol and EDL, respectively. Ilyina-Kakueva [28] found an increase of 39 and 40% in the number of functional capillaries in the Sol and EDL after a 12.5-day flight (Cosmos 1887). No significant change was observed in the QF. Ilyina-Kakueva [27] found no change in the number of functional capillaries in the Sol, Gastroc, QF, or BB after 7 days of flight (Cosmos 1667). These data indicate that the blood supply of slow or fast muscles, at least at the capillary level, is not negatively impacted by these short periods of weightlessness. In fact, because of the decrease in fiber size with spaceflight, these data suggest that the blood supply per unit may actually be higher after, rather than before, flight.

Substrate Content and Use

Based on morphological estimations and biochemical data, it appears that muscle glycogen [30, 45, 60] and triglyceride [45] levels are somewhat increased after spaceflight. After 9 days of flight, the oxidation capacity (in the presence of nonlimiting amounts of substrate or cofactors) for pyruvate was unchanged, whereas the maximum rate of palmitate oxidation was decreased (~33%) in regions of the VL comprised predominantly of either high oxidative or low oxidative fibers [6]. These data suggest that there may be a shift toward increased use of carbohydrates as a source of energy during and immediately after spaceflight. The functional consequences of these metabolic shifts with respect to muscle fatigue are unknown.

Metabolic Enzymes

MUSCLE HOMOGENATES. The levels of oxidative enzymes appear to be relatively unaffected by weightlessness. For example, Desplanches et al. [13] found similar levels of CS and HAD in the sol after a 7-day flight. CS levels were also unaffected in the EDL, but 3-hydroxyacyl-CoA dehydrogenase (HAD) levels were decreased by 22%. Musacchia et al. [45] found no change in CS activity in the VM after 14 days of flight. Similarly, Baldwin et al. [6] reported no change in CS, HAD, or malate dehydrogenase activity in the VI or VL (in either a region comprised primarily of high-oxidative or a region comprised primarily of low-oxidative fibers) after 9 days of flight.

Data on lactate dehydrogenase (LDH), a glycolytic marker enzyme, has been less consistent. Total LDH activity was unchanged in the Sol and EDL after a 7-day flight [13] and in the QF and MG after a 20.5-day flight [20]. Similarly, the LDH isozyme pattern was unchanged in the Plt after 22 days of flight [51, 52]. However, both the total LDH and the relative proportion of muscle type LDH was elevated in the Sol after flights lasting about 20 days [21, 51, 52]. In addition, total LDH activity was elevated by 52% in the VM after a 14-day flight [45]. These data suggest that isozyme forms of LDH in a slow muscle change, toward that found in fast muscles (increase in muscle type LDH) after flight. This adaptation is consistent with the observations that slow muscles show other type-related changes toward "faster" properties and enhance their glycolytic potential after flight. Changes in the LDH activity in fast muscles are less clear, although it appears that the isoform pattern or total enzyme activity are minimally affected. Clearly, more work is necessary to resolve this issue.

SINGLE FIBER DATA. Most of the available metabolic data from spaceflight rats are at the single-fiber level. Based on quantitative histochemical procedures, mean succinate dehydrogenase (SDH) values for either fast or slow fibers in the Sol (i.e., enzyme concentration) were not changed significantly after 4 [32], 7 [41], 12.5 [42], or 14 [49] days of flight. However, when the decreases in mean fiber size were considered, the total amount of enzyme was decreased in both fast and slow fibers (e.g., see ref. 42).For a variety of predominantly fast muscles from the same rats [31, 41, 42], mean or total SDH activities were not significantly altered in any fiber type. Using single-fiber microchemical techniques, Manchester et al. [38] and Chi et al. [10] reported no change in the concentration (on a per dry weight per unit length basis) of a number of oxidative enzymes (termed enzymes that are normally high in the Sol muscle) in Sol muscle fibers (not identified by type) after 12.5 and 14 days of flight, respectively. Hexokinase, on the other hand, was elevated by 47 and 138% after 12.5 and 14 days of flight, respectively. When calculated per dry weight per unit length (i.e., taking into consideration the changes in muscle mass), the absolute levels of hexokinase were 50% higher after 12.5 days and were unchanged after 14 days of flight. The oxidative enzyme levels were decreased by ~10–45%. In the TA, the oxidative enzyme concentrations increased from 53 to 193% after 12.5 days [38] but were not significantly affected after 14 days [10] of flight. It should be noted, however, that the analyses by Manchester et al. [38] and Chi et al. [10] were based on fibers from only one or two flight rats, depending on the availability of the tissue. Thomason et al. [69] reported a 36% decrease in cytochrome c mRNA in the VI after 14 days of flight. No change was observed in the LG or the TB in the same rats or in the TB after a 7-day flight. Thus, there appear to be alterations in the pretranslational control of some proteins related to oxidative metabolism associated with spaceflight. Together, these data indicate that the oxidative capacity of the small fibers after flight is similar to that observed in ground-based control rats. However, because of the atrophy associated with weightlessness, the total number of enzyme units per fiber (or per muscle) decreases after flight.

An analysis of the changes in the intracellular distribution of SDH activity in Sol fibers after 12.5 days (Cosmos 1887) of flight was made, using quantitative histochemistry and "pixel-peeling" technique [8]. This analysis allows one to measure the mean SDH activity in concentric rings from the outermost periphery of the fiber to the innermost concentric ring of consecutive pixels. In the fast fibers of the Sol, SDH activity was reduced in the subsarcolemmal but not in the intermyofibrillar region after spaceflight. In contrast, the slow fibers from flight rats had a higher SDH activity than those of controls throughout the entire fiber diameter, with the largest differences found in the center of the fibers. Because most fibers in the Sol are the slow type histochemically, the overall SDH activity was higher after flight. Riley et al. (Cosmos 1887) [61] reported a 31% decrease in mitochondria (ultrastructural measures) and in SDH and nicotinamide adenine dinucleotide (NADH) staining (qualitative histochemistry) in the subsarcolemmal region of some fibers of another slow muscle, the AL, in the same rats studied by Bell et al. [8]. Riley et al. also observed a 50% decrease in subsarcolemmal mitochondria and a decrease in NADH staining of some fibers in the Sol after a 7-day flight (SLS-3) [60]. No apparent changes in mitochondrial content or distribution were observed in EDL fibers after flight [61]. These ultrastructural changes, however, were not analyzed relative to the myosin type of fibers. The results from these ultrastructural analyses would be consistent with the quantitative histochemical results of Bell et al. [8] if the majority of the fibers analyzed were of the fast type. However, this seems unlikely, given that most fibers remain slow after flight.

The physiological significance of the distribution or redistribution of mitochondria across the diameter of a fiber is unknown. However, a close association among the pattern of mitochondrial distribution, motor unit type, and fatigability has been demonstrated in a cat fast muscle [40]. In any case, these muscle and fiber type-specific adaptations in the content or distribution of mitochondria or SDH activity clearly demonstrate the complexity of the adaptive response.

Adaptations in the glycolytic potential of single fibers have been studied quite extensively. Martin et al. [41] reported that the α-glycerophosphate dehydrogenase (GDP) activity approximately doubled in both fast and slow fibers of predominantly slow muscles (Sol and AL) after a 7-day flight. However, the mean GPD activity of Sol fibers was similar to that of controls after either a 12.5-day [42] or a 14-day [49] flight. No significant changes were observed in predominantly fast muscles after 7 (EDL, Plt, and MG) [41], 12.5 (MG) [42], or 14 (MG and TA) [31] days of flight. In addition, total GPD activities were unchanged in fibers of the Sol or MG after 12.5 days of flight [42]. Manchester et al. [38] and Chi et al. [10] found increases ranging from 20 to 56% in enzymes normally high in fast muscles in the Sol fibers of 12.5- and 14-day flight rats. When calculated on a fiber-length basis, however, the enzyme levels actually decreased by 10–40%. In the TA, these enzymes' concentrations were unchanged (12–25% decreased), whereas the absolute amounts decreased by an average of 50%. In general, these results suggest that the concentration of glycolytic-related enzymes increases or is maintained but that the total amount of these enzymes decreases in both fast and slow muscles after spaceflight. The increases in glycolytic enzymes may be a reflection of the close link between the type of myosin expressed and the glycolytic potential of a fiber.

MORPHOLOGICAL ADAPTATIONS

In addition to decreases in fiber size, it appears that some of the loss in muscle mass and force-producing potential results from fiber damage. Since the early Cosmos flights, signs of muscle fiber damage have been observed after flight (e.g. see refs 12, 27, 30, 54, and 59–61). Based on both visual and some quantitative observations, the extent of fiber damage appears to be much more extensive in predominantly slow (Sol and AL) than in predominantly fast (EDL, Plt, Gastroc, QF, diaphragm, and BB) muscles. Assessment of the damage has been made at both the light and the electron microscope level. Some of the most common observations made almost exclusively in slow muscles include the following: 1) segmental necrosis to include extensive cellular infiltration by mononucleated cells; 2) sarcomere disorientation to include decreased Z-line width and Z-band streaming; 3) signs of degeneration-regeneration to include centrally placed nuclei and an increased number of satellite cells; 4) degeneration in capillary structure; 5) eccentric contraction-like lesions of the sarcomeres; and 6) regional interstitial edema. In addition, elevated concentrations of two proteases, calcium-activated protease and tripeptidylaminopeptidase, were observed in the Sol, but not in the EDL, of rats flown from 7 days on SLS-3 [60]. The increase in calcium-activated protease, which is involved in the initial breakdown of protein, suggests a role of this protease in the atrophic response.

Based on comparative data from Riley and co-workers [59–61], the authors have suggested that the type and extent of damage is related to the time interval between landing and the removal of the muscles. For example, about 7 and 4% of the fibers examined in the Sol and AL muscles, respectively, from Cosmos 1887 (removed ~48 hr after landing) showed severe forms of ultrastructural damage, such as segmental necrosis, signs of regeneration, phagocytosis, and interstitial edema [61]. In contrast, the AL from Cosmos 2044 was removed within 8–12 hr after landing, and the fiber damage was less severe, i.e., the predominant observation was eccentric-like lesions of the sarcomeres [59]. Furthermore, only about 1% of the fibers in the Sol showed some necrosis after a 7-day flight (muscles were removed within 11–17 hr) [60]. It should be noted, however, that D'Amelio and Daunton [12] found extensive and severe damage in the AL of the younger group of rats flown on Cosmos 2044. In fact, these authors estimated that ~60% of the fibers showed one or more abnormalities, and ~10% showed segmental necrosis in flight rats. Whether this difference in the amount of damage was attributable simply to the age of the rats is unknown.

Thus, it appears that some fibers are negatively impacted during the launch-flight-reentry-recovery sequence. Whether the fiber damage is related to the increased force levels reached during launch and reentry, the decreased forces during weightlessness, the increased forces on a weakened muscle during the interval between landing and muscle removal, or a combination of these factors is unknown. In addition, the reported severity and amount of damage is somewhat surprising, because the specific tension at the whole muscle and single-fiber levels appear to be relatively unaffected in flight rats (see above, Contractile Properties). Certainly, more correlative data on the extent of the muscle damage observed and on the functional capability of these muscles from flight rats are needed to assess the possible impact of these adaptations during more prolonged flights.

In this light, it is interesting to note that myofiber repair during a 14-day flight (Cosmos 2044) after a crush injury to the Gastroc 3 days before flight appeared to follow the initial pattern of processes observed at 1g [64]. However, these processes were somewhat delayed, and the presence of increased vascularity and number of macrophages at the repair site indicated a possible development of granulation. If granulation were to occur and form scar tissue, then a less than optimal repair of the muscle tissue would be expected. Thus, if muscle fiber injury were to occur during spaceflight (especially at the rate suggested by the morphological data discussed above), the functional capability of the muscle could be several impacted. Data from more prolonged flights are needed, however, to determine the possibility of this scenario.

The myotendinous junction also appears to be negatively impacted by spaceflight. The area of myotendinous junction membrane folding, a measure closely correlated with the strength of the junction site, was decreased significantly in the Plt of rats flown for only 4 days (STS-41) [70]. The membrane area decreased more than the cross-sectional area of the adjacent muscle fibers, resulting in a weaker junction, one that may be adequate for the loads encountered at 0g but inadequate for the weight-bearing loads at 1g. The appearance of occasional lesions in the extracellular matrix near the myotendinous region of flight rats (~4–6 hr after landing), but not in control rats, supports this contention. Thus, the connective tissue elements at the site of insertion of the muscle fibers can adapt rapidly to spaceflight, and these adaptations may negatively affect the functional capability of the muscles (especially weight-bearing extensor muscles) when returning to 1g.

ADAPTATIONS IN THE NEURAL ELEMENTS

Krasnov [35] has recently published a review on the morphological analyses of neural tissues following spaceflight (microgravity) and chronic centrifugation (hypergravity). In particular, results from early Russian flights are discussed in detail in the review by Krasnov [35]. In addition, Newberg [46] has recently published a review describing the changes in the central nervous system associated with spaceflight. Thus, the next part of this chapter will focus only on the reported adaptations of the spinal cord and peripheral neural elements of the neuromuscular unit, i.e., the neuromuscular junction, the ventral horn neurons, and spinal ganglia neurons, and will concentrate primarily on the results from the most recent flights.

Neuromuscular Junctions

Disruptive adaptations at the neuromuscular junction have been observed in rats from several flights. The changes appear to be quite severe in predominantly slow muscles and resemble the structural changes associated with total or partial denervation. For example, Baranski et al. [7] reported a 62% decrease in the number of synaptic vescicles and the presence of swollen mitochondria at the axonal endings in the Sol muscles of rats flown for 18.5 days (Cosmos 936). Similarly, Pozdnyakov et al. [55] and Babakova et al. [3] found signs of regeneration (restructuring of the presynaptic structures) in the neuromuscular synapses of the Sol after flights of 7 (Cosmos 1667) or 12.5 (Cosmos 1887) days. Much less severe effects were observed in the Gastroc or diaphragm of the same rats. In the most thorough analysis to date, D'Amelio and Daunton [12] studied the ultrastructural features of 38 and 40 neuromuscular junctions from the AL of control and 14-day flight rats (Cosmos 2044). The frequency of junctions showing abnormalities was 11% for control and 89% for flight rats. The most salient changes included the following: 1) a decrease in the number of synaptic vesicles; 2) a degeneration of axonal terminals; 3) axonal sprouting (a sign of regeneration); and 4) a presence of Schwann cell processes between pre- and postsynaptic sites. Riley et al. [61] observed similar changes in 2 of 12 neuromuscular junctions studied from the AL of rats flown for 12.5 days. Adaptations at the neuromuscular junction of the predominantly fast EDL [61], Gastroc [3, 55], or diaphragm [3,55] were either less severe or not present.

These data indicate that some neuromuscular junctions, particularly those located in predominantly slow muscles, show denervation-like characteristics after spaceflight. The extremely high incidence of abnormalities (89%) observed in the AL is quite noteworthy, particularly since flight duration was only 14 days. These findings raise several intriguing questions. First, how representative are the results of all neuromuscular junctions? For example, the ultrastructural examination of 78 neuromuscular junctions is a tedious and difficult task, but the data represent only a few junctions per muscle. Were the structures selected on a random basis, or were they chosen because those that looked abnormal were more interesting to study? These results also lead to the obvious questions of why these marked disruptions would occur and what functional impact they would have. For example, the maintenance of the specific tension of muscles and muscle fibers after flight is inconsistent with a large proportion of the fibers being denervated. Certainly, correlative functional and morphological data are needed to adequately address this issue.

Ventral Horn Neurons of the Spinal Cord

There is a paucity of data related to the adaptation of spinal neurons to spaceflight. Thus, the available data are from a mixture of ventral horn neurons, most likely including alpha and gamma motoneurons and interneurons. Mean SDH activity (quantitative histochemistry) and some size of ventral horn neurons from the upper portion of the lumbar enlargement were unaffected after a 14-day flight [33]. However, there was an increase in the frequency of relatively small cells with high SDH activities. After a recent 14-day flight, a population of neurons located at L5 also showed no change in mean SDH activity or soma size, although there appeared to be a decrease in SDH activity in medium-sized cells and an increase in small cells (A. Ishihara, R. R. Roy, and V. R. Edgerton, unpublished observations, 1995).

Minimal changes in a population of ventral horn neurons in the lower lumbar portion of the spinal cord of rats flown on Cosmos 2044 have been observed [35–37, 50]. The changes included a 12% decrease in nucleolar volume, a decrease in the RNA content of the neurons (an absence in the initial segments of the dendrites), and a 33% increase in the number of perineuronal glia per neuron. None of the changes in soma volume, nuclear volume, cytochrome oxidase activity, acetylcholinesterase activity, or number of active capillaries present with alkaline phosphatase activity were observed. In contrast, following 12. 5 days of flight, Polyakov et al. [50] found an 11% increase in the volume of the nuclei and nucleoli, a 25% increase in the number of "active" capillaries, an appearance of RNA in the initial segments of the dendrites, and a maintenance of the number of perineuronal nuclei per neuron. The authors suggest that the differences in the response of the neurons across flights may be related to factors other than the spaceflight itself, e.g., the rats were exposed to either 48 (Cosmos 1887) or 8–11 (Cosmos 2044) hr of $1g$ conditions before removal of the tissues. The authors further suggest that the longer period of recovery at $1g$ may have allowed for a reestablishment of afferent flow from the periphery and an elevated recruitment of motoneurons, thus resulting in adaptations that reflect an increased activity of the neurons.

Interestingly, more severe adaptations have been observed in the neurons located in the ventral horn of the cervical portion of the spinal cord, compared to those in the lumbar region [35–37]. In Cosmos 2044 rats, neurons in the cervical enlargement showed ~15% decreases in nucleolar and nuclear volumes, a 7% decrease in acetylcholinesterase activity, a 25% decrease in functional capillaries, and a decrease in RNA content in the initial segments of the dendrites. The authors related these findings to the larger impact of "hypoactivity" associated with spaceflight on the more precise and complex movements of the forelimbs, compared to those of the hindlimbs.

Together, these data indicate that specific populations (based on differences in the responsiveness of neurons of various sizes) of the ventral horn cells may be responsive to spaceflight conditions. However, to date no study has identified the portion of the neuronal pool being studied, i.e., no retrograde labeling of specific pools has been possible in these animals. Such studies are needed to determine whether there are any muscle-specific adaptations, i.e., based on the specificity of the muscle adaptations associated with spaceflight, one might expect the largest changes to occur in the motor pools innervating the slow muscles. In addition, the role that factors related to reloading of the hindlimbs associated with reentry and "down-time" before removing the spinal cord from the rats needs to be addressed.

Spinal Ganglia Neurons

Very little is known about the effects of spaceflight on the sensory elements of the neuromuscular unit. In one of the early Cosmos missions (Cosmos 605), Gorbunova and Portugalov (22) and Portugalov et al. [53] reported a decrease in RNA (13%) and protein (14%) content in large but not in small- or medium-sized spinal ganglia cells after 22 days of weightlessness. The ganglia studied were at the level of the lumbar enlargement and, thus, the data were interpreted by the authors to indicate a decreased afferent input from the unloaded hindlimb muscles. However, as pointed out by Krasnov [35], because the rats were at $1g$ for 24 hr before the tissues were removed, the decreased RNA and protein levels could have been a reflection of elevated afferent activation during this period. In addition, the significance of only the large dorsal root ganglia cells being affected is unknown.

More recently, Polyakov et al. [50] studied large, medium, and small cells in spinal ganglia at the L3/L5 levels in rats flown for 12.5 (Cosmos 1887) and 14 (Cosmos 2044) days. After the 14-day flight, the large cells had decreased soma volume (31%), nuclear volume (25%), nucleolar volume (13%), the number of capsular glial cells per neuron (27%), and alkaline phosphatase staining in glia cells and capillary endothelium (reflecting the number of "active" capillaries). The medium-sized cells only had decreases in nuclear volume and number of glial cells per neuron, whereas the small cells were unaffected. The changes in the large cells reflect a decrease in the functional activity of the primary afferent cells, most likely emanating from the hindlimb musculature. In contrast, there was no change in either the soma volume or number of glial cells per neuron, an 11% increase in the nuclear and nucleolar volumes, and a 25% increase in the number of "active" capillaries in the large cells of the spinal ganglia in the rats flown for 12.5 days. The differences in the response of the ganglia cells appear to be related to the time interval between landing and the removal of the ganglia. The rats from Cosmos 2044 were at $1g$ for only ~6–8 hr, whereas those flown on Cosmos 1887 were at $1g$ for at least 48 hr before tissue removal. Thus, the results from Cosmos 1887 could reflect an increased afferent flow that reached the spinal ganglia neurons during the 2 days at $1g$.

SUMMARY

Despite the inherent limitations placed on spaceflight investigations, much has been learned about the adaptations of the neuromuscular system to weightlessness from studies of rats flown for relatively short periods (~4–22 days). Below is a summary of the major effects of spaceflight observed in muscles of rats that are not in their rapid growth stage:

1. Skeletal muscles atrophy rapidly during spaceflight; significant atrophy is observed as early as after 4 days of flight.
2. The atrophic response appears to be related to the primary function of the muscle. In the hindlimb, the relative amount of atrophy can be characterized as slow extensors > fast extensors > fast flexors. This pattern of relative atrophy does not appear to be occurring in the forelimb; however, not enough data are available to draw any definitive conclusions at this time.
3. Both slow and fast fibers atrophy during spaceflight, with the largest fibers within an individual muscle generally showing the greatest atrophic response. Interestingly, the amount of fiber atrophy appears to reach a plateau after about 14 days of flight.
4. Adaptations have been observed in the concentration and content of all muscle proteins pools, with the protein pools in slow muscles the most affected.
5. Some slow and fast fibers in predominantly slow and fast muscles show shifts in their histochemical and biochemical properties, toward those observed in a "faster" phenotype.
6. Some fibers, presumably expressing slow MHC isoforms before flight, begin to express fast MHC isoforms during flight.
7. The oxidative capacity of the muscles or fibers is relatively unaffected by spaceflight, particularly in the slow muscles. Any change in whole-body fatigability associated with spaceflight most likely reflects the loss in muscle and fiber mass.
8. The glycolytic capacity of the muscles and muscle fibers is enhanced after spaceflight. This metabolic adaptation seems to be related to the shift in the contractile proteins towards "faster" isoforms.
9. The vascularity of muscles appears to be maintained after flight, based, at least, on histological observations of capillarity.
10. The force capabilities of the muscles and fibers appear to decrease in parallel with the decreases in size, i.e., the specific tension is not significantly affected after flight.
11. Changes in the speed-related properties of the slow muscles are consistent with the adaptations in the myosin molecule, i.e., the slow muscles and some fibers in the slow muscles become "faster."
12. Some muscle fiber and neuromuscular junction damage has been observed after flight, particularly in the slow muscles. The extent of damage may be related to the amount of time that the muscles are allowed to reload before removal, i.e., in general, shorter intervals result in less fiber damage.
13. Adaptations in the motor (ventral horn) and sensory (spinal ganglia) neurons have been quite variable, but this may be related to the amount

of time that the muscles are allowed to reload before removal. Morphological adaptations after relatively short periods of reloading may reflect a decrease in the activation of the neural elements during flight.

CONCLUSIONS AND RECOMMENDATIONS

1. Spaceflight, to include recovery, appears to be an excellent model to study the mechanisms involved in the rapid remodeling of the neuromuscular unit in the absence of disease or direct neural trauma.
2. The mechanisms responsible for the neuromuscular adaptations associated with periods of weightlessness described above are unknown. However, it is highly likely that the muscle and neural adaptations reflect changes in the activity, i.e., in both activation and loading, patterns of the neuromuscular unit during the spaceflight experience. Activation (e.g., EMG) and loading (e.g., tendon force) data are needed from both slow and fast muscles before flight; during launch, flight and reentry; and after landing to adequately address the role of these factors on the observed adaptations. Furthermore, the interaction of these electrical and mechanical stimuli with growth factors, such as growth hormone, should be investigated in the context of the "unloaded" or weightless state.
3. Because the interval between the time of landing and the removal of neuromuscular tissues appears to have an effect on some of the adaptations in the tissues, effort must be made to minimize and/or control these time intervals to distinguish between flight and postflight effects.
4. The interpretation of many of the results from these spaceflight missions has been limited because of the small number of rats per group flown on individual missions or because too many investigators were required to share animals and tissues from the same flight. An effort should be made either to increase the number of rats flown or to decrease the number of investigators sharing the same tissues.
5. Investigators must have the opportunity to design specific studies that are not limited by inherent compromises when multiple experiments and hypotheses are being tested on the same animals.
6. Finally, future research concerning skeletal muscle plasticity in response to microgravity needs to become more mechanistic concerning the causes of the adaptations in fiber morphology, protein turnover, contractile protein phenotype, and muscle metabolism.

ACKNOWLEDGMENTS

We thank Dr. Richard E.Grindeland from the NASA Ames Research Center for his contribution in verifying, as thoroughly as possible, the information in Table 13.1 We thank C. Rigmaiden and M. K. Day for assistance in

preparing the paper and R. Monti for proofreading this chapter. This work
has been supported in large part by NIH Grant NS16333 and NASA Grants
NCA-1R 390-502, NAG2-555, and NAG2-450.

REFERENCES

1. Allen D. L., W. Yasui, T. Tanaka, et al. Myonuclear number and myosin heavy chain expression in rat soleus single muscle fibers following spaceflight. *J. Appl. Physiol.* in press, 1995.
2. Armstrong, R. B., and R. O. Phelps. Muscle fiber type composition of the rat hindlimb. *Am. J. Anat.* 171:259–272, 1984.
3. Babakova, L. L., M. S. Demorzhi, and O. M. Pozdnyakov. Dynamics of structural changes in skeletal muscle neuromuscular junctions of rats under the influence of the space flight factors. *Physiologist* 35:S224–S225, 1992.
4. Backup, P., K. Westerlind, S. Harris, T. Spelsberg, B. Kline,and R. Turner. Spaceflight results in reduced mRNA levels for tissue-specific proteins in the musculoskeletal system. *Am. J. Physiol.* 266:E567–E573, 1994.
5. Baldwin, K. M., R. E. Herrick, E. Ilyina-Kakueva, and V. S. Oganov. Effects of zero gravity on myofibril content and isomyosin distribution in rodent skeletal muscle. *FASEB J.* 4:79–83, 1990.
6. Baldwin, K. M., R. E. Herrick, and S. A. McCue. Substrate oxidation capacity in rodent skeletal muscle: effects of exposure to zero gravity. *J. Appl. Physiol.* 75:2466–2470, 1993.
7. Baranski, S., W. Baranska, M. Marciniak and E. I. Ilyina-Kakueva. Ultrasonic investigations of the soleus muscle after space flight on the Biosputnik 936. *Aviat. Space Environ. Med.* 50:930–934, 1979.
8. Bell, G. J., T. P. Martin, E. I. Ilyina-Kakueva, V. S. Oganov, and V.R. Edgerton. Altered distribution of mitochondria in rat soleus muscle fibers after spaceflight. *J. Appl. Physiol.* 73:493–497, 1992.
9. Caiozzo, V. J., M. J. Baker, R. E. Herrick, M. Tao, and K. M. Baldwin. Effect of spaceflight on skeletal muscle: mechanical properties and myosin isoform content of a slow muscle. *J. Appl. Physiol.* 76:1764–1773, 1994.
10. Chi, M. M., R. Choksi, P. Nemeth, et al. Effects of microgravity and tail suspension on enzymes of individual soleus and tibialis anterior fibers. *J. Appl. Physiol.* 73:66S–73S, 1992.
11. Chui, L. A., and K. R. Castleman. Morphometric analysis of rat muscle fibers following space flight and hypogravity. *Physiologist* 23:S76–S78, 1980.
12. D'Amelio, F., and N. G. Daunton. Effects of spaceflight in the adductor longus muscle of rats flown in the Soviet Biosatellite COSMOS 2044. A study employing neural cell adhesion molecule (N-CAM) immunocytochemistry and conventional morphological techniques (light and electron microscopy). *J. Neuropathol. Exp. Neurol.* 51:415–431, 1992.
13. Desplanches, D., M. H. Mayet, E. I. Ilyina-Kakueva, B. Sempore, and R. Flandrois. Skeletal muscle adaptation in rats flown on Cosmos 1667. *J. Appl. Physiol.* 68:48–52, 1990.
14. Edgerton, V. R., and R. R. Roy. Adaptations of skeletal muscle to spaceflight. S. Churchill (ed). *Fundamentals of Space Life Sciences,* in press, 1995.
15. Edgerton, V. R., and R. R. Roy. Nervous system and sensory adaptation: neural plasticity associated with chronic neuromuscular activity. C. Bouchard, R. J. Shephard, and T. Stephens (eds). *Physical Activity, Fitness and Health. The International Proceeding and Consensus Statement,* Champaign, IL: Human Kinetics, 1994, chapt. 34, pp.
16. Edgerton, V. R., and R. R. Roy. Neuromuscular adaptation to actual and simulated weightlessness. S. L. Bonting (eds). *Advances in Space Biology and Medicine.* Greenwich, CT: JAI Press, 1994, pp. 33–67.
17. Edgerton, V. R., and R. R. Roy. Neuromuscular adaptations to actual and simulated spaceflight. M. J. Fregly and C. M. Blatteis (eds). *Handbook of Physiology, Environmental Physiology,*

Vol. III: *The Gravitational Environment.* New York: Oxford University Press, 1995, pp. 721–763.

18. Esser, K. A., and E.C. Hardeman. Changes in contractile protein mRNA accumulation in response to spaceflight. *Am. J. Physiol.* 268:C466–471, 1995.

19. Fox, R. A., M. Corcoran, N. G. Daunton, and E. Morey-Holton. Effects of spaceflight and hindlimb suspension on the posture and gait of rats. K. Taguchi, M. Igarashi, and S. Mori (eds). *Vestibular and neurological Front.* Amsterdam: Elsevier, 1994, pp. 603–607.

20. Gayevskaya M. S., R. A. Belitskaya, N. S. Kolganova, Y. V. Kolchina, L. M. Kurkina, and Y. A. Nosova. Tissular metabolism in mixed type fibers of rat skeletal muscles after flight aboard cosmos-690 biosatellite. *Kosm. Biol. Aviakosm. Med.* 3:28–31, 1979.

21. Gayevskaya M. S., N. S. Veresotskaya, N. S. Kolganova, Y. V. Kolchina, L. M. Kurkina, and Y. A. Nosova. Changes in metabolism of soleus muscle tissues in rats following flight aboard the Kosmos-690 biosatellite. *Kosm. Biol. Aviakosm. Med.* 1:16–19, 1979.

22. Gorbunova, A. V., and V. V. Portugalov. Cytochemical investigations of proteins and RNA in spinal motoneurons and neurons of spinal ganglia of the rat after space flight. *Aviat. Space Environ. Med.* 47:708–710, 1976.

23. Grindeland, R., T. Fast, and M. Ruder, et al. Rodent body, organ, and muscle weight responses to seven days of microgravity (Abstract). *Physiologist* 28:375, 1985.

24. Haddad, F., R. E. Herrick, G. R. Adams, and K. M. Baldwin. Myosin heavy chain expression in rodent skeletal muscle: effects of exposure to zero gravity. *J. Appl. Physiol.* 75:2471–2477, 1993.

25. Henriksen, E. J., M. E. Tischler, C. R. Woodman, K. A. Munoz, C. S. Stump, and C. R. Kirby. Elevated interstitial fluid volume in soleus muscles unweighted by spaceflight or suspension. *J. Appl. Physiol.* 75:1650–1653, 1993.

26. Holy, X., and Y. Mounier. Effects of short spaceflights on mechanical characteristics of rat muscles. *Muscle Nerve* 14:70–78, 1991.

27. Ilyina-Kakuyeva, Y. Study of skeletal muscles of rats after a short-term space flight on the cosmos-1667 biosatellite. *Kosm. Biol. Aviakosm. Med.* 21:31–35, 1987.

28. Ilyina-Kakuyeva, Y. Morphohistochemical investigation of the skeletal muscles of rats in an experiment on biosatellite COSMOS-1887. *Kosm. Biol. Aviakosm. Med.* 24:22–25, 1990.

29. Ilyina-Kakueva, E. I., and V. V. Portugalov. Combined effect of space flight and radiation on skeletal muscles of rats. *Aviat. Space Environ. Med.* 48:115–119, 1977.

30. Ilyina-Kakueva, E. I., V. V. Portugalov, and N. P. Krivenkova. Space flight effects on the skeletal muscles of rats. *Aviat. Space Environ. Med.* 47:700–703, 1976.

31. Jiang, B., Y. Ohira, R. R. Roy, et al. Adaptation of fibers in fast-twitch muscles of rats to spaceflight and hindlimb suspension. *J. Appl. Physiol.* 73:58S–65S, 1992.

32. Jiang, B., R. Roy, C. Navarro, and V. Edgerton. Atrophic response of rat soleus fibers subjected to a 4-day spaceflight. *J. Appl. Physiol.* 74:527–531, 1993.

33. Jiang, B., R. R. Roy, I. V. Polyakov, I. B. Krasnov, and V. R. Edgerton. Ventral horn cell responses to spaceflight and hindlimb suspension. *J. Appl. Physiol.* 73:107S–111S, 1992.

34. Kozlovskaya, I., Y. V. Kreidich, V.S. Oganov, and O. P. Koserenko. Pathophysiology of motor functions in prolonged manned space flights. *Acta Astronautica* 8:1059–1072, 1981.

35. Krasnov, I. B. Gravitational neuromorphology. S. L. Bonting (ed). *Advances in Space Biology and Medicine.* Greenwich, CT: JAI Press, 1994, pp. 111–126.

36. Krasnov, I. B., I. V. Polyakov, and V. I. Drobyshev. Neuron-glia-capillary system in spinal cord of rats after 14-day space flight. *Physiologist* 35:S218–S219, 1992.

37. Krasnov, I. B., I. V. Polyakov, and V. I. Drobyshev. The effect of spaceflight and head-down suspension on the motoneuron-glia-capillary system of rat spinal cord. *Aviakos Ecol. Med.* 27:38–42, 1993.

38. Manchester, J. K., M. M. Chi, B. Norris, et al. Effect of microgravity on metabolic enzymes of individual muscle fibers. *F.A.S.E.B. J.* 4:55–63, 1990.

39. Martin, T. P. Protein and collagen content of rat skeletal muscle following space flight. *Cell Tissue Res.* 254:251–253, 1988.

40. Martin, T. P., and V. R. Edgerton. Intrafibre distribution of succinate dehydrogenase in cat tibialis anterior motor units. *Can. J. Physiol. Pharmacol.* 70:970–976, 1992.
41. Martin, T. P., V. R. Edgerton, and R. E. Grindeland. Influence of spaceflight on rat skeletal muscle. *J. Appl. Physiol.* 65:2318–2325, 1988.
42. Miu, B., T. P. Martin, R. R. Roy, et al. Metabolic and morphologic properties of single muscle fibers in the rat after spaceflight, Cosmos 1887. *F.A.S.E.B. J.* 4:64–72, 1990.
42. Miu, B., T. P. Martin, R. R. Roy, et al. Metabolic and morphologic properties of single muscle fibers in the rat after spaceflight, Cosmos 1887. *F.A.S.E.B. J.* 4:64–72, 1990.
43. Musacchia, X. J., J. M. Steffen, and R. D. Fell. Disuse atrophy of skeletal muscle: animal models. *Exerc. Sport Sci. Rev.* 16:61–87, 1988.
44. Musacchia X. J., J. M. Steffen, R. D. Fell, and M. J. Drombrowski. Skeletal muscle response to spaceflight, whole body suspension, and recovery in rats. *J. Appl. Physiol.* 69:2248–2253, 1990.
45. Musacchia, X. J., J. M. Steffen, R. D. Fell, M. J. Dombrowski, V. W. Oganov, and E. I. Ilyina-Kakueva. Skeletal muscle atrophy in response to 14 days of weightlessness: vastus medialis. *J. Appl. Physiol.* 73:44S–50S, 1992.
46. Newberg, A. B. Changes in the central nervous system and their clinical correlates during long-term spaceflight. *Aviat. Space Environ. Med.* 65:562–572, 1994.
47. Oganov, V.S. Neurotrophic influences in the adaption of skeletal muscles and motor functions to weightlessness. G. A. Nasledov (ed). *Mechanisms of Neural Regulation of Muscle Function.* Leningrad: Nauka, 1988, pp. 107–136.
48. Oganov, V. S. and A. N. Potapov. On the mechanisms of changes in skeletal muscles in the weightless environment. *Life Sci. Space Res.* 15:137–143, 1976.
49. Ohira Y., B. Jiang, R. R. Roy, et al. Rat soleus muscle fiber responses to 14 days of spaceflight and hindlimb suspension. *J. Appl. Physiol.* 73:51S–57S, 1992.
50. Polyakov, I. V., V. I. Drobyshev and I. B. Krasnov. Morphological changes in the spinal cord and intervertebral ganglia of rats exposed to different gravity levels. *Physiologist* 34:S187–188, 1991.
51. Portugalov, V. V., A. V. Gorbunova, and N. V. Petrova. Cytochemical changes in the structures of the spinal reflex arc of rats after space flight. *Cell Mol. Biol.* 22:73–77, 1977.
52. Portugalov, V. V., and N. V. Petrova. LDH isoenzymes of skeletal muscles of rats after space flight and hypokinesia. *Aviat. Space Environ. Med.* 47:834–838, 1976.
53. Portugalov, V. V., E. A. Savina, A. S. Kaplansky, et al. Effect of space flight factors on the mammal: experimental-morphological study. *Aviat. Space Environ. Med.* 47:813–816, 1976.
54. Pozdnyakov, O. M., L. L. Babakova, and M. S. Demorzhi. Changes in the ultrastructure of striated muscle in response to space flight factors. *Kosm. Biol. Aviakosm. Med.* 12:746–749, 1988.
55. Pozdnyakov, O. M., L. L. Babakova, M. S. Demorzhi, and Y. Ilyina-Kakuyeva. Change in the ultrastructure of striated muscle and neuromuscle synapses of rats in response to a 13-day space flight. *Kosm. Biol. Aviakosm. Med.* 24:38–42, 1990.
56. Rapcsak, M., V. S. Oganov, L. M. Murashko, T. Szilagyi, and A. Szoor. Effect of short-term spaceflight on the contractile properties of rat skeletal muscles with different functions. *Acta Physiol Hung.* 76:13–20, 1990.
57. Rapcsak, M., V. S. Oganov, A. Szoor, S. A. Skuratova, T. Szilagyi, and O. Takacs. Effect of weightlessness on the function of rat skeletal muscles on the biosatellite "Cosmos-1129." *Acta Physiol Hung.* 62:225–228, 1983.
58. Riley, D. A., and S. Ellis. Research on the adaptation of skeletal muscle to hypogravity: past and future directions. *Adv. Space. Res.* 3:191–197, 1983.
59. Riley, D. A., S. Ellis, C. S. Giometti, et al. Muscle sarcomere lesions and thrombosis after spaceflight and suspension unloading. *J. Appl. Physiol.* 73:33S–43S, 1992.
60. Riley, D. A., S. Ellis, G. R. Slocum, T. Satyanarayana, J. L. Bain, and F. R. Sedlak. Hypogravity-induced atrophy of rat soleus and extensor digitorum longus muscles. *Muscle Nerve* 10:560–568, 1987.

61. Riley, D. A., E. I. Ilyina-Kakueva, S. Ellis, J. L. Bain, G. R. Slocum, and F. R. Sedlak. Skeletal muscle fiber, nerve, and blood vessel breakdown in space-flown rats. *F.A.S.E.B. J.* 4:84–91, 1990.

62. Rokhlenko, K. D., and Z. F. Savik. Effect of space flight factors on skeletal muscle ultrastructure. *Kosm. Biol. Aviakosm. Med.* 15:72–77, 1981.

63. Roy, R. R., K. M. Baldwin, and V. R. Edgerton. The plasticity of skeletal muscle: effects of neuromuscular activity. *Exerc. Sport Sci. Rev.* 19:269–312, 1991.

64. Stauber, W. T., V. K. Fritz, T. E. Burkovskaya, and E. I. Ilyina-Kakueva. Effect of spaceflight on the extracellular matrix of skeletal muscle after a crush injury. *J. Appl. Physiol.* 73:74S–81S, 1992.

65. Steffen, J. M. and X. J. Musacchia. Spaceflight effects on adult rat muscle protein, nucleic acids, and amino acids. *Am. J. Physiol.* 251:R1059–1063, 1986.

66. Stevens, L., Y. Mounier, and X. Holy. Functional adaptation of different rat skeletal muscles to weightlessness. *Am. J. Physiol.* 264:R770–R776, 1993.

67. Takacs, O., M. Rapcsak, A. Szoor, et al. Effect of weightlessness on myofibrillar proteins of rat skeletal muscles with different functions in experiment of biosatellite "Cosmos-1129." *Acta Physiol. Hung.* 62:229–233, 1983.

68. Thomason, D. B., and F. W. Booth. Atrophy of the soleus muscle by hindlimb unweighting. *J. Appl. Physiol.* 68:1–12, 1990.

69. Thomason, D. B., P. R. Morrison, V. Oganov, E. Ilyina-Kakueva, F. W. Booth, and K. M. Baldwin. Altered actin and myosin expression in muscle during exposure to microgravity. *J. Appl. Physiol.* 73:90S–93S, 1992.

70. Tidball, J. G., and D. M. Quan. Reduction in myotendinous junction surface area of rats subjected to 4-day spaceflight. *J. Appl. Physiol.* 73:59–64, 1992.

71. Tischler, M., E. Henriksen, S. Jacob, S. Satarug, and P. Cook. Problems in analysis of data from muscles of rats flown in space. *Physiologist* 31:S10–54, 1988.

72. Tischler, M. E., E. J. Henriksen, K. A. Munoz, C. S. Stump, C. R. Woodman and C. R. Kirby. Spaceflight on STS-48 and earth-based unweighting produce similar effects on skeltal muscle of young rats. *J. Appl. Physiol.* 74:2161–2165, 1993.

14
Muscle Mechanics: Adaptations with Exercise-Training

ROBERT H. FITTS, Ph.D.
JEFFREY J. WIDRICK, Ph.D.

Muscle mechanics can be defined as the basic functional properties of muscles that allows them to produce movements with a characteristic force, velocity, and power. Understanding these properties and how they adapt to programs of regular exercise is essential if we hope to optimize human performance, and delay the deterioration of performance associated with the aging process. Although the basic functional properties of limb skeletal muscle have been known for some time [26], a few of the important cellular and molecular mechanisms of contraction are still not fully elucidated [42, 72, 89, 107, 122]. In particular, the processes of excitation-contraction (E-C) coupling, whereby the depolarization of the surface (sarcolemma) and t-tubular membranes leads to the release of Ca^{2+} from the adjacent terminal cisternae region of the sarcoplasmic reticulum (SR), and the interaction of the contractile proteins actin and myosin with the subsequent generation of force and filament movement (cross-bridge kinetics) are two important muscle cell functions for which we currently lack a complete understanding. Nevertheless, in recent years, considerable progress has been made in these fields, and a complete understanding of these processes appears eminent [72, 107]. In this chapter, it is our intent to review the isometric and isotonic contractile properties of limb skeletal muscle and, to whatever extent possible, to discuss the underlying cellular mechanisms. A second objective is to provide a summary of the published data concerning how the mechanical properties of muscle adapt to various programs of regular exercise-training. We will not discuss muscle fatigue in any detail, as this topic has recently been reviewed [44].

MUSCLE FIBER TYPE COMPOSITION

The mechanical properties of muscle are highly dependent on the fiber type composition of the muscle. Adult mammalian skeletal muscles contain at least three distinct fiber types, classified on the basis of their functional and metabolic properties as fast glycolytic (FG), fast oxidative glycolytic (FOG), and slow oxidative (SO). The FG and FOG fiber types are fast-twitch fibers, characterized by high SR and myofibrillar adenosine triphosphatase

(ATPase) activities and correspondingly short isometric twitch durations and high maximal shortening velocities (V_0) [4, 26, 47, 104]. In contrast, the SO fiber possesses low SR and myofibrillar ATPase activities, prolonged twitch duration, and low V_0, compared with those of fast-twitch fiber types [47, 117]. Each fiber type contains a specific isozyme for the contractile protein myosin, and fibers are frequently identified on the basis of their histochemically determined myosin ATPase activity as Type I, IIa, or IIb [15, 21]. Recently, adult skeletal muscle has been shown to contain a fourth fiber type containing a specific isozyme identified as IIx or IId [15, 16]. Rat skeletal muscle has been shown to express all four of the myosin isozymes. Slow muscles, such as the soleus, contain primarily the Type I fiber (Table 14.1), while fast-twitch muscles (extensor digitorum longus (EDL), gastrocnemius, vastus lateralis) are composed primarily of a mixture of the fast myosin isozymes. Different regions of a muscle may contain a particularly high percentage of a given isozyme. For example, the superficial region of the vastus lateralis (SVL) contains primarily Type IIb fibers, whereas the superficial region of the medial head of the gastrocnemius contains a mixture of Type IIb and hybrid fibers containing Type IIb and IIx myosin (Table 14.1). The percentage distribution of fast Types IIb, IIx, hybrid IIb-IIx, and IIa fibers can be altered by programs of regular exercise training (see Muscle Mechanics: Adaptations with Exercise Training below). In contrast to that of rodents, adult human muscle appears to express only three types of myosin—a slow Type I, a fast Type IIa, and a second fast myosin that is frequently identified as Type IIb but has recently been shown to display the greatest degree of homology with the rodent Type IIx myosin heavy chain [40, 118]. For historical reasons, we will refer to this fiber as fast Type IIb, but the reader should realize that the human IIb fiber discussed in this text is likely to be identical to the recently discovered Type IIx fiber. It seems that human muscle contains little or no Type IIb myosin. The myosin heavy-chain profile of an individual single fiber can be easily identified by sodium dodecyl sulfate (SDS) gel electrophoresis [117]. Figure 14.1 shows an example of human muscle fibers identified on 5% SDS gels. Fourteen individual fibers are shown in Lanes 3–16, and the three fiber types (Types I, IIa, and IIb) are clearly identifiable.

KINETIC MODEL OF CROSS-BRIDGE CYCLING

Since the sliding filament theory of muscle contraction was first proposed by Huxley [74], the molecular mechanism of cross-bridge cycling has been a topic of intense study [53]. Numerous models have been developed [39, 53, 67, 116, 123]; however, the exact molecular events of the cross-bridge interaction responsible for tension development and sarcomere shortening are as yet unknown. Figure 14.2 presents a schematic model of the kinetics of the cross-bridge cycle (actomyosin ATP hydrolysis reaction) in skeletal muscle. The scheme was published by Metzger and Moss [97] and repre-

TABLE 14.1.
Fiber Type Distribution Determined by 5% SDS-PAGE Analysis[a]

Group	n	(I)	(IIa)	(I + IIa)	(I + IIx)	(IIx)	(IIb)	(IIb + IIx)	(IIa + IIx)
				% Fiber Type					
Soleus									
Control	107	92		7	1				
2-hr ET	182	80	4	9	4				2
Red Gastroc									
Control	76	62	22	16					
2-hr ET	55	62	20	18					
White Gastroc									
Control	146					1	62	35	1
2-hr ET	113[b]					18	19	55	8

[a]Data were taken from ref. 117. Sodium dodecyl sulphate-polyacrylamide gel electrophoresis 2-hr ET, 2-hr exercise-trained group; red Gastroc fibers were isolated from deep region of the lateral head of the gastrocnemius; white gastroc fibers were isolated from the superficial region of the medial head of the gastrocnemius.
[b]2-hr ET group was significantly different from the controls.

FIGURE 14.1.

Myosin heavy-chain (MHC) profile of human single fibers run on 5% SDS-PAGE gels. The fibers were isolated from the gastrocnemius muscle. Lanes 1 and 2 contain myosin standards for the slow Type I and fast Type IIb MHC. Lanes 3–16 contain individual fiber segments 5 mm long. The fibers in Lanes 3 and 5–13 are slow Type I fibers, with maximal velocities ranging from 0.228 to 0.423 fiber lengths. Lanes 14–16 show a fast Type IIb, a fast Type IIa, and a slow Type I fiber, respectively, with maximal velocities of 2.387, 1.586, and 0.510 FL/s. PAGE, polyacrylamide gel elecrophoresis.

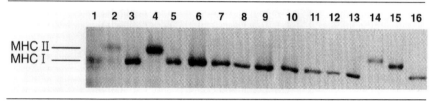

sents their adaptation of the current models of ATP hydrolysis which, in turn, were derived from modifications of the model originally proposed by Lymn and Taylor [91].

The production of force depends on the binding of the myosin head (M) to actin (A). P_i release (Fig. 14.2, Step 5) is thought to be coupled to the transition in actomyosin binding from a weakly bound, low-force state (AM-ADP-P_i) to the strongly bound, high-force state (AM-ADP). This latter state is likely the dominant cross-bridge form during a peak isometric contraction [97]. Brenner [17] and Metzger et al. [95] have suggested that the peak rate of tension development (dP/dt) is limited by the time required for this transition.

The maximal velocity of shortening in skeletal muscle (V_o) is obtained during maximal unloaded contractions, where the need for the strongly bound, high-force states of the cross-bridge (Fig. 14.2, the AM'-ADP state) is low, and the overall cycle rate is maximal. In contrast to dP/dt, in which the rate of cross-bridge attachment appears to be limiting, V_o is highly correlated with the rate of ATP hydrolysis by myosin, and both V_o and ATPase activity are thought to be limited by the rate of cross-bridge dissociation [7, 53]. The rate-limiting step in cross-bridge detachment is not known, but the possibilities include Steps 6, 7, 1, and 2 of the scheme shown in Figure 14.2.

ISOMETRIC CONTRACTILE PROPERTIES

Isometric Twitch Contraction

When a muscle is held isometric (no length change is allowed) and is activated via a single maximal stimulus (either via the nerve or direct stimula-

FIGURE 14.2.

Schematic model of the actomyosin ATP hydrolysis reaction during contraction in skeletal muscle, where A is actin and M is myosin. The scheme is adapted from current models of ATP hydrolysis. Reproduced from ref. 97.

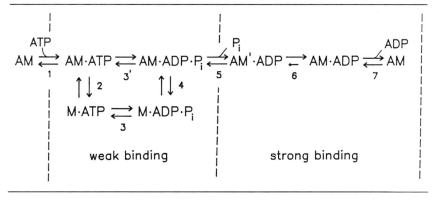

tion of the muscle), it responds with a characteristic pattern of force development that depends on the fiber type composition and temperature of the muscle (26, 48). Figure 14.3 shows a representative drawing of a twitch response for the slow-twitch soleus and fast-twitch EDL. The contraction time (CT) and one-half relaxation time (1/2 RT) are 3- to 4-fold longer in the slow muscle [47, 49]. Another obvious difference is the peak rate of tension development ($+dP/dt$) and decline ($-dP/dt$), in which the fast EDL displays 44 and 7-fold higher values, respectively compared to the slow soleus (Table 14.2). The time course of the twitch duration is thought to reflect and be dependent on the time course of the increase in intracellular Ca^{2+} [14]. Thus, the short relaxation time in fast, compared to slow muscle, has been attributed to the higher activity and concentration of the SR in fast muscle. We have observed the quantity (mg/g muscle) of SR to be 2- to 3-fold higher in fast muscle [47], and we [47] and others [20, 41] have found the SR ATPase activity ($\mu mol\ P_i/min$) and the maximal Ca^{2+} uptake rate to be 3-fold higher and, in some cases, for the latter to be up to 6-fold higher in fast, as compared to slow, skeletal muscle. The data in Table 14.3 demonstrate that the highest SR yields, enzyme activity, and Ca^{2+} uptake capacity are found in muscles containing primarily Type IIb fibers (see data for the superficial region of the vastus lateralis (SVL)), whereas mixed fast muscles such as the EDL (Types IIb and IIa) show SR activity somewhat less than the pure IIb muscle but considerably higher than the predominantly Type I soleus. If data were available for the Type IIx fiber, it would likely display an SR function and isometric twitch duration intermediate between the Type IIb and Type IIa fiber type.

FIGURE 14.3.

Representative isometric twitch contractions for the EDL and the soleus (SOL). The drawings are reproductions of twitch responses at 22°C. The time line on the x-axis is divided into 40-ms segments. The CT of the fast EDL averaged 37 ms, while the slow SOL CT averaged 111 ms. The 1/2 RT averaged 30 and 109 ms, respectively for the EDL and SOL. Reproduced from ref. 49.

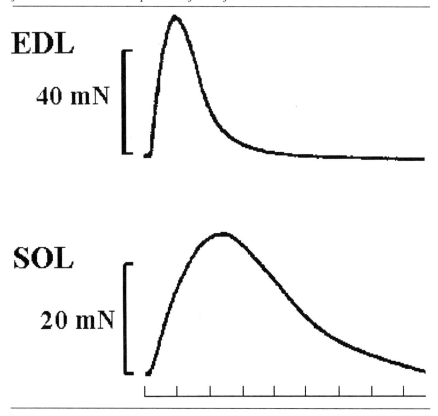

Isometric Tetanic Contraction

The peak force and power output of a muscle depend on numerous factors to include: 1) muscle and fiber size and length; 2) architecture, to include the angle and physical properties of the fiber-tendon attachment, as well as the fiber to muscle length ratio; 3) fiber type; 4) number of cross-bridges in parallel; 5) force per cross-bridge; 6) peak dP/dt; 7) force-velocity relationship; 8) fiber V_o; 9) force-pCa relationship (where pCa= -log $[Ca^{2+}]$); and 10) the force-frequency relationship. Additionally, neural events, such as cortical drive, afferent inputs to the central nervous system, and alpha motoneuron recruitment patterns, affect the force and power of a muscle or muscle group. Figure 14.4 shows a representative drawing of an isomet-

TABLE 14.2.
Isometric Twitch and Tetanic Contractile Properties at 22° C

			Twitch		Tetanus			
Muscle	CT (ms)	1/2RT (ms)	Pt ($kN \cdot M^{-2}$)	P_0 ($kN \cdot m^{-2}$)	$+dP/dt$ ($kN \cdot m^{-2} \cdot ms^{-1}$)	$-dP/dt$ ($kN \cdot m^{-2} \cdot ms^{-1}$)	Pt/Po
SO	111 ± 7	118 ± 3	34 ± 3	243 ± 20	1.57 ± 0.20	2.26 ± 0.39	0.14
EDL	42 ± 2	30 ± 1	62 ± 4	235 ± 17	6.57 ± 0.20	8.63 ± 2.55	0.26

[a]CT and 1/2RT data taken from ref. 130 and remaining data from ref. 47. Values are mean ± SE.

TABLE 14.3.
Sarcoplasmic Reticulum Yield, ATPase activity, and Ca²⁺ Uptake Rate in Fast- and Slow-Twitch Skeletal Muscle

Muscle	SR Yield ($mg \cdot g^{-1}$ tissue)	SR ATPase Activity ($\mu mol\ P_i \cdot min^{-1}$)	Ca²⁺ Uptake Kinetics (V_{max}, $\mu mol \cdot g^{-1} \cdot min^{-1}$)
SO	0.81 ± 0.05[a]	0.220 ± 0.036	8.19 ± 1.05
EDL	1.78 ± 0.14	0.683 ± 0.041	ND
SVL	1.88 ± 0.17	0.711 ± 0.079	56.64 ±4.65

[a]SR yield and ATPase data are from ref. 47, and Ca²⁺ uptake data are from ref. 83. Values are mean ± SE. All experiments were conducted at 25°C.

FIGURE 14.4.
Representative isometric tetanic contractions for the EDL and the soleus (SOL). The drawings are reproductions of tetanic responses at 22°C. The peak rate of tension (dP/dt) is approximately 4-fold higher in the EDL, as compared to that in the SOL. Relaxation occurs in two phases—an initial slow phase (indicated by the 1), followed by a faster exponential decline (indicated by the 2).

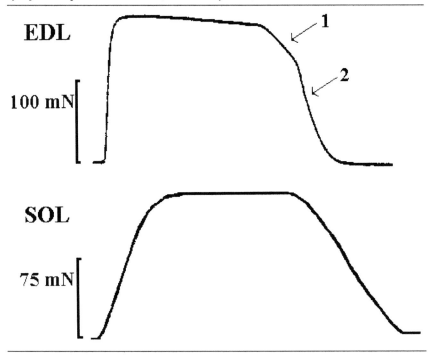

ric tetanic contraction for the slow soleus and fast EDL. As with the twitch, the slow soleus develops tension ($+dP/dt$) 4- to 7-fold slower than the fast EDL. As stated above, $+dP/dt$ is thought to be limited by the rate of binding of actin to myosin or, more specifically, by the rate of cross-bridge transition from a weakly bound, low-force state (AM-ADP-P_i) to the strongly bound, high-force state (AM-ADP), or Step 5 in Figure 14.2. Peak $+dP/dt$ can be measured experimentally by determining the rate of tension redevelopment after an imposed slack-unslack (shortening followed by reextension to the initial optimal length) in a fully activated fiber [19]. Using this technique, Metzger and Moss [98] showed a 7-fold higher rate constant of tension redevelopment (k_{tr}) in fast, as compared to slow-twitch, fibers. The k_{tr} has also been shown to be Ca^{2+}-sensitive; thus, the peak k_{tr} was reduced at suboptimal Ca^{2+} concentrations [18, 98]. The mechanism of the Ca^{2+} sensitivity is not totally understood, but it may result from a direct affect of Ca^{2+} on the forward apparent rate constant or Step 5 of the cross-bridge reaction scheme (Fig. 14.2).

The peak force obtained in a maximal isometric contraction is dependent on the number of cross-bridges acting in parallel that are in the high force state. In nonfatigued fibers, it is dependent on fiber size, as well as the density of cross-bridges per cross-sectional area (CSA). In humans, we have on occasion observed the fast Type II fibers to be larger than the slow Type I fibers; however, this difference was small and often not significant (Table 14.4). In rodents, the fast Type IIa fiber is significantly smaller than the other fiber types (Table 14.4). Consequently, this fiber type would develop less absolute force in newtons (N) (Table 14.4). However, intact slow and fast skeletal muscles, when corrected for varying fiber:muscle length ratios, generate approximately the same amount of relative force or tension between 200 and 250 $kN{\cdot}m^{-2}$, (Table 14.2) [26, 47]. Consistent with these data, if the peak force of individual fibers is expressed as $kN{\cdot}m^{-2}$ little or no difference is observed between the fast and slow fiber types (Table 14.4). Given the similar amounts of myofibrillar protein per unit volume in fast and slow muscle, this finding suggests that the force production per cross-bridge is not different between fiber types.

Muscle length has a direct effect on peak force [58]. The optimal muscle or fiber length (L_o) at which peak tetanic tension (P_o) is elicited occurs between sarcomere lengths (S_L) 2.2 and 2.6 μm [2]. At L_o, optimal overlap exists between the thick (myosin) and thin (actin) filaments, producing the maximal number of cross-bridges and, thus, peak tension. Below S_L, 2.0 μm (defined as the ascending limb of the S_L-tension relationship) tension during an isometric contraction falls because of overlap of the thin filaments from opposite ends of the sarcomere and to an increase in the filament lattice spacing [2]. Stretching a muscle or fiber beyond L_o (defined as the descending limb of the S_L-tension relationship) causes isometric tension to

TABLE 14.4.
Contractile Properties of Single Slow- and Fast-Twitch Gastrocnemius Fibers at 15°C

Fiber Type	Species	Diameter (μm)	Peak Force (mN)	Peak Tension ($kN \cdot m^{-2}$)	V_o ($FL \cdot s^{-1}$)	Peak Power ($\mu N \cdot FL \cdot s^{-1}$)
Type 1	Rat	77 ± 3	0.58 ± 0.04	125 ± 5	1.38 ± 0.07	22.7 ± 1.5
	Human	82 ± 3	0.76 ± 0.05	144 ± 4	0.45 ± 0.02	8.6 ± 0.5
Type IIa	Rat	65 ± 1	0.42 ± 0.02	126 ± 4	4.21 ± 0.18	48.6 ± 3.4
	Human	88 ± 3	0.92 ± 0.07	154 ± 8	2.11 ± 0.10	49.1 ± 5.3
Type IIb	Rat	87 ± 3	0.63 ± 0.03	106 ± 5	8.68 ± 0.21	160.3 ± 12.6
	Human	85 ± 2	0.95 ± 0.03	166 ± 4	5.86 ± 0.43	87.1 ± 3.9

[a]Values are mean $\pm$ SE. FL, fiber lengths$\cdot s^{-1}$.

fall because of a reduced thick and thin filament overlap, producing fewer cross-bridges. Resting muscle lengths in vivo are generally at or slightly shorter than L_o [26]. Consequently, the force output of a muscle in vivo can generally be increased by a slight stretch preceding activation.

As shown in Figure 14.4, relaxation generally occurs in two phases, an initial slow linear phase, followed by a faster exponential decline [132]. The initial linear phase (Fig. 14.4, Point 1) has been shown to be completely isometric. However at the transition to the exponential phase (Fig. 14.4, Point 2), portions of the fiber are less activated than others and, consequently, intrafiber movement occurs [132]. The peak rate of relaxation ($-dP/dt$) is at least 4-fold slower and, thus, the duration of the relaxation transient is considerable longer in slow, as compared to fast, skeletal muscle (Fig. 14.4).The $-dP/dt$ may be limited by the speed of cross-bridge detachment, but the duration of the relaxation transient is correlated with and thought to be established by the density and activity of the SR pump proteins which, in an ATP-dependent process, transport the Ca^{2+} ions back into the SR lumen [20, 47, 50].

The twitch:tetanus ratio ranges from 0.15 to 0.45, with higher values obtained as the muscle temperature declines. Despite having faster rates of inactivation, fast muscles generally have higher twitch:tetanus ratios than slow muscles (Table 14.2), which is a direct result of the faster rate of activation (dP/dt) in fast muscles, such that a higher percent of peak force is obtained in response to a single stimulus. The optimal frequency for force development is dependent on fiber type and temperature. At in vivo muscle temperatures (30–35°C), stimulation frequencies of approximately 100 and 200 Hz are required to elicit a peak tetanic contraction (P_o) for slow and fast muscles, respectively [26]. Since alpha motoneurons show in vivo firing rates of 10–40 Hz, it is clear that skeletal muscle rarely, if at all, contract with maximal tetanic force [37].

ISOTONIC CONTRACTILE PROPERTIES

Maximal Velocity of Shortening

The maximal velocity of shortening can be determined by the slack test method [38] or from extrapolation of the force-velocity relation to zero load [68]. The velocity obtained by the slack test method is generally higher than that obtained by the extrapolation technique, and it is abbreviated V_o to indicate that the measurement represents an unloaded or zero-load velocity. The lower values obtained with the force-velocity technique may result from the development of sarcomere nonuniformity during the loaded contractions, and/or the technique may miss the initial fastest phase of shortening [81]. Values obtained from the extrapolation technique are generally abbreviated as V_{max}.

In the slack test, a fiber or muscle is first fully activated to produce a peak tetanic contraction (P_o) and is then rapidly slacked to a shorter length, such that tension declines to baseline. The fiber(s) shortens, taking up the slack, after which tension redevelops. To determine V_o, a fiber(s) is activated and slacked five to six times, and the duration of unloaded shortening (time between onset of slack and redevelopment of tension) is plotted against the slack distance. V_o is determined from the slope of the fitted straight line. Figure 14.5 shows representative plots for fast- and slow-twitch fibers. Two slow fibers are shown, one from the gastrocnemius muscle of a sedentary subject and the other from the gastrocnemius of a world-class marathon runner. The inset provides the original records used to generate the plot. To express V_o in fiber lengths (FL)/s or, in the case of whole muscles, in muscle lengths/s, the slope of the fitted line is divided by the fiber or muscle length. The fiber V_o is highly correlated with and thought to be dependent on the specific activity of the myosin or myofibrillar ATPase activity [7], which is clearly seen in Figure 14.6 where fiber V_o is plotted against the fiber ATPase activity. The hierarchy for V_o is Type IIb>IIx>IIa>I (Table 14.4) [15, 117]. This functional difference for the fast fiber types explains the higher V_o observed in the predominantly Type IIb SVL vs. the mixed fast Type IIa and IIb EDL muscle [49]. Fast twitch muscles have been reported to be three- to fourfold faster than slow muscles [47, 49]. Single-fiber data show that the fast type IIa fiber is on the low end of this range, whereas the V_o of the fast type IIb fiber is 5- to 6-fold higher than the slow Type I fiber (15, 46, R. H. Fitts and J. J. Widrick unpublished data). The V_o of a given fiber type varies somewhat from muscle to muscle within a species. For example, the Type I fiber in rat soleus and gastrocnemius averaged 1.3 and 1.5 fiber lengths/s, which represented a small but significant difference in maximal shortening velocity. In man, this relationship appears to be reversed, as we have observed the slow soleus Type I fiber to have an average V_o of 0.62, whereas the gastrocnemius slow type I fiber averaged 0.43. A plot of V_o vs. species size for data collected in our laboratory on rat, monkey, and

FIGURE 14.5.

*Slack test methodology for the determination of maximal unloaded shortening veloc-
ity. The inserts in the lower right display original force-time recordings obtained from
three single human gastrocnemius fibers. Each insert consists of five superimposed
force-time recordings, illustrating the redevelopment of force after imposed slack
lengths, ranging from 150 to 400 μm. Note the different time scale in the Type I fiber
recording. All fibers were obtained from sedentary middle-aged males. In the main figure, the time required for force redevelopment is plotted against slack length for each
individual fiber. The points are fit by a least-squares regression line ($R^2 \geq .995$ for
all fibers). The slope of each line is the maximal unloaded shortening velocity, or V_o,
of the individual fiber in $mm \cdot s^{-1}$. The velocity is expressed in terms of fiber lengths $\cdot s^{-1}$
($FL \cdot s^{-1}$). V_o values for Type IIb, Type IIa, and Type I fibers were 4.46, 2.31, and
0.45 $FL \cdot s^{-1}$, respectively. The open symbols and dotted line show the data for a slow
Type I fiber from the gastrocnemius of an elite middle-aged male distance runner. Note
that at each imposed slack distance, this fiber required less time to redevelop force, in
comparison to the sedentary Type I fiber. The fiber V_o was 0.55 $FL \cdot s^{-1}$, which is approximately 20% greater than the V_o of the sedentary Type I fiber.*

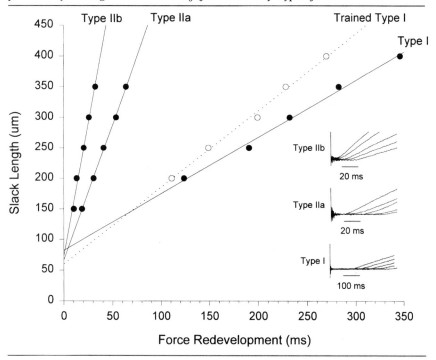

FIGURE 14.6.

Relationship between fiber V_o and ATPase activity. Results of individual experiments. Open symbols represent control fibers; filled symbols represent trained fibers as follows: ○, soleus (Type I); ▽, red gastrocnemius (Type I); □, red gastrocnemius (Type IIs); △, white gastrocnemius (Type IIb). Correlation coefficient (r) for all data points = .88; r, for type I, IIa, and IIb fibers = .56, .72, and .65, respectively. fl/s, fiber lengths/s. (Reproduced from ref. 117.)

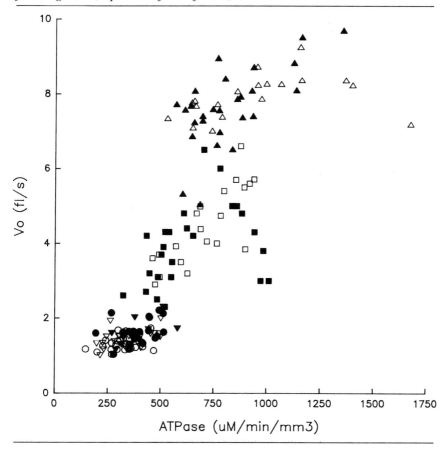

man demonstrates that an inverse relationship exists between V_o and body mass (Fig. 14.7). These data are for the slow Type I fiber only, and the slope of the relationship agrees well with the published data of Rome et al. [109]. The data of Rome et al. [109] suggest that the relationship may be considerably less steep (indicative of less difference between species) for the fast Type II fibers. However, the data for the IIb fibers likely contained some IIx fibers, and the relationship was not plotted for the Type IIa fiber. Thus, the relationship between V_o and body mass for the fast fibers may become more

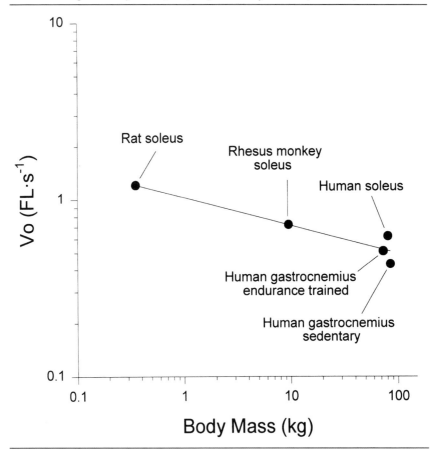

440 | *Fitts, Widrick*

FIGURE 14.7.

Effect of body mass on maximal shortening velocity of the Type I fiber in mammalian hindlimb muscles. The mean maximal unloaded shortening velocity (V_o, in fiber lengths·s^{-1}) is plotted against species body mass. Note logarithmic scaling of axis. All fibers were tested in our laboratory under identical experimental conditions. Observe that fibers from smaller mammals possess higher intrinsic V_o than similar fibers from larger mammals. In this example, V_o of soleus and gastrocnemius fibers were found to scale with species body mass (BM) as follows: $V_o = 1.03 (BM^{-0.16})$.

apparent when the comparison is restricted to a particular isozyme (Type IIa, IIx, or IIb).

Force-Velocity Relationship

During locomotion, the limb skeletal muscles are required to perform concentric (shortening) and eccentric (lengthening) contractions against a load of varying magnitude, but in no phase of a movement cycle are the muscles totally unloaded. Consequently, it is important to evaluate the force-velocity relationship for skeletal muscles. Since the early work of A. V. Hill [68], it has been known that this relationship for both fast- and slow-twitch skeletal muscle is hyperbolic with the maximal velocity of shortening obtained at zero load. The curvature or concavity of the force-velocity relationship can be determined from the $a:P_o$ ratio, where a is a constant of the Hill equation [68], and P_o is the peak tetanic tension. The greater the concavity of the force-velocity curve, the lower the $a:P_o$ ratio [26]. For mammalian muscle this ratio ranges from 0.15 to 0.30, with fast-twitch muscles having higher ratios than slow-twitch muscles [26]. Thus, fast muscles not only have higher maximal shortening speeds, compared to those of slow muscles, but they are capable of maintaining a higher percent of their peak speed as the load increases. This is clearly seen in Figure 14.8, which shows representative force-velocity curves for slow Type I, fast Type IIa, and fast Type IIb fibers isolated from the human gastrocnemius muscle. Because the velocity of muscle shortening depends on the relative load (load/P_o), the rate of cross-bridge activation or force development (dP/dt) may affect the shortening speed in the initial few milliseconds of a phasic contraction. As a consequence of these factors, body speed is directly related to the ratio of fast:slow twitch fibers involved in a given movement.

Peak Power and the Power-Force Relationship

From the standpoint of work capacity or the ability to move a load, the important functional property is power output. Power curves can be constructed from force-velocity curves, but few studies have actually calculated the power spectrum and determined the optimal speed for peak power. Both animal and human studies of individual muscles indicate that peak power is obtained at loads considerably below 50% of P_o [33, 35]. In man, peak power during knee extension has been shown to be correlated with the percentage of fast-twitch fibers in the vastus lateralis [30]. As described above, muscle tension (torque) decreases as the velocity of movement increases. Because of the shape of the force-velocity relationship, individuals with a high percentage of fast-twitch fibers generate a greater torque and higher power at a given velocity than individuals with predominantly slow-twitch fibers [30, 127].

We have recently studied the peak power and power-force relationship in individual slow and fast fibers isolated from the gastrocnemius muscle of man (R. H. Fitts and J. J. Widrick, unpublished data). Figure 14.9 shows representative power curves for the fast Type IIb, fast Type IIa, and slow Type I fibers. Mean peak power, expressed in either absolute or normalized terms, occurred in a ratio of 10:5:1 for the Type IIb, IIa, and I fibers, respectively. The relative load at which peak power was elicited ranged from 15% of P_o in the slow Type I fiber up to 30% of P_o in the fast Type IIb fiber.

FIGURE 14.8.

Force-velocity relationships of single Type I, Type IIa, and Type IIb human gastrocnemius fibers. Individual force-velocity data points were determined from analysis of fiber force and length recordings obtained during a series of isotonic force steps. Maximal shortening velocity (in FL·s⁻¹), defined as the intercept of each regression line with the y axis, and a/Po, a unitless parameter specifying the curvature of the relationship, were subsequently determined by nonlinear regression analysis ($r^2 \geq .992$ for all fibers). V_{max} and a/Po were 0.56 FL·s⁻¹ and 0.024, 1.10 FL·s⁻¹ and 0.085, and 1.63 FL·s⁻¹ and 0.102, for the Type I, Type IIa, and Type IIb fibers, respectively. Note that individual fibers displaying higher V_{max} are associated with higher a/Po values, indicating that they have less curvature to their force-velocity relationship.

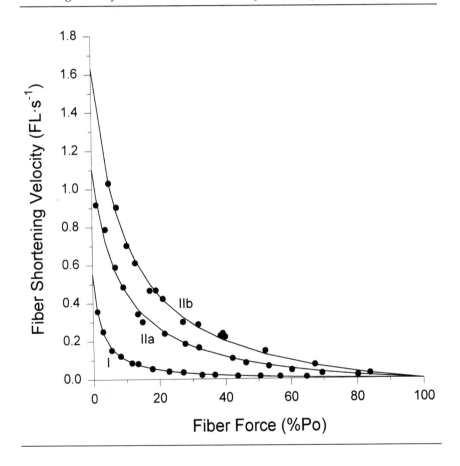

FIGURE 14.9.

The solid regression lines denote the force-power relationships of the three single fibers described previously in Figure 14.8. The peak power of these single Type I, Type IIa, and Type IIb fibers were 7.9 μN·FL·s⁻¹, 48.8 μN·FL·s⁻¹, and 79.8 μN·FL·s⁻¹, respectively. Note that peak power of Type I, Type IIa, and Type IIb fibers occurred at progressively greater external loads (14, 22, and 23% of peak isometric tension, respectively). The dashed regression lines illustrate the force-power relationships for a Type I and a Type IIa fiber obtained from an endurance trained subject. The peak power produced by these fibers was 7.1 μN·FL·s⁻¹ (Type I) and 30.1 μN·FL·s⁻¹ (Type IIa). These values are 10–38% less than the peak power produced by corresponding single fibers from the sedentary subject. The lower peak power output of the fibers obtained from the endurance-trained individuals was attributable to their smaller diameters and lower peak isometric force production.

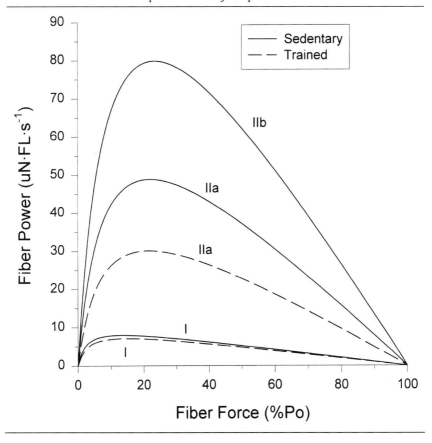

The Force-pCa Relationship

We [52] and others [96] have observed that slow-twitch fibers require significantly lower free Ca^{2+} (higher pCa) to reach an activation threshold and that the force-pCa relationship is less steep, compared to that of fast-twitch fibers. The force-pCa curves for the fast fibers are shifted to the right, compared to those of slow-twitch fibers. Thus, fast-twitch fibers require a higher free Ca^{2+} level to reach a given percent of P_o. The steeper force-pCa curve in fast-twitch fibers is indicative of greater cooperativity in Ca^{2+} activation of tension, compared to that of slow-twitch fibers. Although the exact mechanism of this effect is unknown, it is thought to be at least, in part, attributable to differences in the Ca^{2+} binding characteristics of the slow and fast isoforms of troponin, as well as to the effect of neighboring cross-bridges on the affinity of Ca^{2+} for the thin filament [96, 138].

Effect of Temperature on Muscle Mechanics (Q_{10})

Both the isometric and isotonic contractile properties are highly dependent on temperature, and the fast- and slow-twitch muscles demonstrate somewhat different Q_{10} characteristics [27]. Consequently, it is important to monitor muscle temperature when studying muscle mechanics, and comparisons of studies done at different temperatures need to be corrected for the Q_{10} effect. For in vitro studies, muscle temperature should be maintained at 35°C or less. For example, peak force (P_o) has been shown to increase with temperature between 22 and 30°C, to plateau between 30 and 35°C, and to decline at temperatures above 35°C [99, 106]. Above 35°C, protein degradation increases faster than synthesis and, thus, a net catabolic effect could contribute to the decline in contractile function. An increase in temperature causes twitch tension (P_t) to decrease and increase in fast- and slow-twitch muscle, respectively [27]. The maximal isotonic shortening velocity (V_{max}) responds to temperature in a manner similar to P_o. The increased V_{max} with temperature is undoubtedly caused by an increased myofibrillar ATPase activity and cross-bridge cycle rate. The isometric twitch duration (CT and 1/2 RT) shortens as temperature increases, and this is thought to be caused by an increased rate of SR Ca^{2+} reuptake. As a result of the shortened twitch duration, the force-frequency relationship shifts to the right, such that, higher stimulation frequencies are required to elicit P_o.

IN VIVO DETERMINATION OF CONTRACTILE FUNCTION

Relationship between In Vivo and In Vitro Mechanical Properties

In 1949, A. V. Hill theorized that the in vivo contractile properties of a muscle were directly related to the functional demands placed on the muscle [69]. Based on his earlier work on the force-velocity relationship of the in vitro amphibian muscle preparation [68], Hill proposed that intact muscles were designed to shorten at a specific velocity, V, which optimized power output. Furthermore, because the relationship between force and contractile efficiency closely parallels the force-velocity relationship, a muscle producing maximal power output would also be contracting at near optimal efficiency. Based on the in vitro force-velocity relationship, these conditions would be satisfied when the ratio of V to the muscles maximal shortening velocity, V_{max}, approximates 0.3.

Verification of this theory requires knowledge of muscle V and V_{max}. Recently, Rome and associates [108] have succeeded in establishing these parameters for swimming carp by determining which muscles were active during various swimming speeds, estimating V of these muscles from high-speed cinematography and muscle fixation, and quantifying muscle V_{max} from work conducted on in vitro preparations. The results of this study demonstrate that the red and white muscles of the carp possess unique isotonic contractile properties that make each ideally suited for a specific swimming function. At 15°C, the V_{max} of red and white muscle were 4.65 and 12. 88 muscle lengths/s, respectively. During slow, steady swimming at this temperature, the red muscle shortened at a V between 0.73 and 1.67 muscle lengths/s, or at a V/V_{max} of 0.16 to 0.36. During maximal swimming, the white muscle shortened at 4.85 muscle lengths/s, or a V/V_{max} of 0.38. Thus, power output was optimized by both red and white muscle, each of which was recruited during distinctly different swimming activities.

The carp is an excellent model in which to examine in vivo muscle function, because red and white muscle are located in distinct anatomical locations. Furthermore, the red fibers run parallel to the spine, and the white fibers form helical bundles orientated along the long axis of the fish [108]. These relatively simple, well-characterized architectural properties facilitate the determination of muscle fiber V. Applying a similar approach to the study of human muscle function requires quantification of the V_{max} of those fibers comprising a particular muscle and the V of these fibers during a specific movement or activity. The V_{max} of human skinned muscle fibers has been determined for single fibers, expressing each of the adult myosin heavy-chain isoforms [46, 88; and R. H. Fitts and J. J. Widrick, unpublished data, 1995]. However, methodological and interpretational problems arise in estimating in vivo fiber V during human movement, because the primary extensors and flexors in humans have a mixed fiber composition [78] and possess complex architectural characteristics [65, 66,115, 135]. Consequently, in vivo measurements of limb torque and angular velocity during extension and flexion provide limited information about the actual force and shortening velocity of the contracting muscle fibers.

To address this problem, Wickiewicz et al. [135] studied the morphology of the human lower limb to establish architectural parameters for the major antigravity and locomotor muscles. Based on their architectural properties, lower limb muscles could be classified into two broad categories:

muscles designed to develop high tension at the expense of velocity and those designed to shorten at high velocity at the expense of force production. Muscles in the first group, notably, the soleus and gastrocnemius, had relatively short fiber lengths, which maximized their physiological cross-sectional areas. For example, the physiological cross-sectional areas of the plantarflexors were more than twice that of the dorsiflexors. The greater physiological cross-sectional area of the extensors is presumably advantageous, because these muscles must oppose the forces of gravity during standing and locomotion. Muscles in the second category, for example, the adductors, had a greater number of sarcomeres arranged in series, biasing their function toward displacement. In a subsequent article, Wickiewicz et al. [136] concluded that these architectural properties played a large role in determining in vivo muscle function. For instance, the in vivo estimated V_{max} of the knee extensors and flexors was found to be two to three times greater than the V_{max} of the ankle flexors and extensors. Because fibers from these muscle groups had similar histochemical characteristics, it was difficult to explain these variations in V_{max} solely on intermuscular fiber-type differences. However, the architectural properties of the muscle groups clearly differed with the extensors and flexors of the knee, having longer muscle fibers lengths than the muscles comprising the ankle flexors and extensors. Thus, the greater number of sarcomeres in series contributed to the higher in vivo V_{max} of the muscles of the upper leg.

Wickiewicz and colleagues were aware of a number of limitations inherent in their approach. Because architectural properties were determined from cadavers, the calculated physiological cross-sectional areas were most likely biased because of tissue shrinkage. These authors also assumed that the pennation angles in resting muscle were representative of pennation angles during muscular activity. Recently, ultrasonography has been used to noninvasively measure pennation angles in intact human muscle [65, 66, 111]. It has been demonstrated that the angle of pennation can double or even triple during an isometric contraction and that this change occurs in a nonlinear manner with muscle torque output [66]. Consequently, the relationship between the angle of pennation and muscle torque is likely to be complex. These dynamic architectural properties will complicate future efforts to accurately model in vivo muscle function.

In Vivo Torque-Velocity Relationships

It should be clear from the preceding discussion that human torque-velocity data collected during isokinetic or isotonic dynamometry may not be representative of the contractile properties of the individual fibers comprising the muscles under study. Nevertheless, in vivo torque-velocity relationships quantify the ability of the intact neuromuscular system to function under various loading conditions, data which is very valuable in the assessment and understanding of human performance.

Currently, there is controversy regarding whether in vivo torque-velocity curves established using isokinetic or isotonic dynamometry are similar to the force-velocity relationships obtained on isolated muscles contracting in vitro. The resolution of this issue is important, because deviations between in vivo and in vitro relationships could signal the influence of neural factors that modulate muscular function in the intact neuromuscular system. At moderate to high velocities of limb extension or flexion, ~2.0–5.0 rad/s, torque-velocity and force-velocity curves have very similar shapes and, if scaled appropriately, will coincide, [136]. However, there are conflicting reports as to the relationship between in vivo muscle torque and angular velocity as velocity approaches, and, finally, reaches zero. Wilkie [137] studied maximal isotonic forearm flexion against various external loads and after correcting for the inertial effects of the limb and dynamometer and converting angular measurements into linear parameters, he concluded that the data could be adequately described by Hill's equation for isolated muscle. His general conclusion, that in vivo torque-velocity relationships were similar to those of in vitro relationships, has been supported by a number of researchers, using both isotonic and isokinetic testing protocols [13, 34, 76, 102, 125, 127, 129, 133, 134]. In contrast, Edgerton and colleagues have observed a marked deviation between the in vivo torque-velocity relationship and the relationship observed for isolated muscles studied in vitro [23, 60, 103, 136]. They have observed that peak angle-specific torque is substantially lower at angular velocities < 2.0 rad/s, including 0 rad/s, in comparison to the values predicted by Hill's equation. This relationship has been observed, even after torque and angular velocity were converted to linear measurements of muscle force and shortening velocity [136]. Their general results have been replicated by at least one independent laboratory [51].

These apparent deviations between in vivo torque-velocity and in vitro force-velocity relationships have led Edgerton and colleagues to propose that a neural mechanism modulates in vivo torque output at zero and low velocities of movement [23, 60, 103, 136]. However, the general consensus is that little central inhibition of peak torque output can be observed in most individuals. Healthy subjects are able to achieve maximal activation of the quadriceps [12, 79, 101, 134], tibialis anterior [11], first dorsal interosseus [110], and adductor pollicis [94, 110] during well-motivated, voluntary isometric contractions. These conclusions are based on the observations that 1) no increase in maximal voluntary torque is noted after the imposition of single superimposed twitches and 2) when the muscle, either directly or via the motor nerve, is electrically stimulated to produce a tetanic contraction, the force is the same as that obtained with a maximal voluntary contraction. For the soleus, one group has reported no central inhibition of maximal voluntary force [12], whereas another group observed that superimposed twitches exceeded voluntary efforts by an average of 7% in half of their subjects [11]. Based on the twitch superimposition technique, approximately 25% of the subjects could not voluntarily achieve maximal activation of their biceps, although the degree of inhibition was small [112].

There are less data concerning the possible influence of neural inhibition during maximal isokinetic movements. Newham et al. [101] reported that during concentric isokinetic knee extensions performed at 0.2 and 2.6 rad/s, a small number of subjects (22 and 9% of the total subjects, respectively) displayed some inhibition in peak torque production. However, this inhibition changed the total mean torque by only 2.0 and 0.7%, respectively, which is considerably less than the reductions reported by Edgerton and colleagues [23, 60, 103, 136]. Westing et al. [134] found that angle-specific torque produced during maximal voluntary concentric isokinetic knee extensions at velocities ≤6.3 rad/s, was slightly greater than torque produced when percutaneous electrical stimulation was superimposed on maximal voluntary contractions, suggesting that there was no central neural inhibition in their subjects. It is noteworthy that their subjects were all very physically active individuals. Similar results have been obtained for velocities up to 2.1 rad/s, when concentric isokinetic contractions are induced by femoral nerve stimulation [77].

In contrast to concentric contractions, there may be substantial inhibition of peak torque output during eccentric muscular activity. Westing and colleagues [134] have observed that when maximal voluntary eccentric contractions were performed with superimposed electrical stimulation, peak angle-specific torque was 20–23% greater than that measured during voluntary efforts at all velocities between 1.05 and 6.28 rad/s. This inhibition may serve a protective function by attenuating the high muscle forces that could be experienced during lengthening contractions [133, 134].

Although there continues to be debate over the exact relationship between torque and velocity during in vivo movements, there is general agreement as to the relationship between these variables and muscle fiber-type distribution. Most studies have reported no correlation between fiber-type distribution, expressed either as a percentage of total fiber number or total fiber area, and peak isometric torque [92, 102, 113]. In contrast, positive relationships have been observed between the percentage of fast fibers, or the relative area occupied by these fibers, and relative peak torque output at moderate to high angular isokinetic velocities [30, 60, 127–129]. A similar relationship has been reported between fiber-type distribution or relative area and maximal velocity of contraction, measured either directly with a light dynamometer lever or estimated by extrapolation of the torque-velocity relationship to zero load [127, 129]. Consequently, peak power output is substantially greater in subjects possessing a predominance of fast fibers [30, 76, 121, 129]. Nevertheless, it should be noted that intersubject differences in fiber-type composition can account for only ~25% of the variability in relative peak torque or power; thus additional factors must play a substantial role in determining intersubject variations in muscle performance.

MUSCLE MECHANICS: ADAPTATIONS WITH EXERCISE TRAINING

In 1967, Holloszy [70] demonstrated, in his now classic work, that regular endurance exercise-training can induce an increase in limb skeletal muscle mitochondria and tissue oxidative capacity. Furthermore, in subsequent work, Holloszy and his colleagues showed that endurance exercise increased the oxidative capacity of all three fiber types by approximately 2-fold (5). These data suggested that, at least from a metabolic point of view, regular exercise did not result in fiber transformations. By the mid 1970s, the biochemical adaptations in limb skeletal muscle to regular endurance exercise were well established [71]. However, considerably less was known about whether or not programs of regular exercise altered the mechanical or contractile properties of skeletal muscle. In this section, we will address this topic by considering studies evaluating the effects of exercise-training on 1) whole limb skeletal muscles of animals; 2) the contractile function of human skeletal muscle in vivo, and 3) the contractile function of individual single fibers isolated from rat and man. It should be kept in mind that exercise-induced adaptations in contractile function and fiber-type characteristics depend on the type of exercise program used. Factors such as the duration, intensity, and frequency of the exercise are all important in determining the extent and nature of the adaptation in a given fiber type. Regardless of the type of exercise, the cellular changes are restricted to the muscle fibers recruited for the exercise task.

Animal Studies on Limb Skeletal Muscle

Many of the early studies evaluating the effects of regular exercise on muscle mechanics used muscles composed of a mixed fiber type (both fast- and slow-twitch fibers) and, perhaps for that reason, much of the data was negative [9, 45]. Barnard et al. [9] found a combined endurance-sprint treadmill running program to have no effect on the isometric contractile properties of the gastrocnemius-plantaris muscle in male guinea pigs. In agreement with these results, Fitts and his colleagues [45] observed that neither endurance nor sprint programs of treadmill exercise-training affected the isometric contractile properties of the tibialis anterior in miniature pigs. Both Barnard et al. [9] and Fitts et al. [45] found the exercise programs to improve the endurance capacity of the in situ contracting muscles. This increased fatigue resistance was undoubtedly caused by the increased tissue aerobic capacity induced by the training program. In the mid-1970s, Baldwin et al. [6] reported that endurance treadmill running in rats caused a small but significant increase and decrease, respectively, in the actomyosin

ATPase activity of the slow soleus and the deep predominantly fast-twitch Type IIa region of the vastus lateralis (DVL). Because it has been proposed that ATP hydrolysis by means of actomyosin was the rate-limiting step that determines the velocity of muscle shortening [7], these results suggest that regular endurance exercise should increase slow and decrease fast muscle V_o. In 1977, Fitts and Holloszy [48] demonstrated that at least the former was true, as endurance exercise-training induced a 20% increase in the V_o of the soleus. Unfortunately, the fiber alignment of the DVL prevented reliable measurements of contractile function and, thus, we were unable to determine whether endurance exercise depressed the shortening speed of this muscle. The increased V_o was correlated to, and likely caused by, the increased actomyosin ATPase activity. At the time, we hypothesized that these changes could be attributed to either 1) a small increase in V_o for all or most of the fibers or 2) a conversion of a few fibers from slow to fast. We believed then, and now, that the former is correct, as there is no evidence that exercise training significantly increases the proportion of fast-twitch fibers [8, 55, 75, 117]. That slow- to fast-twitch fiber transformations do not occur in response to exercise has been shown by both enzyme histochemical analysis of muscle cross-sections and SDS gel analysis of individual fibers. Recent single-fiber data suggest that the exercise-induced increase in myofibrillar ATPase and V_o in the soleus may be caused by the expression of fast myosin light chains (MLC) in the slow Type I fibers (see Single-Cell Studies of Contractile Function below).

In addition to the increased V_o, Fitts and Holloszy [46] found that endurance exercise decreased peak tetanic force (P_o), increased twitch dP/dt, and shortened the isometric CT and 1/2 RT of the soleus. The mechanism for the exercise-induced decline in P_o is unknown. Recently, we have observed a similar decline in the peak force of single slow Type I fibers isolated from the soleus of rats endurance trained by 2 or 3.5 hr of daily running (R. H. Fitts and L. V. Thompson, unpublished data). These data on single fibers document that the reduced force was not caused by an increase in the extracellular connective tissue or water but, rather, by an actual reduction in the contractile protein per unit area. Consequently, the number of cross-bridges acting in parallel per cross-sectional area declined as a result of the exercise program. Peak dP/dt is thought to be limited by the rate of actin and myosin binding or, specifically, the rate of the transition from the low-force to the high-force state of the cross-bridge (Fig. 14.2, Step 5). The mechanism of the exercise training-induced increase in dP/dt in the slow soleus is unknown, but it could relate to the expression of the fast MLC in the slow Type I fiber. This hypothesis is based on the fact that light chains have been shown to be involved in the power stroke, and removal of light chains depresses force as well as velocity [89, 122]. The shortened twitch duration in the soleus after endurance exercise was most likely caused by a reduction in the duration of the Ca^{2+} transient, which suggests that the activity of the SR pump protein may have increased. However, we have been unable to detect a significant change in the rate of SR Ca^{2+} uptake by crude homogenates prepared from the soleus of exercise-trained rats [83].

What do we know about the effects of high-intensity exercise on muscle mechanics? In evaluating this question, it is important to consider whether the exercise involves relatively low-load, high-velocity contractions (high-speed running) or high-load, low-velocity (to include zero velocity isometric) contractions. In animals, there is very little information on the effects of high-intensity exercise on muscle mechanics. Weight-lifting programs have been shown to increase fiber size in both slow and fast muscles, and this alone would result in an increased force production. Klitgaard et al. [85] observed weight training to increase the P_o of the rat plantaris, such that muscle force was higher in 24-mo exercise-trained vs. 9-mo control animals. They also found the strength training to decrease both CT and 1/2 RT in the plantaris, as well as CT in the slow soleus. Gonyea and Bonde-Petersen [57] also reported weight training to increase tetanic tension in the wrist flexor muscles of the cat but, in contrast to the study of Klitgaard et al. [85], they observed a prolonged CT and 1/2 RT in the muscles from the weight-trained animals. The latter results are particularly difficult to understand, in that the authors reported an increase in the number of fast glycolytic fibers—a fiber type known to have the shortest twitch duration.

In contrast to weight training, programs of high-speed treadmill running have little or no affect on fiber size [43]. Increasing the speed of running from that requiring 70–120% of maximal oxygen uptake has been shown to increase the extent of the oxidative enzyme increase in the fast-twitch SVL [36]. Consequently, one might hypothesize that high-speed training would be more effective than endurance running in altering the mechanical properties of fast muscles. However, to date, there is very little evidence to support or reject this hypothesis. Troup et al. [130] did observe sprint training to induce a small reduction in the CT and increase the twitch dP/dt and the isotonic shortening speed at low loads in the fast EDL. This training program also resulted in similar changes in the slow-twitch soleus, while the P_o was not affected in either muscle. Staudte et al. [119] did find an increased peak torque in the slow soleus, but not in the fast rectus femoris, after a high-intensity training program.

In Vivo Studies on Human Limb Skeletal Muscle

In this section, we will review the exercise-induced adaptations in human skeletal muscle mechanics, as assessed by in vivo technology. Presumably, the altered in vivo contractile properties after periods of exercise training can be attributed to the chronic changes in muscular activity that occurred during the training period. Results from studies using high-intensity isometric or moderate-intensity dynamic exercise protocols demonstrate that each of the parameters describing the torque-velocity relationship, i.e., peak isometric torque, V_{max}, and the curvature of the relationship, are altered by exercise training.

PEAK ISOMETRIC TORQUE. An increase in muscle strength [measured either by maximal voluntary contraction (MVC) or free weights] is a consistent observation after high-intensity exercise training in humans [43]. In many cases, the magnitude of the increase is considerably larger (by 50% or more) than can be explained by Type II fiber hypertrophy [100]. The integrated electromyographic activity (IEMG) also increases, which has led several laboratories to conclude that an elevated neural drive is in part responsible for the exercise-induced increase in strength [61–63, 100]. An increased neural drive may be important in obtaining full activation of the fast-twitch fibers during high-intensity (particularly high-load) exercise. Nevertheless, gains in peak torque after exercise-training have been documented in the absence of changes in neural drive. Three months of isometric training have been reported to increase the peak isometric force of the adductor pollicis by 20% [35] and the peak isometric torque of the quadriceps by 35% [79]. In both of these studies, pre- and postpeak torque values were induced by electrical stimulation of the motor nerve or muscle. Consequently, the observed adaptations in peak torque output were independent of any neural, motivational, or learning effects that may have occurred during the training programs. The mechanisms behind these increases in peak isometric torque are not completely clear. In one of the above studies, the anatomical area of the quadriceps was determined from CAT scans performed before and after training [79]. These data indicated that no relationship existed between training-induced changes in quadriceps cross-sectional area, which increased an average of 5%, and improvements in peak isometric torque. This finding is consistent with that of a number of studies that have reported little or no relationship between muscle fiber hypertrophy and gains in voluntary strength [29, 61, 63, 100]. Consequently, mechanisms in addition to muscle hypertrophy appear to contribute to the training-induced increase in peak torque.

One mechanism could involve training-induced alterations in the cross-sectional area occupied by various muscle fiber types. Dynamic resistance training has been reported to selectively increase the cross-sectional area or the relative area occupied by the Type IIa fibers [29, 31, 61, 63, 93] whereas short-term detraining has been observed to selectively reduce Type II fiber area [73]. It has been proposed that Type II fibers may produce greater in vivo tension, or force per fiber cross-sectional area, than slow Type I fibers [124, 139]. Consequently, an increase in fibers with a greater potential for tension production would increase in vivo peak isometric torque output. Although this is an attractive hypothesis, several studies have demonstrated that there is no relationship between muscle fiber composition and in vivo peak isometric torque output [92, 102, 113]. Furthermore, most studies performed on single fibers isolated from human muscle have concluded that there is no difference in the peak Ca^{2+}-activated force of slow and fast fibers [46, 88], although recent data from our laboratory indicates that fast fibers may produce greater peak isometric tension than slow fibers (R. H. Fitts and J. J. Widrick) unpublished data 1995; Table 14.4).

It is important to note that peak isometric torque is a function of the physiological cross-sectional area of the muscle, but the variable measured by most current noninvasive imaging techniques is the muscle's anatomical cross-sectional area. As Gollnick et al. [56] pointed out, any increase in the weight of a mature muscle at a constant length must be accompanied by a change in the fiber pennation angle and, consequently, the muscle's physiological cross-sectional area. It is, therefore, conceivable that changes in the physiological cross-sectional area of the muscle occur during training and that these changes are not apparent when measuring the anatomical cross-sectional area of the muscle. In an attempt to address this question, Rutherford and Jones [111] measured the angle of pennation of the quadriceps using ultrasonography. Despite a 14% increase in quadriceps torque, they reported that the training program had no effect on the angle of pennation of the quadriceps fibers. Nevertheless, the effect of resistance exercise on muscle physiological cross-sectional area is an open issue, because the ultrasound technique may not have the sensitivity required to detect small changes in fiber angle. It has been estimated that a change in pennation of only 1° would change force acting along the muscle tendon by ~6% [100].

Narici et al. [100] found that not all of the muscles comprising the quadriceps displayed the same degree of hypertrophy after 60 days of strength training. The anatomical cross-sectional areas of the vastus intermedius and medialis increased considerably more than the areas of the vastus lateralis or rectus femoris. Furthermore, the greatest degree of hypertrophy was noted in the proximal fractions of these muscles. These findings suggests that multiple cross-sectional area determinations are required to gain a valid indication of muscle hypertrophy after exercise training. Studies relying on a single image made at the midpoint of the muscle may underestimate gains in muscle area.

The confounding effect that antagonist muscle activity may have on in vivo muscle function has been recognized for quite some time [137]. Recently, Carolan and Cafarelli [24] reported that coactivation of the hamstrings during maximal isometric knee extension decreased by ~20% during the first week of isometric training. Based on the relationship between EMG and torque, the authors estimated that this decrease in hamstring coactivation could account for approximately one-third and 10% of the increase in knee extension torque observed at the end of the 1st and 8th weeks of training, respectively. These data demonstrate the degree to which reductions in antagonist coactivation, which appear to be most important during the early stages of training, may confound measurement of training-induced changes in peak isometric torque.

Several cellular mechanisms could contribute to the increased torque output observed after resistance training. First, there may be an increase in the myofibrillar density of muscle fibers after resistance training so that the number of cross-bridges acting in parallel increases independently of any increase in fiber diameter. This idea is supported by the finding of a greater radiological density of the human quadriceps after 12 wk of strength training [79]. However, Claassen et al. [25] found no difference in the linear distance between myosin filaments, despite significant increases in both muscle cross-sectional area and radiological density after 6 wk of training. A second cellular mechanism that would increase fiber force production independently of fiber size is an increase in the average force generated by each cross-bridge, a possibility that has not been experimentally tested.

Increases in peak isometric torque observed after isotonic training are considerably lower than those observed after isometric training. Using electrical stimulation of the muscle or motor nerve, it was confirmed that isotonic exercise conducted at torques between 30 and 80% of peak isometric torque produced improvements in peak isometric torque that ranged from 11 to 15%, or only 33 to 55% of the improvement observed after a similar period of isometric training [35, 79]. The smaller improvement in peak isometric torque under these training conditions is presumably attributable to the lower likelihood that Type II fibers are recruited during the submaximal isotonic contractions. Because of the maintained nature of the contractions, dynamic training performed isokinetically may have substantially different effects. For instance, Coyle et al. [31] reported an 11% increase in Type II fiber area after 6 wk of isokinetic exercise performed at only 25% of peak isometric torque. Exercise protocols incorporating maximal eccentric actions have been reported to produce greater fiber hypertrophy and gains in voluntary peak isometric torque than protocols using maximal concentric contractions exclusively [87]. Häkkinen et al. [61] observed a 27% increase in maximal isometric leg extension force after a 24-wk training program that included an eccentric component, and Hather et al. [64] reported higher strength gains in subjects trained by concentric/eccentric exercise than by concentric work alone. Furthermore, in the latter study, although both exercise programs induced Type II fiber hypertrophy, Type I fiber hypertrophy was elicited only by the concentric/eccentric program. It is thought that the higher forces experienced during eccentric exercise may provide a greater training stimulus. During maximal lengthening contractions, the torque produced by the muscle may be ~10% greater than peak isometric force [133]. Thus, the tension produced by a particular muscle fiber may be greater than that produced during a maximal isometric contraction. In a recent study, the power outputs performed during eccentric-only and concentric-only exercise were matched such that the same amount of work was done over a 4-wk training period [93]. Results indicated that the concentric-only exercise was superior in producing gains in peak isometric torque and hypertrophy of Type II fiber area. These results support the hypothesis that whatever benefits can be ascribed to maximal eccentric exercise are related to the higher level of work that can be performed by the muscle or muscle fibers during eccentric exercise. However, it is also possible that differences between concentric and eccentric exercise protocols may be attributable to neural mechanisms. When pre- and posttraining peak torque values were confirmed by superimposed percutaneous twitches, there was no advantage in an eccentric vs. a concentric protocol in improving the maximal isometric force output of the quadriceps [79]. This result occurred despite the fact that the resistance was 45% greater during eccentric training.

Both isometric and dynamic training are known to increase the muscle's peak rate of tension development, or dP/dt [35, 63]. Häkkinen et al.[63] reported that the decreased CT and increased dP/dt after exercise training was correlated with an elevation in the IEMG activity and the increased CSA of the fast-twitch, as compared to the slow-twitch, fibers. Additionally, the subjects with the greatest percentage of fast-twitch fibers showed the largest change in both CT and dP/dt. The data support the hypothesis that at least part of the change in these functional properties can be attributed to the increased fast-twitch fiber area and the relative contribution of this fiber type to the functional capacity of the whole muscle.

MAXIMAL SHORTENING VELOCITY (V_{MAX}). The in vivo measurement of the force-velocity relationship and V_{max} in human muscle is difficult because of limitations inherent in the equipment (particularly deficiencies in the frequency response of the torque recording systems) and the inability to study the large limb muscles independently [80]. Additionally, the most frequently studied quadriceps muscles are composed of a mixture of slow- and fast-twitch fibers, which makes fiber type-specific responses difficult to detect. Nevertheless, it is a consistent finding that dynamic, but not isometric, exercise-training increases V_{max}. For example, 3 mo of isometric training at peak voluntary force failed to alter V_{max}, but a similar period of dynamic training performed at a resistance equivalent to 30–40% of peak force increased V_{max} by 21% [35]. Thus, whereas both isometric and dynamic training increase peak torque, only dynamic training appears to have an effect on the maximal shortening velocity measured in vivo. Whether this represents a shift in the fiber type composition of the trained muscle and/or an increase in the V_{max} of individual fibers expressing a specific myosin heavy-chain isoform is unknown. Current evidence suggests that the latter of these two possibilities is more likely, because strength training increases the number of fibers expressing Type IIa MHC at the expense of fibers expressing Types IIx or IIb MHC [1, 86]. Because human skeletal muscle fibers expressing Type IIb or IIx MHC have a greater maximal shortening velocity than fibers expressing Type IIa MHC [88; R. H. Fitts and J. J.Widrick, unpublished data 1995; Table 14.4), these changes would be expected to reduce the V_{max} of the whole muscle.

CURVATURE OF THE TORQUE-VELOCITY RELATIONSHIP. Training-induced changes in the curvature of the in vivo torque-velocity relationship are a function of the characteristics of the training stimulus. In general, the greatest gains in torque occur at velocities at or near those experienced during the training program [23, 31]. However, small increases have been observed at other velocities [23, 31]. The training-induced increase in peak torque would, in itself, explain some of the effect. This is true, as a given absolute load would represent a lower percentage of P_o (lower relative load), and due to the shape of the force-velocity relationship higher shortening velocities. In addition to this, increases in fiber shortening speed would contribute to the higher velocities, particularly at low loads.

Alterations in the torque-velocity relationship occur independently of the training mode, i.e., whether dynamic contractions are performed eccentrically or concentrically. In fact, there appears to be a considerable degree of crossover in training adaptations. Training solely with concentric actions increases torque at angular velocities between 0.52 and 2.62 rad/s during both shortening and lengthening movements [28]. A similar crossover effect has been observed for eccentric-only training [28]. However, there is evidence that training-induced alterations in the shape of the torque-velocity curve are greater when eccentric movements are incorporated into the training program [28], which is likely a direct result of the fact that eccentric training results in a greater increase in peak torque, as compared to concentric exercise.

PEAK POWER. Peak power output is a function of peak torque, V_{max}, and the curvature of the torque-velocity relationship. Consequently, an increase in any of these variables will increase power output. It appears that isometric or low-to-intermediate velocity isokinetic training is more effective in improving peak power output than dynamic high-velocity training. Apparently, isometric or low-velocity training results in greater improvements in peak torque output than low torque-high velocity training and greater changes in the torque-velocity relationship at velocities or loads associated with peak power. For example, Duchateau and Hainaut [35] reported that isometric training produced a 51% increase in peak power, in comparison to a 19% increase after dynamic training. Even though the isometric training program had no effect on V_{max}, it was superior in improving peak power, because the increase in peak isometric torque was considerably greater than that observed after dynamic exercise. These results are in general agreement with the observations of Kanehisa and Miyashita [82], who found that subjects who trained at slow (1.05 rad/s) or intermediate (3.14 rad/s) isokinetic velocities improved peak power at low, intermediate, and high isokinetic testing velocities. In contrast, subjects who trained at relatively high velocities (5.24 rad/s) displayed improvements only at high testing velocities.

Single-Cell Studies of Contractile Function

Recently, our laboratory has begun to evaluate the mechanisms by which individual fibers (slow Type I and fast Type IIa, IIb, and IIx) adapt to regular programs of exercise-training [46, 52, 117]. This work used the skinned fiber preparation, which has the advantage of being stable for 4–5 wk (stored at $-20°$). Consequently, a large number of fibers from a given muscle biopsy can be studied. After the measurement of contractile function, each fiber was typed based on its MHC isoform, as determined from SDS gel analysis. An example of the fiber typing by gel analysis is shown in Figure 14.1. In sections to come, we will review our results regarding the effects of exercise-training on the contractile properties of individual slow- and fast-twitch fibers. Where possible, we will provide the cellular and molecular mechanisms for the exercise-induced changes in cell function. To our knowledge, there is no information as to how strength or weight training effects the functional capacity of individual slow- and fast-twitch fibers. Consequently, our review will focus primarily on results from endurance exercise-training programs.

ALTERATIONS IN MAXIMAL SHORTENING VELOCITY. As mentioned above, the histochemical evidence suggests that regular exercise does not change the percentage of the slow-twitch type I fibers [8, 55, 75, 117]. Thus, the question remains: What causes the 20% increase in the soleus muscle V_o? Our single-fiber analysis showed 2-hr of treadmill running, 5 days/wk to significantly increase the rat soleus Type I fiber V_o from 1.3 ± 0.03 to 1.6 ± 0.04 fiber lengths (fl/s) (Table 14.5). This represents a 23% increase in V_o, which agrees well with the 20% increase observed in the intact soleus [48]. A histogram analysis suggests that essentially all of the fibers adapted. In the control group, the majority of fibers displayed V_o's between 1 and 1.5 fl/s, whereas after the training there was a shift right, such that, the majority of the fibers fell between 1.3 and 1.8 fl/s. These fibers contained only the slow MHC and, thus, the increased V_o could not be attributed to coexpression of a small amount of fast MHC. However, the fibers did show an increased expression of the fast myosin light chains (Fig. 14.10). Because myosin light chains are known to influence fiber-shortening speed, Schluter and Fitts hypothesized that the exercise-induced increase in the speed of the Type I fiber could be caused by the incorporation of the fast myosin light chains [117]. The increased V_o was correlated to an increased myofibrillar ATPase activity (Fig. 14.6). Taken together, these observations suggest that the fast myosin light chain increased fiber ATPase and the cross-bridge cycle rate and, consequently, fiber V_o. Although the total number of slow fibers remained unchanged, the treadmill running program did induce a small increase in the number of hybrid slow fibers (those containing Type I and IIa

TABLE 14.5.
V_o *and ATPase Activities for Fibers from Control and Exercise-trained Groups*

Fiber Type	V_o Fiber Lengths/s	ATPase Activity ($\mu M \cdot min^{-1} \cdot mm^{-3}$)
Rat slow Type I		
Control	1.3 ± 0.03[a]	326 ± 14
2-hr ET	1.6 ± 0.04[b]	403 ± 14[b]
Rat fast Type IIa		
Control	4.4 ± 0.21	760 ± 60
2-hr ET	3.9 ± 0.19	688 ± 48
Rat fast Type IIb		
Control	7.9 ± 0.22	927 ± 70
2-hr ET	7.7 ± 0.18	820 ± 38
Human Type I		
Control	0.86 ± 0.04	ND
Swim ET	1.03 ± 0.15[b]	ND
Human Type II		
Control	4.85 ± 0.50	ND
Swim ET	2.68 ± 0.58[b]	ND

[a]Rat data were taken from ref. 117, and human data were taken from ref. 46. Values are means $\pm$ SE. 2-hr ET, rats were trained for 2 hr/day for 10 wk; swim ET, collegiate male swimmers who trained intensely for 6 mo.; ND, not determined.
[b]Values were significantly different from those of controls, P < .05.

or I and IIx myosin). Thus, the soleus from both control and trained animals contained approximately 90% slow Type I fibers; however, after exercise-training, only 80% of the fibers contained the slow type I MHC exclusively (Table 14.1). It should be emphasized here, that although almost all slow fibers showed an increase in the fast myosin light-chain content, approximately only 10% showed an increased fast MHC content.

The increased Type I fiber V_o is not unique to rat muscle or to treadmill running, as we observed a similar effect in humans after swim exercise-training. We examined the effects of a typical collegiate swim-training program on the contractile properties of fast and slow fibers isolated from biopsies of the deltoid muscle [46]. The slow Type I fibers showed a significant increase in V_o from 0.86 ± 0.04 to 1.03 ± 0.04 fl/s which, similar to rat muscle, represents a 20% increase induced by the exercise program (Table 14.5). In both the rat and human studies, the exercise programs decreased the V_o of the fast fibers [47, 117]. However, in the rat study, the decline in the V_o of the fast Type IIa and IIb fibers was not significant, whereas in the swim study, Type II fiber velocity decreased from 4.85 ± 0.50 to 2.68 ± 0.58 fl/s (Table 14.5). Even in the rat study, the histogram demonstrated that some of the fast Type IIa fibers shifted to a lower V_o after the exercise training. This observation was consistent with a lower mean fiber ATPase activity (Table 14.5). Recently, we studied the contractile properties of single fibers isolated from the gastrocnemius of elite master runners (R. H. Fitts

FIGURE 14.10.

Myosin light-chain (MLC) profile of rat single fibers run on 12% SDS-PAGE. Fibers were isolated from the soleus of control (A) and exercise-trained (B) rats. Beside each gel lane is a densitometric scan, illustrating the relative concentration of the light-chain species. LC, myosin light chain; s, slow; f, fast. The exercise-trained fiber contained significantly more fast type myosin light chains. Reproduced from ref. 117.

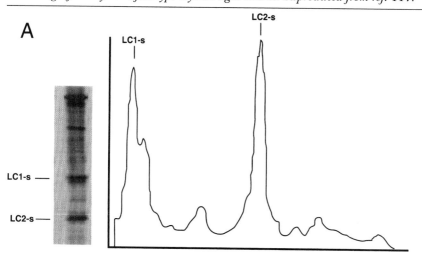

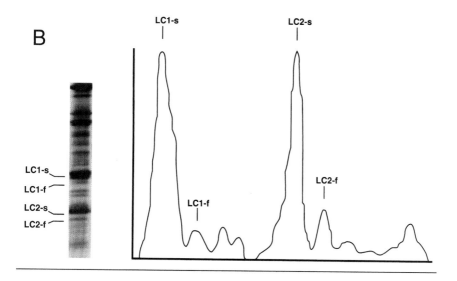

and J. J. Widrick, unpublished data 1995). Compared to that of age-matched controls, the Type I fiber V_o of the elite runner was 19% higher, whereas we observed no differences in either of the two fast fiber types. The difference in slow fiber velocity can be seen from the analysis of the slack test data shown in Figure 14.5. The slope of the plot of the slack imposed on the fiber (in micrometers) vs. time for the redevelopment of force represents the maximal shortening speed. From the figure, it is clear that the slow Type I fiber from the elite runner has a higher velocity than the slow fiber from an age-matched control; however, the velocity is still considerably less than that observed for fast fibers (Fig. 14.5).

ALTERATIONS IN FIBER SIZE AND PEAK FORCE. The adaptability of fiber size in response to altered loading patterns is well documented [71,126]. Both slow and fast-twitch fibers have the capacity to hypertrophy when overloaded. For example, weight training and surgical overloading by tenotomy of synergistic muscles both produce fiber hypertrophy [54, 131]. In contrast, endurance and high-speed running, in rat has no effect on fiber size for any fiber type. Even after 3.5 hr/day of treadmill running, 5 days/wk for 12 wk, we did not observe any change in fiber size in the rat (R. H. Fitts and L. V. Thompson unpublished data 1995). However, under certain conditions muscle fiber diameter has been shown to decline in response to prolonged activity. For example, chronic electrical stimulation of the rabbit EDL for 28 days at 40 Hz significantly reduced the mean fiber size from 72 ± 1 to 65 ± 1 μm [22]. Perhaps more relevant to our discussion of exercise-induced effects, we have recently observed that the slow Type I and fast Type IIa fibers isolated from the gastrocnemius of elite master runners were significantly smaller than those of age-matched controls (R. H. Fitts and J. J. Widrick, unpublished observations 1995). A smaller fiber coupled with an increased capillary number would be advantageous to an endurance athlete, as it would decrease the diffusion distance for oxygen from the capillary to the mitochrondria.

In both whole-muscle and single-fiber studies, we have found programs of endurance running to reduce peak tension ($kN \cdot m^{-2}$), but in our published work, the decline never reached significance [48, 117]. However, we recently observed 3.5 hr/day of endurance treadmill running in rat to significantly reduce the P_o of the slow Type I and fast Type IIa fiber (R. H. Fitts and L. V. Thompson, unpublished data 1995). The reduced tension was accompanied by a reduced fiber stiffness, which suggests that the decline in force was caused by fewer cross-bridges per CSA. One interpretation would be that prolonged endurance activity triggered a small but significant decline in the amount of contractile protein. In the elite master runners, peak force (mN) of the slow Type I and fast Type IIa fiber was significantly lower than those of the age-matched controls. This decline was attributable entirely to the reduced fiber size, as peak tension ($kN \cdot m^{-2}$) was the same in both groups.

As described above, the force-pCa relationship is shifted to the right in fast, as compared to slow fibers, and fast fibers show significantly greater co-operativity. After endurance exercise-training, the force-pCa relationship of the slow Type I fiber of the rat soleus shifted right, toward that observed for the fast Type IIa fiber (R. H. Fitts and L. V. Thompson, unpublished data 1995). For example, after 3.5 hr of daily treadmill running, the activation threshold of the Type I fiber increased from a value of $pCa = 7.22$ to 6.93, whereas the slope of the relationship below pCa_{50} (n_2) increased from 2.03 to 2.51. Although these represented significant increases, they were still distinctively different from those of the fast Type IIa fiber, for which the activation threshold value averaged $pCa = 6.60$, and the $n_2 = 4.24$. Similar adaptations were observed in the Type I fibers of humans after swim exercise-training [46]. Although the activation threshold did not change, the curve shifted right, as shown by a decline in the pCa_{50} from 5.61 to 5.54 and an increase in n_2 from 2.18 to 3.17 (see Fig. 14.7 of ref. 47). These changes in the force-pCa relationship with exercise-training are small, and the mechanism or cause of the change is unknown. The possibility exists that the exercise program induced a small amount of fast troponin C in the slow fiber type and/or the increased expression of fast MLCs increased dP/dt which, in turn, increased cooperativity in the Ca^{2+} activation of tension. Finally, it should be noted that in comparing the elite master runners with age-matched controls, we observed no differences in the force-pCa relationship.

ALTERATIONS IN FORCE-VELOCITY AND POWER RELATIONSHIPS. From the standpoint of the ability to do work, an important consideration is: How does regular exercise affect the force-velocity and force-power relationships? Also, is peak power altered? There is very little published information concerning these questions but, recently, we have collected considerable data from investigations of both rats and humans that address these questions. In one published report, we found a swim exercise program in humans to have no significant effects on the force-velocity relationship, in either the slow Type I or fast Type II fiber [46]. In rats, we observed peak power to significantly decline in both the Type I and IIa fibers in response to 3.5 hr/day of treadmill running. The decline in peak power was primarily, if not entirely, attributable to the reduced force-generating capacity of the fiber. We observed similar results when comparing elite master runners with age-matched controls. The force-velocity relationships were not significantly different and, thus, no differences existed in either V_{max} or the a:P_o ratio. However, when expressed as $\mu N \cdot FL \cdot s^{-1}$, peak power was significantly depressed in the Type I (8.2 ± 0.3 to 7.1 ± 0.3) and Type IIa (42.2 ± 3.6 to 30.8 ± 1.8) fibers (Fig. 14.9). When we expressed the data corrected for differences in cross-sectional area ($kN \cdot m^{-2} \cdot FL \cdot s^{-1}$), there were no significant differences in either peak power or the force-power relationship between fibers from the elite athlete or control group. These data show that the reduced absolute peak power of the fibers from the exercise-trained athletes was simply a result of the smaller diameter and correspondingly lower peak force in the exercised group.

FUNCTIONAL SIGNIFICANCE OF THE EXERCISE-INDUCED ADAPTATIONS. The data reviewed above allow us to make a few general conclusions regarding the effects of regular endurance exercise on single-cell function and to provide working hypotheses about the importance of the observed changes. It is reasonable to expect that regular endurance exercise would induce changes directed toward optimizing cells' ability to work for prolonged periods and that such adaptations may negatively impact on the cells' ability to perform high-intensity exercise. It is well documented that endurance exercise improves the oxidative capacity of all fibers, both slow- and fast-twitch [71]. The slow type I fiber is designed for slow tonic activities, such as the maintenance of posture. Consequently, it is characterized by a slow but efficient cross-bridge cycling rate. When faced with a phasic activity, such as running, the slow cycling speed and V_o of the slow fiber may limit muscle speed and, thus, body speed. In the case of mixed muscles (composed of fast and slow fibers), the slow fiber may place a significant internal drag (load) on the fast-twitch fibers and, in this way, lowers muscle V_o. Thus, to meet the speed requirements of the exercise bout, the slow fiber must adapt by becoming faster. However, if it were to switch completely to a fast Type IIa fiber, it would be faster, but less efficient, and the velocity acquired would be far in excess of that needed for the exercise task [32, 117]. Thus, it makes sense that the slow Type I fibers respond to regular endurance exercise with a modified myosin (slow MHC combined with slow and fast MLCs), producing a fiber more suited for the rapid phasic patterns of exercise, while maintaining the efficiency required of tonic activity [117]. The exercise-induced decrease in the V_o of the fast-twitch fiber at first seems to be a detrimental or negative effect of endurance exercise. However, the net result is a fiber with higher efficiency (higher force/ATPase rate), with still more than the required velocity for the running task. The tendency to develop smaller fibers with less force and power also fits what one might expect of a fiber designed for prolonged endurance activity. The fiber's small size facilitates oxygen diffusion, and the reduction in force and power is a direct result of the reduced fiber size. For strictly endurance events, the loss in peak power would not likely limit performance; however, this adaptation would present problems for any athlete competing in events requiring a high power component. It will be important for future research to determine whether the reduction in peak power can be prevented by combining programs of strength and endurance exercise.

The Relationship between Programs of Regular Exercise Training and
Fiber Type Switching

It has long been debated whether or not programs of regular exercise induce the transformation of one fiber type to another [71, 105]. One complication is that the criteria used to assess fiber type (oxidative potential, myosin isozyme profile) will in itself have an effect on the conclusion drawn. For example, it is well known that treadmill running elicits a 2-fold increase in the mitochondrial content of all three fiber types [5, 71]. Thus, using on these criteria, one would conclude that exercise training did not cause transformation of one fiber type to another, as the percent of each fiber type and their relative difference in oxidative capacity remained the same. However, when fiber typing is based on qualitative, rather than quantitative, changes in cell protein (for example, the type of MHC expressed), different conclusions will likely be reached. An additional problem in the resolution of this question is that typing is frequently carried out, using enzyme histochemical procedures on samples obtained from a portion of the selected muscle. The former is a qualitative procedure and, consequently it is difficult to unequivocally assign a fiber to a particular type. The latter can lead to an erroneous conclusion, as sampling only slightly different regions of a given muscle can result in significantly different fiber type distributions. This would be true particularly for human studies in which the samples were obtained by the needle biopsy technique, as the portion assayed is extremely small, relative to total muscle cross-sectional area.

Despite the limitations stated above, the published data demonstrates that MHC transformations do occur in response to exercise training. It seems clear that certain transformations occur more easily and at a higher frequency than others. Many of the older histochemical studies have demonstrated endurance exercise to increase the percentage of the Type IIa fiber while causing a decline in the Type IIb population [3, 10, 75]. However, these studies were conducted before the discovery of the fast Type IIx myosin and before it was possible to distinguish the Type IIx fiber from the type IIa fiber. Consequently, the transformation elicited may have been from a Type IIb to IIx or a IIx to IIa, rather than from a type IIb to IIa. Recent data suggest that human muscle contains little or no type IIb myosin [40, 118]. One possibility is that the conversion from Type IIb to IIx requires only minimal recruitment of the Type IIb fiber type and, thus, that the muscle of even sedentary individuals contains little or no Type IIb myosin. Like endurance training, strength training has also been reported to increase and decrease the number of fast Type IIa and IIb fibers, respectively, in both men and women [1, 3, 64, 86]. This transformation from IIb to IIa was based not only on classical enzyme histochemistry but also on MHC composition, assessed by SDS gel electrophoresis [1]. We showed that the white region of the rat gastrocnemius contained 62% Type IIb, 35% hybrid Type IIb-IIx, and 1% Type IIx fibers. With 2 hr of treadmill running, 5 days/wk for 10 wk, the Type IIb population declined to 19%, whereas the hybrid and type IIx population increased to 55 and 18%, respectively (Table 14.1) [117]. When the duration of daily running was increased from 2 to 3.5 hr, the population of Type IIb fibers remained unchanged. However, the Type IIx population showed an additional increase to 36%, while the hybrid IIb-IIx fibers declined to 37% of the total (R. H. Fitts and L. V. Thompson, unpublished data 1995). Additionally, Sugiura et al. [120] reported 1 hr of daily swimming to increase and decrease the percentage of Type IIx and Type IIb fibers, respectively, in the rat EDL. Consequently, at least in the rat, it can be concluded that endurance exercise-training converts the fast Type IIb fiber to the hybrid Type IIb-IIx fiber and then to the fast Type IIx fiber. It is apparent, from the data reviewed here, that any activity, regardless of its nature (endurance or strength), induces transformation of the fast Type IIb MHC to fast Type IIx and/or fast Type IIa MHC.

The question of whether fast Type IIa fibers can be switched to slow Type I fibers with exercise training is still controversial [59, 117]. Green et al. [59] found 3.5 hr/day of treadmill running to significantly increase the percentage of slow Type I fibers in the deep region of the rat vastus lateralis (DVL) from 10 ± 5 to $27 \pm 11\%$, while the fast Type II fibers declined from 90 ± 5 to $73 \pm 11\%$. Additionally, Luginbuhl et al. [90] found sprint treadmill running (55 m/min) to significantly increase and decrease the Type I and Type II fibers, respectively, in the rat plantaris and DVL. In humans, Schantz and Dhoot [114] analyzed the triceps brachii muscle of cross-country skiers and reported an increased expression of slow-type proteins in the fast fibers. These data suggest that at least the endurance training increased the percentage of hybrid fibers. However, many of the early histochemical studies found exercise-training to have no effect on the percentage of slow Type I fibers [8, 55, 75]. If a significant fiber transformation from Type II to Type I had occurred, these authors would have observed an increase in the percentage of slow Type I fibers. We recently studied this question by using SDS gel electrophoresis to analyze the myosin isozyme profile of single fibers isolated from the deep region of the lateral head of the rat gastrocnemius muscle (117; R. H. Fitts and L.V. Thompson unpublished data 1995.) The percentage of slow Type I fibers in the trained groups (2 and 3.5 hr/day of treadmill running) was not significantly altered from the control value of 62% (Table 14.1). These data suggest that fiber type transformations from fast to slow did not occur as a result of exercise training. At this point, we would conclude that the question of whether fast-to-slow transitions occur in response to programs of exercise training remains unanswered. The data in support of fast-to-slow transformations are based on qualitative enzyme histochemical techniques and, in the case of the DVL, regional sampling of a muscle. Sampling of the DVL is particularly problematic, as small differences in the region assayed (pre- vs. post) could explain the observed difference in fiber types. However, our single-fiber analyses can also be criticized because the tedious nature of the analysis limits the number of fibers that can be sampled. The possibility exists that the switch (fast to slow) can only be detected with a considerably larger sample size than that used in our studies. Based on the data discussed, it seems reasonable to conclude that when exercise training does induce fast-to-slow fiber type transitions, these transitions occur at a low frequency, relative to the Type IIb to IIx transition.

The final point in this discussion is whether or not exercise training can switch the slow Type I fiber to the fast Type IIa fiber. The observation described above that many studies showed exercise training to have no effect on the percentage of slow Type I fibers argues not only that there is no fast-to-slow transition but also no significant slow-to-fast conversion. Our SDS gel analysis suggests that the percentage of fibers in the rat soleus containing slow myosin is approximately 95% and that this number is unaffected by 2 or 3.5 hr of daily treadmill running (117; R. H. Fitts and L. V. Thompson unpublished data 1995). However, the percentage of fibers containing only slow myosin declined with exercise training from 92 to 80% after the exercise training programs (Table 14.1). The exercise training caused a small increase in the percentage of fibers containing both slow and fast myosin. The percentage of fibers containing I–IIa and I–IIx both increased. These data suggest that endurance exercise training does not cause a switch from slow to fast fibers but that a small population of slow fibers is induced to coexpress fast-type MHCs. Klitgaard et al. [84] observed that fibers from the vastus lateralis of endurance athletes contained a considerably higher percentage of hybrid (I–IIa) fibers, compared to those of sedentary controls. However, they concluded that the primary isoform was the Type I, with the hybrid fibers containing only minute amounts of the Type IIa isoform. From a quantitative standpoint, we would conclude that the most important exercise-induced change in the slow fiber is the increased expression of fast light chains, as this occurs in essentially all fibers, whereas only a few percent show coexpression of the fast Type IIa MHC [117].

SUMMARY

Based on the MHC isoform pattern, adult mammalian limb skeletal muscles contain two and, in some species, three types of fast fibers (Type IIa, IIx, and IIb), and one slow fiber (Type I). Slow muscles, such as the soleus, contain primarily the slow Type I fiber, whereas fast-twitch muscles are composed primarily of a mixture of the fast myosin isozymes. Force generation involves cross-bridge interaction and transition from a weakly bound, low-force state (AM-ADP-P_i) to the strongly bound, high-force state (AM-ADP). This transition is thought to be rate limiting in terms of dP/dt, and the high-force state is the dominant cross-bridge form during a peak isometric contraction. Intact fast and slow skeletal muscles generate approximately the same amount of peak force (P_o) of between 200 and 250 kN·m^{-2}. However, the rate of transition from the low- to high-force state shows Ca^{2+} sensitivity and is 7-fold higher in fast-twitch, as compared to slow-twitch, skeletal muscle fibers. Fiber V_o or the maximal cross-bridge cycle rate is highly correlated with and thought to be dependent on the specific activity of the myosin or myofibrillar ATPase. The hierarchy for V_o is the Type IIb>IIx>IIa>I. This functional difference for the fast fiber types explains the higher V_o observed in the predominantly Type IIb SVL vs. the mixed fast Type IIa and IIb EDL muscle. A plot of V_o vs. species size demonstrates that an inverse relationship exists between V_o and body mass. From the standpoint of work capacity, the important property is power output. An analysis of individual muscles indicates that peak power is obtained at loads considerably below 50% of P_o. Individuals with a high percentage of fast-twitch fibers generate a greater torque and higher power at a given velocity than those with predominantly slow-twitch fibers. In humans, mean peak power occurred in a ratio of 10:5:1 for the Type IIb, IIa, and I fibers.

The in vivo measurement of the torque-velocity relationship and V_{max} in human muscle is difficult because of limitations inherent in the equipment used and the inability to study the large limb muscles independently. Nevertheless, the in vivo torque-velocity relationships are similar to those measured in vitro in animals. This observation suggests that little central nervous system inhibition exists and that healthy subjects are able to achieve maximal activation of their muscles. Although peak isometric tension is not dependent on fiber type distribution, a positive correlation exists between the percentage of fast fibers and peak torque output at moderate-to-high angular isokinetic velocities. Consequently, peak power output is substantially greater in subjects possessing a predominance of fast fibers.

The mechanical properties of slow and fast muscles do adapt to programs of regular exercise. Endurance exercise training has been shown to increase the V_o of the slow soleus by 20%. This increase could have been caused by either a small increase in all, or most, of the fibers, or to a conversion of a few fibers from slow to fast. Recently, the increase was shown to be caused by the former, as the individual slow Type I fibers of the soleus showed a 20% increase in V_o, but there was little or no change in the percentage of fast fibers. The increased V_o was correlated with, and likely caused by, an increased fiber ATPase. We hypothesize that the increased ATPase and cross-bridge cycling speed might be attributable to an increased expression of fast MLCs in the slow Type I fibers (Fig. 14.10). This hypothesis is based on the fact that light chains have been shown to be involved in the power stroke, and removal of light chains depresses force and velocity. Regular endurance exercise training had no effect on fiber size, but with prolonged durations of daily training it depressed P_o and peak power. When the training is maintained over prolonged periods, it may even induce atrophy of the slow Type I and fast Type IIa fibers. This hypothesis is based on the observation that the elite master athletes had significantly smaller fibers than age-matched controls.

In contrast to endurance exercise, strength training is known to cause fiber hypertrophy, particularly of fast Type II fibers. Isometric exercise is more effective than isotonic contractions in stimulating gains in P_o, and eccentric contractions have been reported to produce greater fiber hypertrophy and gains in peak torque than protocols using exclusively maximal concentric contractions. On the other hand, dynamic or isotonic but not isometric exercise has been shown to increase V_{max}. In general, the maximal gains in torque at a given velocity occur at velocities at or near the velocities experienced during the training program. Because peak power is obtained at velocities between 15 and 30% of V_{max}, isometric or low to intermediate isokinetic training is more effective in improving peak power than dynamic high-velocity training.

It is clear from this review that the contractile properties (and, although not reviewed here, the biochemical properties) of the individual fiber types show extensive plasticity and, consequently, a high ability to adapt to varying functional demands. With regular endurance exercise, slow fibers do not switch to fast fibers but, rather, they express fast MLCs. This adaptation allows the slow Type I fiber to be more suited for the rapid phasic patterns of exercise while maintaining the efficiency required of tonic activity. It is well documented that in the rat, the fast Type IIb fiber transforms to the hybrid fast Type IIb-IIx and, to a significant degree, to the fast Type IIx fiber in the response to endurance exercise training. In humans there is evidence that strength as well as endurance exercise induces a Type IIb to IIa switch. It appears to be more difficult to induce a fast Type IIa to slow Type I switch, and indeed it remains controversial whether or not this switch occurs in response to regular exercise.

ACKNOWLEDGMENTS

We thank Dr. Jane Schluter, Dr. LaDora Thompson, Ms. Carol Vergoth, and Mr. Paul Gardetto for conducting some of the single-fiber studies reviewed in this manuscript, and Ms. Shannon Knuth for her help in the preparation of the figures and for her careful reading of the manuscript. This work was supported in part by National Institute of Health Research Grant AR39894.

REFERENCES

1. Adams, G. R., B. M. Hather, K. M. Baldwin, and G. A. Dudley. Skeletal muscle myosin heavy chain composition and resistance training. *J. Appl. Physiol.* 74:911–915, 1993.
2. Allen, J. D., and R. L. Moss. Factors influencing the ascending limb of the sarcomere length-tension relationship in rabbit skinned muscle fibres. *J. Physiol. (Lond.)* 390:119–136, 1987.
3. Andersen, P., and J. Henriksson. Training induced changes in the subgroups of human type II skeletal muscle fibres. *Acta Physiol. Scand.* 99:123–125, 1977.
4. Armstrong, R. B., and R. O. Phelps. Muscle fiber type composition of the rat hindlimb. *Am. J. Anat.* 171:259–272, 1984.

5. Baldwin, K. M., G. H. Klinkerfuss, R. L. Terjung, P. A. Molé, and J. O. Holloszy. Respiratory capacity of white, red, and intermediate muscle: adaptive response to exercise. *Am. J. Physiol.* 222:373–378, 1972.

6. Baldin, K. M., . W. W. Winder, and J. O. Holloszy. Adaptations of actomyosin ATPase in different types of muscle to endurance exercise. *Am. J. Physiol.* 229:422–426, 1975.

7. Bárány, M. ATPase activity of myosin correlated with speed of muscle shortening. *J. Gen. Physiol.* 50:197–218, 1967.

8. Barnard, R. J., V. R. Edgerton, and J. B. Peter. Effect of exercise on skeletal muscle. I. Biochemical and histochemical properties. *J. Appl. Physiol.* 28:762–766, 1970.

9. Barnard, R. J., V. R. Edgerton, and J. B. Peter. Effect of exercise on skeletal muscle. II. Contractile properties. *J. Appl. Physiol.* 28:767–770, 1970.

10. Baumann, H., M. Jäggi, F. Soland, H. Howald, and M. C. Schaub. Exercise training induces transitions of myosin isoform subunits within histochemically typed human muscle fibres. *Pflügers Arch.* 409:349–360, 1987.

11. Belanger, A. Y., and A. J. McComas. Extent of motor unit activation during effort. *J. Appl. Physiol.* 51:1131–1135, 1981.

12. Bigland-Ritchie, B., F. Furbush, and J. J. Woods. Fatigue of intermittent submaximal voluntary contractions: central and peripheral factors. *J. Appl. Physiol.* 61:421–429, 1986.

13. Binkhorst, R. A., L. Hoofd, and A. C. A. Vissers. Temperature and force-velocity relationship of human muscles. *J. Appl. Physiol.* 42:471–475, 1977.

14. Blinks, J. R., R. Rüdel, and S. R. Taylor. Calcium transients in isolated amphibian skeletal muscle fibres: detection with aequorin. *J. Physiol. (Lond.)* 277:291–323, 1978.

15. Bottinelli, R., R. Betto, S. Schiaffino, and C. Reggiani. Unloaded shortening velocity and myosin heavy chain and alkali light chain isoform composition in rat skeletal muscle fibres. *J. Physiol (Lond.)* 478:341–349, 1994.

16. Bottinelli, R., S. Schiaffino, and C. Reggiani. Force-velocity relations and myosin heavy chain isoform compositions of skinned fibers from rat skeletal muscle. *J. Physiol. (Lond.)* 437:655–672, 1991.

17. Brenner, B. Mechanical and structural approaches to correlation of cross-bridge action in muscle with actomyosin ATPase in solution. *Annu. Rev. Physiol.* 49:655–672, 1987.

18. Brenner, B. Effect of Ca^{2+} on cross-bridge turnover kinetics in skinned single psoas fibers: implications for regulation of muscle contraction. *Proc. Natl. Acad. Sci. U.S.A.* 85:3265–3269, 1988.

19. Brenner, B., and E. Eisenberg. Rate of force generation in muscle: correlation with actomyosin ATPase in solution. *Proc. Natl. Acad. Sci. U.S.A.* 83:3542–3546, 1986.

20. Briggs, F. N., J. L. Poland, and R. J. Solaro. Relative capabilities of sarcoplasmic reticulum in fast and slow mammalian skeletal muscles. *J. Physiol. (Lond.)* 266:587–594, 1977.

21. Brooke, M. H., and K. K. Kaiser. Muscle fiber types: how many and what kind? *Arch. Neurol.* 23:369–379, 1970.

22. Brown, M. D., M. A. Cotter, O. Hudlická, and G. Vrbová. The effects of different patterns of muscle activity on capillary density, mechanical properties and structure of slow and fast rabbit muscles. *Pflügers Arch.* 361:241–250, 1976.

23. Caiozzo, V. J., J. J. Perrine, and V. R. Edgertn. Training-induced alterations of the in vivo force-velocity relationship of human muscle. *J. Appl. Physiol.* 51:750–754, 1981.

24. Carolan, B., and E. Cafarelli. Adaptions in coactivation after isometric resistance training. *J. Appl. Physiol.* 73:911–917, 1992.

25. Claassen, H., C. Gerber, H. Hoppeler, J-M. Luthi, and P. Vock. Muscle filament spacing and short-term heavy-resistance exercise in humans. *J. Physiol. (Lond.)* 409:491–495, 1989.

26. Close, R. I. Dynamic properties of mammalian skeletal muscles. *Physiol. Rev.* 52:129–197, 1972.

27. Close, R. I., and J. F. Y. Hoh. Influence of temperature on isometric contractions of rat skeletal muscles. *Nature* 217:1179–1180, 1968.

28. Colliander, E. B., and P. A. Tesch. Effects of eccentric and concentric muscle actions in resistance training. *Acta Physiol. Scand.* 140:31–39, 1990.
29. Costill, D. L., E. F. Coyle, W. F. Fink, G. R. Lesemes, and F. A. Witzmann. Adaptions in skeletal muscle following strength training. *J. Appl. Physiol.* 46:96–99, 1979.
30. Coyle, E. F., D. L. Costill, and G. R. Lesmes. Leg extension power and muscle fiber composition. *Med. Sci. Sports* 11:12–15, 1979.
31. Coyle, E. F., D. C. Feiring, T. C. Rotkis, R. W. Cote III, F. B. Rody, W. Lee, and J. H. Wilmore. Specificity of power improvements through slow and fast isokinetic training. *J. Appl. Physiol.* 51:1437–1442, 1981.
32. Coyle, E. F., L. S. Sidossis, J.F. Horowitz, and J. D. Beltz. Cycling efficiency is related to the percentage of type I muscle fibers. *Med. Sci.Sports Exerc.* 24:782–788, 1992.
33. de Haan, A., D. A. Jones, and A. J. Sargeant. Changes in velocity of shortening, power output and relaxation rate during fatigue of rat medial gastrocnemius muscle. *Pflügers. Arch.* 413:422–428, 1989.
34. de Koning, F. L., R. A. Binkhorst, J. A. Vos, and M. A. van't Hof. The force-velocity relationship of arm flexion in untrained males and females and arm-trained athletes. *Eur. J. Appl. Physiol.* 54:89–94, 1985.
35. Duchateau, J., and K. Hainaut. Isometric or dynamic training: differential effects on mechanical properties of a human muscle. *J. Appl. Physiol.* 56:296–301, 1984.
36. Dudley, G. A., W. A. Abraham, and R. L. Terjung. Influence of exercise intensity and duration on biochemical adaptations in skeletal muscle. *J. Appl. Physiol.* 53:844–850, 1982.
37. Edgerton, V. R. Neuromuscular adaptation to power and endurance work. *Can. J. Appl. Sport Sci.* 1:49–58, 1976.
38. Edman, K. A. P. The velocity of unloaded shortening and its relation to sarcomere length and isometric force in vertebrate muscle fibres. *J. Physiol. (Lond.)* 291:143–159, 1979.
39. Eisenberg, E., and T. L. Hill. Muscle contraction and free energy transduction in biological systems. *Science* 227:999–1006, 1985.
40. Ennion, S., J. Sant'Ana Pereira, A. J. Sargeant, A. Young, and G. Goldspink. Characterization of human skeletal muscle fibres according to the myosin heavy chains they express. *J. Muscle Res. Cell Motil* 16:35–43, 1995.
41. Fiehn, W., and J. B. Peter. Properties of the fragmented sarcoplasmic reticulum from fast twitch and slow twitch muscles. *J. Clin. Invest.* 50:570–573, 1971.
42. Fischer, A. J., C. A. Smith, J. Thoden, R. Smith, K. Sutoh, H. M. Holden, and I. Rayment. Structural studies of myosin:nucleotide complexes: a revised model for the molecular basis of muscle contraction. *Biophys. J.* 68:19s–28s, 1995.
43. Fitts, R. H. Substrate supply and energy metabolism during brief high intensity exercise: importance in limiting performance. D. R. Lamb and C. V. Gisolfi (eds). *Perspectives in Exercise Science and Sports Medicine. Energy Metabolism in Exercise and Sport, Vol. 5.* Brown and Benchmark, 1992, Dubuque, IA pp. 53–106.
44. Fitts, R. H. Cellular mechanisms of muscle fatigue. *Physiol. Rev.* 74:49–94, 1994.
45. Fitts, R. H., D. Campion, F. J. Nagle, and R. Cassens. Contractile properties of skeletal muscle from trained miniature pig. *Pflügers Arch.* 343:133–141, 1973.
46. Fitts, R. H., D. L. Costill, and P. R. Gardetto. Effect of swim exercise training on human muscle fiber function. *J. Appl. Physiol.* 66:465–475, 1989.
47. Fitts. R. H., J. B. Courtright, D. H. Kim, and F. A. Witzmann. Muscle fatigue with prolonged exercise: contractile and biochemical alterations. *Am. J. Physiol. 242 (Cell Physiol. 11):* C65–C73, 1982.
48. Fitts, R. H., and J. O. Holloszy. Contractile properties of rat soleus muscle: effects of training and fatigue. *Am. J. Physiol. 233 (Cell Physiol. 2):* C86–C91, 1977.
49. Fitts, R. H., J. M. Metzger, D. A. Riley, and B. R. Unsworth. Models of disuse: a comparison of hindlimb suspension and immobilization. *J. Appl. Physiol.* 60:1946–1953, 1986.

50. Fleischer, S., and M. Inui. Biochemistry and biophysics of excitation-contraction coupling. *Annu. Rev. Biophys. Chem.* 18:333–364, 1989.

51. Froese, E. A., and M. E. Houston. Torque-velocity characteristics and muscle fiber type in human vastus lateralis. *J. Appl. Physiol.* 59:309–314, 1985.

52. Gardetto, P. R., J. M. Schluter, and R. H. Fitts. Contractile function of single muscle fibers after hindlimb suspension. *J. Appl. Physiol.* 66:2739–2749, 1989.

53. Goldman, Y. E., and B. Brenner. Special topic: molecular mechanisms of muscle contraction. *Annu. Rev. Physiol.* 49:629–636, 1987.

54. Goldspink, G., and K. F. Howells. Work-induced hypertrophy in exercised normal muscles of different ages and the reversibility of hypertrophy after cessation of exercise. *J. Physiol. (Lond.)* 239:179–193, 1973.

55. Gollnick, P. D., R. B. Armstrong, B. Saltin, C. W. Saubert IV, W. L. Sembrowich, and R. E. Shepherd. Effect of training on enzyme activity and fiber composition of human skeletal muscle. *J. Appl. Physiol.* 34:107–111, 1973.

56. Gollnick, P. D., B. F. Timson, R. L. Moore, and M. Riedy. Muscular enlargement and number of fibers in skeletal muscles of rats. *J. Appl. Physiol.* 50:936–943, 1981.

57. Gonyea, W., and F. Bonde-Petersen. Alterations in muscle contractile properties and fiber composition after weight-lifting exercise in cats. *Exp. Neurol.* 59:75–84, 1978.

58. Gordon, A. M., A. F. Huxley, and F. J. Julian. The variation in isometric tension with sarcomere length in vertebrate muscle fibres. *J. Physiol. (Lond.)* 184:170–192, 1966.

59. Green. H. J., G. A. Klug, H. Reichmann, U. Seedorf, W. Wiehrer, and D. Pette. Exercise-induced fibre type transitions with regard to myosin, parvalbumin, and sarcoplasmic reticulum in muscles of the rat. *Pflügers Arch.* 400:432–438, 1984.

60. Gregor, R. J., V. R. Edgerton, J. J. Perrine, D. S. Campion, and C. DeBus. Torque-velocity relationships and muscle fiber composition in elite female athletes. *J. Appl. Physiol.* 47:388–392, 1979.

61. Häkkinen, K., M. Alén, and P. V. Komi. Changes in isometric force- and relaxation-time, electromyographic and muscle fibre characteristics of human skeletal muscle during strength training and detraining. *Acta Physiol. Scand.* 125:573–585, 1985.

62. Häkkinen, K., and P. V. Komi. Electromyographic changes during strength training and detraining. *Med. Sci. Sports Exerc.* 15:455–460, 1983.

63. Häkkinen, K., P. V. Komi, and M. Alén. Effect of explosive type strength training on isometric force- and relaxation-time, electromyographic and muscle fibre characteristics of leg extensor muscles. *Acta Physiol. Scand.* 125:587–600, 1985.

64. Hather, B. M., P. A. Tesch, P. Buchanan, and G. A. Dudley. Influence of eccentric actions on skeletal muscle adaptations to resistance training. *Acta Physiol. Scand.* 143:177–185, 1991.

65. Henriksson-Larsen, K., M-L. Wretling, R. Lorentzon, and L. Oberg. Do muscle fibre size and fibre angulation correlate in pennated human muscles? *Eur. J. Appl. Physiol.* 64:68–72, 1992.

66. Herbert, R. D., and S. C. Gandevia. Changes in pennation with joint angle and muscle torque: in vivo measurements in human brachialis muscle. *J. Physiol. (Lond.)* 484:523–532, 1995.

67. Hibberd, M. G., and D. R. Trentham. Relationships between chemical and mechanical events during muscular contraction. *Annu. Rev. Biophysics Biophys. Chem.* 15:119–161, 1986.

68. Hill, A. V. The heat of shortening and dynamic constants of muscle. *Proc. R. Soc. London, Ser. B.* 126:136–195, 1938.

69. Hill, A. V. The dimensions of animals and their muscular dynamics. *Proc. R. Inst. Great Britain* 34:450–471, 1949.

70. Holloszy, J. O. Biochemical adaptations in muscle. Effects of exercise in mitochondrial oxygen uptake and respiratory enzyme activity in skeletal muscle. *J. Biol. Chem.* 242: 2278–2282, 1967.

71. Holloszy, J. O., and F. W. Booth. Biochemical adaptations to endurance exercise in muscle. *Annu. Rev. Physiol.* 38:273–291, 1976.

72. Holmes, K. C. The actomyosin interaction and its control by tropomyosin. *Biophys. J.* 68:2s–7s, 1995.

73. Hortobágyi, T., J. A. Houmard, J. R. Stevenson, D. D. Fraser, R. A. Johns, and R. G. Israel. The effects of detraining on power athletes. *Med. Sci. Sports Exerc.* 25:929–935, 1993.

74. Huxley, A. F. Muscle structure and theories of contraction. *Prog. Biophys.* 7:255–318, 1957.

75. Ingjer, F. Effects of endurance training on muscle fibre ATP-ase activity, capillary supply and mitochondrial content in man. *J. Physiol. (Lond.)* 294:419–432, 1979.

76. Ivy, J. L., R. T. Withers, G. Brose, B. D. Maxwell, and D. L. Costill. Isokinetic contractile properties of the quadriceps with relation to fiber type. *Eur. J. Appl. Physiol.* 47:247–255, 1981.

77. James, C., P. Sacco, M. V. Hurley, and D. A. Jones. An evaluation of different protocols for measuring the force-velocity relationship of the human quadriceps muscles. *Eur. J. Appl. Physiol.* 68:41–47, 1994.

78. Johnson, M. A., J. Polgar, D. Weightman, and D. Appleton. Data on the distribution of fibre types in thirty-six human muscles. An autopsy study. *J. Neurol. Sci.* 18:111–129, 1973.

79. Jones, D. A., and O. M. Rutherford. Human muscle strength training: the effects of three different regimes and the nature of the resultant changes. *J. Physiol. (Lond.)* 391:1–11, 1987.

80. Jones, D. A., O. M. Rutherford, and D. F. Parker. Physiological changes in skeletal muscle as a result of strength training. *Q. J. Exp. Physiol.* 74:233–256, 1989.

81. Julian, F. J., and R. L. Moss. Effects of calcium and ionic strength on shortening velocity and tension development in frog skinned muscle fibres. *J. Physiol. (Lond.)* 311:179–199, 1981.

82. Kanehisa, H., and M. Miyashita. Specificity of velocity in strength training. *Eur. J. Appl. Physiol.* 52:104–106, 1983.

83. Kim, D. H., G. S. Wible, F. A. Witzman, and R. H. Fitts. The effect of exercise-training on sarcoplasmic reticulum function in fast and slow skeletal muscle. *Life Sci.* 28:2671–2677, 1981.

84. Klitgaard, H., O. Bergman, R. Betto, G. Salviati, S. Schiaffino, T. Clausen, and B. Saltin. Co-existence of myosin heavy chain I and IIa isoforms in human skeletal muscle fibres with endurance training. *Eur. J. Physiol.* 416:470–472, 1990.

85. Klitgaard, H., R. Marc, A. Brunet, H. Vandewalle, and H. Monod. Contractile properties of old rat muscles: effect of increased use. *J. Appl. Physiol.* 67:1401–1408, 1989.

86. Klitgaard, H., M. Zhou, and E. A. Richter. Myosin heavy chain composition of single fibres from m. biceps brachii of male body builders. *Acta Physiol. Scand.* 140:175–180, 1990.

87. Komi, P. V., and E. R. Buskirk. Effect of eccentric and concentric muscle conditioning on tension and electrical activity of human muscle. *Ergonomics* 15:417–434, 1972.

88. Larsson, L., and R. L. Moss. Maximum velocity of shortening in relation to myosin isoform composition in single fibers from human skeletal muscles. *J. Physiol. (Lond.)* 472:595–614, 1993.

89. Lowey, S., and K. M. Trybus. Role of skeletal and smooth muscle myosin light chains. *Biophys. J.* 68:120s–127s, 1995.

90. Luginbuhl, A. J., G. A. Dudley, and R. S. Staron. Fiber type changes in rat skeletal muscle after intense interval training. *Histochemistry* 81:55–58, 1984.

91. Lymn, R. W., and E. W. Taylor. Mechanism of adenosine triphosphate hydrolysis by actomyosin. *Biochemistry* 10:4617–4624, 1971.

92. Maughan, R. J., and M. A. Nimmo. The influence of variations in muscle fibre composition on muscle strength and cross-sectional area in untrained males. *J. Physiol. (Lond.)* 351:299–311, 1984.

93. Mayhew, T. P., J. M. Rothstein, S. D. Finucane, and R. L. Lamb. Muscular adaption to concentric and eccentric exercise at equal power levels. *Med. Sci. Sports Exerc.* 27:868–873, 1995.

94. Merton, P. A. Voluntary strength and fatigue. *J. Physiol. (Lond.)* 123:553–564, 1954.

95. Metzger, J. M., M. L. Greaser, and R. L. Moss. Variations in cross-bridge attachment rate and tension with phosphorylation of myosin in mammalian skinned skeletal muscle fibers. *J. Gen. Physiol.* 93:855–883, 1989.

96. Metzger, J. M., and R. L. Moss. Greater H$^+$ ion-induced depression of tension and velocity in single skinned fibers of rat fast versus slow muscles. *J. Physiol. (Lond.)* 393: 727–742, 1987.

97. Metzger, J. M., and R. L. Moss. pH modulation of the kinetics of a Ca^{2+}-sensitive cross-bridge state transition in mammalian single skeletal muscle fibers. *J. Physiol. (Lond.)* 428:751–764, 1990.

98. Metzger, J. M., and R. L. Moss. Calcium-sensitive cross-bridge transitions in mammalian fast and slow skeletal muscle fibers. *Science* 247:1088–1090, 1990.

99. Metzger, J. M., K. B. Scheidt, and R. H. Fitts. Histochemical and physiological characteristics of the rat diaphragm. *J. Appl. Physiol.* 58:1085–1091, 1985.

100. Narici, M. V., G. S. Roi, L. Landoni, A. E. Minetti, and P. Cerretelli. Changes in force-cross-sectional area and neural activation during strength training and detraining of the human quadriceps. *Eur. J. Appl. Physiol.* 59:310–319, 1989.

101. Newham, D. J., T. McCarthy, and J. Turner. Voluntary activation of human quadriceps during and after isokinetic exercise. *J. Appl. Physiol.* 71:2122–2126, 1991.

102. Nygaard, E., M. Houston, Y. Suzuki, K. Jorgensen, and B. Saltin. Morphology of the brachial biceps muscle and elbow flexion in man. *Acta Physiol. Scand.* 117:287–292, 1983.

103. Perrine, J. J., and V. R. Edgerton. Muscle force-velocity and power-velocity relationships under isokinetic loading. *Med. Sci. Sports* 10:159–166, 1978.

104. Peter, J. B. Histochemical, biochemical, and physiological studies of skeletal muscle and its adaptation to exercise. R. J. Podolsky (ed.) *Contractility of Muscle Cells and Related Processes.* Englewood Cliffs, N.J.: Prentice-Hall, 1971, pp. 151–173.

105. Pette, D. Activity-induced fast to slow transitions in mammalian muscle. *Med. Sci. Sports Exerc.* 16:517–528, 1984.

106. Ranatunga, K. W. Temperature-dependence of shortening velocity and rate of isometric tension development in rat skeletal muscle. *J. Physiol. (Lond.)* 329:465–483, 1982.

107. Rios, E., and G. Pizarro. The voltage sensor of excitation-contraction coupling in skeletal muscle. *Physiol. Rev.* 71:849–908, 1991.

108. Rome, L. C., R. P. Funke, R. M. Alexander, G. Lutz, H. Aldridge, F. Scott, and M. Freadman. Why animals have different muscle fibre types. *Nature* 335:824–827, 1988.

109. Rome, L. C., A. A. Sosnicki, and D. O. Goble. Maximal velocity of shortening of three fibre types from horse soleus muscle: implications for scaling with body size. *J. Physiol. (Lond.)* 431:173–185, 1990.

110. Rutherford, O. M., and D. A. Jones. Contractile properties and fatiguability of the human adductor pollicis and first dorsal interosseus: a comparison of the effects of two chronic stimulation patterns. *J. Neurol. Sci.* 85:319–331, 1988.

111. Rutherford, O. M., and D. A. Jones. Measurement of fibre pennation using ultrasound in the human quadriceps in vivo. *Eur. J. Appl. Physiol.* 65:433–437, 1992.

112. Rutherford, O. M., D. A. Jones, and D. J. Newham. Clinical and experimental application of the percutaneous twitch superimposition technique for the study of human muscle activation. *J. Neurol. Neurosurg. Psychiatry* 49:1288–1291, 1986.

113. Sale, D. G., J. D. MacDougall, S. E. Alway, and J. R. Sutton. Voluntary strength and muscle characteristics in untrained men and women and male bodybuilders. *J. Appl. Physiol.* 62:1786–1793, 1987.

114. Schantz, P. G., and G. K. Dhoot. Coexistence of slow and fast isoforms of contractile and regulatory proteins in human skeletal muscle fibres induced by endurance training. *Acta Physiol. Scand.* 131:147–154, 1987.

115. Scott, S. H., C. M. Engstrom, and G. E. Loeb. Morphology of human thigh muscles. Determination of fascile architecture by magnetic resonance imaging. *J. Anat.* 182:249–257, 1993.

116. Sleep, J. A., and S. J. Smith. Actomyosin ATPase and muscle contraction. *Curr. Top. Bioenergetics* 11:239–286, 1981.

117. Schluter, J. M., and R. H. Fitts. Shortening velocity and ATPase activity of rat skeletal mus-

cle fibers: effect of endurance exercise training. *Am. J. Physiol. 266 (Cell Physiol. 35)*: C1699–C1713, 1994.

118. Smerdu, V., I. Karsch-Kizrachi, M. Campione, L. Leinwand, and S. Schiaffino. Type IIx myosin heavy chain transcripts are expressed in type IIb fibers of human skeletal muscle. *Am. J. Physiol. 267 (Cell Physiol. 36)*: C1723–C1728, 1994.

119. Staudte, H. W., G. U. Exner, and D. Pette. Effects of short-term high intensity (sprint) training on some contractile and metabolic characteristics of fast and slow muscle of the rat. *Pflügers Arch.* 344:159–168, 1973.

120. Sugiura, T., A. Morimoto, Y. Sakata, T. Watanabe, and N. Murakami. Myosin heavy chain isoform changes in rat diaphragm are induced by endurance training. *Jpn. J. Physiol.* 40:759–763, 1990.

121. Suter, E., W. Herzog, J. Sokolosky, J. P. Wiley, and B. R. MacIntosh. Muscle fiber type distribution as estimated by Cybex testing and by muscle biopsy. *Med. Sci. Sports Exerc.* 25:363–370, 1993.

122. Sweeney, H. L. Function of the N terminus of the myosin essential light chain of vertebrate striated muscle. *Biophys. J.* 68:112s–119s, 1995.

123. Taylor, E. W. Mechanism of actomyosin ATPase and the problem of muscle contraction. *CRC Crit. Rev. Biochem. Mol. Biol.* 6:103–164, 1979.

124. Tesch, P., and J. Karlsson. Isometric strength performance and muscle fibre type distribution in man. *Acta Physiol. Scand.* 103:47–51, 1978.

125. Thomas, D. O., M. J. White, G. Sagar, and C. T. M. Davies. Electrically evoked isokinetic plantar flexor torque in males. *J. Appl. Physiol.* 63:1499–1503, 1987.

126. Thomason, D. B., and F. W. Booth. Atrophy of the soleus muscle by hindlimb unweighting. *J. Appl. Physiol.* 68:1–12, 1990.

127. Thorstennsson, A., G. Grimby, and J. Karlsson. Force-velocity relations and fiber composition in human knee extensor muscles. *J. Appl. Physiol.* 40:12–16, 1976.

128. Thorstensson, A., L. Larsson, P. Tesch, and J. Karlsson. Muscle strength and fiber composition in athletes and sedentary men. *Med. Sci. Sports* 9:26–30, 1977.

129. Tihanyi, J., P. Apor, and G. Fekete. Force-velocity-power characteristics and fiber composition in human knee extensor muscles. *Eur. J. Appl. Physiol.* 48:331–343, 1982.

130. Troup, J. P., J. M. Metzger, and R. H. Fitts. Effect of high-intensity exercise training on functional capacity of limb skeletal muscle. *J. Appl. Physiol.* 60:1743–1751, 1986.

131. Tsika, R. W., R. E. Herrick, and K. M. Baldwin. Time course adaptations in rat skeletal muscle isomyosins during compensatory growth and regression. *J. Appl. Physiol.* 63:2111–2121, 1987.

132. Westerblad, H., and J. Lännergren. Slowing of relaxation during fatigue in single mouse muscle fibres. *J. Physiol. (Lond.)* 434:323–336, 1991.

133. Westing, S. H., J. Y. Seger, E. Karlson, and B. Ekblom. Eccentric and concentric torque-velocity characteristics of the quadriceps femoris in man. *Eur. J. Appl. Physiol.* 58:100–104, 1988.

134. Westing, S. H., J. Y. Seger, and A. Thorstensson. Effects of electrical stimulation on eccentric and concentric torque-velocity relationships during knee extension in man. *Acta Physiol. Scand.* 140:17–22, 1990.

135. Wickiewicz, T. L., R. R. Roy, P. L. Powell, and V. R. Edgerton. Muscle architecture of the human lower limb. *Clin. Orthop. Related Res.* 179:275–283, 1983.

136. Wickiewicz, T. L., R. R. Roy, P. L. Powell, J. J. Perrine, and V. R. Edgerton. Muscle architecture and force-velocity relationships in humans. *J. Appl. Physiol.* 57:435–443, 1984.

137. Wilkie, D. R. The relation between force and velocity in human muscle. *J. Physiol. (Lond.)* 110:249–280, 1950.

138. Wilkinson, J. M. Troponin C from rabbit slow skeletal and cardiac muscle is the product of a single gene. *Eur. J. Biochem.* 103:179–188, 1980.

139. Young, A. The relative strength of type I and type II muscle fibres in human quadriceps. *Clin. Physiol.* 4:23–32, 1984.

15
Magnetic Resonance Imaging and Spectroscopy in Studying Exercise in Children

DAN MICHAEL COOPER, M.D.
THOMAS J. BARSTOW, Ph.D.

The widely held but largely intuitive notion that vigorous physical activity occurs more frequently in children and adolescents than in adults is increasingly supported by scientific investigation [20, 51]. Moreover, there are intriguing data suggesting that physical activity of childhood and adolescence influences the very process of growth and development by modulating anabolic agents at the cellular level [22]. Despite the unique and important role of exercise in the lives of children, our understanding of developmental aspects of cardiorespiratory responses to exercise is limited.

Methodological difficulties are, of course, a major stumbling block in probing mechanisms of adaptation to exercise in children and young adults. Only minimally invasive studies are ethically acceptable in this population, and even simple tasks like breathing on a mouthpiece and/or pedaling on an ergometer at a regular frequency require a level of cooperation and attention often beyond the developmental capabilities of many otherwise willing and enthusiastic subjects. Magnetic resonance imaging (MRI) and spectroscopy (MRS) provide researchers with powerful noninvasive tools that can be used in children. In this chapter, we review recent insights into structural and functional adaptive responses to exercise during the period of growth and development. Our focus is on application of MRI techniques to this specific biological question, rather than on the mechanics of MRI itself. We refer the interested reader to published review for further discussion of exactly how MRI works (e.g., see ref. 57).

GROWTH AND DEVELOPMENT OF CARDIORESPIRATORY RESPONSES TO EXERCISE

The adaptation to physical activity in children represents the unique interaction of two distinct biological processes, human development and physical exercise, each of which is characterized by tissue plasticity. Physical activity plays a profound role in tissue anabolism, growth, and development. Yet, surprisingly little is understood about the mechanisms linking exercise with muscle hypertrophy [60], increased capillarization and mitochondrial capacity [12], stronger bones [43], changes in body composition [4, 5], and improved cardiorespiratory dynamics [15].

475

The interaction between physical activity and growth is not limited to individuals engaged in competitive sports and athletics. Disuse atrophy—the reduction in muscle mass and bone density that accompanies bed rest, limb immobilization, or neural injury—occurs even in sedentary individuals [13]. This implies that a sizeable anabolic stimulus arises from the relatively modest physical activity of daily living. Moreover, the existence of the "training effect"—the ability to improve performance with repeated exercise—suggests a "dose-response" relationship between activity and anabolic effect.

There is increasing evidence suggesting that the metabolic pathways essential for physical activity mature during growth in children. The gas exchange response (measured at the mouth, breath by breath) to high-intensity exercise in children has been shown to be qualitatively and quantitatively different from that of adults. The oxygen cost of high-intensity exercise normalized to the actual work done (O_2/J) is higher in children, suggesting less dependence on anaerobic metabolism [77] (Fig. 15.1). After vigorous exercise, blood and muscle lactate concentrations are lower in children, reflected by lower levels of metabolic acidosis [32, 59]. Consistent with this phenomenon is our recent observation that the early exponential increase in $\dot{V}O_2$ during constant work rate, high-intensity exercise is greater in children than in adults, but the slower additional $\dot{V}O_2$ (which has been shown to correlate with the magnitude of blood lactate [64] is less [2]. The growth-related differences in the adaptive response to high-intensity exercise might be related to maturation of muscle metabolic pathways, but no definitive mechanism has been established.

The use of phosphorus nuclear magnetic resonance spectroscopy (^{31}P MRS) now provides safe and noninvasive means of monitoring intraceulluar inorganic phosphate (P_i), phosphocreatine (PCr), adenosine triphosphate (ATP), and pH [18] (Fig. 15.2) that are acceptable for studies in children. These variables, in turn, allow the assessment of muscle oxidative metabolism and intramuscular glycolytic activity [18]. As leg muscle work rate increases, adenosine diphosphate (ADP) and P_i are released from the breakdown of ATP and PCr. One current theory holds that ADP and P_i may regulate the rate of oxidative phosphorylation exactly, so that homeostasis of the ATP concentration is obtained until very heavy levels of exercise are encountered [7, 8, 18]. As ATP hydrolysis approaches the maximal rate of oxidative phosphorylation, glycolysis (similarly activated by ADP and P_i) assumes an increasing proportion of the metabolic burden [18].

We hypothesized that the growth-related changes in whole-body O_2 uptake and O_2 cost of exercise observed during high-intensity exercise reflect a maturation of the kinetics of high-energy phosphate metabolites in muscle tissue. This hypothesis was tested by comparing P_i, PCr, and pH kinetics in calf muscles during progressive incremental exercise in children and adults [76].

In adult healthy subjects, the relationship between P_i:PCr and work rate is characterized by an initial, almost linear portion. The slope of P_i:PCr to

FIGURE 15.1.
*Cumulative O_2 cost per joule at different work intensities in adults and children. Values are means ± SD. Cumulative O_2 cost was not affected by increasing work intensity in children and adults. However, cost was significantly higher in children than in adults at higher work rates. 50% Δ refers to a work rate above the subject's anerobic threshold (AT) by exactly 50% of the difference between the AT and $\dot{V}O_{2max}$. 100% max and 125% max refer to the subject's $\dot{V}O_{2max}$. (*P < .001; **, P < .01). Reproduced from ref. 77.*

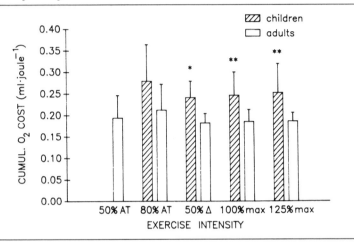

work rate is a function of mitochondrial density and reflects the sensitivity of respiratory control [27] (Fig. 15.3), which is followed by a second steeper slope that is associated with acceleration of glycolysis and increased lactic acid production suggestive of anerobic metabolism [18]. Production of lactic acid, which is dissociated at physiological pH, results in increasing [H$^+$]. Therefore, ^{31}P MRS can indirectly monitor glycolyic activity by measuring intracellular pH.

We found that during progressive exercise, muscle P_i:PCr ratio increases to a smaller extent in children, compared with that in adults, even when the data are related to work rate normalized to body weight (Fig. 15.4). In addition, children showed a smaller drop in intramuscular pH. A slow and fast phase of P_i:PCr increase and pH decrease was noted in 75% of adults and 50% of children. The initial linear slope was the same in children and adults, suggesting a similar rate of mitochondrial oxidative metabolism during low-intensity exercise. However, the different responses of the P_i:PCr ratio and pH during high-intensity exercise in children, compared with those in adults, indicate growth-related differences in energy metabolism (limited primarily to the high-intensity exercise range).

Our data might suggest that children may either deliver O_2 more effec-

FIGURE 15.2.

³¹P MRS spectra from right calf of an 8-yr-old boy at rest, during incremental exercise, and recovery. Reproduced from ref. 76.

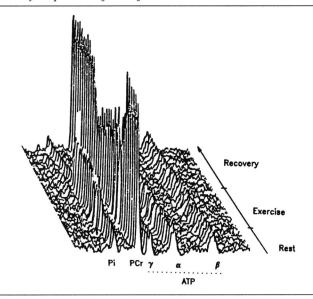

FIGURE 15.3.

P_i:PCr and pH at rest and during incremental exercise in a 33-yr-old man. Arrows transition points between slow and fast phases of P_i:PCr increase and pH reduction. Reproduced from ref. 76.

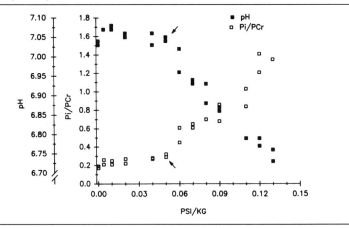

FIGURE 15.4.

P_i:PCr and pH at rest and during incremental exercise in a 9-yr-old girl. Arrows, transition points between slow and fast phases of P_i:PCr and pH changes. Reproduced from ref. 76.

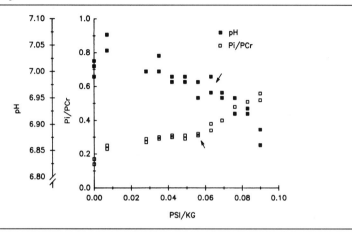

tively to the mitochondria than adults, be less able to facilitate anerobic pathways, or have tissue O_2 requirements during exercise that are not found in adults. More effective O_2 use could result from factors that influence mitochondrial oxidative ATP resynthesis, such as delivery of oxygen from the capillary blood, delivery of substrates, or greater density of mitochondria. Each of these factors might be responsible for a greater oxygen-dependent ATP generation, lower P_i:PCr ratio, and higher pH during exercise in children.

But a more effective oxygen delivery in children alone should not inhibit the glycolytic capability. As work rate increases, children, like adults, will eventually require anaerobic glycolysis, with concomitant lactate production as an additional mechanism of ATP rephosphorylation. This phenomenon is observed in trained athletes: Although anaerobic metabolism occurs at higher work rates than that in untrained subjects, lactate levels ultimately achieved are much higher. It is noteworthy that the threshold in the slope of P_i:PCr to work rate occurred at the same relative work rate in children and adults (0.05 psi/kg), indirect evidence against the idea of greater aerobic capacity in children. It appears, therefore, that when the work rate exceeds a threshold value, the ability to stimulate anaerobic metabolism is less in children, compared to that in adults. Ultimately, the work performed is less in children.

There could be less glycolytic capability in children, so that the rate of glycolysis may not contribute sufficiently to muscle energy requirements, resulting in early muscle exhaustion. The minimal drop in pH seen in children for heavy exercise demonstrates that even after the transition point, i.e., when further energy sources appear to be required, the glycolytic processes play less of a role. Moreover, children achieved an end-exercise P_i:PCr value of 0.54 ± 0.12 (only 27% of adult values), which indicates that soon after the threshold, when the oxidative rate has presumably reached its maximum, children can no longer sustain muscular contraction.

A reduced muscle glycolytic ability during exercise, compared with that of adults, was recently noted by Kuno et al. [47] in trained and untrained boys 12–17 yr old. Using ^{31}P MRS and exhaustive exercise (in the magnet), the findings of these investigators supported the previous results in our laboratory of generally higher intramuscular pH and lower P_i:PCr ratios in children, compared with those in adults (Fig. 15.5). Interestingly, Kuno et al. found no effect of training on end exercise intramuscular pH or P_i:PCr ratios. In contrast, ^{31}P MRS data suggest that training in healthy adults and patients with heart failure tends to reduce the development of intramuscular acidosis [49, 70].

It could also be argued that children do not reach their real maximal work rate, because they simply do not try hard enough. Objective criteria for maximal effort are not easy to define, even for cycle ergometry, let alone single-leg treadle exercise. The children were told that they would be doing a hard exercise and were actively encouraged throughout the test. In addition, a transition in the P_i:PCr to work rate slope, i.e., a critical point in the cellular energy metabolism, was observed in 50% of the children at 62% of the maximal work rate. The same value (62%) was reported for the ratio of anaerobic threshold to $\dot{V}O_{2max}$ in children of comparable age during maximal cycle ergometer exercise [23].

These results are consistent with those of previous studies, which reported growth-related differences in gas exchange response to high-intensity exercise. A higher CO_2:O_2 cost ratio (ie., higher acidosis) for 1 min of heavy exercise was observed in adults, compared to that of with children [3]. Bar-Or reported a lower anaerobic capacity (measured by a supramaximal 30-s cycle ergometer test, the Wingate anaerobic test) in young children, compared to adolescents and adults [6]. In addition, in the few invasive studies that have been done, blood and muscle lactate concentrations at high-intensity exercise are lower in children than in adults [32, 59].

Our results can not be explained by a faster lactate removal or subsequent metabolism in children. If glycolysis had increased with a simultaneous increase in lactate removal, then we ought to have found a more rapid increase in P_i without a parallel drop in pH in children. This was not the case, as the relationship between P_i:PCr and pH was the same in children and adults.

Both phosphofructokinase (PFK) and glycogen phosphorylase are key regulatory enzymes of glycolysis, but little attention has been paid to possible maturational pattern of their activity. Eriksson et al. reported a lower

FIGURE 15.5.

The values of intracellular pH at exhaustion in thigh muscles of well-trained and untrained children and adolescents. All children and adolescent values were significantly greater than those found in adults. There was no effect of training on intramuscular pH at the end of exercise in the children or adolescents. Data redrawn from ref. 47.

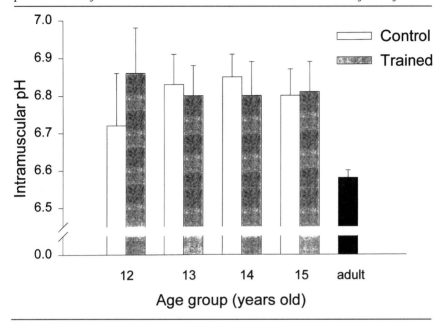

muscle concentration of PFK in 11- to 13-yr-old children, compared to that in adults [31]. In addition, studies in rats showed a 17-fold increase in total PFK activity, occurring during the first 2 mo of age (equivalent to birth to puberty in humans). This was accompanied by a dramatic decrease in C-type PFK subunit and an increase in M-type subunit, the isozyme best suited for glycolysis [30]. Finally, low levels of C-type PFK subunit have been shown to promote increased affinity for fructose-6-phosphate and diminished susceptibility to ATP inhibition [28, 29].

^{31}P MRS was used to study muscle metabolism during exercise in one adult subject with PFK deficiency [1]. A normal slope of the initial linear relationship of P_i:PCr to work rate, no drop in pH, and a gradual increase of phosphomonoester levels were observed during exercise. We did not observe a phosphomonoester peak in any of our children, which might simply reflect a much milder PFK impairment, compared to that of the subject affected by the myopathy.

Maturation of the muscle metabolic response to exercise might be related to the hormonal changes (increase in testosterone, estradiol, growth hormone, and insulin-like growth factor-1) occurring during puberty [52]. To date, little is known about the effect of these hormones on functional and structural muscle growth. Testosterone has been shown to increase sarcotubular and mitochondrial enzymes [65] in mature male subjects. In addition, Kelly et al. demonstrated that testosterone administration stimulated the transition from Type IIa (fast oxidative glycolytic) to Type IIB (fast glycolytic) fibers in guinea pig temporalis muscles [44].

A maturation of skeletal muscle fiber-type pattern might also account for growth-related differences in the metabolic response to high-intensity exercise. The pattern of rise in $\dot{V}O_2$ during heavy exercise in children [2]—large early rise to a greater O_2 cost, with less continued slower rise over time (slow component of $\dot{V}O_2$)—is also observed in adult subjects with a greater percent of slow twitch (Type I) muscle fibers in the vastus lateralis [41] (Fig. 15.6 and 15.7). Moreover, Mizuno et al. [55] recently found, with ^{31}P MRS, that in adults performing forearm exercise, the end exercise pH was inversely related to the percent of slow twitch fibers—i.e., those subjects with less pH drop (which is similar to our finding in children) had greater percent slow-twitch muscle fibers. These observation, coupled with the reduced anaerobic capacity noted in children [6], suggest that a likely underlying explanation for the differences in metabolic and gas exchange responses during heavy exercise between children and adults may be a maturational change in muscle fiber type distribution. As expected, there are very few studies of systematic changes in muscle fiber types from biopsies in

FIGURE 15.6.

Group mean O_2 cost of below anaerobic threshold (AT)-intensity (A, 80% AT) and above-AT (B, 75%Δ) intensity exercise in children and adults. For both low- and high-intensity exercise, average O_2 cost was significantly higher in children. Compare these results with those of adults with different fiber type proportions, shown in Figure 15.7. Reproduced from ref. 2.

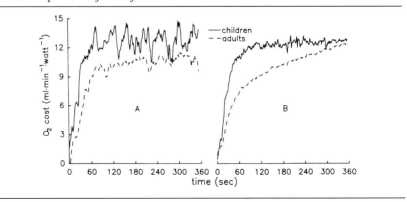

FIGURE 15.7.

Schematic of rise in $\dot{V}O_2$ during heavy exercise, scaled as O_2 cost by dividing by work rate. FT represents a subject with predominance of fast-twitch (Type II) fibers in vastus lateralis, whereas ST is the idealized response of the subject with majority of slow-twitch (Type I) fibers. Data from ref. 41. Compare these results with those of Figure 15.6.

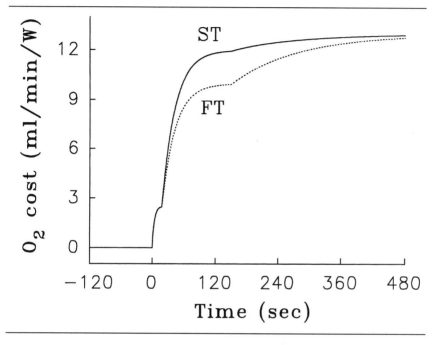

children. However, several studies examining biopsies of human diaphragm [42] and hindlimb muscles [10] demonstrated that fiber-type differentiation occurs relatively early in life, and by 6 yr of age, the skeletal muscle histochemical profile is similar to that of a young adult. Obviously, work is needed to determine the ultimate role of fiber-type maturation in the overall development of the cardiorespiratory response to exercise.

In conclusion, muscle high-energy phosphate kinetics during high-intensity exercise is different between children and adults. In this range of work, children seem to rely less on anaerobic glycolytic metabolism than adults do. ^{31}P MRS has proved to be a noninvasive unique technique to gain sight into muscle metabolism during exercise in children. Our results suggest a potentially important role of ^{31}P MRS spectroscopy during exercise in identifying abnormal muscle metabolism and in assessing the value of therapeutic approaches designed to improve exercise tolerance in children with a variety of disease.

PHOSPHODIESTER PEAK

In our studies, a phosphodiester (PDE) peak between the P_i and PCr peaks (at a chemical shift of 2.9–3 from the PCr) was observed in some of the subjects. In these subjects, PDE area was used to calculate the PDE:PCr ratio. The phosphodiester peak was observed in all adults; this peak was not observed in seven children.

The physiological meaning of this difference is not readily apparent, but it is intriguing to consider the possible mechanisms. We found significantly lower PDE/PCr peaks in girls, as compared to those of the other subjects, and although not statistically different, the value of this ratio in boys was substantially smaller than in adult males. Two previous groups of investigators have also found an age-related increase in the appearance of phosphodiester peaks in resting muscle [67, 75].

The phosphodiester peak in muscles likely represent glycerol-3-phosphorylcholine [14] and/or serine ethanolamine phosphodiester [16]. Age- or sex-related differences in glycerol-3-phosphorylcholine may reflect differences in lipid membrane metabolism or breakdown. The role of serine ethanolamine phosphodiester is not known; however, it has been shown to be characteristic of slow fiber types [17]. Satrústegui and coworkers [67] noted the age-dependence of PDE accumulation and the appearance of another phospholipid breakdown product, lipofuscin, a well-described marker of aging in muscle [26, 40]. Satrústegui and coworkers speculated: "The detection of phosphodiester by MR *in vivo* is one of the few, if not the only, non-invasive biochemical tests of the 'biochemical aging' of a human body organ." Precisely how these phosphodiesters interact with muscle function is not yet known. Whether or not our finding is evidence for fiber type maturation or change during growth, or represents another process related to aging, remains an important topic for future research.

MRI AND STRUCTURE-FUNCTION RESPONSES TO EXERCISE

Body size is a major determinant of maximal physiological function, and allometric equations quantify the relationships of body size (e.g., muscle mass) to metabolic rate (e.g., peak $\dot{V}O_2$ during exercise). Allometric analyses are used to assess size-structure relationships in mature animals of different sizes and species [71] as well as of those in a single species during the period of growth and development [9, 21, 68, 69]. The objective of the following study performed in our laboratory [78] was to examine the relationship between muscle size and the peak $\dot{V}O_2$ ($\dot{V}O_2$ peak) and work rate (WRpeak) in a group of children and adults.

$\dot{V}O_2$peak and WRpeak were measured from a progressive cycle ergometer test. Muscle size was estimated using MRI of the calf musculature. MRI is a noninvasive method not requiring ionizing radiation and is, therefore, more feasible for studies in healthy children. MRI provided a means of measuring muscle cross-sectional area (CSA) and allowed us to account for bone and subcutaneous fat, factors that substantially limit the accuracy of limb diameter alone in estimating muscle size.

Allometric equations have the general form $q \propto a \cdot M^b$, where q indicates a metabolic rate (e.g., $\dot{V}O_2$), M is a parameter related to body dimension (e.g., mass), a is the mass coefficient, and b is the dimensionless mass exponent or the scaling factor [36]. The scaling factor relating body mass to $\dot{V}O_2$ peak in mature mammals of different sizes is about 0.75 [71]. In contrast, in cross-sectional studies of children and young adults performed in our laboratory, the scaling factor was found to be 1.01 [23], a value significantly greater than 0.75.

The observation of different scaling factors implies that the mechanisms accounting for size-function relationships are not entirely the same during growth in children as among mature animals of different sizes. A. V. Hill [39] in 1950 and T. A. McMahon [53] in 1984 reviewed the experimental data and theoretical considerations of size-function relationships during exercise in mature animals. Insight into the mechanisms governing size-function relationships during growth can be gained by testing certain assumptions reached by Hill and McMahon:

1. Peak muscle function $\propto$ muscle CSA^1. The inherent or intrinsic strength of a contracting voluntary muscle fiber is constant and independent of the size of an animal. A bigger muscle is capable of greater work and metabolic rate only because it is bigger, not because its inherent metabolic capacity is greater [39].
2. Peak muscle strength $\propto$ peak metabolic rate. In terms of a progressive exercise test, this could be stated as WRpeak $\propto \dot{V}O_2$ peak.

These assumptions would then predict that: $\dot{V}O_2$ peak $\propto$ muscle CSA^1 and WRpeak $\propto$ muscle CSA^1.

We hypothesized that the scaling factor of 1.0, predicted from studies of mature animals, would not be found experimentally in children and adults. An important implication of finding a scaling factor other than 1 would be that the intrinsic strength and/or metabolic capacity of muscles change during growth and development.

The study population consisted of 20 children (age range, 6–11 yr, 11 boys and 9 girls) and 18 adults (age range, 23–42 yr, 10 men and 8 women). Each subject performed a ramp-type progressive exercise test on an electromagnetically braked cycle ergometer to determine maximal oxygen uptake. MRI was performed on a Picker 1.5-T whole body MRI system. A round (10 cm in diameter) surface coil was used for signal detection, while a proton body coil was used for radiofrequency (RF) transmission for imaging. The subject was positioned with the center of the receive coil at the largest circumference of the calf (as estimated by the investigator). The whole leg was then moved into the isocenter of the magnet bore. Images were obtained from a coronal slice (2 cm in diameter) at isocenter with a 30-cm field of view providing single-slice pictures of muscle, fat, and bone.

Computerized planimetry was used to determine calf muscle CSA. The major muscles included: gastrocnemius, soleus, tibialis anterior and posterior, and peroneus longus and brevis. The investigator traced the circumference of the calf, using a pointing device. These areas were traced as well and, subsequently, were subtracted from the limb CSA to yield the muscle CSA. A similar approach was recently presented by Nishida and coworkers [56].

A log-log transform was used to calculate the scaling factor [36]. Linear regression was performed on the transformed data, and the slope of the regression is equal to the scaling factor. Because work done by all of the calf muscles is a major component of the total work done during cycle ergometry [34, 38], we used the ratios of $\dot{V}O_2$ peak to CSA and WRpeak to CSA as indicators of the relative contribution of this muscle group to maximal metabolic rate and maximal power output. These ratios were analyzed in several ways: first, we calculated the mean value for the four groups: boys, girls, men,and women. Secondly, we calculated the linear regression of the ratios as a function of body weight in all male subjects, all female subjects, and in the group as a whole.

The mean peak $\dot{V}O_2$ normalized to body weight was 39.9 ± 8.6 (SD) ml/min/kg in the adults and 38.8 ± 7.4 in children (not significant).WRpeak per body weight in children (2.9 ± 0.6 W/kg) was significantly lower than in adults (3.9 ± 0.8 W/kg, P < .001). Both peak $\dot{V}O_2$ and WRpeak were similar to values found previously in our laboratory [23, 77].

Scaling Factors

The scaling factors, relating WRpeak and $\dot{V}O_2$ to muscle CSA, are shown in Table 15.1. Table 15.2 summarizes the linear regression analysis for WRpeak/CSA and $\dot{V}O_2$ peak/CSA as a function of body weight in males, females,and in the group as a whole. $\dot{V}O_2$ peak/CSA was not affected by body

TABLE 15.1.
Scaling Factors Relating Indices of Body Mass with Metabolic Function during Exercise

	Females		*Males*		*All Subjects*	
	Factor	*SEM*	*Factor*	*SEM*	*Factor*	*SEM*
WRpeak vs. CSA	1.25	0.22	1.40	0.16	1.37	0.12
$\dot{V}O_2$ peak vs. CSA	0.94	0.21	1.03	0.15	1.04	0.12

TABLE 15.2.
Regression Slope and Constant for the Equation y = a · x + ᵃb

	Slope	Constant	r	P^a
WRpeak/CSA♂	0.043	2.34	0.70	P < 0.005
WRpeak/CSA♀	0.045	2.17	0.57	P < 0.05
WRpeak/CSA, all	0.044	2.26	0.68	P < .0001
$\dot{V}O_2$peak/CSA, ♂	0.13	47.2	0.24	NS
$\dot{V}O_2$peak/CSA, ♀	0.18	41.3	0.25	NS
$\dot{V}O_2$peak/CSA, all	0.17	43.6	0.29	NS

[a]In this equation where y is either WRpeak/CSA or $\dot{V}O_2$peak/CSA; a is the slope, either as in watts per square centimeter per kilogram or milliters per square centimeter per kilogram; x is body weight in kilograms; and b is the constant in either watts per square centimeter or milliliter per minute per square centimeter. The correlation coefficient is r and P values are calculated for significance of the difference of the slope from the value 0.

weight, but the WRpeak/CSA increased as a function of weight both in males (P < .005) and females (P < .05). No differences in $\dot{V}O_2$ peak/CSA were observed between children and adults. On the contrary, WRpeak/CSA was significantly higher in adults, compared to that in children (Fig. 15.8).

We found, as expected, that WRpeak, $\dot{V}O_2$ peak, and calf muscle CSA all increased with age and body size in this group of children and adults. As hypothesized, the scaling factor relating WRpeak to muscle CSA was significantly greater than 1.0 (Table 15.1), which was corroborated by the observations that the ratio WRpeak/CSA increased significantly with body weight, and that the mean values of WRpeak/CSA were less in boys and girls than in men and women (Fig. 15.8). (Note that these results were confirmed by analysis of covariance of the data as well.) A possible implication of this finding is that inherent muscle metabolic capacity increases with size during growth and maturation.

But we had also hypothesized that the scaling factors for both $\dot{V}O_2$ peak and WRpeak to muscle CSA would be the same because WRpeak $\propto$ $\dot{V}O_2$ peak (Assumption 2). This was not the case: the scaling factor of $\dot{V}O_2$ peak to muscle CSA did not significantly differ from 1.0. This was corroborated by the observation that the ratio $\dot{V}O_2$ peak/CSA did not change with body weight. One implication of the discrepancy between the WRpeak and $\dot{V}O_2$ peak scaling factors is that the coupling of $\dot{V}O_2$ (measured at the mouth) to muscle work and metabolic rate may change during growth and maturation.

It is first necessary to address some of the methodological limitations of this study. Working with children imposes a number of real constraints: these subjects, although enthusiastic and cooperative, can become distracted rather quickly, particularly in the confines of a whole body magnet, and then start moving and fidgeting. Thus, images must be obtained

FIGURE 15.8.

*Peak work rate (WRpeak)/cross-sectional area (CSA) and peak oxygen uptake ($\dot{V}O_2$ peak)/CSA in adults (males and females) and children (boys and girls). *,WRpeak/CSA in men was significantly greater than in boys (P < .05) and girls (P < .05); **,WRpeak/CSA in women was significantly greater than in boys (P < .05). No differences were found in $\dot{V}O_2$ peak/CSA among the four groups. Data are expressed as means ± SD. Reproduced from 78.*

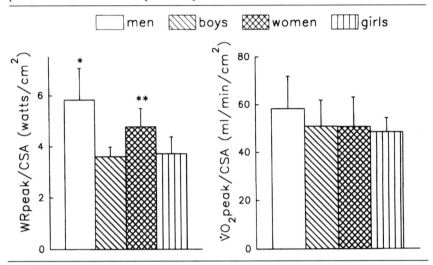

quickly. We chose to image the calf muscle simply because the investigator could easily and quickly identify the prominent gastrocnemius head, which invariably represents the largest diameter of the lower leg.

An inherent assumption of this study was that the calf muscle CSA accurately represents all muscles involved in ergometry exercise. The calf muscles (e.g., soleus and gastrocnemius) are used extensively in cycle ergometry and have electromyographic power spectra during cycle ergometry that are similar to the vastus medialis of the thigh musculature [34, 38], but our results cannot exclude the possibility that the recruitment of thigh and calf muscles in cycle ergometer actually change with age. For example, when children relied on thigh muscles to a greater extent than adults did in the performance of heavy-cycle ergometer exercise, than our results could be explained without necessarily concluding that muscle power per CSA is smaller in children than in adults.

The relative inability of MRI to identify *intramuscular* fat could also add to the error of this technique. When the muscle CSA in children reflected a higher fat-to-muscle ratio than that of adults, then the WRpeak:CSA ratio would likely be lower in children and not necessarily indicate differences in muscle tissue per se. But, in general, children are leaner than adults (note that the BMI in children was $17.5 \pm 2.9 \, \text{kg}/\text{m}^2$, as compared with 23.2 ± 2.2 in adults), which suggests relatively *less* fat than in adults. Thus, if anything, an inability to account for intramuscular fat by MRI would mean that we had *underestimated* the true difference in WRpeak/CSA between adults and children.

As noted, we chose the calf because the prominence of the gastrocnemius heads makes it relatively easy to choose the largest circumference by inspection. But using only a single CSA could lead to possible errors attributable to position of the coil or maturational changes in calf muscle anatomy. MRI may yield other ways of assessing muscle size that could potentially improve this type of analysis. For example, Roman and co-workers [62] recently showed increases in muscle size in elderly men after upper arm resistance training by using 1-cm contiguous MRI-derived CSA and calculating the *volume* of the muscle in question.

Despite these possible confounding features of the methodology, our observations are consistent with previous studies focused on different aspects of muscle function. From our own laboratory, reanalysis of previous progressive exercise data in a large number of children and teenagers revealed that the ratio of WRpeak/kg body weight increased with age in children and teenagers [23, 77]. This was unexpected, because Assumptions 1 and 2 above would suggest that WRmax $\propto$ weight$^{2/3}$, and, therefore, that the ratio of WRmax/weight would *decrease* as body weight increased. Davies and coworkers [25] measured electrically evoked contractile properties of the triceps surae muscle in children and adults. They calculated the mean force per cross-sectional area (estimated by anthropometry and water displacement) to be greater in young adults ($34 \, \text{N}/\text{cm}^2$) than in children ($29 \, \text{N}/\text{cm}^2$), even though the children in their study were not as young (mean age, 13 yr) as those in our study. Finally, Parker and coworkers [58] found that isometric quadriceps strength in boys and male teenagers increased, even when growth in height and body weight had virtually ceased.

Along these lines, Bar-Or and others [6, 33] have suggested that there is an increasing "anerobic capacity" (the ability to produce ATP regeneration for muscular work anerobically) as children mature into adulthood. Whether or not such changes are related to the anabolic effects of puberty is not known; however, it is noteworthy that the increases in WRpeak/CSA were observed in both males and females. To the extent that our observations can be explained by hormonal changes occurring during the process of maturation, the role of *both* estradiol and testosterone—the hormones responsible for the female and male adolescent growth spurts [52]—must be considered.

As noted, unlike the WRpeak, the $\dot{V}O_2$ peak increased in direct proportion with muscle CSA—the scaling factor was not significantly differently from 1.0. Davies and co-workers [24] discovered that $\dot{V}O_2$ peak, when scaled to leg volume (determined by anthropometry and water displacement), actually decreased slightly with increasing age in a cross-sectional study of children and adults. Moreover, in previous studies in this laboratory we found that the oxygen cost of 1 min of high-intensity exercise—normalized to external work performed (in milliliters per minute per joule)—was actually *greater* in children, as compared to that in adults [77].

Maturation of the "anerobic potential" referred to above may shed light on the apparent discrepancy between WRpeak and $\dot{V}O_2$ peak. The $\dot{V}O_2$ during exercise does not necessarily represent the total metabolic cost of the work performed. In particular, ATP rephosphorylation derived from anerobic metabolism and from high-energy phosphagen stores, important components of the total metabolic cost of exercise [73], is simply not accounted for by gas exchange measured at the mouth. Our data may be explained by the following scenario: Muscles grow in size and gain potential for anerobic metabolism as children grow and develop. WRpeak increases out of proportion to the growth in muscle (i.e., the scaling factor for WRpeak and muscle CSA is greater than 1.0), but a greater proportion of the energy required to perform work is anaerobically derived, not reflected in the $\dot{V}O_2$ peak. Consequently, as muscles become bigger, WRpeak scales differently with respect to muscle size than does the $\dot{V}O_2$ peak.

These observations support the notion that the changes in body size and function that occur during growth are not regulated by the same mechanisms that account for size-function relationships among mature mammals of different sizes and species. Moreover, some of the assumptions often used in allometric analyses of size-function relationships during exercise in adult animals of different species do not appear to hold when considering the size changes that occur during normal growth and development within a species such as humans. Our data suggest that the inherent metabolic capacity of muscles increases with age in human beings.

MR ASSESSMENT OF FIBER TYPING

As noted above, the maturation of cardiorespiratory responses to exercise might be explained by fiber type changes; moreover, physical training can profoundly affect fiber type. A number of recent studies indicate that proton MR may be used to noninvasively assess fiber type in skeletal muscles. Kuno et al. [45, 46] studied the effect of strength training on the relationship between T_1 and T_2 relaxation times and muscle fiber composition. T_1 and T_2 relaxation times refer to the time it takes for the tissue to dissipate energy received after RF pulses. Five healthy men underwent a 5-mo heavy-resistance exercise training program and were compared with four control subjects. Needle biopsies from the vastus lateralis muscle were obtained before and after the experimental period, and cross-sectional area of fast-twitch (FT) fibers was significantly increased by training.

Both T_1 and T_2 relaxation times from proton MR analysis of the vastus lateralis muscle significantly increased in the trained subjects. In addition, cross-sectional analysis of data from 21 subjects showed a significant correlation between T_1 and the proportion of FT fibers (Fig. 15.9). While the mechanism of the relationship between relaxation times and fiber type composition is not known, it is possible that the water content of fiber types differ [66]. Water content can be a major determinant of T_1 and T_2.

Noninvasive assessment of fiber type might also be possible, using ^{31}P MRS. Meyer and coworkers [54] used isolated in vitro preparations of cat soleus and biceps muscles to determine possible differences in phosphorus compounds between slow oxidative (SO) and fast-glycolytic (FG) fiber types, respectively. FG muscle had lower P_i and higher PCr, compared to that of SO fibers, these investigators suggested that the relative increase in P_i during muscle contraction would be greater in FG, as compared to that of SO muscles. More recently, Kushmerick et al. [48] studied a variety of surgically excised rat muscles. These workers noted about a 10-fold range in the P_i:PCr ratios in normal resting muscles, from 0.05 in fast-twitch fibers (Types IIa and IIb) to 0.5 in muscles containing predominantly Type I and IIx fibers. Clearly, more work is needed to further explore these intriguing

FIGURE 15.9.

Relationship between magnetic resonance longitudinal relaxation time and muscle fiber composition for a group of healthy subjects with a range of % fast-twitch (FT) fibers, as determined by muscle biopsy. Data redrawn from ref. 45.

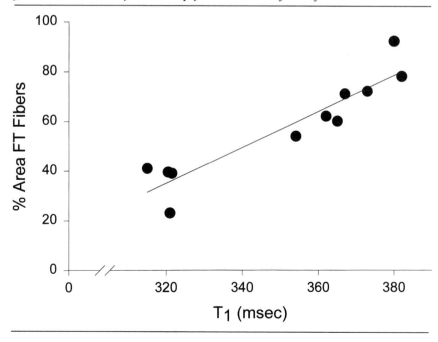

observations; such tools would be of great value in assessing maturation of cardiorespiratory responses to exercise in the growing child.

ASSESSMENT OF BODY COMPOSITION USING MRI

A variety of indirect techniques (e.g., skin-fold thickness or underwater weighing) have been used to estimate muscle mass and/or body fat content. But such techniques cannot quantify changes that occur in fat or muscle tissue at specific anatomical sites, which is important because training programs, for example, might increase the mass of a particular muscle group without measurably affecting overall body composition. Moreover, particular programs of exercise training might influence fat and muscle differently in different anatomical sites. Indeed, tissue-specific effects on adiposity have been documented when growth hormone is replaced in GH-deficient children [63].

FIGURE 15.10.

Mean increase (± SE) increase in the ratio of muscle:adipose tissue area in groups of children with growth impairments (growth hormone deficiency (GHD), Turner's syndrome, and intrauterine growth retardation (IUGR)) treated with GH and in untreated healthy children. The ratios were obtained from MRI of the midthigh. As can be seen, exogenous GH therapy increased the ratio of muscle:adipose tissue in the children with growth impairment. Data redrawn from ref. 50.

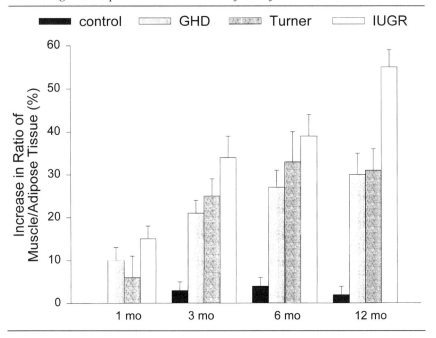

There is increasing use of MR assessment of fat and muscle tissue to guage the effects of hormonal therapy or exercise training. For example, Leger et al. [50] demonstrated a significant increase in muscle tissue and decrease in adipose tissue cross-sectional area from MRI images of thighs in children with growth retardation GH deficiency, Turner's syndrome, and intrauterine growth retardation) (Fig. 15.10). Treuth et al. [72] studied the effects of 16 wk of resistance training on 13 men (mean age, 60 yrs), and found substantial increases in body strength, as well as increases in midthigh muscle cross-sectional area and decreases in midthigh subcutaneous fat, as assessed by MRI. In our own laboratory, we are now using MRI assessment of muscle mass and abdominal fat to determine the effects of aerobic training in a group of 44 healthy female adolescents (Fig. 15.11 and 15.12).

FUTURE DIRECTIONS

The studies outlined above have, hopefully, demonstrated the ways in which these techniques have already substantially improved our ability to gain insight into cardiorespiratory, hormonal, and skeletal muscle adapta-

FIGURE 15.11.
An example of MRI of the abdomen at the umbilicus in a 15-yr-old girl. These images are being used in our laboratory to determine the effect of exercise training on body fat in specific anatomical locations.

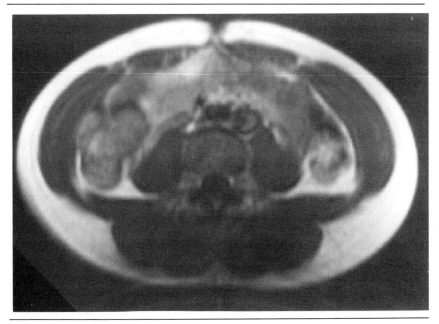

FIGURE 15.12.

An example of MRI of the midthigh in a 15-yr-old girl. These images are being used in our laboratory to determine the effect of exercise training on the mass of specific muscle groups. In addition, these images can be used to estimate the lean:fat ratio in the thigh.

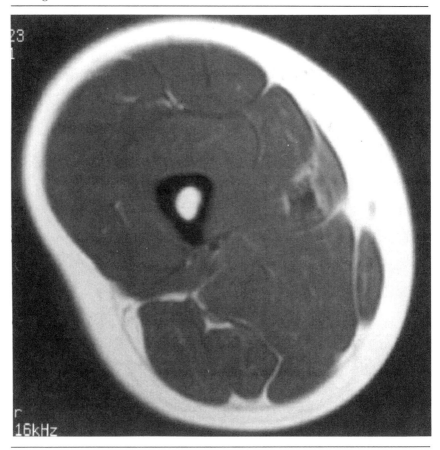

tion to physical activity. It is unfortunate that the development of MR as a research tool is occurring in a period of downsizing in biomedical research. MRI is expensive; even for research purposes, 1 hr of magnet time may be about $500 or more, because of the high clinical load of most MRI centers. MR units can cost over a million dollars, and maintenance is expensive, requiring highly skilled technologists. It is unlikely, therefore, that the use of MRI to explore such questions as the development of high-energy phosphate responses to exercise in muscle tissues will proceed as rapidly as did research tied to new technologies in the 1970s and early 1980s.

Nonetheless, it is worth noting that MR techniques hold the promise of even more dramatic insights. MRI has been used to measure *pulmonary* blood flow in patients having undergone surgical repair of complex congenital heart disease [35, 61, 74] and can be used to measure blood flow to muscle groups as well [11, 19]. MRI studies of cerebral function in humans have yielded new insights into respiratory control [37], and such approaches could be used to focus on neural function during exercise. A number of possible uses of MR have yet to be fully developed; for example, greater understanding of the paramagnetic effects of oxygen to assess blood flow might provide researchers with tools that can be used in children, as well as in adults. In summary, MR is an impressive technological breakthrough with great potential for defining underlying mechanisms of cardiorespiratory adaptation to exercise in health and in disease. Whether or not this potential will be fully exploited in the near future remains to be seen.

ACKNOWLEDGMENTS

This work was supported by NIH Grant HD26939, General Clinical Research Grant RR00425, and by Grant HL11907. D. M. Cooper recently completed the Career Investigator Award of the American Lung Association.

REFERENCES

1. Argov, Z., W. J. Bank, J. Maris, J. S. J. Leigh, and B. Chance. Muscle energy metabolism in human phosphofructokinase deficiency as recorded by 31-P nuclear magnetic resonance spectroscopy. *Ann. Neurol.* 22:46–51, 1987.
2. Armon, Y., D. M. Cooper, R. Flores, S. Zanconato, and T. J. Barstow. Oxygen uptake dynamics during high-intensity exercise in children and adults. *J. Appl. Physiol.* 70:841–848, 1991.
3. Armon, Y., D. M. Cooper, and S. Zanconato. Maturation of ventilatory responses to one-minute exercise. *Pediatr. Res.* 29:362–368, 1991.
4. Astrand, P.-O. and K. Rodahl. *Textbook of Work Physiology,* 2nd ed. New York: McGraw-Hill, 1977, pp. 389–446.
5. Ballor, D. L., L. J. Tommerup, D. B. Smith, and D. P. Thomas. Body composition, muscle and fat pad changes following two levels of dietary restriction and/or exercise training in male rats. *Int. J. Obes.* 14:711–722, 1990.
6. Bar-Or, O. *Pediatric Sports Medicine for the Practitioner.* New York: Springer-Verlag, 1983.
7. Barstow, T. J., S. Buchthal, S. Zanconato, and D. M. Cooper. Muscle energetics and pulmonary oxygen uptake kinetics during moderate exercise. *J. Appl. Physiol.* 77:1742–1749, 1994.
8. Barstow, T. J., C. Buchthal, S. Zanconato, and D. M. Cooper. Changes in potential controllers of human skeletal muscle respiration during incremental calf exercise. *J. Appl. Physiol.* 77:2169–2176, 1994.
9. Belk, K. E., J. D. Tatum, and F. L. Williams, Jr. Deposition and distribution of carcass fat for steers differing in frame size and muscle thickness. *J. Anim. Sci.* 69:609–616, 1991.
10. Bell, R. D., J. D. MacDougall, R. Billeter and H. Howald. Muscle fiber types and morphometric analysis of skeletal muscle in six-year-old children. *Med. Sci. Sports Exerc.* 12:28–31, 1980.

11. Blaak, E. E., M. A. Van Baak, G. J. Kemerink, M. T. Pakbiers, G. A. Heidendal, and W. H. Saris. Total forearm blood flow as an indicator of skeletal muscle blood flow: effect of subcutaneous adipose tissue blood flow. *Clin. Sci.* 87:559–566, 1994.

12. Blomqvist, C. G., and B. Saltin. Cardiovascular adaptations to physical training. *Annu. Rev. Physiol.* 45:169–189, 1983.

13. Booth, F. W., and P. D. Gollnick. Effects of disuse on the structure and function of skeletal muscle. *Med. Sci. Sports Exerc.* 15:415–420, 1983.

14. Burt, C. T., T. Glonek, and M. Barany. Phosphorus-31 nuclear magnetic resonance detection of unexpected phosphodiesters in muscle. *Biochemistry* 15:4850–4853, 1976.

15. Casaburi, R., T. W. Storer, I. Ben-Dov, and K. Wasserman. Effect of endurance training on possible determinants of $\dot{V}O_2$ during heavy exercise. *J. Appl. Physiol.* 62:199–207, 1987.

16. Chalovich, J. M., C. T. Burt, S. M. Cohen, T. Glonek, and M. Barany. The identification of an unknown 31P NMR from dystrophic chicken as L-serine ethanolamine phosphodiester. *Arch. Biochem. Biophys.* 182:683–689, 1977.

17. Chalovich, J. M., C. T. Burt, M. J. Danon, T. Glonek, and M. Barany. Phosphodiesters in muscular dystrophies. *Ann. N.Y. Acad. Sci.* 317:649–668, 1979.

18. Chance, B., J. S. Leigh, J. Kent, and K. McCully. Metabolic control principles and 31-P NMR. *Fed. Proc.* 45:2915–2920, 1986.

19. Chernoff, D. M., A. T. Walker, R. Khorasani, J. F. Polak, and F. A. Jolesz. Asymptomatic functional popliteal artery entrapment: demonstration at MR imaging. *Radiology* 195:176–180, 1995.

20. Cohen, L. A., E. Boylan, M. Epstein, and E. Zang. Voluntary exercise and experimental mammary cancer. M. M. Jacobs (ed). *Exercise, Calories, Fat, and Cancer.* New York: Plenum Press, pp. 41–59, 1992.

21. Cooper, D. M. Development of the oxygen transport system in normal children. O. Bar-Or (ed). *Advances in Pediatric Sport Sciences, Biological Issues,* Vol. 3. Champaign, IL: Human Kinetics, pp. 67–100, 1989.

22. Cooper D. M. Evidence for and mechanisms of exercise modulation of growth. *Med. Sci. Sports Exerc.* 26:733–740, 1994.

23. Cooper, D. M., D. Weiler-Ravell, B. J. Whipp, and K. Wasserman. Aerobic parameters of exercise as a function of body size during growth in children. *J. Appl. Physiol.* 56:628–634, 1984.

24. Davies, D. T. M., C. Barnes, and S. Godfrey. Body composition and maximal exercise performance in children. *Hum. Biol.* 44:195–214, 1972.

25. Davies, C. T. M., M. J. White, and K. Young. Muscle function in children. *Eur. J. Appl. Physiol.* 52:111–114, 1983.

26. Dayan, D., I. Abrahami, A. Buchner, M. Gorsky, and N. Chimovitz. Lipid pigment (lipofuscin) in human perioral muscles with aging. *Exp. Gerontol.* 23:97–102, 1988.

27. Dudley, G. A., P. C. Tullson, and R. L. Terjung. Influence of mitochondrial content on the sensitivity of respiratory control. *J. Biol. Chem.* 262:9109–9114, 1994.

28. Dunaway, G. A., and T. P. Kasten. Physiological implications of the alteration of 6-phosphofructo-1-kinase isozyme pools during brain development and aging. *Brain Res.* 456:310–316, 1988.

29. Dunaway, G. A., T. P. Kasten, S. Crabtree, and Y. Mhaskar. Age-related changes in subunit composition and regulation of hepatic 6-phosphofructo-1-kinase. *Biochem J.* 266:823–827, 1990.

30. Dunaway, G. A., T. P. Kasten, G. A. Nickols, and J. A. Chesky. Regulation of skeletal muscle 6-phosphofructo-1-kinase during aging and development. *Mech. Ageing Dev.* 36:13–23, 1986.

31. Eriksson, B. O., P. B. Gollnick, and B. Saltin. Muscle metabolism and enzyme activity after training in boys 11–13 years old. *Acta Physiol. Scand.* 87:485–487, 1973.

32. Eriksson, B. O., J. Karlsson, and B. Saltin. Muscle metabolites during exercise in pubertal boys. *Acta Paediatr. Scand.* 217(Suppl):154–157, 1971.

33. Falk, B., and O. Bar-Or. Longitudinal changes in peak aerobic and anaerobic mechanical power of circumpubertal boys. *Pediatr. Exerc. Sci.* 5:318–331, 1993.
34. Gamet, D., J. Duchene, C. Garapon-Bar, and F. Goubel. Electromyogram power spectrum during dynamic contractions at different intensities of exercise. *Eur. J. Appl. Physiol.* 61:331–337, 1990.
35. Gefter, W. B., and H. Hatabu. Evaluation of pulmonary vascular anatomy and blood flow by magnetic resonance (Review). *J. Thorac. Imaging* 8:122–136, 1993.
36. Gould, S. J. Allometry and size in ontogeny and physiology. *Biol. Rev. Camb. Philos. Soc.* 41:587–640, 1966.
37. Gozal, D., G. M. Hathout, K. A. Kirlew, et al. Localization of putative neural respiratory regions in the human by functional magnetic resonance imaging. *J. Appl. Physiol.* 76: 2076–2083, 1994.
38. Hanninen, O., O. Airaksinen, M. Karipohja, K. Manninen, T. Sihvonen, and H. Pekkarinen. On-line determination of anaerobic threshold with rms-EMG. *Biomed. Biochim. Acta* 48:S493–S503, 1989.
39. Hill, A. V. The dimensions of animals and their muscular dynamics. *Sci. Prog.* 38:208–230, 1950.
40. Jakobsson, F., K. Borg, and L. Edstrom. Fibre-type composition, structure and cytoskeletal protein location of fibres in anterior tibial muscle. Comparison between young adults and physically active aged humans. *Acta Neuropathol.* 80:459–468, 1990.
41. Jones, A. M., P. H. Nguyen, R. Casaburi, and T. J. Batstow. Slow component of VO₂ during heavy exercise is correlated with % fast twitch muscle fibers. Indianapolis: ACSM Fall Speciality Conference, 1995.
42. Keens, T. G., A. C. Bryan, H. Levison, and C. D. Ianuzzo. Developmental pattern of muscle fiber types in human ventilatory muscles. *J. Appl. Physiol.* 44:900–913, 1978.
43. Kelly, P. J., J. A. Eisman, M. C. Stuart, N. A. Pocock, P. N. Sambrook, and T. H. Gwinn. Somatomedin-C, physical fitness, and bone density. *J. Clin. Endocrinol. Metab.* 70:718–723, 1990.
44. Kelly, A., G. Lyons, B. Gambki, and N. Rubinstein. Influence of testosterone on contractile proteins of the guinea pig temporalis muscle. *Adv. Exp. Med. Biol.* 182:155–168, 1983.
45. Kuno, S., S. Katsuta, M. Akisada, I. Anno, and K. Matsumoto. Effect of strength training on the relationship between magnetic resonance relaxation time and muscle fibre composition. *Eur. J. Appl. Physiol.* 61:33–36, 1990.
46. Kuno, S., S. Katsuta, T. Inouye, I. Anno, K. Matsumoto, and M. Akisada. Relationship between MR relaxation time and muscle fiber composition. *Radiology* 169:567–568, 1988.
47. Kuno, S., H. Takahashi, K. Fujimoto, et al. Muscle metabolism during exercise using phosphorus-31 nuclear magnetic resonance spectroscopy in adolescents. *Eur. J. Appl. Physiol.* 70:301–304, 1994.
48. Kushmerick, M. J., T. S. Moerland, and R. W. Wiseman. Mammalian skeletal muscle fibers distinguished by contents of phosphocreatine, ATP, and Pi. *Proc. Natl. Acad. Sci. U.S.A.* 89:7521–7525, 1992.
49. Laurent, D., H. Reutenauer, J. F. Payen, et al. Discrimination between cross-country and downhill skiers by pulmonary and local ³¹P-NMR evauations. *Med. Sci. Sports Exerc.* 25:29–36, 1993.
50. Leger, J., C. Carel, I. Legrand, A. Paulsen, M. Hassan, and P. Czernichow. Magnetic resonance imaging evaluation of adipose tissue and muscle tissue mass in children with growth hormone (GH) deficiency. Turner's syndrome, and intrauterine growth retardation during the first year of treatment with GH. *J. Clin. Endocrinol. Metab.* 78:904–909, 1995.
51. Livingstone, M. B., W. A. Coward, A. M. Prentice, et al. Daily energy expenditure in free-living children: comparison of heart-rate monitoring with the double labeled water (²H₂¹⁸O) method. *Am. J. Clin. Nutr.* 56:343–352, 1992.
52. Marshall, W. A., and J. M. Tanner. Puberty. F. Falkner, and J. M. Tanner, (eds). *Human Growth,* 2nd ed. New York: Plenum Press, 1986, pp. 171–210.

53. McMahon, T. A. *Muscles, Reflexes, and Locomotion.* Princeton, N.J.: Princeton University Press, 1984.

54. Meyer, R. A., T. R. Brown, and M. J. Kushmerick. Phosphorus nuclear magnetic resonance of fast- and slow-twitch muscle. *Am. J. Physiol.* 248:C279–287, 1985.

55. Mizuno, M., N. H. Secher, and B. Quistorff. ^{31}P-NMR spectroscopy, rsEMG, and histochemical fiber types of human wrist flexor muscles. *J. Appl. Physiol.* 76:531–538, 1994.

56. Nishida, M., H. Nishijima, K. Yonezawa, et al. Phosphorus 31 magnetic resonance spectroscopy of forearm flexor muscles in student rowers using an exercise protocol adjusted for differences in cross-sectional muscle area. *Eur. J. Appl. Physiol.* 64:528–533, 1992.

57. Oldendorf, W., and W. Oldendorf, Jr. *MRI Primer.* New York: Raven Press, 1991.

58. Parker, D. F., J. M. Round, P. Sacco, and D. A. Jones. A cross-sectional survey of upper and lower limb strength in boys and girls during childhood adolescence. *Ann. Hum. Biol.* 17:199–211, 1990.

59. Paterson, D. H., D. A. Cunningham, and L. A. Bumstead. Recovery O_2 and blood lactic acid: longitudinal analysis in boys aged 11 to 15 years. *Eur. J. Appl. Physiol.* 55:93–99, 1986.

60. Pearson, A. M. Muscle growth and exercise. *Crit. Rev. Food Sci. Nutr.* 29:167–196, 1990.

61. Rebergen, S. A., J. Ottenkamp, J. Doornbos, E. E. van der Wall, J. G. Chin, and A. Roos. Postoperative pulmonary flow dynamics after Fontan surgery: assessment with nuclear magnetic resonance velocity mapping. *J. Am. Coll. Cardiol.* 21:123–131, 1993.

62. Roman, W. J., J. Fleckenstein, J. Stray-Gundersen, S. E. Alway, R. Peshock, and W. J. Gonyea. Adaptations in the elbow flexors of elderly males after heavy-resistance training. *J. Appl. Physiol.* 74:750–754, 1993.

63. Rosenbaum, M., J. M. Gertner, and R. L. Leibel. Effects of systemic growth hormone (GH) administration on regional adipose tissue distribution and metabolism in GH-deficient children. *J. Clin. Endo. Metab.* 69:1274–1281, 1989.

64. Roston, W. L., B. J. Whipp, J. A. Davis, D. A. Cunningham, R. M. Effros, and K. Wasserman. Oxygen uptake kinetics and lactate concentrations during exercise in humans. *Am. Rev. Respir. Dis.* 135:1080–1084, 1987.

65. Saborido, A., J. Vila, F. Molano, and A. Megias. Effect of anabolic steroids on mitochondria and sarcotubular system of skeletal muscle. *J. Appl. Physiol.* 70:1038–1043, 1991.

66. Saryan, L. A., D. P. Hollis, J. S. Economou, and J. C. Eggleston. Nuclear magnetic resonance studies of cancer. *J. Natl. Cancer Inst.* 52:599–602, 1974.

67. Satrústegui, J., H. Berkowitz, B. Boden, et al. An in vivo phosphorus nuclear magnetic resonance study of the variations with age in the phosphodiers' content of human muscle. *Mech. Ageing Dev.* 42:105–114, 1988.

68. Siddiqui, R. A., S. N. McCutcheon, H. T. Blair, et al. Growth allometry of organs, muscles and bones in mice from lines divergently selected on the basis of plasma insulin-like growth factor-I. *Growth Dev. Aging* 56:53–60, 1992.

69. Sjodin, B., and J. Svedenhag. Oxygen uptake during running as related to body mass in circumpubertal boys: a longitudinal study. *Eur. J. Appl. Physiol.* 65:150–157, 1992.

70. Stratton, J. R., J. F. Dunn, S. Adamopoulos, G. J. Kemp, A. J. Coats, and B. Rajagopalan. Training partially reverses skeletal muscle metabolic abnormalities during exercise in heart failure. *J. Appl. Physiol.* 76:1575–1582, 1994.

71. Taylor, C. R., G. M. O. Maloiy, E. R. Weibel, et al. Design of the mammalian respiratory system. 3. Scaling maximum aerobic capacity to body mass: wild and domestic mammals. *Resp. Physiol.* 44:25–38, 1981.

72. Treuth, M. S., A. S. Ryan, R. E. Pratley, et al. Effects of strength training on total and regional body composition in older men. *J. Appl. Physiol.* 77:614–620, 1994.

73. Wasserman, K., B. J. Whipp, and J. A. Davis. Respiratory physiology of exercise: metabolism, gas exchange, and ventilatory control. J. G. Widdicombe, (ed). *Respiratory Physiology, III: International Reviews of Physiology Series,* Vol. 23, Baltimore: University Park Press, 1981.

74. Wexler, L., and C. B. Higgins. The use of magnetic imaging in adult congenital heart disease (Review). *Am. J. Cardiac Imaging.* 9:15–28, 1995.

75. Younkin, D. P., P. Berman, J. Slakdy, C. Chee, W. Bank, and B. Chance. 31P NMR studies in Duchenne muscular dystrophy: age-related metabolic changes. Neurology 37:165–169, 1987.

76. Zanconato, S., S. Buchthal, T. J. Barstow, and D. M. Cooper. ^{31}P-magnetic resonance spectroscopy of leg muscle metabolism during exercise in children and adults. *J. Appl. Physiol.* 74:2214–2218, 1993.

77. Zanconato, S., D. M. Cooper, and Y. Armon. Oxygen cost and oxygen uptake dynamics and recovery with one minute of exercise in children and adults. *J. Appl. Physiol.* 71:993–998, 1991.

78. Zanconato, S., G. Reidy, and D. M. Cooper. Calf muscle cross sectional area and maximal oxygen uptake in children and adults. *Am. J. Physiol.* 267:R720–R725, 1994.

Index

*Numbers followed by the letter t indicate tables; numbers followed by the letter f indicate figures.